Methods in Molecular Biology

Series Editor
John M. Walker
School of Life and Medical Sciences
University of Hertfordshire
Hatfield, Hertfordshire, AL10 9AB, UK

For further volumes:
http://www.springer.com/series/7651

Inflammation

Methods and Protocols

Edited by

Björn E. Clausen

Institute for Molecular Medicine, University Medical Center of the Johannes Gutenberg-University Mainz, Mainz, Germany

Jon D. Laman

Section Medical Physiology, Department of Neuroscience, University of Groningen, University Medical Center Groningen, Groningen, The Netherlands

Humana Press

Editors
Björn E. Clausen
Institute for Molecular Medicine
University Medical Center of the Johannes Gutenberg-University Mainz
Mainz, Germany

Jon D. Laman
Section Medical Physiology
Department of Neuroscience
University of Groningen
University Medical Center Groningen
Groningen, The Netherlands

ISSN 1064-3745 ISSN 1940-6029 (electronic)
Methods in Molecular Biology
ISBN 978-1-4939-8300-1 ISBN 978-1-4939-6786-5 (eBook)
DOI 10.1007/978-1-4939-6786-5

Printed on acid-free paper

This Humana Press imprint is published by Springer Nature
The registered company is Springer Science+Business Media LLC
The registered company address is: 233 Spring Street, New York, NY 10013, U.S.A.

Preface

Inflammation is part of a complex defense reaction of live tissues to injury. It is triggered by harmful stimuli, including pathogens, physical trauma, radiation, and chemical irritants. Inflammation is largely mediated by innate and adaptive immune cells in their efforts to eliminate the initial cause of tissue injury, clear out dead or infected cells, and facilitate tissue repair and wound healing. Hence, *acute* inflammation is beneficial to the host and must be tightly regulated. Too little inflammation may lead to progressive tissue destruction, for example, by the invading pathogen and compromise the survival of the host. In contrast, exaggerated and *chronic* inflammation is associated with many diseases ranging from contact allergy and asthma, psoriasis and rheumatoid arthritis, to inflammatory bowel disease, liver fibrosis, and inflammation of the central nervous system. Thus, a better understanding of the intricate interactions of the diverse cellular players and their molecular mediators holds the key to discover novel targets for designing improved immunotherapeutic strategies for the treatment of immune-mediated inflammatory diseases (IMID).

Considering the broad spectrum of IMID and the multidisciplinary scope of inflammation research, any protocol collection such as *Inflammation Protocols* will represent a limited selection of methods and tools to investigate inflammation that is largely biased by the personal choices of the editors. Owing to our strong conviction that the complex nature of an inflammatory reaction can best be studied in vivo, we have focused this volume on relevant animal models of human IMID. While naturally the emphasis lies on mice, we have also included innovative protocols studying zebrafish and nonhuman primates. Another personal flavor we introduced to the book is the combination of state-of-the-art descriptions of standard well-established IMID protocols, with bringing some highly specialized niche protocols such as the isolation and characterization of leukocytes from the aorta or oral mucosa to broader attention. Finally, we sought to incorporate some emerging technologies such as CyTOF and RNA sequencing that are currently being developed to study inflammation. These cutting-edge methods have the high potential to reveal novel targets, which can then be tested in different IMID models for the benefit of treating human diseases.

This volume of *Inflammation Protocols* is divided into four parts: The first three parts describe methods investigating IMID models affecting epithelial barriers to the environment, i.e., the skin (Part I), the lung (Part II), and the intestinal and oral mucosa (Part III). The last part illustrates inflammatory disease models of the brain, joints, and vasculature (Part IV). Despite the established relevance and high significance of in vivo protocols to study inflammation, there is an increasing awareness of issues concerning their reproducibility. Therefore, prior to the detailed descriptions of the various experimental protocols, we provide a viewpoint on how to avoid potential pitfalls in animal inflammation research.

Finally, we are particularly grateful to our friends and colleagues who contributed their favorite inflammation protocol to this collection. All contributing authors are leading experts in their respective fields, and we hope that their unique and comprehensive protocols will inspire the experienced investigator and the young experimenter alike to disentangle the fascinating process of inflammation.

Mainz, Germany — *Björn E. Clausen*
Groningen, The Netherlands — *Jon D. Laman*

Contents

Contributors

NAZIRA J. ALBARGOTHY • *Clinical Neurosciences, Faculty of Medicine, University of Southampton, Southampton, UK*

C.H. ALVES • *Department of Rheumatology and Immunology, Erasmus MC, University Medical Center Rotterdam, Rotterdam, The Netherlands*

P.S. ASMAWIDJAJA • *Department of Rheumatology and Immunology, Erasmus MC, University Medical Center Rotterdam, Rotterdam, The Netherlands*

CALUM C. BAIN • *Centre for Immunobiology, Institute of Infection, Immunity and Inflammation, College of Veterinary, Medical and Life Sciences, University of Glasgow, Scotland, UK; MRC Centre for Inflammation Research, Queens Medical Research Institute, University of Edinburgh, Edinburgh, Scotland, UK*

JACO BAKKER • *Animal Science Department, BPRC, Biomedical Primate Research Center, Rijswijk, The Netherlands*

BURKHARD BECHER • *Institute of Experimental Immunology, University of Zürich, Zürich, Switzerland*

DIOR M.J.M. BEERENS • *Department of Pulmonary Medicine, Erasmus MC Rotterdam, Rotterdam, The Netherlands*

YASMINE BELKAID • *Mucosal Immunology Section, Laboratory of Parasitic Diseases, National Institute of Allergy and Infectious Disease, National Institutes of Health, Bethesda, MD, USA*

L.A. VAN BERKEL • *Laboratory of Pediatrics, Division Gastroenterology and Nutrition, Erasmus University Medical Center, Rotterdam, The Netherlands*

ERIK W.G.M. BODDEKE • *Department of Neuroscience, University of Groningen, University Medical Center Groningen, Groningen, The Netherlands*

TOBIAS BOPP • *Institute for Immunology, University Medical Center of the Johannes Gutenberg-University Mainz, Mainz, Germany*

NICOLAS BOULADOUX • *Mucosal Immunology Section, Laboratory of Parasitic Diseases, National Institute of Allergy and Infectious Disease, National Institutes of Health, Bethesda, MD, USA*

ANNA BRAND • *Institute for Molecular Medicine, University Medical Center of the Johannes Gutenberg-University Mainz, Mainz, Germany*

ELIA BREEDVELD • *Department of Immunobiology, BPRC, Biomedical Primate Research Center, Rijswijk, The Netherlands*

MAARTEN D. BREM • *Department of Pulmonary Medicine, Erasmus MC Rotterdam, Rotterdam, The Netherlands*

NIESKE BROUWER • *Department of Neuroscience, University of Groningen, University Medical Center Groningen, Groningen, The Netherlands*

SYLVIA BRUGMAN • *Animal Sciences Group, Cell Biology and Immunology, Wageningen University, Wageningen, The Netherlands*

A. BRUHS • *Department of Dermatology, University Kiel, Kiel, Germany*

ROXANA O. CARARE • *Clinical Neurosciences, University of Southampton, Southampton, UK*

CHEOLHO CHEONG • *Laboratory of Cellular Physiology and Immunology, Institut de Researches Cliniques de Montréal, Montréal, QC, Canada; Division of Experimental Medicine, Department of Medicine, McGill University, Montreal, QC, Canada; Department of Microbiology, Infectiology, and Immunology, University of Montreal, Montreal, QC, Canada*

JAE-HOON CHOI • *Department of Life Science, College of Natural Sciences, Hanyang University, Seoul, Republic of Korea*

BJÖRN E. CLAUSEN • *Institute for Molecular Medicine, University Medical Center of the Johannes Gutenberg-University Mainz, Mainz, Germany*

CURDIN CONRAD • *Department of Dermatology, University Hospital CHUV, Lausanne, Switzerland*

NINCY DEBEUF • *VIB Inflammation Research Center, University of Ghent, Ghent, Belgium; Department of Internal Medicine, University Hospital Ghent, Ghent, Belgium*

ANDREAS DIEFENBACH • *Research Centre for Immunology and Institute of Medical Microbiology and Hygiene, University Medical Center of the Johannes Gutenberg-University Mainz, Mainz, Germany; Institute of Microbiology, Charité - University Medical Centre Berlin, Hindenburgdamm, Berlin, Germany*

JEREMY DI DOMIZIO • *Department of Dermatology, University Hospital CHUV, Lausanne, Switzerland*

SANDRINE DUBRAC • *Epidermal Biology Laboratory, Department of Dermatology, Venereology and Allergology, Medical University of Innsbruck, Innsbruck, Austria*

GYOHEI EGAWA • *Department of Dermatology, Kyoto University Graduate School of Medicine, Kyoto, Japan*

BART J.L. EGGEN • *Department of Neuroscience, University of Groningen, University Medical Center Groningen, Groningen, The Netherlands*

HENRIKE FLEIGE • *Institute of Immunology, Hannover Medical School, Hannover, Germany*

EDWIN F. FLORENCIA • *Department of Dermatology, Erasmus University Medical Center, Rotterdam, The Netherlands*

REINHOLD FÖRSTER • *Institute of Immunology, Hannover Medical School, Hannover, Germany*

THAIS F. GALATRO • *Department of Neurology, School of Medicine, University of São Paulo, São Paulo, Brazil*

MAUREEN GATHERER • *Clinical Neurosciences, University of Southampton, Southampton, UK*

BEN N.G. GIEPMANS • *Department of Cell Biology, University Medical Center Groningen, University of Groningen, Groningen, The Netherlands*

MICHEL GILLIET • *Department of Dermatology, University Hospital CHUV, Lausanne, Switzerland*

KONRAD GRONKE • *Research Centre for Immunology and Institute of Medical Microbiology, University Medical Center of the Johannes Gutenberg-University Mainz, Mainz, Germany; Max-Planck-Institute for Immunobiology and Epigenetics, Freiburg, Germany*

BERNHARD HAID • *Department for Pediatric Urology, Hospital of the Sisters of Charity, Linz, Austria*

TJAKKO J. VAN HAM • *Department of Clinical Genetics, Erasmus MC, University Medical Center Rotterdam, Rotterdam, The Netherlands*

HAMIDA HAMMAD • *VIB Inflammation Research Center, University of Ghent, Ghent, Belgium; Department of Internal Medicine, University Hospital Ghent, Ghent, Belgium*

FELIX J. HARTMANN • *Institute of Experimental Immunology, University of Zürich, Zürich, Switzerland*

ELINE HASPESLAGH • *VIB Inflammation Research Center, University of Ghent, Ghent, Belgium; Department of Biomedical Molecular Biology, University of Ghent, Ghent, Belgium*

CHERYL HAWKES • *Department of Life, Health and Chemical Sciences, The Open University, Milton Keynes, UK*

INEKE M. HEKKING-WEIJMA • *Department of Plastic Surgery, Erasmus University Medical Center, Rotterdam, The Netherlands*

RUDI W. HENDRIKS • *Department of Pulmonary Medicine, Erasmus MC Rotterdam, Rotterdam, The Netherlands*

CLOTILDE HENNEQUIN • *Centre d'Immunologie de Marseille-Luminy, Aix Marseille Université, Inserm, CNRS, Marseille, France*

SANDRINE HENRI • *Centre d'Immunologie de Marseille-Luminy, Aix Marseille Université, Inserm, CNRS, Marseille, France*

LAURA HESSE • *Department of Pathology and Medical Biology, Laboratory of Experimental Pulmonology and Inflammation Research (EXPIRE), University Medical Center Groningen, University of Groningen, Groningen, The Netherlands; Groningen Research Institute for Asthma and COPD (GRIAC), University Medical Center Groningen, University of Groningen, Groningen, The Netherlands*

AVI-HAI HOVAV • *Institute of Dental Sciences, Faculty of Dental Medicine, Hebrew University, Jerusalem, Israel*

MARCEL F. JONKMAN • *Center for Blistering Diseases, Department of Dermatology, University Medical Center Groningen, University of Groningen, Groningen, The Netherlands*

KENJI KABASHIMA • *Department of Dermatology, Kyoto University Graduate School of Medicine, Kyoto, Japan*

MEREI KEEHNEN • *Animal Science Department, BPRC, Biomedical Primate Research Center, Rijswijk, The Netherlands*

YONG OOK KIM • *Institute of Translational Immunology, and Research Center for Immune Therapy (FZI) University Medical Center, Johannes Gutenberg-University Mainz, Mainz, Germany*

MATTHIAS KLEIN • *Institute for Immunology, University Medical Center of the Johannes Gutenberg-University Mainz, Mainz, Germany*

RIANNE KLOMP • *Department of Immunobiology, BPRC, Biomedical Primate Research Center, Rijswijk, The Netherlands*

MICHAEL KOFOED-NIELSEN • *Research Centre for Immunology and Institute of Medical Microbiology, University Medical Center of the Johannes Gutenberg-University Mainz, Mainz, Germany; Max-Planck-Institute for Immunobiology and Epigenetics, Freiburg, Germany*

SUSANNE M. KOOISTRA • *Section Medical Physiology, Department of Neuroscience, University of Groningen, University Medical Center Groningen, Groningen, The Netherlands*

SABINE KOSSMANN • *Center for Thrombosis and Hemostasis Mainz, University Medical Center Mainz, Mainz, Germany; Center for Cardiology, University Medical Center Mainz, Mainz, Germany*

A.E. KOZIJN • *Laboratory of Pediatrics, Division Gastroenterology and Nutrition, Erasmus University Medical Center, Rotterdam, The Netherlands*

LAURA E. KUIL • *Department of Clinical Genetics, Erasmus MC, University Medical Center Rotterdam, Rotterdam, The Netherlands*

JEREMY LAGRANGE • *Center for Thrombosis and Hemostasis Mainz, University Medical Center Mainz, Mainz, Germany*

JON D. LAMAN • *Section Medical Physiology, Department of Neuroscience, University of Groningen, University Medical Center Groningen, Groningen, The Netherlands*

BART N. LAMBRECHT • *VIB Inflammation Research Center, University of Ghent, Ghent, Belgium; Department of Internal Medicine, University Hospital Ghent, Ghent, Belgium*

JUN SEONG LEE • *Laboratory of Cellular Physiology and Immunology, Institut de Recherches Cliniques de Montréal, Montréal, QC, Canada; Department of Microbiology, Infectiology and Immunology, University of Montreal, Montreal, QC, Canada*

BOBBY W.S. LI • *Department of Pulmonary Medicine, Erasmus MC Rotterdam, Rotterdam, The Netherlands*

ERIK LUBBERTS • *Department of Rheumatology and Immunology, Erasmus MC, University Medical Center Rotterdam, Rotterdam, The Netherlands*

BERNARD MALISSEN • *Centre d'Immunologie de Marseille-Luminy, Aix Marseille Université, Inserm, CNRS, Marseille, France*

CAMILLE MALOSSE • *Centre d'Immunologie de Marseille-Luminy, Aix Marseille Université, Inserm, CNRS, Marseille, France*

GABRIEL MIZRAJI • *Department of Periodontology, Faculty of Dental Medicine, Hebrew University-Hadassah Medical Center, Jerusalem, Israel; Institute of Dental Sciences, Faculty of Dental Medicine, Hebrew University, Jerusalem, Israel*

M. MOLENDIJK • *Department of Rheumatology and Immunology, Erasmus MC, University Medical Center Rotterdam, Rotterdam, The Netherlands*

VERENA MOOSBRUGGER-MARTINZ • *Epidermal Biology Laboratory, Department of Dermatology, Venereology and Allergology, Medical University of Innsbruck, Innsbruck, Austria*

ALAN MORRIS • *Clinical Neurosciences, Faculty of Medicine, University of Southampton, Southampton, UK*

ALLAN MCI MOWAT • *Centre for Immunobiology, Institute of Infection, Immunity and Inflammation, College of Veterinary, Medical and Life Sciences, University of Glasgow, Glasgow, Scotland, UK*

DUNJA MRDJEN • *Institute of Experimental Immunology, University of Zürich, Zürich, Switzerland*

A.M.C. MUS • *Department of Rheumatology and Immunology, Erasmus MC, University Medical Center Rotterdam, Rotterdam, The Netherlands*

MARTIJN C. NAWIJN • *Department of Pathology and Medical Biology, Laboratory of Experimental Pulmonology and Inflammation Research (EXPIRE), University Medical Center Groningen, Groningen, The Netherlands; Groningen Research Institute for Asthma and COPD (GRIAC), University Medical Center Groningen, University of Groningen, Groningen, The Netherlands*

EDWARD E.S. NIEUWENHUIS • *Department of Pediatrics, Wilhelmina Children's Hospital, UMC Utrecht, University Medical Center Utrecht, Utrecht, The Netherlands*

MIRANDA NIJENHUIS • *Center for Blistering Diseases, Department of Dermatology, University Medical Center Groningen, University of Groningen, Groningen, The Netherlands*

JULIA L. OBER-BLÖBAUM • *Institute for Molecular Medicine, University Medical Center of the Johannes Gutenberg-University Mainz, Mainz, Germany*

Armanda J. Onderdijk • *Department of Dermatology, Erasmus University Medical Center, Rotterdam, The Netherlands*
Nynke Oosterhof • *Department of Clinical Genetics, Erasmus MC, University Medical Center Rotterdam, Rotterdam, The Netherlands*
Daniela Ortner • *Department of Dermatology, Venereology & Allergology, Division of Experimental Dermatology, Medical University of Innsbruck, Innsbruck, Austria*
Anton Page • *Biomedical Imaging Unit, University of Southampton, Southampton, UK*
Hendri H. Pas • *Center for Blistering Diseases, Department of Dermatology, University Medical Center Groningen, University of Groningen, Groningen, The Netherlands*
Yury Popov • *Division of Gastroenterology, Beth Israel Deaconess Medical Center, Harvard Medical School, Boston, MA, USA*
M.F. du Pré • *Laboratory of Pediatrics, Division Gastroenterology and Nutrition, Erasmus University Medical Center, Rotterdam, The Netherlands*
Errol P. Prens • *Department of Dermatology, Department of Dermatology, Rotterdam, The Netherlands*
W. Razawy • *Department of Rheumatology and Immunology, Erasmus MC, University Medical Center Rotterdam, Rotterdam, The Netherlands*
Sonja Reißig • *Institute for Molecular Medicine, University Medical Center of the Johannes Gutenberg-University Mainz, Mainz, Germany*
Janneke N. Samsom • *Laboratory of Pediatrics, Division Gastroenterology and Nutrition, Erasmus University Medical Center, Rotterdam, The Netherlands*
Edgar Schmitt • *Institute for Immunology, University Medical Center of the Johannes Gutenberg-University Mainz, Mainz, Germany*
Matthias Schmuth • *Epidermal Biology Laboratory, Department of Dermatology, Venereology and Allergology, Medical University of Innsbruck, Innsbruck, Austria*
Detlef Schuppan • *Institute of Translational Immunology and Research Center for Immune Therapy (FZI), University Medical Center of the Johannes Gutenberg-University Mainz, Mainz, Germany; Division of Gastroenterology, Beth Israel Deaconess Medical Center, Harvard Medical School, Boston, MA, USA*
Thomas Schwarz • *Department of Dermatology, University Kiel, Kiel, Germany*
Charlotte L. Scott • *Centre for Immunobiology, Institute of Infection, Immunity and Inflammation, College of Veterinary, Medical and Life Sciences, University of Glasgow, Scotland, UK; Inflammation Research Centre (IRC), Laboratory of Immunoregulation, Inflammation Research Centre (IRC), VIB Ghent University, Ghent (Zwijnaarde), Belgium*
Hafez Sharawi • *Institute of Dental Sciences, Faculty of Dental Medicine, Hebrew University, Jerusalem, Israel*
Matthew MacGregor Sharp • *Clinical Neurosciences, University of Southampton, Southampton, UK*
Dahee Shim • *Department of Life Science, College of Natural Sciences, Hanyang University, Seoul, Republic of Korea*
Klaas A. Sjollema • *Department of Cell Biology, University Medical Center Groningen, University of Groningen, Groningen, The Netherlands*
Ena Sokol • *Department of Cell Biology, University Medical Center Groningen, University of Groningen, Groningen, The Netherlands; Center for Blistering Diseases, Department of Dermatology, University Medical Center Groningen, University of Groningen, Groningen, The Netherlands*

PATRIZIA STOITZNER • *Department of Dermatology, Venereology & Allergology, Division of Experimental Dermatology, Medical University of Innsbruck, Innsbruck, Austria*
YAARA TABIB • *Institute of Dental Sciences, Faculty of Dental Medicine, Hebrew University, Jerusalem, Israel*
CHRISTOPH TRIPP • *Department of Dermatology, Venereology & Allergology, Division of Experimental Dermatology, Medical University of Innsbruck, Innsbruck, Austria*
ALEXANDER ULGES • *Institute for Immunology, University Medical Center of the Johannes Gutenberg-University Mainz, Mainz, Germany*
ILIA D. VAINCHTEIN • *Department of Neuroscience, University of Groningen, University Medical Center Groningen, Groningen, The Netherlands*
S. VEENBERGEN • *Laboratory of Pediatrics, Division Gastroenterology and Nutrition, Erasmus University Medical Center, Rotterdam, The Netherlands*
MICHEL P.M. VIERBOOM • *Department of Immunobiology, BPRC, Biomedical Primate Research Center, Rijswijk, The Netherlands*
BENNO WEIGMANN • *Department of Medicine 1, University of Erlangen-Nuremberg, Erlangen, Germany*
ROY O. WELLER • *Clinical Neurosciences, University of Southampton, Southampton, UK*
PHILIP WENZEL • *Center for Cardiology—Cardiology I, German Center for Cardiovascular Research (DZHK), Mainz, Germany; Center for Thrombosis and Hemostasis, German Center for Cardiovascular Research (DZHK), Mainz, Germany*
ASAF WILENSKY • *Department of Periodontology, Faculty of Dental Medicine, Hebrew University-Hadassah Medical Center, Jerusalem, Israel*
TAE JIN YUN • *Laboratory of Cellular Physiology and Immunology, Institut de Recherches Cliniques de Montréal, Montréal, QC, Canada; Division of Experimental Medicine, Department of Medicine, McGill University, Montreal, QC, Canada*

Chapter 1

Reproducibility Issues: Avoiding Pitfalls in Animal Inflammation Models

Jon D. Laman, Susanne M. Kooistra, and Björn E. Clausen

Abstract

In light of an enhanced awareness of ethical questions and ever increasing costs when working with animals in biomedical research, there is a dedicated and sometimes fierce debate concerning the (lack of) reproducibility of animal models and their relevance for human inflammatory diseases. Despite evident advancements in searching for alternatives, that is, replacing, reducing, and refining animal experiments—the three R's of Russel and Burch (1959)—understanding the complex interactions of the cells of the immune system, the nervous system and the affected tissue/organ during inflammation critically relies on in vivo models. Consequently, scientific advancement and ultimately novel therapeutic interventions depend on improving the reproducibility of animal inflammation models. As a prelude to the remaining hands-on protocols described in this volume, here, we summarize potential pitfalls of preclinical animal research and provide resources and background reading on how to avoid them.

Key words Animal models, Reproducibility, Repeatability, Replication, Statistics, Randomization, Research assessment, Publication bias, Robustness, Transgenic artifact, Microbiome, Microbiota, Immunity, Inflammation, Lymphocytes, Myeloid cells

1 General Background

Reproducibility of experimental findings is a cornerstone to scientific progress, as well as to the rational development of novel medical interventions. Although the scientific discourse on this theme is longstanding, during the past 5 years this has developed into an intense societal debate. A well-researched article in The Economist (2013) titled "*Trouble at the lab*", attracted broad attention, following up on scientific papers demonstrating disappointingly low replicability of a selection of major scientific breakthroughs. For instance, researchers at the *Amgen* company could replicate not more than six out of 53 studies on cancer biology [1], a result highly similar to an analysis performed by *Bayer* [2].

The importance of this debate is paramount as reproducibility issues impair true progress, drain limited resources and can negatively

Björn E. Clausen and Jon D. Laman (eds.), *Inflammation: Methods and Protocols*, Methods in Molecular Biology, vol. 1559, DOI 10.1007/978-1-4939-6786-5_1, © Springer Science+Business Media LLC 2017

affect public and political support for research. On the positive side, a wide array of publications, guidelines, checklists, and online resources has flourished from the discussions. These will eventually improve the quality of future studies and data, although it remains a continuous challenge to not stifle scientific progress with an overload of administration.

A strong and creative voice in the debate and the development of improvements is that of epidemiologist John Ioannidis and colleagues such as Steven Goodman. Several of their central contributions are referred to in this chapter. They recently initiated the Meta-Research Innovation Center at Stanford University (METRICS) to perform "*rigorous evaluation of research practices and find ways to optimize the reproducibility and efficiency of scientific investigations.*" Although the emphasis in this effort lies more on clinical studies and epidemiology, very worthwhile investigations were also done into animal work [3–6]. Several such papers contain very practical tables, boxes and checklists for enhancing reproducibility [7, 8]. Notably, the latter two papers (and also others) emphasize that the current scientific reward systems require improvements: "*Scientists may continue publishing and getting grants, without making real progress, if more publications and more grants are all that matters*".

Similarly, microbiologist Ferric Fang and immunologist Arturo Casadevall have made several constructive and critical contributions to both the scientific and societal debate on the organization of the scientific enterprise, including publication bias, scientific integrity, reward systems, and how these could be improved [9–15].

2 Aims and Outline of this Chapter

It is quite conceivable that for young researchers focusing on their individual projects and experiments, it can be difficult to select relevant items from the seemingly bewildering array of publications and resources. This may also be true for some more experienced and seasoned investigators who are often much pressed for time, and who by definition were trained in other times.

Hence, this chapter aims to do just that, namely to provide an accessible toolbox and starter kit, with a particular focus on inflammation in animal models, the theme of this volume. The core of this chapter is formed by four boxes on definitions (Boxes 1 and 2), distinct resources (Box 3), and practical tips (Box 4). With this in hand, we hope junior researchers will be able to avoid a considerable series of potential pitfalls. In addition, we provide an extensive reference list, highlighting a number of central publications we regard particularly informative. Note that not all references are individually discussed and cited in the text [16–36]. We would like to recommend that junior researchers starting to work with animal models read at least the following key publications: On being a scientist [37], the ARRIVE guidelines [38, 39], Reproducibility in science [7], A call for transparent reporting to optimize the predictive value of preclinical research [40], How to make more published research true [8], The Leiden Manifesto [41], and The fickle p-value [42]. This amounts to a few-hour investment that will pay off from a scientific, an ethical, and an educational perspective.

Box 1. Definitions and (mis)understandings

Repeatability, replicability, and reproducibility are terms used to describe the expected outcome of further experimentation under different conditions. As the terms are often used interchangeably, it is advised to describe precisely what is meant, instead of assuming that they are self-explanatory. These three terms are referred to with different and sometimes conflicting meanings, both between fields (e.g., engineering versus biomedicine), and even within fields, biomedicine being no exception.

Repeatability—Getting the same results over and over again, without changing anything in the experimental setup (including the experimenter). This does not exclude that the results are due to an unknown factor. For example: a method for staining samples gave highly consistent results, until a new bottle of a standard ingredient was obtained. It later appeared that the ingredient had to be aged 6 months or more in order to get the desired result.

Replicability—Reproducing results on other samples, or using other methods.

Reproducibility—Results obtained by different people in redoing an experiment.

For instance, in animal behavior experiments, introducing systematic variation of experimental conditions, termed heterogenization, limited spurious results and improved reproducibility [43]. This seems counterintuitive since one would expect standardization to be beneficial. Heterogenization is a powerful tool to detect the sensitivity of experiments for unwanted but often unavoidable variations in conditions, by applying systematic changes that are larger than the expected random fluctuations. Variations should be carefully planned, and use of experimental design methods is highly recommended. A statistician's advice is needed for all but the most simple setups.

Statistical generalizability—Inferring from a sample to a population. Statistical generalization is based on sampling theory. This implies that if a sample is not really random (as is often the case) statistical generalizability is not guaranteed. Especially case control designs where allele frequencies are compared between groups are vulnerable for random bias due to inadequate matching, because allele frequencies are subject to exponential variation in closed populations. Inbred strains can have very different properties from wild type animals. One reason for this is that natural selection in inbred strains could eliminate all variants with strong and lethal effects that could survive in a random breeding population.

The results of significance testing (P values) can vary considerably between random samples. Reporting of results by computing confidence intervals is therefore strongly advised.

Scientific generalizability—Applying the theoretical model based on a particular set of conditions to other situations.

Largely based on [44] and discussions with Dr. G.J. te Meerman.

Box 2. A core set of reporting standards for rigorous study design

Randomization

- Animals should be assigned randomly to the various experimental groups, and the method of randomization reported.
- Data should be collected and processed randomly or appropriately blocked.

Blinding

- Allocation concealment: the investigator should be unaware of the group to which the next animal taken from a cage will be allocated.
- Blinded conduct of the experiment: animal caretakers and investigators conducting the experiments should be blinded to the allocation sequence.
- Blinded assessment of outcome: investigators assessing, measuring, or quantifying experimental outcomes should be blinded to the intervention.

Sample-size estimation

- An appropriate sample size should be computed when the study is being designed and the statistical method of computation reported.
- Statistical methods that take into account multiple evaluations of the data should be used when an interim evaluation is carried out.

Data handling

- Rules for stopping data collection should be defined in advance.
- Criteria for inclusion and exclusion of data should be established prospectively.
- How outliers will be defined and handled should be decided when the experiment is being designed, and any data removed before analysis should be reported.
- The primary end point should be prospectively selected. If multiple end points are to be assessed, then appropriate statistical corrections should be applied.
- Investigators should report on data missing because of attrition or exclusion.
- Pseudo replicate issues need to be considered during study design and analysis.
- Investigators should report how often a particular experiment was performed and whether results were substantiated by repetition under a range of conditions.

Reproduced with permission from [40].

Box 3. Selection of online reproducibility resources and checklists

Resources	Refs
General	
The reproducibility initiative aims to identify and reward reproducible research	[45]
Transparency and Openness promotion (*TOP*) guidelines	[46, 47]
Reporting checklist for Life Sciences articles (*Nature*)	[26, 48]
Meta-Research Innovation Center at Stanford (*METRICS*)	[49]
Protocol exchange (*Nature*)	[50]
Reducing IrreProducibility in labOratory STudiEs (*RIPOSTE*)	[51]
Laboratory Quality Management System Training Toolkit (*World Health Organization*)	[52]

(continued)

Box 3. (continued)

Authorship Guidelines (*International Committee of Medical Journal Editors*)	[53]
Reporting guidelines for health research (*EQUATOR*)	[54]
Guidelines from the Federation of American Societies for Experimental Biology (FASEB)	[55]
On being a scientist (NIH)	[37]
Pipetting techniques	
Several manufacturers of manual pipettes (Including *Gilson*, *Mettler Toledo* and *Eppendorf*) have published online tutorials	[56–58]
Animal experimental setup	
Animal Research: Reporting of In Vivo Experiments (*ARRIVE* guidelines)	[38, 59]
Guidance for the Description of Animal Research in Publications from ILAR	[60]
A gold standard publication checklist to improve the quality of animal studies	[61]
SYRCLE tool to reduce bias in animal studies	[62]
International mouse phenotyping consortium (IMPC)	[63]
Experimental design assistant (*EDA*) from the National Centre for the Replacement, Refinement & Reduction of Animals in Research (NC3R^s)	[64]
In vitro cell culture	
International Cell Line Authentication Committee (*ICLAC*)	[65, 66]
Guidelines for the use of cell lines in biomedical research	[67, 68]
Downstream analyses	
Immunohistochemistry	[69, 70]
Image acquisition	[71]
Digital image analysis do's and don'ts	[72]
Quantification of Western blots using *densitometry*	[73]
Design and reporting of qPCR data: Minimum Information for Publication of Quantitative Real-Time PCR Experiments *(MIQE)* guidelines	[74]
Identification of functional elements in the genome (e.g., Chromatin Immunoprecipitation, whole genome bisulphite sequencing, DNase sequencing, FAIRE sequencing): *ENCODE* guidelines and the *Roadmap Epigenomics Project*	[75–77]
Minimum Information for Biological and Biomedical Investigations (*MIBBI*), including guidelines for flow cytometry, cellular assays and many others	[78]

Box 4. Selection of pitfalls/pointers/tips/red flags from authors experiences

Awareness/Training and preparation
Many widely used cell lines have been reported to be contaminated. This does not allow for rigorous testing of hypotheses (an example: when sequencing data from HeLa cells contain sequences covering the Y-chromosome). However, it is not only old cell lines that have been passaged for many generations, also newly generated cell lines can be subject to contamination issues. A recent example is the reported identification of STAP cells [79], a high profile finding that was not reproducible [80] and involved cell contamination.
Use of siRNA/shRNA strategies to deplete a protein of interest can result in quite severe off target effects [81]. Using at least 2 independent hairpin sequences and rescue experiments using a cDNA that is not targeted by the hairpin helps to avoid this. Especially certain cell types, including embryonic stem cells, appear to be prone to phenotypic changes that are not related to the downregulation of the gene of interest.
The product sheets depicted on supplier websites are often not updated when new batches of the reagent are made available. For example in case of polyclonal antibodies targeting posttranslationally modified proteins, new batches could be less/nonspecific and should always be tested.
The choice of mouse strain can greatly influence results: Inbred vs. outbred, but also more specifically FVB, C57BL/6, BALB/c, DBA, etc.
Insufficient preparatory reading prior to design of the animal experiment—"*Half a year in the lab can save half an hour in the library*". This point is also made in the SYRCLE recommendations for animal studies: a systematic analysis of the literature on the topic should be performed [62].
Lack of formal and high level biostatistics training of junior and experienced researchers. In conjunction, expert advice of certified statisticians is not sought sufficiently, both for experimental design and data interpretation.
Exceptional features of individual mouse strains used, including strong bias towards C57Bl/6 mice due to compatibility with transgenesis. This problem may be alleviated by rapid spread of CRISPR/Cas technologies pioneered by Jennifer Doudna [82, 83].
Thorough power analysis is required in the design of any animal experiment. Button and colleagues state that "*small studies consistently give more favorable (that is "positive") results than larger studies and that study quality [rigour] is inversely related to effect size*" [84].
Transgenic artifacts: Insufficient awareness of and reporting on the limitations of the transgenic model used, e.g., leakiness, promoter activity in other than anticipated cell type, the effect of usually strong viral promoters driving resistance cassettes on nearby genes, or the effect of an inserted reporter gene as compared to a clean knockout.
Execution
Use of PBS for solutions and in controls results in effects due to the phosphates present in PBS. 0.9% NaCl is a better alternative.
The presence of chicken ovalbumin (OVA) in standard commercial mouse chow can be a serious confounder in experiments where OVA is used as a model immunogen and tolerogen, for instance by oral administration.
In the analysis of knockout mice, littermates (wild type and heterozygotes) should be used as controls, in contrast to wild type animals obtained from commercial or in-house suppliers.
All experimental animals should be genotyped, as well as re-genotyped after termination of the experiment.

(continued)

Many aspects of mouse housing can influence experimental outcome. Examples are: the climate in housing facilities, the effect of specific housing conditions, including bedding material and cage enrichment, the effect of individual housing, the need of animals to acclimatize after transport, the effect of circadian rhythm on behavioral experiments, the exact type of food used, or unawareness of how high-fat food goes rancid quickly, thereby influencing food intake, and, as is becoming increasingly clear differences in the microbiome between different animal facilities.
Stress can influence experimental outcome and can be induced in animals in response to the skill-level of the researcher, the presence of other researchers in the facility, fighting or when animals are used in multiple studies.
Reproducibility can be improved by thorough standardization of experimental procedures, including the time of injection and sampling etc.
LPS potency can vary greatly between batches. Ideally the same batch/lot should be used throughout experiments.
A single inbred animal strain formally represents only a single individual in biological terms, including MHC haplotype.
Animal gender: insufficient systematic use of both male and female animals. Obviously, there are many scientific and pragmatic reasons why both genders cannot always be used. There is also enjoyable anecdotal evidence that some regulatory bodies can have overshoot reflexes, for instance in demanding that female animals are included in prostate research.
Underestimation of irradiation artifacts in experiments to generate bone marrow chimeras (e.g., large scale inflammation due to damage in the intestines).
Animals should be formally randomized over groups and rooms.
The observers in animal experiments should be blinded to animal treatment. This is essential, and logistically not trivial. The coding scheme should be officially secured and locked away from the observers. Treatment agents should be coded such that their functional identity is not known.
Antigen-adjuvant preparations are critical to all vaccination studies and most autoimmune animal models. Procedures used are vastly different from lab to lab, and they are often only minimally described in publications. Sources of variation and confusion include: Poorly characterized peptide and protein batches, often with contaminations such as LPS and containing protein/peptide fragments; Highly unreliable weighing of powder-form protein or peptide since this is very hygroscopic; Inoculum preparation by simple mixing (at different temperatures), versus mixing using connected syringes providing high shear stress and completely different colloidal properties; Complete Freund's Adjuvant (CFA) containing different types of mycobacterium species, e.g., *M. tuberculosis* versus *M. butyricum*; Addition of extra mycobacterium to commercial CFA, and incomplete mention of this in the Materials and Methods section.
For autoimmune disease models, with EAE as the prime example, it can be advised to in vivo titrate larger batches of self proteins/peptides, in conjunction with the appropriate adjuvant and additional treatments, such as pertussis toxin (PTX). This allows to calibrate disease course and severity such that both upmodulation and downmodulation is possible for a large series of future experiments. Some companies now offer pre-titrated self-antigen/adjuvant emulsions, excluding at least some sources of variation.
For investigators new to in situ analysis, it is often useful to stress the importance and difference between tissue controls (e.g., untreated versus treated animals) and positive and negative staining controls (e.g., First antibody/reagent omission control; For new antibodies an isotype matched positive control antibody that is sure to work in the tissue under investigation; An isotype/subclass matched negative control antibody; Confirmatory check that substrate solution is active by mixing with final step enzyme-linked reagent present in off-flow from sections.

(continued)

Box 4. (continued)

Tissue-endogenous peroxidase, for instance in neutrophils, is often a confounding factor in HRP enzyme immunohistochemistry. Addition of low percentage of H_2O_2 in the acetone used for fixation of frozen sections alleviates this issue, but not always completely. This problem can be conveniently circumvented by visualizing endogenous peroxidase activity with chloronaphthol, resulting in a blue-black precipitate.
LPS contamination of glassware, reagents, synthetic peptides, and (recombinant) proteins, such as ovalbumin. There is evidence that also Ficoll and Percoll can contain unduly high levels of LPS.
Injection of cells or compound into the mouse brain should take into account that very small volumes should be used, in the order of 0.5 μL. 4 μL is already too much, leading to undue damage and leakage into other compartments.
Mouse splenic red pulp macrophages contain so much iron from effete erythrocytes, that the group of Kurts turned an initial artifactual finding into an experimental procedure: even without addition of magnetic beads, these macrophages can be magnetically isolated [85].
Affinity purification of monoclonal antibodies for in vivo treatment: surprisingly, it does happen that researchers do not correctly match the biological species in which the antibody was made (large majority mouse, rat, hamster) with either Protein-A or Protein-G. In addition, an alternative approach is the classic method of thiophilic agarose. When optimized, this method allows to isolate 100–150 mg of antibody from 3 to 4 l of culture medium [86].
Isotype controls for in vivo treatment studies: We have argued previously [87] that the use of antibody isotype controls has very serious limitations and should be discouraged. (1) Undue crossbinding of the control antibody, to an unknown epitope in the target animal model should be completely excluded, and this is very difficult to do with certainty. (2) When an antibody isotype control yields an unexpected outcome, in practice often another one is selected which behaves as predicted. Hence, there is selection of the isotype control. Strictly speaking, isotype control treatment could be regarded as a waste of animals and resources since it introduces an uncontrolled parameter into the experiment [86].
Biased survival of only a fraction of mouse couples joined by parabiosis surgery.
Commercial reagents can be a source of contamination, for instance in microbiome sequencing [88].
Microbiota typing: We predict that different levels of routine gut microbiota typing of animal models for inflammation will soon become commonplace. This will be followed by mandatory typing imposed by top tier journals. Dependent on the application of the model, routine microbiota typing for other organs and anatomical locations will be implemented (e.g., skin, eye, lungs).
Analysis/Reporting
Insufficient mention in publications of animal housing conditions, including light/dark regime, (acidified) water, composition of and variation in mouse chow, sound conditions (including radio music for benefit of investigators and animal care takers), measures to prevent infection.
To prevent publication bias, negative outcomes (i.e., lack of effects) should be published in a way that data are available to the international community. Fortunately, more types of outlets for such publications are becoming available, including new journals, and (institutional) server resources.
In silico artifacts: we argue that this is an underestimated source of problems. Examples include: Uncritical adoption of other investigators spreadsheet designs, including mathematical formulas for analysis; In addition, experimenters generate large NGS datasets that they often cannot analyze themselves, whereas bioinformaticians sometimes lack biological background. As a result unintended mistakes in analysis can go unnoticed.

Box 4 represents a selection of tips, recommendations, challenges, potential pitfalls, and red flags that we experienced in our own experiments, and that were collected from some of the authors in this volume. Especially, here we aim to provide original and practical information to enhance the quality and success rate of your experiments.

3 Are Animal Models Useful to Model Human Conditions Anyway?

The validity of animal models for human conditions including inflammatory diseases is a topic of heated and controversial debate as well as detailed conflicting reviews. For the purpose of this book, we restrict ourselves to a number of premises:

- The discussion is often confused by insufficient separation of the distinct aims of dissecting basic biology, versus uncovering mechanisms of pathogenesis, versus drug development.
- The famous quote "*All models are wrong, but some are useful*" by statistician George Box referring to statistical models was explained by him in 1979 as "*Now it would be very remarkable if any system existing in the real world could be exactly represented by any simple model. However, cunningly chosen parsimonious models often do provide remarkably useful approximations.* [.....] *For such a model there is no need to ask the question* "*Is the model true?*". *If* "*truth*" *is to be the* "*whole truth*" *the answer must be* "*No*". *The only question of interest is* "*Is the model illuminating and useful?*". Hence, in animal models of inflammation, it should be defined very strictly what aspect of the distinct human conditions the system should mimic.
- The interactions between the highly diverse and mobile immune cell subsets with complex organ systems cannot be reliably mimicked with human and in vitro studies only.
- Therefore, the calls by some to replace all animal testing by human studies are ill-founded since the consequence would be an inacceptable slowing of the pace of discovery, and many immunological questions would become completely intractable.
- However, there is no doubt that the high attrition rate of candidate drugs should be reduced by major improvements and extension of the current animal models. This entire volume strives to attain such improvements. Several of the chapters contribute to the three R's of animal studies, i.e., reduction, replacement and refinement [89].

- One such improvement could entail an intermediary step between human trials and the basic research performed in inbred, genetically modified and SPF-housed mice. These models are invaluable, allow for rigorous testing and have resulted in the discovery of many mechanistic insights into the development of inflammatory diseases. However, recent reports indicate that the exposure of laboratory mouse strains to pathogens results in an immune system that is more comparable to the human situation [90, 91]. Mice with such a 'normalized microbial environment' could prove highly useful in the future to validate promising therapeutic candidates from "clean" mouse models prior to clinical trials in patients.

4 Study Design and Statistics

It has been recognized for a while now that the quality and rigor of statistical methods in (bio)medical publications is often inadequate or even poor, both in clinical and in animal studies. Interestingly, recent papers highlight the (mis)interpretations of what the p-value represents, and what it can or should not be used for [42, 92]. A series of measures at different levels aims to mitigate this issue, including: More attention for statistics training of young investigators; Early engagement of certified statisticians in study design, execution and analysis; Development of guidelines for statistical reporting that can be adopted by all journals; Within-study replication of the findings in an independent cohort (now mostly for human genetics studies); And enhanced statistic rigor in the review process, with some journals employing independent statisticians for that purpose.

In animal research, some hot topics on study design include:

- Optimal balancing of animal number based on ethical and financial considerations in relation to statistical power analysis.
- Robust randomization of experimental animals; Blinding of researchers to treatment; Publication of neutral or negative outcomes.
- The tendency of some methodologists and, in particular, animal ethics committees to claim that a single experiment with relatively large animal groups is to be preferred over replicate experiments. This is a fundamental issue, and the prestigious *Journal of Experimental Medicine* in an editorial quite rightly stated "*Although this is a laudable practice [using large animal groups] that should apply to all experiments, it has no bearing on the issue of experimental reproducibility*" [93].

- The fact that experimental animals are most often housed under specified pathogen free (SPF), or otherwise relatively artificial conditions, with very limited exposure to environmental pathogens. Moreover, the SPF status differs between different animal facilities.
- The genetic background (e.g., C57BL/6 or BALB/c) can have a strong influence on phenotype. In addition, for understandable economic reasons, most often (very) young adult animals of the same sex are used.

The discussion on the usefulness of animal models for inflammation research recently got much confused by an initial paper bluntly claiming that animal models do not appropriately mimic human conditions [94]. Subsequently, other researchers reached exactly the opposite conclusions using the very same data set [95]. This controversy was followed by an extensive debate in a series of papers. We would like to recommend the commentary by Christoph Benoist [96] as particularly informative. Another constructive contribution to the discussion is the concise and very balanced review on the use of animal models for research on aging (in which inflammation is essential) with oftentimes quite subtle pros and cons [97].

An influential effort to improve the quality of animal models is the establishment of the ARRIVE guidelines [38, 39]. Even if the ARRIVE guidelines are not compulsory under national conditions, it is still highly recommended to refer to them in detail for the design, execution and reporting of animal experiments. A core set of reporting standards can be found in Box 2. Ioannidis and colleagues have also detailed useful recommendations on animal experimentation [5, 7]. Another approach is the SYRCLE tool to reduce bias in animal studies employing systematic review [62]. It employs an adaptation of the Cochrane Risk of Bias analytical tool for randomized clinical trials. For many animal models of inflammation, extensive recent recommendations have been made, for instance: Experimental autoimmune encephalomyelitis (EAE) as a model for multiple sclerosis [98, 99]. Also in a recent effort, a consortium of six independent research centers analyzed the effect of a potential stroke therapy using a coordinated, randomized, and blinded approach [100].

5 Pipetting Techniques, Standard Procedures and Accreditation Systems

Surprisingly, many formal education programs in life sciences and medicine do not provide systematic and formal training in pipetting skills, however critical to safety, accuracy, and precision of laboratory research. Sequential pipetting errors in complex and long experiments can jointly result in dramatic errors. As an example, many researchers are not familiar with the technique of reverse pipetting and its applications. Occasionally, homemade instruction materials on pipetting such as YouTube tutorials even spread non-trivial errors. Several international companies provide good instruction materials free of charge, and Box 3 lists a selection of those. Optimally, pipetting skills of new recruits at any career stage should be validated, and lab policies on calibration and servicing of pipettes should be clearly communicated.

On a more general note, concise but complete standard operating procedures (SOP) are crucial for improving reproducibility within a given department. Laboratory researchers are often understandably reluctant to implement formalized quality and accreditation programs such as based on ISO criteria and requiring independent auditing. However, we argue from experience, that when executed pragmatically, accreditation strongly improves reliability of the work, and saves time and costs associated with suboptimal lab organization.

6 Reproducibility of Individual Techniques: qPCR and FACS as Examples

As it is obviously not possible to discuss the myriads of techniques used in animal experimentation, we use quantitative PCR as an example. There are examples in the literature where two groups reach diametrically opposite conclusions based on different qPCR routines. This has stimulated the design of the MIQE [74, 101]. Even if one does not fully adopt the 30-odd MIQE items to be reported in publications, it does provide a highly useful checklist.

A technique commonly used in immunology is flow cytometry and Fluorescence Activated Cell Sorting (FACS). Considering the complexity of the technology and the great number of variables, standardization of experiments and their reporting can greatly improve reproducibility [102]. Due to the increasing use of FACS for clinical purposes, the International Council for Standardization of Haematology and International Clinical Cytometry Society has also recently published guidelines for cell-based fluorescence assays [103].

7 Cell Line Authentication and Mycoplasma Contamination

There is a tendency to underestimate or even ignore the importance of cell line authentication, and verification that mycoplasma does not contaminate cell lines and primary cultures [67, 104–108]. There are notorious and unfortunate examples of how misidentification and cross-contamination of cell lines negatively affected research fields [109–113]. Attempting to ban cell-line contaminants from future literature, many journals now require authors to verify the source and validity of cell lines at the time of manuscript submission. Other positive developments include the establishment of the Institute for Cell Line Authentication, novel guidelines and technologies for such authentication, and for improved detection and eradication of mycoplasma (*see* Box 3).

8 Research Assessment and Animal Work Robustness

In parallel to the reproducibility debate, discussion on how to rate the importance and value of research efforts (research assessment) is recently intense. We raise this issue here briefly since many (young) researchers trying to select the best publications from the ocean of literature use the journal impact factor (JIF) as a proxy for quality of the studies presented in papers. In other words, highly cited scientific journals would be expected to publish the best-designed and controlled studies. In a well-phrased paper, Brembs, Button, and Munafo argue that using journal rank as an assessment tool is bad scientific practice and that journal rank is a poor indicator of methodological soundness [114]. Their evidence leads to four conclusions: "*1. Journal rank is a weak to moderate predictor of utility and perceived importance. 2. Journal rank is a moderate to strong predictor of both intentional and unintentional scientific unreliability. 3. Journal rank is expensive, delays science and frustrates researchers, and, 4. Journal rank as established by impact factor violates even the most basic scientific standards, but predicts subjective judgments of journal quality.*" Hence, it is clearly a misconception to assume that the JIF correlates well with study quality. A recent insightful and forward-looking commentary in *Nature* issues positive guidelines for more appropriate means of research assessment [41].

9 Concluding Remarks

We hope this chapter will raise the awareness of reproducibility issues concerning animal inflammation research and, at the same time, provides a practical resource for both junior and more experienced researchers to further improve both the standardization and innovation of animal models for inflammatory diseases. The authors welcome any critical comments and suggestions to be incorporated into future resources on this topic.

Acknowledgments

The authors thank Dr. C.M.A. Thuring and Drs. M. van der Meulen-Frank, veterinarians at the UMC Groningen animal facility (CDP) for textual contributions on animal work and Box 3, and

Dr. G.J. te Meerman for contributing to Box 1. In addition, we are grateful to several people for providing items for Box 3, including Drs. Janneke Samsom, Bart Eggen, Louis Boon, Nieske Brouwer and Chaitali Paul. Funding was partly provided by NWO VENI (#016.161.072) to S.M.K., and by the Dutch MS Research Foundation (program grant to the MS Center Noord Nederland, MSCNN). B.E.C. was an NWO VIDI fellow (#917.76.365) and is currently supported by the DFG (CL 419/2-1) and the Research Center for Immunotherapy (FZI) Mainz.

References

1. Begley CG, Ellis LM (2012) Drug development: raise standards for preclinical cancer research. Nature 483:531–533
2. Prinz F, Schlange T, Asadullah K (2011) Believe it or not: how much can we rely on published data on potential drug targets? Nat Rev Drug Discov 10:712
3. Lara-Pezzi E, Menasche P, Trouvin JH, Badimon L, Ioannidis JP, Wu JC et al (2015) Guidelines for translational research in heart failure. J Cardiovasc Transl Res 8:3–22
4. Tsilidis KK, Panagiotou OA, Sena ES, Aretouli E, Evangelou E, Howells DW et al (2013) Evaluation of excess significance bias in animal studies of neurological diseases. PLoS Biol 11:e1001609
5. Ioannidis JP (2012) Extrapolating from animals to humans. Sci Transl Med 4:151ps15
6. Kitsios GD, Tangri N, Castaldi PJ, Ioannidis JP (2010) Laboratory mouse models for the human genome-wide associations. PLoS One 5:e13782
7. Begley CG, Ioannidis JP (2015) Reproducibility in science: improving the standard for basic and preclinical research. Circ Res 116:116–126
8. Ioannidis JP (2014) How to make more published research true. PLoS Med 11:e1001747
9. Casadevall A, Fang FC (2012) Reforming science: methodological and cultural reforms. Infect Immun 80:891–896
10. Casadevall A, Fang FC (2013) Is the nobel prize good for science? FASEB J 27:4682–4690
11. Casadevall A, Fang FC (2014) Causes for the persistence of impact factor mania. mBio 5:e00064–14
12. Casadevall A, Fang FC (2015) Impacted science: impact is not importance. mBio 6:e01593–15
13. Fang FC, Casadevall A (2011) Retracted science and the retraction index. Infect Immun 79:3855–3859
14. Fang FC, Casadevall A (2012) Reforming science: structural reforms. Infect Immun 80:897–901
15. Fang FC, Casadevall A (2015) Competitive science: is competition ruining science? Infect Immun 83:1229–1233
16. Mullane K, Winquist RJ, Williams M (2014) Translational paradigms in pharmacology and drug discovery. Biochem Pharmacol 87: 189–210
17. Bacchetti P, Deeks SG, McCune JM (2011) Breaking free of sample size dogma to perform innovative translational research. Sci Transl Med 3:87ps24
18. Macleod MR, Lawson McLean A, Kyriakopoulou A, Serghiou S, de Wilde A, Sherratt N et al (2015) Risk of bias in reports of in vivo research: a focus for improvement. PLoS Biol 13:e1002273
19. Mazumdar M, Banerjee S, Van Epps HL (2010) Improved reporting of statistical design and analysis: guidelines, education, and editorial policies. Methods Mol Biol 620:563–598
20. Plant AL, Locascio LE, May WE, Gallagher PD (2014) Improved reproducibility by assuring confidence in measurements in biomedical research. Nat Methods 11:895–898
21. Schooler JW (2014) Metascience could rescue the 'replication crisis'. Nature 515:9
22. Baker M (2015) Reproducibility crisis: blame it on the antibodies. Nature 521:274–276
23. Iorns E, Chong C (2014) New forms of checks and balances are needed to improve research integrity. F1000Res 3:119
24. Couchman JR (2014) Peer review and reproducibility. Crisis or time for course correction? J Histochem Cytochem 62:9–10
25. Mullane K, Williams M (2015) Unknown unknowns in biomedical research: does an inability to deal with ambiguity contribute to issues of irreproducibility? Biochem Pharmacol 97:133–136
26. Anon (2013) Announcement: reducing our irreproducibility. Nature 496:398
27. Munafo M, Noble S, Browne WJ, Brunner D, Button K, Ferreira J et al (2014) Scientific rigor and the art of motorcycle maintenance. Nat Biotechnol 32:871–873

28. Button KS, Munafo MR (2014) Incentivising reproducible research. Cortex 51:107–108
29. Shoda LK, Young DL, Ramanujan S, Whiting CC, Atkinson MA, Bluestone JA et al (2005) A comprehensive review of interventions in the NOD mouse and implications for translation. Immunity 23:115–126
30. Frye SV, Arkin MR, Arrowsmith CH, Conn PJ, Glicksman MA, Hull-Ryde EA et al (2015) Tackling reproducibility in academic preclinical drug discovery. Nat Rev Drug Discov 14:733–734
31. Katsnelson A (2010) Biologists tackle cells' identity crisis. Nature 465:537
32. Tittel AP, Heuser C, Ohliger C, Llanto C, Yona S, Hammerling GJ et al (2012) Functionally relevant neutrophilia in CD11c diphtheria toxin receptor transgenic mice. Nat Methods 9:385–390
33. Bennett CL, Clausen BE (2007) DC ablation in mice: promises, pitfalls, and challenges. Trends Immunol 28:525–531
34. Walter A, Schafer M, Cecconi V, Matter C, Urosevic-Maiwald M, Belloni B et al (2013) Aldara activates TLR7-independent immune defence. Nat Commun 4:1560
35. Davis J, Maillet M, Miano JM, Molkentin JD (2012) Lost in transgenesis: a user's guide for genetically manipulating the mouse in cardiac research. Circ Res 111:761–777
36. Geghman K, Li C (2011) Practical considerations of genetic rodent models for neurodegenerative diseases. Methods Mol Biol 793:185–193
37. National Academy of Sciences, National Academy of Engineering (US) and Institute of Medicine (US) Committee on Science, Engineering, and Public Policy (2009) On being a scientist: a guide to responsible conduct in research. The National Academies Press, Washington (DC), USA
38. Kilkenny C, Browne WJ, Cuthill IC, Emerson M, Altman DG (2010) Improving bioscience research reporting: the ARRIVE guidelines for reporting animal research. PLoS Biol 8:e1000412
39. Kilkenny C, Browne WJ, Cuthill IC, Emerson M, Altman DG (2012) Improving bioscience research reporting: the ARRIVE guidelines for reporting animal research. Osteoarthritis Cartilage 20:256–260
40. Landis SC, Amara SG, Asadullah K, Austin CP, Blumenstein R, Bradley EW et al (2012) A call for transparent reporting to optimize the predictive value of preclinical research. Nature 490:187–191
41. Hicks D, Wouters P, Waltman L, de Rijcke S, Rafols I (2015) Bibliometrics: the Leiden manifesto for research metrics. Nature 520:429–431
42. Halsey LG, Curran-Everett D, Vowler SL, Drummond GB (2015) The fickle P value generates irreproducible results. Nat Methods 12:179–185
43. Richter SH, Garner JP, Auer C, Kunert J, Wurbel H (2010) Systematic variation improves reproducibility of animal experiments. Nat Methods 7:167–168
44. Kenett RS, Shmueli G (2015) Clarifying the terminology that describes scientific reproducibility. Nat Methods 12:699
45. The Reproducibility Initiative. Available from: http://validation.scienceexchange.com/ - /reproducibility-initiative.
46. Nosek BA, Alter G, Banks GC, Borsboom D, Bowman SD, Breckler SJ et al (2015) SCIENTIFIC STANDARDS. Promoting an open research culture. Science 348:1422–1425
47. TOP guidelines. Available from: https://cos.io/top/
48. Nature author policies. Available from: http://www.nature.com/authors/policies/checklist.pdf
49. METRICS. Available from: http://metrics.stanford.edu/
50. Protocol Exchange. Available from: http://www.nature.com/protocolexchange
51. Masca NG, Hensor EM, Cornelius VR, Buffa FM, Marriott HM, Eales JM et al (2015) RIPOSTE: a framework for improving the design and analysis of laboratory-based research. ELife 4:e05519
52. World Health Organization. Available from: http://www.who.int/ihr/training/laboratory_quality/doc/en/
53. ICMJE. Available from: http://www.icmje.org/recommendations/browse/roles-and-responsibilities/defining-the-role-of-authors-and-contributors.html
54. EQUATOR. Available from: http://www.equator-network.org/reporting-guidelines/
55. FASEB guidelines. Available from: http://www.faseb.org/Science-Policy-and-Advocacy/Science-Policy-and-Research-Issues/Research-Reproducibility.aspx
56. Gilson pipetting guide. Available from: http://www.gilson.com/en/GilsonProducts/PipetteAccessories/GilsonGuidetoPipetting-ThirdEdition.aspx - .Vq30km_2aUk
57. Mettler Toledo pipetting technique. Available from: https://http://www.youtube.com/watch?v=X73R_4cntpA
58. Eppendorf pipetting guidelines. Available from: en/155258_SOP.pdf
59. ARRIVE guidelines. Available from: https://http://www.nc3rs.org.uk/arrive-guidelines
60. ILAR (2011) Guidance for the description of animal research in scientific publications. The National Academies Collection: Reports

funded by National Institutes of Health. Washington (DC), USA

61. Hooijmans CR, Leenaars M, Ritskes-Hoitinga M (2010) A gold standard publication checklist to improve the quality of animal studies, to fully integrate the Three Rs, and to make systematic reviews more feasible. Altern Lab Anim 38:167–182
62. Hooijmans CR, Rovers MM, de Vries RB, Leenaars M, Ritskes-Hoitinga M, Langendam MW (2014) SYRCLE's risk of bias tool for animal studies. BMC Med Res Methodol 14:43
63. IMPC. Available from: http://www.mousephenotype.org/
64. Nc3Rs design assistant. Available from: https://eda.nc3rs.org.uk/
65. ICLAC. Available from: http://iclac.org/resources/
66. Capes-Davis A, Theodosopoulos G, Atkin I, Drexler HG, Kohara A, MacLeod RA et al (2010) Check your cultures! A list of cross-contaminated or misidentified cell lines. Int J Cancer 127:1–8
67. Yu M, Selvaraj SK, Liang-Chu MM, Aghajani S, Busse M, Yuan J et al (2015) A resource for cell line authentication, annotation and quality control. Nature 520:307–311
68. Geraghty RJ, Capes-Davis A, Davis JM, Downward J, Freshney RI, Knezevic I et al (2014) Guidelines for the use of cell lines in biomedical research. Br J Cancer 111:1021–1046
69. Ward JM, Rehg JE (2014) Rodent immunohistochemistry: pitfalls and troubleshooting. Vet Pathol 51:88–101
70. Hewitt SM, Baskin DG, Frevert CW, Stahl WL, Rosa-Molinar E (2014) Controls for immunohistochemistry: the Histochemical Society's standards of practice for validation of immunohistochemical assays. J Histochem Cytochem 62:693–697
71. North AJ (2006) Seeing is believing? A beginners' guide to practical pitfalls in image acquisition. J Cell Biol 172:9–18
72. J. Immunol. Available from: http://www.jimmunol.org/site/misc/DigitalImageDosandDonts.pdf
73. Gassmann M, Grenacher B, Rohde B, Vogel J (2009) Quantifying Western blots: pitfalls of densitometry. Electrophoresis 30:1845–1855
74. Bustin SA, Benes V, Garson JA, Hellemans J, Huggett J, Kubista M et al (2009) The MIQE guidelines: minimum information for publication of quantitative real-time PCR experiments. Clin Chem 55:611–622
75. ENCODE guidelines. Available from: https://http://www.encodeproject.org/about/experiment-guidelines/
76. Roadmap Epigenomics. Available from: http://www.roadmapepigenomics.org/protocols/type/data/
77. Landt SG, Marinov GK, Kundaje A, Kheradpour P, Pauli F, Batzoglou S et al (2012) ChIP-seq guidelines and practices of the ENCODE and modENCODE consortia. Genome Res 22:1813–1831
78. MIBBI. Available from: https://biosharing.org/standards/?selected_facets=isMIBBI:true
79. Obokata H, Wakayama T, Sasai Y, Kojima K, Vacanti MP, Niwa H et al (2014) Stimulus-triggered fate conversion of somatic cells into pluripotency. Nature 505:641–647
80. De Los Angeles A, Ferrari F, Fujiwara Y, Mathieu R, Lee S, Tu HC, Ross S, Chou S, Nguyen M, Wu Z, Theunissen TW, Powell BE, Imsoonthornruksa S, Chen J, Borkent M, Krupalnik V, Lujan E, Wernig M, Hanna JH, Hochedlinger K, Pei D, Jaenisch R, Deng H, Orkin SH, Park PJ, Daley GQ (2015) Failure to replicate the STAP cell phenomenon. Nature 525(7570):E6–E9. doi: 10.1038/nature15513
81. Stainier DY, Kontarakis Z, Rossi A (2015) Making sense of anti-sense data. Dev Cell 32:7–8
82. Sternberg SH, Doudna JA (2015) Expanding the biologist's toolkit with CRISPR-Cas9. Mol Cell 58:568–74
83. Doudna JA, Charpentier E (2016) Genome editing. The new frontier of genome engineering with CRISPR-Cas9. Science 346:1258096
84. Button KS, Ioannidis JP, Mokrysz C, Nosek BA, Flint J, Robinson ES et al (2013) Power failure: why small sample size undermines the reliability of neuroscience. Nat Rev Neurosci 14:365–376
85. Franken L, Klein M, Spasova M, Elsukova A, Wiedwald U, Welz M et al (2015) Splenic red pulp macrophages are intrinsically superparamagnetic and contaminate magnetic cell isolates. Sci Rep 5:12940
86. Boon L, Brok HP, Bauer J, Ortiz-Buijsse A, Schellekens MM, Ramdien-Murli S et al (2001) Prevention of experimental autoimmune encephalomyelitis in the common marmoset (Callithrix jacchus) using a chimeric antagonist monoclonal antibody against human CD40 is associated with altered B cell responses. J Immunol 167:2942–2949
87. Boon L, den Hartog MT, Laman JD (2002) Antagonistic CD40 Mab 5D12 on its way to the clinic. In: Korte R, Vogel F, Weinbauer GF (eds) Primate models in pharmaceutical drug development. Waxmann, Munster, Germany, pp 127–146
88. Salter SJ, Cox MJ, Turek EM, Calus ST, Cookson WO, Moffatt MF et al (2014) Reagent and laboratory contamination can

critically impact sequence-based microbiome analyses. BMC Biol 12:87
89. Russell WMS, Burch LR (1959) The principles of humane experimental technique. Universities Federation for Animal Welfare. Wheathampstead, England (reprinted in 1992)
90. Beura LK, Hamilton SE, Bi K, Schenkel JM, Odumade OA, Casey KA et al (2016) Normalizing the environment recapitulates adult human immune traits in laboratory mice. Nature 532:512–516
91. Reese TA, Bi K, Kambal A, Filali-Mouhim A, Beura LK, Burger MC et al (2016) Sequential infection with common pathogens promotes human-like immune gene expression and altered vaccine response. Cell Host Microbe 19:713–719
92. Nuzzo R (2014) Scientific method: statistical errors. Nature 506:150–152
93. Van Epps HL (2009) JEM's 2009 tune-up. J Exp Med 206:968–969
94. Seok J, Warren HS, Cuenca AG, Mindrinos MN, Baker HV, Xu W et al (2013) Genomic responses in mouse models poorly mimic human inflammatory diseases. Proc Natl Acad Sci U S A 110:3507–3512
95. Takao K, Hagihara H, Miyakawa T (2015) Reply to Warren et al. and Shay et al.: Commonalities across species do exist and are potentially important. Proc Natl Acad Sci U S A 112:E347–E348
96. Shay T, Lederer JA, Benoist C (2015) Genomic responses to inflammation in mouse models mimic humans: we concur, apples to oranges comparisons won't do. Proc Natl Acad Sci U S A 112:E346
97. Mitchell SJ, Scheibye-Knudsen M, Longo DL, de Cabo R (2015) Animal models of aging research: implications for human aging and age-related diseases. Annu Rev Anim Biosci 3:283–303
98. Amor S, Baker D (2012) Checklist for reporting and reviewing studies of experimental animal models of multiple sclerosis and related disorders. Mult Scler Relat Disord 1:111–115
99. Baker D, Amor S (2014) Experimental autoimmune encephalomyelitis is a good model of multiple sclerosis if used wisely. Mult Scler Relat Disord 3:555–564
100. Llovera G, Hofmann K, Roth S, Salas-Perdomo A, Ferrer-Ferrer M, Perego C et al (2015) Results of a preclinical randomized controlled multicenter trial (pRCT): anti-CD49d treatment for acute brain ischemia. Sci Transl Med 7:299ra121
101. Bustin SA, Benes V, Garson J, Hellemans J, Huggett J, Kubista M et al (2013) The need for transparency and good practices in the qPCR literature. Nat Methods 10:1063–1067
102. Herzenberg LA, Tung J, Moore WA, Herzenberg LA, Parks DR (2006) Interpreting flow cytometry data: a guide for the perplexed. Nat Immunol 7:681–685
103. Bene MC, Marti GE (2013) ICSH/ICCS practice guidelines special issue. Cytometry B Clin Cytom 84:279–280
104. Grens K (2015) The great big clean-up. Scientist 29:50–55
105. Masters JR (2012) Cell-line authentication: end the scandal of false cell lines. Nature 492:186
106. Lorsch JR, Collins FS, Lippincott-Schwartz J (2014) Cell biology. Fixing problems with cell lines. Science 346:1452–1453
107. Hughes P, Marshall D, Reid Y, Parkes H, Gelber C (2007) The costs of using unauthenticated, over-passaged cell lines: how much more data do we need? Biotechniques 43:575
108. Callaway E (2014) Contamination hits cell work. Nature 511:518
109. Di Girolamo N, Chow S, Richardson A, Wakefield D (2016) Contamination of primary human corneal epithelial cells with an SV40-transformed human corneal epithelial cell line: a lesson for cell biologists in good laboratory practice. Invest Ophthalmol Vis Sci 57:611–616
110. Nelson-Rees WA, Daniels DW, Flandermeyer RR (1981) Cross-contamination of cells in culture. Science 212:446–452
111. Clément V, Marino D, Cudalbu C, Hamou MF, Mlynarik V, de Tribolet N, Dietrich PY, Gruetter R, Hegi ME, Radovanovic I (2010) Marker-independent identification of glioma-initiating cells. Nat Methods 7(3):224–228. doi:10.1038/nmeth.1430
112. Van Bergen NJ, Wood JP, Chidlow G, Trounce IA, Casson RJ, Ju WK et al (2009) Recharacterization of the RGC-5 retinal ganglion cell line. Invest Ophthalmol Vis Sci 50:4267–4272
113. Anon (2015) STAP revisited. Nature 525:426
114. Brembs B, Button K, Munafo M (2013) Deep impact: unintended consequences of journal rank. Front Hum Neurosci 7:291

Part I

Skin Inflammation

Chapter 2

Hapten-Specific T Cell-Mediated Skin Inflammation: Flow Cytometry Analysis of Mouse Skin Inflammatory Infiltrate

Nicolas Bouladoux, Clotilde Hennequin, Camille Malosse, Bernard Malissen, Yasmine Belkaid, and Sandrine Henri

Abstract

Hapten-specific T cell-mediated skin inflammation also known as contact hypersensitivity (CHS) is characterized by a strong influx of $CD8^+$ cytotoxic T cells within the skin upon reexposure of sensitized individuals to the same hapten. As many other leukocytes are also recruited during this elicitation phase, we attempted to revisit the skin infiltrate and characterize the inflammatory pattern. Recent improvement in the isolation in conventional as well as inflammatory dendritic cell and macrophage subsets from tissues and in the use of appropriate surface markers unraveling their heterogeneity should allow to determinate their specific functions in the CHS model. Here, we describe procedures to extract those cells from the skin and to analyze them by flow cytometry using a combination of appropriate surface markers allowing further transcriptomic analysis and functional assays.

Key words Skin, Contact hypersensitivity (CHS), Dendritic cell subsets, Monocyte-derived cells, Macrophages, Neutrophils, $CD4^+$ T cells, $CD8^+$ T cells, γδ T cells, Flow cytometry

1 Introduction

Hapten-specific T cell-mediated skin inflammation is known under various names: contact hypersensitivity (CHS), allergic contact dermatitis (ACD) or delayed-type hypersensitivity (DTH). This inflammatory skin disease is common in industrialized countries [1] and can be mimicked with animal models by painting a hapten onto the skin allowing the dissection of the pathophysiology of CHS. Using the strong contact sensitizer 2,4-dinitro-1-fluorobenzene (DNFB), it was shown that optimal CHS was a two-step reaction with two temporally and spatially dissociated phases [2, 3]. The first contact with the hapten on the skin is referred to as the sensitization phase also called afferent or induction phase. During this phase, the innate immune system is stimulated leading to the activation of skin dendritic cells (DCs) that migrate to the skin draining lymph nodes and prime naïve T cells

Björn E. Clausen and Jon D. Laman (eds.), *Inflammation: Methods and Protocols*, Methods in Molecular Biology, vol. 1559, DOI 10.1007/978-1-4939-6786-5_2, © Springer Science+Business Media LLC 2017

to become skin-tropic, hapten-specific effector T cells. Upon reexposure to the same hapten, those specific T lymphocytes are rapidly activated within the skin, triggering a strong inflammatory process within 24–72 h characterizing the elicitation phase that is also called efferent or challenge phase [4]. At steady-state, the skin contains many cell types of the hematopoietic system including conventional DCs, monocytes, monocyte-derived DCs, macrophages, γδ T cells, αβ T cells mainly CD4$^+$ T lymphocytes and very few neutrophils. Conventional DCs were firstly described in lymphoid organs in the early seventies [5], but due to their low numbers and the difficulty to extract them, extensive studies assessing their functions were primarily performed using bone marrow- or monocyte-derived DCs [6–8]. With the use of a few key markers, we could disentangle the complexity of the skin DC network allowing to distinguish phenotypically and functionally distinct subsets [9–11]. Moreover, for many years, there was confusion in the field of DC characterization in tissues as many studies were often mixing conventional tissue DCs derived from DC precursors with monocyte-derived DCs and even tissue macrophages. Such confusion was even worse during inflammatory conditions. Indeed, in models such as CHS, both phases are characterized by a strong influx of neutrophils and monocytes, which will differentiate into inflammatory monocyte-derived DCs, commonly called Tip-DCs for TNF and iNOS producing DCs. We and others contributed to improve cell extraction from mouse skin and unravel the combination of specific surface markers to stain the immune skin infiltrate and distinguish the different conventional DC subsets, the monocytes, monocyte-derived DCs and the macrophages by flow cytometry [12–14]. Upon inflammation, the analysis of the inflammatory response can be completed with the same gating strategy [14, 15]. In the present protocol, we explain how to thoroughly analyze the immune skin infiltrate in a DNFB-induced CHS model. Not only we show how to distinguish the innate cells from the neutrophils to the DC subsets and macrophages but we also show how to follow the adaptive T cell immune response as it ultimately plays a major role within the tissue [16–18].

2 Materials

2.1 Induction of DNFB-Mediated CHS

1. 6–9-week-old, sex- and weight-matched C57BL6 mice.
2. Shaving device and hair depilation cream.
3. Acetone/olive oil vehicle (4:1).
4. 2,4-dinitro-fluorobenzene (DNFB).

2.2 Analysis of the Leukocyte Skin Infiltrate by Flow Cytometry

Keep all the solutions sterile. Do not add sodium azide to the solutions.

1. Basic medium: To 500 mL of RPMI 1640, add 5 mL of penicillin–streptomycin solution (10,000 I.U, 10,000 μg/mL), 5 mL of 100 mM sodium pyruvate, 5 mL of MEM nonessential amino acids (100×), 5 mL of 200 mMl-glutamine, 500 μL of 55 mM βME, and 10 mL of 1 M HEPES. Store at 4 °C.
2. Complete medium: Basic medium complemented with 10% FBS.
3. FACS Buffer: PBS, 2% FBS, 5 mM EDTA (combine 100 mL of 10× PBS, 10 mL of 0.5 M EDTA (pH8.0), 20 mL of inactivated FBS and complete to 1 L with ultrapure water). Filter through a 0.2 μm filter and store at 4 °C.
4. Sorting FACS Buffer: PBS, 10% FBS, 5 mM EDTA (combine 100 mL of 10× PBS, 10 mL of 0.5 M EDTA (pH8.0), 100 mL of inactivated FBS and complete to 1 L with ultrapure water). Filter through a 0.2 μm filter and store at 4 °C.
5. DNase stock solution (deoxyribonuclease I from bovine pancreas): 10 mg/mL solution in basic medium (resuspend 100 mg of powder in 10 mL of basic medium). Aliquot (1 mL aliquots) and store at −20 °C.
6. DNase working solution: on the day of the experiment, take 500 μL of DNase stock solution at 10 mg/mL and complete to 10 mL with basic medium. Keep the solution on ice.
7. Liberase TL stock solution: 25 mg/mL solution in sterile water (resuspend 5 mg of powder in 200 μL of sterile water). Aliquot (50 μL aliquots) and store at −20 °C.
8. Liberase TL-DNase working solution: on the day of the experiment, combine 100 μL of Liberase TL stock solution at 25 mg/mL and 500 μL of DNase stock solution at 10 mg/mL and complete to 10 mL with basic medium. Keep the solution on ice.
9. Forceps, scissors.
10. Petri dishes.
11. 24-well plates.
12. Automated mechanical disaggregation system (Medimachine).
13. 50 μm sterile disposable chambers (Medicons) to be used on the Medimachine and allowing an efficient cutting of the tissue (microblades).
14. 50 μm sterile syringe filters (Filcon).
15. 20 mL sterile syringes and 19G needles.
16. 10 mL sterile pipettes.
17. 70 μm sterile cell strainers.

18. 15 mL sterile polypropylene (PP) tubes.
19. 1.5 mL sterile Eppendorf tubes.
20. Fc block (clone 24G2).
21. RLT Plus Buffer: Lysis buffer for lysing cells prior to RNA isolation.

3 Methods

3.1 Induction of DNFB-Mediated CHS (See Fig. 1)

1. Firstly, 2 cm^2 of fur is removed on dorsal skin using the shaving device and the hair depilation cream.
2. 24 h later, mice are sensitized by epicutaneous application of 25 μl of 0.5 % DNFB diluted in acetone/olive oil (4:1), using a 200 μl pipette tip.
3. Five days later, mice are challenged on the ear by epicutaneous application of 25 μl of 0.2 % DNFB diluted in acetone/ olive oil (4:1), using a 200 μl pipette tip. This group is called CHS in Figs 1–6 and Table 4 (*see* **Note 1**).

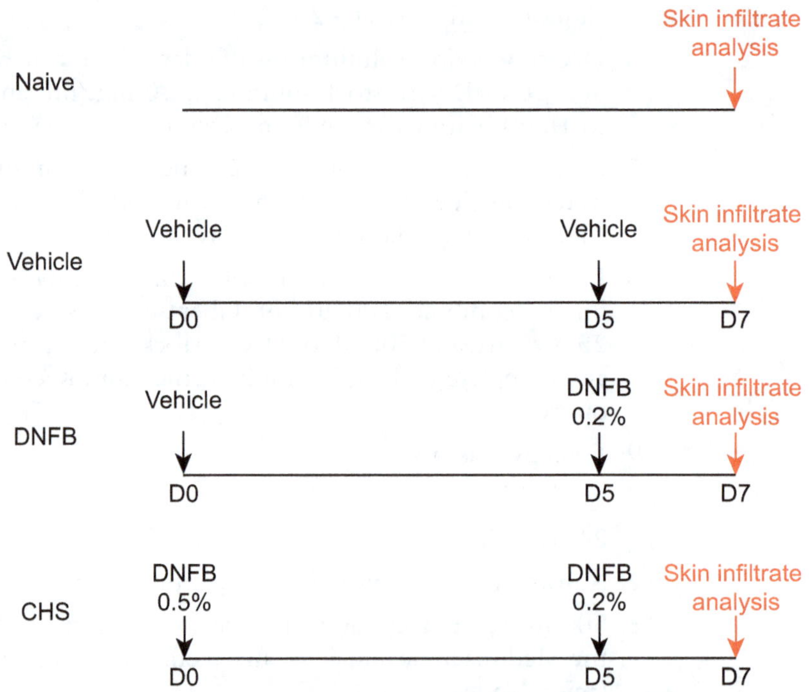

Fig. 1 CHS induction model CHS was induced as follows: firstly mice were sensitized by topical application of 0.5 % DNFB on the dorsal skin. Five days later, animals were challenged on the ear by topical application of 0.2 % DNFB and the ear skin infiltrate was analyzed 2 days later. Ear skin infiltrate analysis was realized comparing naïve mice (Naïve) to mice that received the vehicle only (Vehicle), to mice that received first the vehicle and then DNFB 0.2 % on the ears (DNFB) and to mice which were sensitized and challenged with DNFB (CHS)

3.2 Tissues Collection

1. Two days after the challenge, sacrifice the mice.
2. Using forceps and small surgery scissors, cut the ears 2 mm from their basis to avoid including hair from the scalp.
3. Add 1 mL of PBS in 24-well plates, place the ears on the PBS and keep on ice.

3.3 Enzymatic Treatment

1. In a 24-well plate, distribute 750 μL Liberase TL-DNase working solution per well. You will need 2 wells per mouse (if collecting both ears) (*see* **Note 2**).

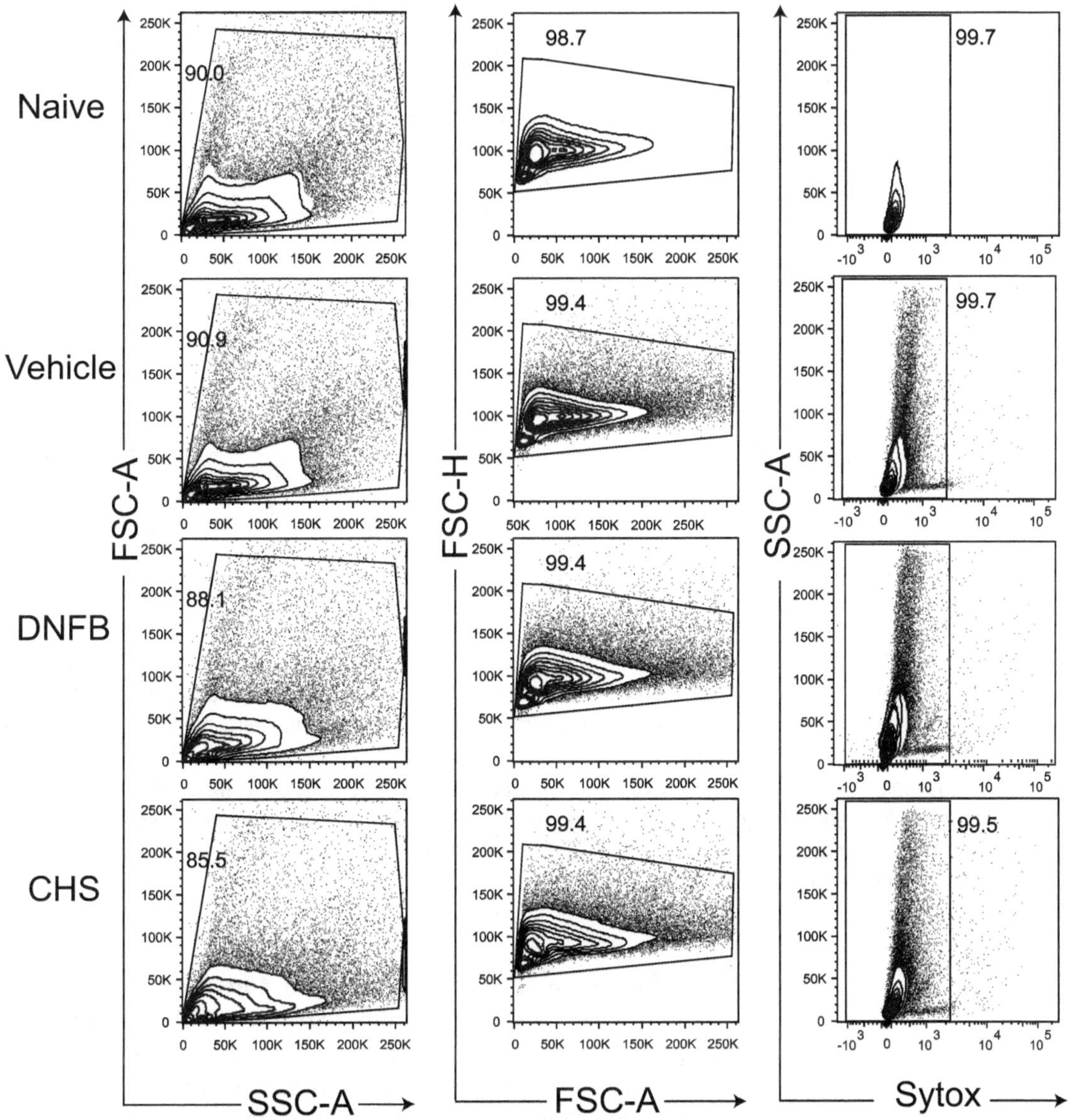

Fig. 2 Pre-gating strategy of living cells. Cells were prepared from skin and analyzed by flow cytometry. Cells are pre-gated according to their size (FSC-A/SSC-A). Doublets and dead cells are excluded using FSC-H and Sytox *blue* respectively

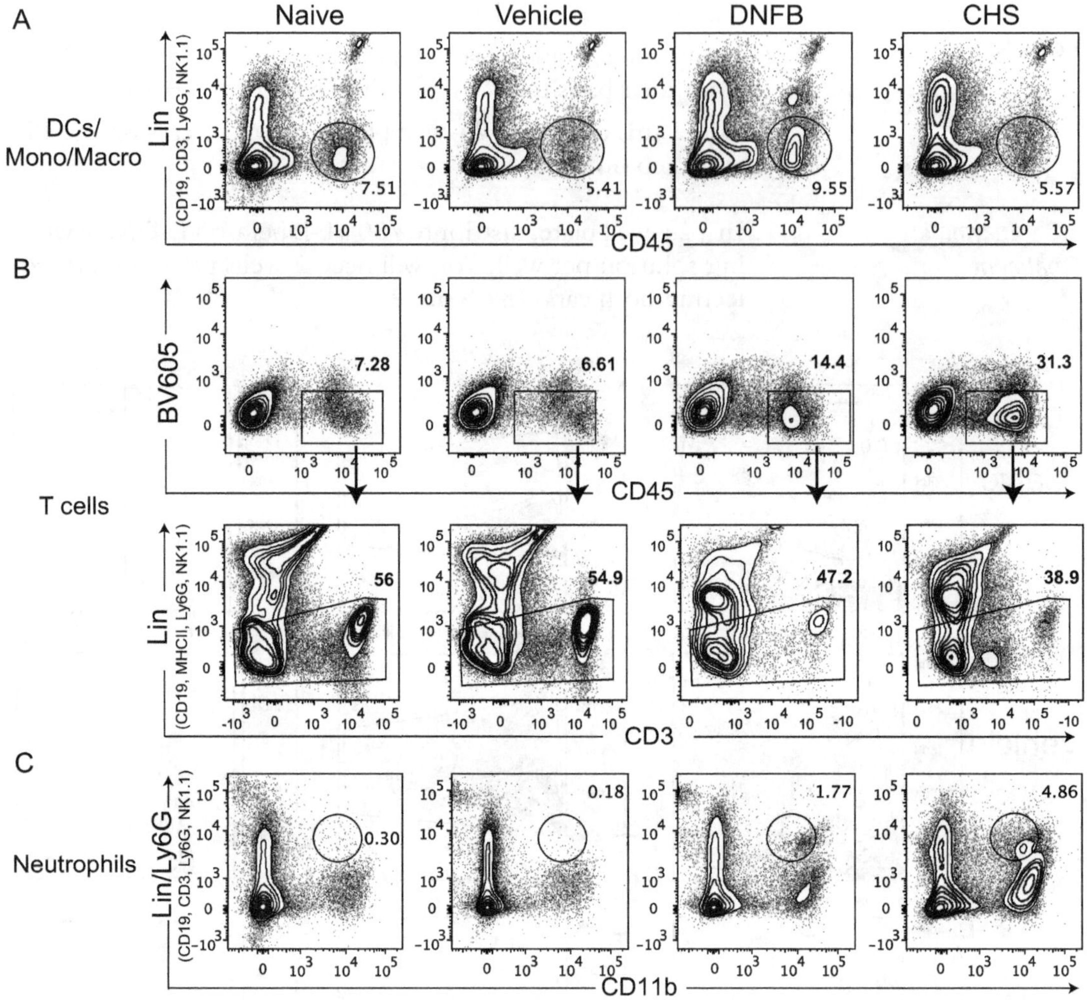

Fig. 3 Pre-gating strategy of hematopoietic cells of myeloid or lymphoid lineage Cells were prepared from skin, run on a flow cytometer, pre-gated on live cells as described in Fig. 1 and further gated to analyze myeloid populations or T lymphocytes or neutrophils. (**a**) Myeloid cells including dendritic cells, monocytes, and macrophages (DCs/Mono/Macro) were selected as hematopoietic cells (CD45⁺) with further exclusion of NK cells, B cells, T cells, and neutrophils (Lin⁻) according to the staining presented in Table 1. (**b**) T lymphocytes were selected as hematopoietic cells (CD45⁺) with further exclusion of NK cells, B cells, myeloid cells and neutrophils (Lin⁻) according to the staining presented in Table 3. (**c**) Neutrophils were selected as CD11b⁺ and Ly6G⁺, which is included in the Lin channel according to the staining presented in Table 2

2. With forceps, separate the internal and external faces of the ears (the internal face will come with the cartilage) and lay it down flat on 750 μL Liberase TL-DNase working solution. The "outside" (epidermis) of each skin layer should be up, whereas the "inside" (dermis) should be in contact with the solution (*see* **Note 3**).

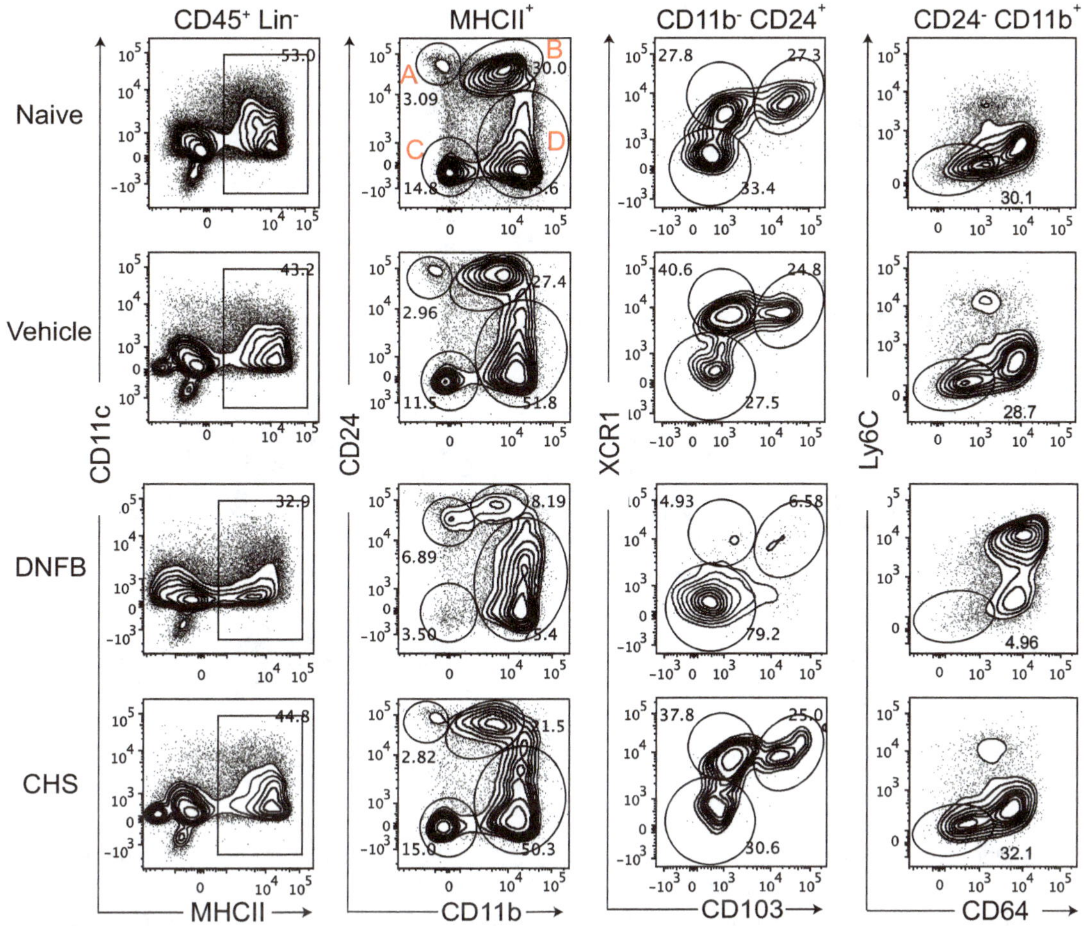

Fig. 4 Conventional DC subset gating strategy Cells were prepared from skin and analyzed by flow cytometry (*see* Table 1). After pre-gating on CD45⁺ Lin⁻, MHCII⁺ CD11c$^{low\ to\ +}$ cells were selected. Conventional DC subsets can then be discriminated using CD24 versus CD11b. CD24⁺CD11b⁻, which correspond to CD24/CD207 dermal DCs can be further divided according to their expression of XCR1 and CD103. CD24⁺CD11b⁺ correspond to the Langerhans cells (LCs). The CD24⁻CD11b⁻ population is often referred to as DN DCs and finally, within the CD24⁻CD11b⁺ population, only the Ly6C⁻CD64⁻ cells correspond to the conventional CD11b⁺ dermal DC subset

3. Incubate for 1:45 h at 37 °C in a cell culture incubator (5 % CO_2).
4. To stop the enzymatic treatment, at the end of the incubation, add 750 μL of DNase working solution and 15 μl of 0.5 M EDTA.
5. Using fine forceps, collect the ear halves and place them in the Medicon tissue grinder. Add 1.5 mL of DNase working solution.
6. Place the Medicon in the Medimachine and turn it on for 8 min.

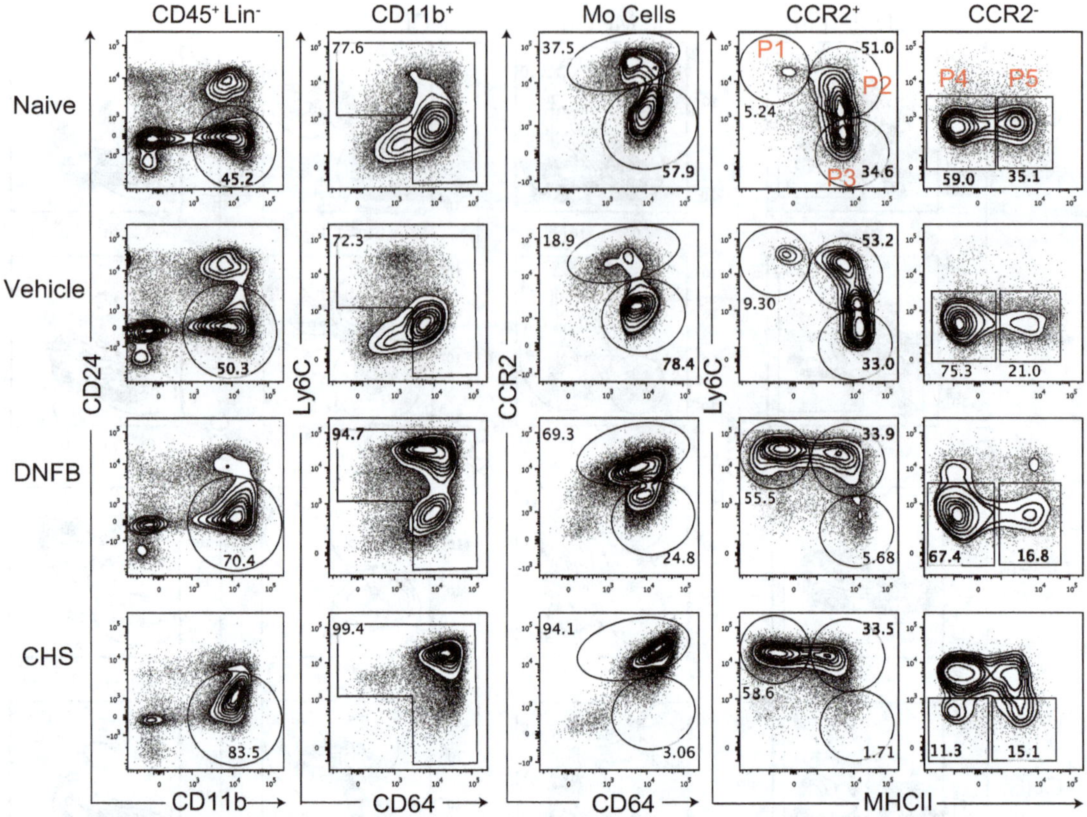

Fig. 5 Monocyte, monocyte-derived DC, macrophages gating strategy Cells were prepared from skin and analyzed by flow cytometry (*see* Table 2). After pre-gating on CD45⁺ Lin⁻, total CD11b⁺ cells were selected. Conventional CD11b⁺ DC subset was excluded using Ly6C and CD64. Monocyte-derived cells (Mo-cells) were selected based on their expression of Ly6C and CD64. This population can be further divided into CCR2⁺ and CCR2⁻. CCR2⁺ cells include dermal monocytes (P1, Ly6C⁺MHCII⁻) and dermal monocyte-derived DCs (P2, Ly6C⁺MHCII⁺ and P3, Ly6C⁻MHCII⁺). CCR2⁻ cells correspond to the dermal macrophages and can be divided into two populations P4 and P5, which are Ly6C⁻MHCII⁻ and Ly6C⁻MHCII⁺, respectively

7. Collect the cell suspension from the Medicon using a 20 mL syringe and rinse the Medicon with 8 mL of DNase working solution.
8. Proceed to the filtration in a 15 mL tube using 50 μm syringe filter (Filcon).
9. Centrifuge for 5 min at 450 × *g* and 4 °C.
10. Resuspend the pellet with 1 mL of FACS Buffer and proceed to counting and staining (*see* **Note 4**).

3.4 FACS Staining (See Note 5)

1. Prepare the antibody mix as described in Tables 1, 2 and 3 (without the Sytox blue) (*see* **Note 6**). The antibodies are diluted in FACS Buffer and require to be titrated before use.

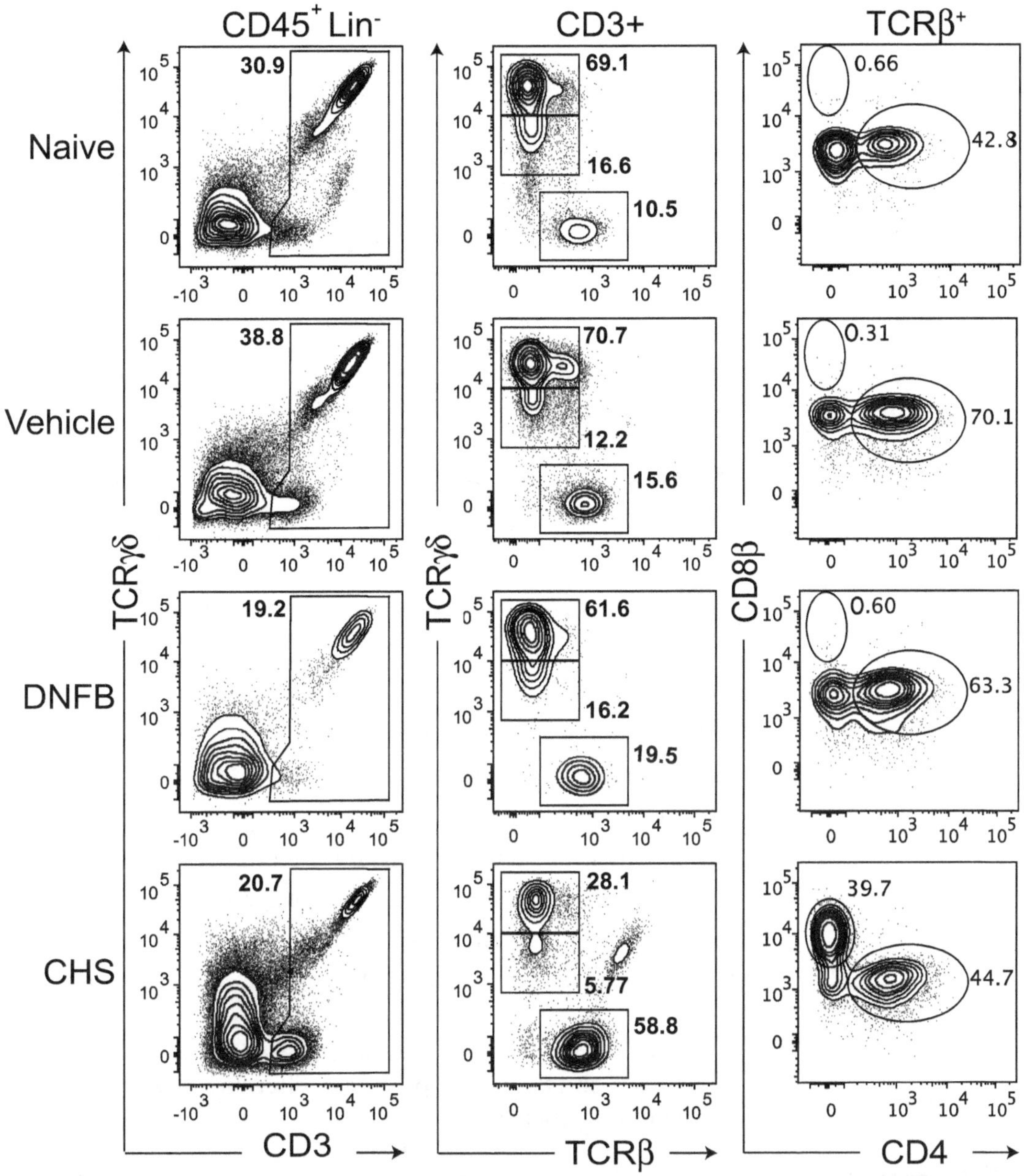

Fig. 6 T cell gating strategy Cells were prepared from skin and analyzed by flow cytometry (*see* Table 3). After pre-gating on CD45⁺ Lin⁻, T cell subsets were further divided according to their expression of γδ and β TCR. DETC correspond to TCRγδ^{high}, whereas dermal γδ cells correspond to TCRγδ^{intermediate}. Conventional CD4⁺ and CD8⁺ T cells are found after pre-gating on TCRβ expressing cells

2. Cells are distributed in 1.5 mL Eppendorf tubes for staining (with a maximum of 1 million cells per tube).
3. Centrifuge for 5 min at 400 × *g*.
4. Add Fc block (0.025 μg/mL).

Table 1
mAbs used for FACS analysis of conventional DC subsets

	Conjugate	Name	Clone	Purchased from
Violet laser (405 nm)	SytoxBlue	Viability		Lifetechnologies
	BV610	CD11c	N418	Biolegend
	BV711	CD11b	M1/70	Pharmingen
Blue laser (488 nm)	FITC	Ly6C	AL-21	Pharmingen
Green-Yellow laser (561 nm)	Biotin	CD103	M290	Pharmingen
	PECF594	Streptavidin		Pharmingen
	PECy5	CD24	M1/69	Biolegend
	PECy5.5	CD45	30-F11	eBioscience
	PE	XCR1	ZET	Biolegend
Red laser (633 nm)	Alexa700	MHCII	M5/114.15.2	Biolegend
	APCCy7	Ly6G	HK1.4	Biolegend
	APCCy7	CD19	6D5	Biolegend
	APCCy7	NK1.1	PK136	Biolegend
	APCCy7	CD3	145-2C11	Biolegend
	APC	CD64	X54-5/7.1	BD

5. Incubate for 10 min on ice.
6. Centrifuge for 5 min at 400 × *g*.
7. Add 100 μL of antibody mix.
8. Incubate for 30 min on ice and protected from light.
9. Add 1 mL of FACS buffer to wash the cells.
10. Centrifuge for 5 min at 400 × *g*.
11. Resuspend the cell pellet in Sytox blue diluted (1/1000) in FACS buffer.
12. Cells are ready to be run on the FACS or cell sorter (*see* **Notes 7** and **8**). If clumps appear, filter one more time using a 70 μm cell strainer.

3.5 Gating Strategy for FACS Analysis or Cell Sorting

1. Gate cells according to their size using FSC and SSC, excluding debris (*see* Fig. 2).
2. Remove dead cells by gating on Sytox blue negative cells (*see* Fig. 2).
3. Gate on hematopoietic cells as $CD45^+$ cells (*see* Fig. 3).
4. Gate on DCs and monocyte-related cells as dump channel negative cells ($APCCy7^-$) within $CD45^+$ cells (*see* Fig. 3a).
5. DC subsets are gated as follows (*see* Fig. 4 and Tables 1 and 4): within $CD45^+$ Lin^- cells, select $MHCII^+$ $CD11c^{\text{low to high}}$. Then plot them using CD24 versus CD11b (*see* **Note 6**).

Table 2
mAbs used for FACS analysis of monocytes, monocytes derived DC, macrophages, and neutrophils

	Conjugate	Name	Clone	Purchased from
Violet laser (405 nm)	SytoxBlue	Viability		Life Technologies
	BV610	CD11c	N418	BioLegend
	BV711	CD11b	M1/70	Pharmingen
Blue laser (488 nm)	FITC	Ly6C	AL-21	Pharmingen
Green-yellow laser (561 nm)	Biotin	CD103	M290	Pharmingen
	PECF594	Streptavidin		Pharmingen
	PECy5	CD24	M1/69	Biolegend
	PECy5.5	CD45	30-F11	eBioscience
	PE	CCR2	475301	R&D
Red laser (633 nm)	Alexa700	MHCII	M5/114.15.2	BioLegend
	APCCy7	Ly6G	HK1.4	BioLegend
	APCCy7	CD19	6D5	BioLegend
	APCCy7	NK1.1	PK136	BioLegend
	APCCy7	CD3	145-2C11	BioLegend
	APC	CD64	X54-5/7.1	BD

Table 3
mAbs used for FACS analysis of T cell subsets

	Conjugate	Name	Clone	Purchased from
Violet laser (405 nm)	SytoxBlue	Viability		Life Technologies
	BV650	CD4	RM4-5	Pharmingen
	BV421	TCRγδ	GL3	BioLegend
Blue laser (488 nm)	FITC	TCRβ	H57-597	Pharmingen
Green-yellow laser (561 nm)	PECy5.5	CD45	30-F11	eBioscience
	PE	CD8β	H35-17.2	eBioscience
Red laser (633 nm)	APCCy7	MHCII	M5/114.15.2	BioLegend
	APCCy7	Ly6G	HK1.4	BioLegend
	APCCy7	CD19	6D5	BioLegend
	APCCy7	NK1.1	PK136	BioLegend
	Alexa700	CD3ε	500A2	Pharmingen

Four distinct populations should be found: (a) the dermal $CD24^+CD11b^-$ cells which can be further divided using XCR1 and CD103 (*see* **Note 9**), (b) The $CD24^+CD11b^+$ cells which correspond to the Langerhans cells (LCs), (c) the $CD24^-CD11b^-$ cells and (D) the $CD24^-CD11b^+$ cells which

Table 4
Absolute numbers of cells (10^3) and standard deviation per mouse (two ears)

			cDCs			Mono	Mo DCs		Macro		T cells			
	Neutro	LCs	$CD24^+$ $CD11b^-$	$CD24^-$ $CD11b^-$	$CD24^-$ $CD11b^+$	P1	P2	P3	P4	P5	$CD4^+$	$CD8^+$	$\gamma\delta^{low}$	DETC
Naïve	3.6 ± 1	17 ± 6	2 ± 0.03	9 ± 3	16 ± 1	0.8 ± 0.09	5.2 ± 2.9	6.7 ± 2.5	17 ± 2.3	7 ± 3.3	0.6 ± 0.4	0.007 ± 0.004	1.9 ± 1.6	8.5 ± 5.8
Vehicle	11 ± 5.2	24 ± 3	3 ± 0.3	10 ± 978	30 ± 3	1.3 ± 0.1	4.8 ± 0.8	9.5 ± 1.4	49 ± 11	15 ± 2.8	5.2 ± 2.7	0.03 ± 0.0002	5.3 ± 2.9	37 ± 8
DNFB	62 ± 3.8	11 ± 3	7 ± 0.3	3 ± 0.6	63 ± 13	83 ± 9.6	53 ± 13	9.3 ± 3.2	32 ± 1.8	8.3 ± 2.1	4.2 ± 2.4	0.2 ± 0.2	4.1 ± 0.7	16 ± 7
CHS	144 ± 36	19 ± 0.5	2 ± 0.7	12 ± 1.5	21 ± 13	407 ± 31	231 ± 26	10 ± 2.4	4 ± 2.6	3.4 ± 1.1	26 ± 8.6	19 ± 6.8	10 ± 3.1	23 ± 14

should be further separated using CD64 and Ly6C. The conventional $CD24^-CD11b^+$ dermal DCs correspond to the $Ly6C^-CD64^-$ cells (*see* **Note 10**).

6. Monocyte-related cells are gated as follows (*see* Fig. 5 and Tables 2 and 4): within $CD45^+$ Lin^- cells, select $CD24^-CD11b^+$ cells. Then plot them using Ly6C versus CD64. Remove the $Ly6C^-CD64^-$ cells, which correspond to the conventional $CD11b^+$ dermal DCs. On the remaining cells, plot CD64 versus CCR2 and select $CCR2^+CD64^{low}$ and $CCR2^-CD64^+$ populations. Within $CCR2^+CD64^{low}$ cells, by plotting Ly6C versus MHCII, you can distinguish the monocytes (P1, $Ly6C^{hi}MHCII^-$) and monocyte-derived DCs (P2 and P3, $Ly6C^+MHCII^+$ and $Ly6C^-MHCII^+$ respectively), whereas within $CCR2^-CD64^+$ cells, the macrophage populations (P4, $Ly6C^{low}MHCII^-$ and P5, $Ly6C^{low}MHCII^+$) can be distinguished.
7. T cells are gated as follows: Remove non T cells using dump channel negative cells ($APCCy7^-$) within $CD45^+$ cells (*see* Fig. 3b). γδ and αβ T cells can be separated by plotting TCRβ versus TCRγδ (*see* Fig. 6 and Tables 3 and 4). $TCR\gamma\delta^{hi}$ correspond to the dendritic epidermal T cells (DETC), $TCR\gamma\delta^{intermediate}$ correspond to the dermal γδ T cells and $TCR\beta^+$ correspond to the conventional αβ T lymphocytes. Conventional αβ T lymphocytes can be further divided into $CD4^+$ and $CD8^+$ T cells (*see* Fig. 6 and Tables 3 and 4).
8. Neutrophils are gated as follows: As Ly6G was included in the dump channel (*see* Table 2), within $CD45^+$ cells, neutrophils can be discriminated as $CD11b^+$ $Ly6G^+/Dump^+$ cells (*see* Fig. 3c and Tables 2 and 4).

4 Notes

1. Appropriate controls should be added such as vehicle only for sensitization and elicitation (called Vehicle group on the figures and Table 4), DNFB 0.2% on ear skin with previous sensitization with vehicle on the dorsal skin (called DNFB group on Figs. 1–6 and Table 4) as well as untouched skin (called Naïve in Figs. 1–6 and Table 4).
2. If you wish to separate the dermis from the epidermis prior to the digestion treatment, ears can be treated with dispase II (from *Bacillus polymyxa* grade 2). Briefly, internal and external faces of the ears are separated with forceps and laid on 1 mL of 0.4 mg/mL (or 1000 CU/mL) dispase (diluted in PBS) and incubated 1–2 h at 37 °C or on 1 mL of 0.2 mg/mL dispase and incubated overnight at 4 °C. Take each ear half from the dispase solution, dry it on a paper towel and using forceps pull

off the epidermis from the dermis as well as the cartilage layer from the internal face, before proceeding to the digestion step. To digest further, the epidermis and dermis are laid on 500 μl of collagenase D/4 from *Clostridium histolyticum* (5 mg/mL in RPMI with 0.05% DNase) and incubated 1–2 h at 37 °C. Then tissues are processed using the Medimachine.

3. If your experiments require that you extract cells from flank or back skin of mice, we recommend shaving the skin. Then on a 1 cm^2 piece of skin, remove the subcutaneous fat using fine forceps and a scalpel. Using a 300 μl insulin microneedle, inject the skin biopsy five to ten times with Liberase TL-DNase working solution and place it on 1 mL of Liberase TL-DNase working solution in a 24-well plate (dermal side down). Incubate for 2 h at 37 °C in a cell culture incubator (5% CO_2) and proceed with the grinding as described for the ears (*see* step 3.3).
4. If the cells need to be restimulated in vitro to assess cytokine production, at this step the cell pellet should be resuspended with 1 mL of complete medium (basic medium complemented with 10% FBS). Cytokine-producing T cell subsets can be easily distinguished using intracellular FACS staining to detect IL-17 and IFN-γ cytokines [16, 17].
5. The antibody mix provided in Tables 1, 2 and 3 can be used with the appropriate FACS device with four lasers. In our case, most of the experiments are done using an LSRII for analysis and a FACS-ARIA for sorting.
6. In the past we have used CD207 to discriminate DC subsets but as it requires intracellular staining, we now use CD24 whose expression correlates perfectly with CD207 and whose staining is extracellular. This allows further ex vivo functional assays as well as transcriptomic analysis.
7. For ex vivo functional assays, cells are sorted using a flow cytometer and collected in 5 mL tubes containing 2 mL of Sorting FACS buffer (10%FCS EDTA-PBS).
8. For microarray analysis, cells are sorted using a flow cytometer and collected in RNAse free Eppendorf tubes containing 90 μL of RLT plus buffer for further RNA extraction using a Qiagen microkit plus.
9. XCR1 allows to distinguish cross-presenting DCs in all tissues and lymphoid organs including the skin [19–21]. Until very recently, there was no antibody to track them and instead we were staining them with a dimeric molecule containing XCL1, which is the ligand for XCR1 fused with the fluorescent molecule mCherry (XCL1-vaccibody) which can also be used for very efficient targeting-based vaccine [21, 22].

10. Part of the Ly6C⁻CD64⁻ cells may produce aldehyde dehydrogenase (ALDH), which is involved in Treg induction [23, 24].

Acknowledgment

This work is supported by CNRS, INSERM and PIOF-GA-2013-625328-MeTaPATH to S.H.

References

1. Peiser M, Tralau T, Heidler J, Api AM, Arts JH, Basketter DA, English J, Diepgen TL, Fuhlbrigge RC, Gaspari AA et al (2012) Allergic contact dermatitis: epidemiology, molecular mechanisms, in vitro methods and regulatory aspects. Current knowledge assembled at an international workshop at BfR, Germany. Cell Mol Life Sci 69(5):763–781
2. Saint-Mezard P, Krasteva M, Chavagnac C, Bosset S, Akiba H, Kehren J, Kanitakis J, Kaiserlian D, Nicolas JF, Berard F (2003) Afferent and efferent phases of allergic contact dermatitis (ACD) can be induced after a single skin contact with haptens: evidence using a mouse model of primary ACD. J Invest Dermatol 120(4):641–647
3. Vocanson M, Hennino A, Rozieres A, Poyet G, Nicolas JF (2009) Effector and regulatory mechanisms in allergic contact dermatitis. Allergy 64(12):1699–1714
4. Kehren J, Desvignes C, Krasteva M, Ducluzeau MT, Assossou O, Horand F, Hahne M, Kagi D, Kaiserlian D, Nicolas JF (1999) Cytotoxicity is mandatory for CD8(+) T cell-mediated contact hypersensitivity. J Exp Med 189(5):779–786
5. Steinman RM, Cohn ZA (1973) Identification of a novel cell type in peripheral lymphoid organs of mice. I. Morphology, quantitation, tissue distribution. J Exp Med 137(5):1142–1162
6. Brasel K, De Smedt T, Smith JL, Maliszewski CR (2000) Generation of murine dendritic cells from flt3-ligand-supplemented bone marrow cultures. Blood 96(9):3029–3039
7. Inaba K, Inaba M, Romani N, Aya H, Deguchi M, Ikehara S, Muramatsu S, Steinman RM (1992) Generation of large numbers of dendritic cells from mouse bone marrow cultures supplemented with granulocyte/macrophage colony-stimulating factor. J Exp Med 176(6):1693–1702
8. Xu Y, Zhan Y, Lew AM, Naik SH, Kershaw MH (2007) Differential development of murine dendritic cells by GM-CSF versus Flt3 ligand has implications for inflammation and trafficking. J Immunol 179(11):7577–7584
9. Henri S, Guilliams M, Poulin LF, Tamoutounour S, Ardouin L, Dalod M, Malissen B (2010) Disentangling the complexity of the skin dendritic cell network. Immunol Cell Biol 88(4):366–375
10. Henri S, Poulin LF, Tamoutounour S, Ardouin L, Guilliams M, de Bovis B, Devilard E, Viret C, Azukizawa H, Kissenpfennig A et al (2010) CD207+ CD103+ dermal dendritic cells cross-present keratinocyte-derived antigens irrespective of the presence of Langerhans cells. J Exp Med 207(1):189–206
11. Kissenpfennig A, Henri S, Dubois B, Laplace-Builhe C, Perrin P, Romani N, Tripp CH, Douillard P, Leserman L, Kaiserlian D et al (2005) Dynamics and function of Langerhans cells in vivo: dermal dendritic cells colonize lymph node areas distinct from slower migrating Langerhans cells. Immunity 22(5):643–654
12. Gautier EL, Shay T, Miller J, Greter M, Jakubzick C, Ivanov S, Helft J, Chow A, Elpek KG, Gordonov S et al (2012) Gene-expression profiles and transcriptional regulatory pathways that underlie the identity and diversity of mouse tissue macrophages. Nat Immunol 13(11):1118–1128
13. Malissen B, Tamoutounour S, Henri S (2014) The origins and functions of dendritic cells and macrophages in the skin. Nat Rev Immunol 14(6):417–428
14. Tamoutounour S, Guilliams M, Montanana Sanchis F, Liu H, Terhorst D, Malosse C, Pollet E, Ardouin L, Luche H, Sanchez C et al (2013) Origins and functional specialization of macrophages and of conventional and monocyte-derived dendritic cells in mouse skin. Immunity 39(5):925–938
15. Terhorst D, Chelbi R, Wohn C, Malosse C, Tamoutounour S, Jorquera A, Bajenoff M,

Dalod M, Malissen B, Henri S (2015) Dynamics and transcriptomics of skin dendritic cells and macrophages in an imiquimod-induced, biphasic mouse model of psoriasis. J Immunol 195(10):4953–4961

16. Naik S, Bouladoux N, Linehan JL, Han SJ, Harrison OJ, Wilhelm C, Conlan S, Himmelfarb S, Byrd AL, Deming C et al (2015) Commensal-dendritic-cell interaction specifies a unique protective skin immune signature. Nature 520(7545):104–108
17. Naik S, Bouladoux N, Wilhelm C, Molloy MJ, Salcedo R, Kastenmuller W, Deming C, Quinones M, Koo L, Conlan S et al (2012) Compartmentalized control of skin immunity by resident commensals. Science 337(6098): 1115–1119
18. Ramirez-Valle F, Gray EE, Cyster JG (2015) Inflammation induces dermal Vgamma4+ gammadeltaT17 memory-like cells that travel to distant skin and accelerate secondary IL-17-driven responses. Proc Natl Acad Sci U S A 112(26):8046–8051
19. Bachem A, Guttler S, Hartung E, Ebstein F, Schaefer M, Tannert A, Salama A, Movassaghi K, Opitz C, Mages HW et al (2010) Superior antigen cross-presentation and XCR1 expression define human CD11c+CD141+ cells as homologues of mouse CD8+ dendritic cells. J Exp Med 207(6):1273–1281
20. Crozat K, Guiton R, Contreras V, Feuillet V, Dutertre CA, Ventre E, Vu Manh TP, Baranek T, Storset AK, Marvel J et al (2010) The XC chemokine receptor 1 is a conserved selective marker of mammalian cells homologous to mouse CD8alpha+dendritic cells. J Exp Med 207(6):1283–1292
21. Crozat K, Tamoutounour S, Vu Manh TP, Fossum E, Luche H, Ardouin L, Guilliams M, Azukizawa H, Bogen B, Malissen B et al (2011) Cutting edge: expression of XCR1 defines mouse lymphoid-tissue resident and migratory dendritic cells of the CD8alpha+type. J Immunol 187(9):4411–4415
22. Terhorst D, Fossum E, Baranska A, Tamoutounour S, Malosse C, Garbani M, Braun R, Lechat E, Crameri R, Bogen B et al (2015) Laser-assisted intradermal delivery of adjuvant-free vaccines targeting XCR1+ dendritic cells induces potent antitumoral responses. J Immunol 194(12):5895–5902
23. Guilliams M, Crozat K, Henri S, Tamoutounour S, Grenot P, Devilard E, de Bovis B, Alexopoulou L, Dalod M, Malissen B (2010) Skin-draining lymph nodes contain dermis-derived CD103(−) dendritic cells that constitutively produce retinoic acid and induce Foxp3(+) regulatory T cells. Blood 115(10):1958–1968
24. Sun CM, Hall JA, Blank RB, Bouladoux N, Oukka M, Mora JR, Belkaid Y (2007) Small intestine lamina propria dendritic cells promote de novo generation of Foxp3 T reg cells via retinoic acid. J Exp Med 204(8):1775–1785

Chapter 3

Monitoring Skin Dendritic Cells in Steady State and Inflammation by Immunofluorescence Microscopy and Flow Cytometry

Julia L. Ober-Blöbaum, Daniela Ortner, Bernhard Haid, Anna Brand, Christoph Tripp, Björn E. Clausen*, and Patrizia Stoitzner*

Abstract

Skin dendritic cells (DC) are strategically positioned at the body's second largest epithelial border to the environment. Hence they are the first antigen presenting cells that encounter invading pathogens and environmental antigens, including contact sensitizers and carcinogens penetrating the skin. Moreover, DC have the unique ability to induce immunity or tolerance and thus take center stage in regulating innate and adaptive immune responses. Skin DC can be divided into several phenotypically and functionally distinct subtypes. The three main subsets are Langerin$^+$ epidermal Langerhans cells (LC) and Langerin$^+$ as well as Langerin^{neg} dermal DC. In the steady state skin DC form a dense network to survey the periphery for pathogens and harmful substances breaching the cutaneous barrier. During inflammation DC become rapidly activated and start their migration to skin-draining lymph nodes where they initiate antigen-specific T cell responses. The homeostasis and mobilization of DC in the skin can be visualized by immunofluorescent staining of epidermal and dermal sheet preparations or skin sections. Here, we describe in detail how inflammation can be induced in the skin with tape stripping or FITC painting and how the skin DC network can be monitored using immunofluorescence microscopy and flow cytometry.

Key words Dendritic cells, Epidermal and dermal sheets, FITC painting, Immunofluorescence microscopy, Langerhans cells, Skin inflammation, Skin cryosections, Tape stripping

1 Introduction

The skin can be divided into an outer epidermis and the underlying dermis that are separated by a basement membrane. Together they form a strong mechanical barrier that protects the host from physical stress and a wide variety of environmental threats, including chemicals and pathogens. In addition, the skin harbors a heterogeneous population of dendritic cells (DC), professional antigen presenting

Note: In the printed book and online version of chapter 3, an asterisk (*) was mistakenly omitted after the author Patrizia Stoitzner's name. It has now been inserted to show that she and Björn E. Clausen have contributed equally to this chapter.

Björn E. Clausen and Jon D. Laman (eds.), *Inflammation: Methods and Protocols*, Methods in Molecular Biology, vol. 1559, DOI 10.1007/978-1-4939-6786-5_3, © Springer Science+Business Media LLC 2017

cells that orchestrate the immunological barrier and are central regulators of innate and adaptive immune responses [1, 2]. In the steady state, DC continuously scrutinize the skin for invading pathogens and along the way sample self- and environmental antigens. Through an unknown mechanism a small fraction of the cells undergoes spontaneous maturation, facilitating their chemokine receptor CCR7-mediated migration to the T cell areas of skin-draining lymph nodes. During migration, the DC upregulate the expression of surface MHC/peptide complexes and cell adhesion molecules enabling efficient recognition and interaction with naïve antigen-specific T cells. Encounter of these *phenotypically mature* DC with T cells recognizing self- or harmless environmental antigens leads to T cell anergy, deletion or induction of regulatory T cells (Treg) (*tolerizing function*) [3, 4]. Pathogen invasion together with proinflammatory signals trigger the *functional maturation* of DC, which now also upregulate expression of costimulatory molecules and, importantly, proinflammatory cytokines. Together, these mediate the activation and proliferation of naïve antigen-specific T cells as well as their polarization towards appropriate T helper (Th) type-1, Th2 or Th17 effector cells (*sensitizing function*) [5–7].

To date, we can distinguish five phenotypically distinct subsets among the CD11c$^+$MHC-II$^+$ DC that reside in healthy mouse skin using multi-color flow cytometry [8, 9]. The only DC population present in the epidermis are Langerhans cells (LC), which are characterized by the expression of the C-type lectin Langerin (CD207), the β_2-integrin CD11b and the cell adhesion molecule EpCam. In addition to transmigrating LC, the dermis contains a small population of Langerin$^+$ DC that can be unambiguously recognized by expression of the chemokine receptor XCR1, lack CD11b and EpCam, and can be further subdivided into a CD103$^+$ and negative subset. The by far largest population of DC present in the skin are Langerin^{neg}CD11b$^+$ dermal DC and, finally, the dermis harbors a minor population of Langerin^{neg}XCR1^{neg} DC that are uniquely identified by high expression levels of the chemokine receptor CX$_3$CR1. During their low-level migration to skin-draining lymph nodes in the steady state, emigrating LC are replaced from a local precursor, while dermal DC are replenished from blood-borne precursors [10, 11]. To compensate for the increased loss of cutaneous DC due to their enhanced mobilization during inflammation, large numbers of monocytes infiltrate the skin where they differentiate into CD11c$^{neg\text{-}low}$CD11b$^+$CD64$^+$ monocyte-derived DC as well as LC [9, 12]. However, these cells mainly activate skin-resident T cells and disappear after resolution of the inflammation.

In light of their phenotypic diversity, major research efforts have been aimed at dissecting the unique functions of the different skin DC subsets in balancing immunity and tolerance (reviewed in [1]). While there is overwhelming evidence for a functional specialization of the various skin DC populations (*division of labor*) [13], it is becoming increasingly clear that a given DC subset exerts a particular function that may differ depending on the context, i.e., the type of inflammation. For example, the different skin DC populations exhibit functional redundancy during contact hypersensitivity [14, 15], while LC act as negative regulators of the anti-*Leishmania* immune response [16], are essential to induce antigen-specific Th17 responses after epicutaneous *Candida albicans* infection [17], and mediate cross-tolerance towards epicutaneously applied ovalbumin [18]. On the other hand, Langerin$^+$ dermal DC promote *C. albicans*-specific Th1 and efficiently cross-present fungal antigens to activate cytotoxic T cell (CTL) responses [17]; they are also responsible for cross-priming CTL responses following deposition of the model antigen ovalbumin in the skin [18].

In all of these studies, advanced multi-color flow cytometry is essential to distinguish and analyze the small number of cells of individual DC subsets that can be purified from/are present in the skin [8, 9, 11]. However, during their life cycle, the morphology, tissue distribution, mobilization, and migration are important parameters of skin DC function, which can only be visualized by immunofluorescence microscopy. Here we describe in detail how to monitor the skin DC network in the steady state and during inflammation induced by tape stripping or FITC painting.

2 Materials

2.1 Tape Stripping of Murine Ear Skin

1. Sex- and weight-matched mice (*see* **Notes 1** and **2**).
2. Ketamine, xylazine for anesthesia.
3. Syringes.
4. 25–30 gauge needles.
5. 3 M™ Transpore™ Surgical Tape.

2.2 FITC Painting

1. Sex- and weight-matched mice (*see* **Notes 1** and **2**).
2. Ketamine, xylazine for anesthesia.
3. FITC (Fluorescein isothiocyanate isomer I).
4. Dimethyl sulfoxide (DMSO).
5. Dibutyl phthalate (DBP).
6. Acetone.
7. Syringes.
8. 25–30 gauge needles.

2.3 Epidermal and Dermal Sheet Preparation from Murine Ear Skin

2.3.1 Preparation of Epidermal and Dermal Skin Biopsies

1. Sex- and weight-matched mice (*see* **Notes 1** and **2**).
2. Carbon dioxide (CO_2) for euthanizing animals.
3. Scissors.
4. Two surgical splinter forceps.
5. 24-well plates.

6. 0.1 M phosphate buffer (8.9 g $Na_2HPO_4 \times 2\ H_2O$ plus 6.8 g KH_2PO_4 in 500 ml distilled water, pH 6.8).
7. 0.5 M ammonium thiocyanate solution (ATC) (1.9 g ATC in 50 ml 0.1 M phosphate buffer, pH 6.8).
8. Two surgical fine curved forceps.
9. Phosphate buffered saline (PBS).
10. Glass petri dishes.
11. Acetone.
12. PBS supplemented with 1 % bovine serum albumin (1 % BSA/PBS, dissolve 1 g BSA in 100 ml PBS).

2.3.2 Epidermal Sheet Preparation of Whole Ear on Tape

1. Sex- and weight-matched mice (*see* **Notes 1** and **2**).
2. Carbon Dioxide (CO_2) for euthanizing animals.
3. Scissors.
4. Two surgical fine curved forceps.
5. Depilation cream.
6. 15 ml Falcon tubes.
7. 12-well plates.
8. 20 mM EDTA solution (372 mg in 50 ml phosphate buffer, pH 7.2).
9. Phosphate buffered saline (PBS).
10. 5 cm petri dishes.
11. Tesa tape "crystal clear" (*see* **Note 3**).
12. Optional: Acetone.
13. Glycine solution (3 % BSA/200 mM glycine/PBS, dissolve 3 g BSA and 1.5 g glycine in 100 ml PBS).
14. Optional: 0.1 % Sudan black in 70 % ethanol.

2.4 Immunofluorescence Staining of Murine Ear Skin Sheets

2.4.1 Immunofluorescence Staining of Epidermal and Dermal Sheets

1. Freshly prepared or thawed epidermal and dermal sheets.
2. One fine curved forceps.
3. 96-well plate.
4. Primary and secondary antibodies for immunofluorescence staining.
5. 1 % BSA/PBS.
6. VECTASHIELD® Antifade Mounting Medium (Vector Laboratories).
7. Glass microscopic slides and coverslips.

2.4.2 Immunofluorescent Staining of Epidermal Sheets on Tape

1. Epidermal sheets on tape, prepared fresh or taken from the fridge.
2. Fine curved forceps (Dumont 7).
3. Phosphate buffered saline (PBS).

4. Glycine solution (3% BSA/200 mM glycine/PBS, dissolve 3 g BSA and 1.5 g glycine in 100 ml PBS).
5. Fc-block.
6. Saponin solution (10% w/v saponin in PBS).
7. Parafilm.
8. Humid chamber (an airtight, lightproof plastic box with a wet tissue at the bottom).
9. Blocking solution: 1× PBS containing 3% FCS and 0.02% Tween 20.
10. Staining solution: 1× PBS containing 1% BSA and 0.25% saponin (saponin is only necessary for intracellular staining, for example, for Langerin).
11. Primary and secondary antibodies for immunofluorescence staining.
12. ProLong® Gold Antifade Mountant with DAPI.
13. Microscope slides, superfrost and coverslips.

2.5 Preparation and Immunofluorescent Staining of Cryosections of Murine Skin

1. Sex- and weight-matched mice (*see* **Notes 1** and **2**).
2. Carbon dioxide (CO_2) for euthanizing animals.
3. Scissors.
4. One splinter forceps.
5. Freezing microtome.
6. Colorless Neg50-Frozen-Section-Medium (Thermo Fischer Scientific).
7. Poly-L-lysine coated slides.
8. Humid chamber.
9. Glass cuvette.
10. Acetone.
11. Hydrophobic slide marker (PAP-pen, Sigma-Aldrich).
12. 1% BSA/PBS.
13. Primary and secondary antibodies for immunofluorescence staining.
14. VECTASHIELD® Antifade Mounting Medium (Vector Laboratories).
15. Glass microscopic slides and coverslips.

2.6 Preparation of Migratory Skin DC from Lymph Nodes for FACS Analysis

1. Fine curved forceps (Dumont 7).
2. Fine scissors.
3. 1× phosphate buffered saline (PBS).
4. 1× PBS containing 2 mM EDTA.
5. 500 mM EDTA solution.

6. Digestion mix (RPMI 1640, containing 200 U/ml collagenase IV and 0.5 U/ml DNase I).
7. FACS buffer (PBS containing 2 mM EDTA, 3% FCS, and 0.02% thimerosal).
8. 1.5 ml Eppendorf tubes.
9. 50 ml Falcon tubes.
10. 15 ml Falcon tubes.
11. 70 μm cell strainer.
12. Fc-block.
13. Primary antibodies to stain for skin-derived DC subsets in lymph nodes.

3 Methods

3.1 Induction of Skin Inflammation by Tape Stripping

Mice are anesthetized with a mixture of 80–120 mg/kg ketamine and 5–10 mg/kg xylazine in PBS. The dorsal side of the ear is tape stripped by repeated application and removal of 3 M™ Transpore™ Surgical Tape. For each stripping a fresh piece of tape is lightly pressed onto the ear and pulled off [19]. Tape stripping causes

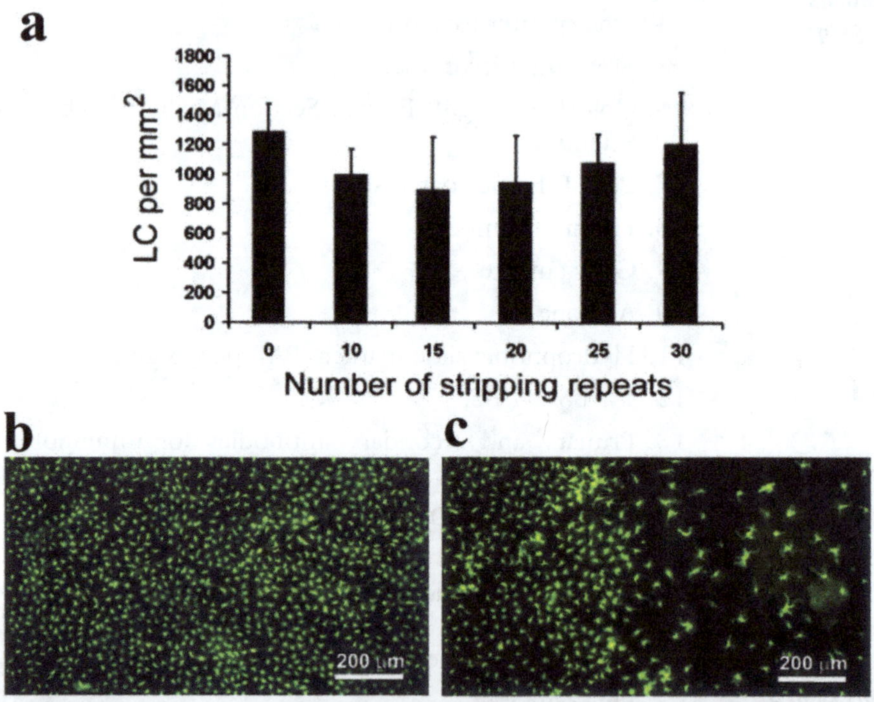

Fig. 1 Tape stripping induces emigration of LC from epidermis. (**a**) Number of stripping repeats affects the network of LC in the epidermis. (**b, c**) Epidermal sheets from steady state skin (**b**) and tape stripped skin (**c**) were stained with antibodies against MHC-class II. Tape stripping induces emigration of LC from epidermis. [Reproduced from Holzmann S, J Invest Dermatol, 2004 with permission from Nature Publishing Group.]

inflammation in the skin and emigration of immune cells like LC and dermal DC (Fig. 1). Experimental parameters e.g., kind of tape and number of stripping repeats, are crucial to the outcome of the procedure. For induction of mild inflammation we recommend 8 strippings, for strong inflammation 12 strippings (*see* **Note 4**).

3.2 Induction of Skin Inflammation by FITC Painting

5 mg FITC are dissolved in 100 ml DMSO. Acetone and DBP are mixed in a 1:1 ratio. The DMSO/FITC is diluted 10-fold in the Acetone/DBP mixture and mixed well. Mice are anesthetized with a mixture of 80–120 mg/kg ketamine and 5–10 mg/kg xylazine in PBS. Both ears (and optional the back) are shaved carefully and painted with 25 μl FITC solution each (optional: paint 100 μl FITC solution on the back, i.e., on the posterior flank, lateral to the spine). After the FITC solution has dried mice are put back into their cages. After 24, 48, 72, and/or 96 h (*see* **Note 5**) mice are sacrificed and the ears are cut off to prepare epidermal sheets as depicted in Fig. 2 (*see* Subheading 3.3 and 3.4), cryosections

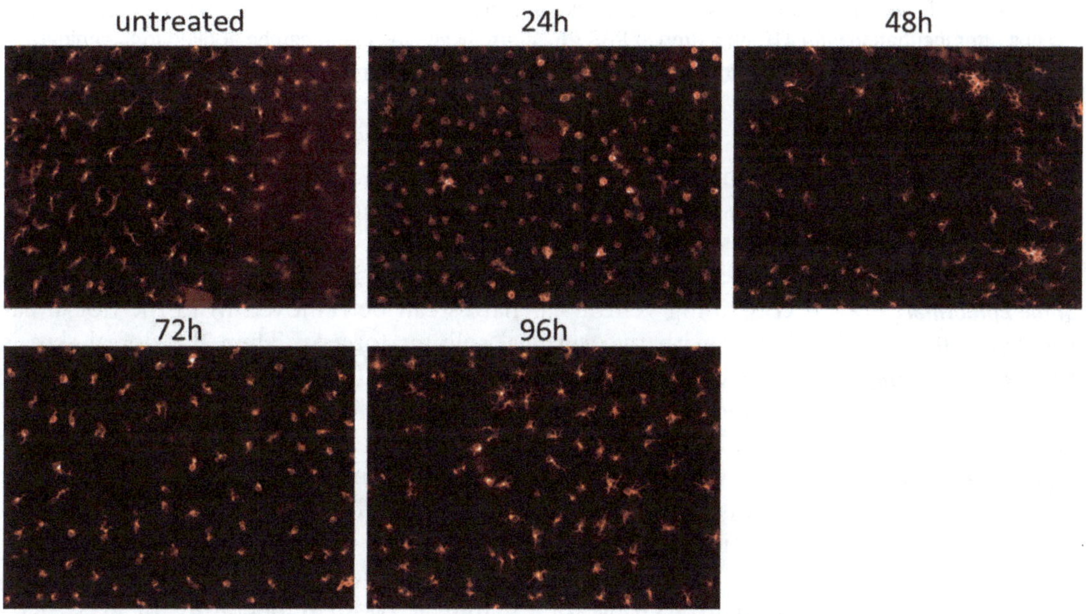

Fig. 2 LC emigration from epidermis after FITC painting. After 24 h LC (stained with MHC-class II in *red*) round up and start to leave the epidermis. 48 h after FITC painting most of the LC have left, while new LC start to repopulate the epidermis. After 72 h new LC have filled in most of the blanks and after 96 h new LC close the gaps by extending their dendrites. The LC network is re-established and the epidermis appears comparable to untreated control samples

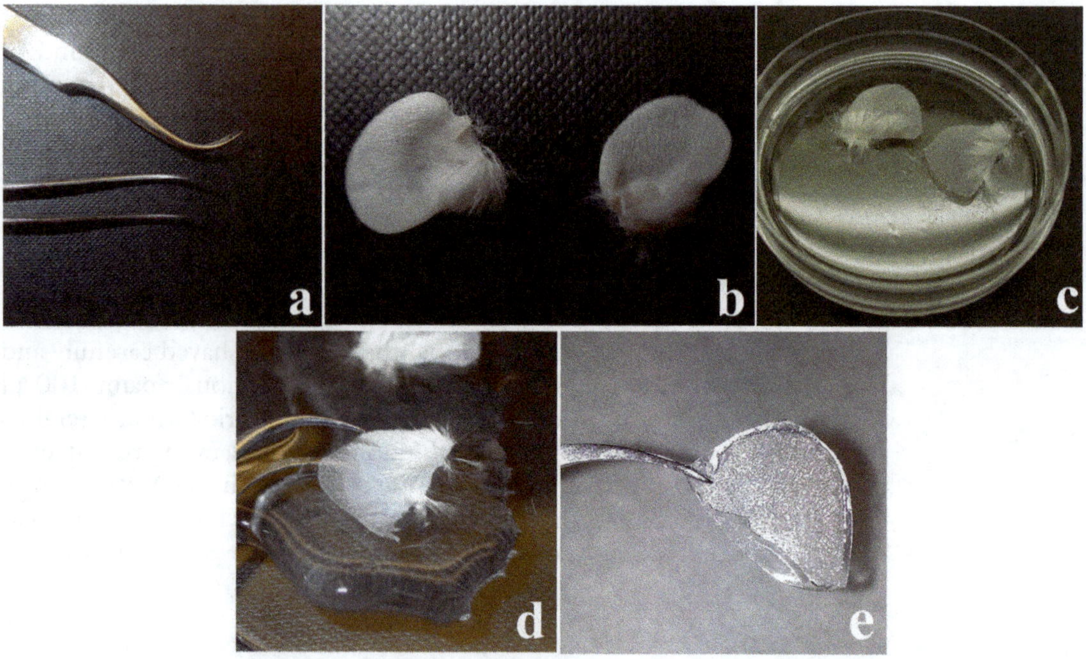

Fig. 3 Epidermal and dermal sheet preparation. Sheets are prepared with thin curved forceps (**a**) from ear skin (**b**). Dorsal ear halves are floated on ATC to split epidermis from dermis (**c**). Epidermis can be peeled off with forceps after incubation with ATC on a drop of PBS (**d**). Alternatively, Tesa tape can be applied to the epidermis before separating from the dermis to obtain whole ear specimens for immune-fluorescence staining (**e**)

(Subheading 3.5) or migratory skin DC from skin-draining lymph nodes for FACS analysis (*see* Subheading 3.6).

3.3 Monitoring of the Epidermal and Dermal DC Network—Epidermal and Dermal Sheet Preparation: Two Alternative Techniques

3.3.1 Preparation of Epidermal and Dermal Sheets

Mice are sacrificed and ears are cut off at their base. The cartilage-containing ventral ear halves can be removed from the dorsal ear halves with two surgical splinter forceps. Then the dorsal skin is floated epidermal side up on 500 μl 0.5 M ammonium thiocyanate solution for 20 min at 37 °C in a 24-well plate (one ear per well) (Fig. 3a–c). This chemically digests the basement membrane and allows the separation of epidermis and dermis [20]. Thereafter the skin is transferred onto a drop of PBS in a petri dish and the epidermis is separated from the dermis using two surgical curved forceps (Fig. 3d, *see* **Note 6**). The epidermal and dermal tissues are fixed in acetone for 20 min at room temperature in glass petri dishes. After fixation tissues are washed in a 24-well plate for 10 min twice in PBS and twice in 1% BSA/PBS to remove the acetone. Epidermal and dermal sheets can be used instantly for immunofluorescence staining or can be frozen in a drop of PBS and wrapped in aluminum foil for storage at −20 °C (*see* **Note 7**).

3.3.2 Epidermal Sheet Preparation of Whole Ear on Tape

Mice are sacrificed and the ears are cut off at their base. Depilation cream is applied onto both sides of the ears and incubated for 3 min at room temperature. Subsequently the ears are washed twice in 10 ml PBS by vortexing vigorously (*see* **Note 8**). Blot the ears on paper to dry and remove any remaining hair. The ears are split into the cartilage-containing ventral side and the dorsal side using two forceps (Fig. 3a–c). Both halves are stretched out on a reversed 5 cm petri dish with the dermal side facing downwards. A small piece (~3–4 cm) of tape is applied onto the epidermal side of each half and rubbed on (*see* **Note 9**). Next, the tape—with the dorsal or ventral half of the ear sticking to it—is carefully taken off the petri dish and is trimmed to leave only a small rim around the ear (Fig. 3e). Now the halves are floated with the dermal sides facing down on 500 μl of 20 mM EDTA solution for 1.5 h at 37 °C in a 12-well plate (one half per well) to digest the basement membrane and to allow the separation of epidermis and dermis. Thereafter, the tape—with the ear halves sticking to it—is transferred with the tape side down into a 5 cm petri dish filled with ~2 ml PBS. The dermis can now be detached from the epidermis by carefully peeling it off. The epidermis remains glued to the tape. For fixation the epidermis is floated—epidermis side down—on 500 μl of either 4% PFA or ice-cold acetone for 20 min at room temperature (PFA) or −20 °C (acetone) in a 12-well plate (one half per well). After fixation the epidermal sheets are washed twice in PBS. Afterwards 500 μl of Glycine solution is added per well and the sheets are incubated for at least 1 h (and up to 1 week) at 4 °C to reduce potential background fluorescence prior to immunofluorescence staining (*see* **Note 10**).

3.4 Monitoring of the Epidermal and Dermal DC Network—Immunofluorescent Staining of Epidermal Sheets: Two Alternative Techniques

Freshly prepared or thawed epidermal and dermal sheets are cut into smaller pieces of 5 × 5 mm and used for immunofluorescence staining. Stained sheets can be preserved on microscopic slides in VECTASHIELD® Antifade Mounting Medium for long-term storage at 4 °C for up to 1–2 years.

3.4.1 Immunofluorescence Staining of Epidermal and Dermal Sheets

One-Step Staining Procedure/Direct Staining

Sheets can be incubated with one or a mixture of primary antibodies, which are directly conjugated with different fluorescence dyes. Antibody staining solutions are prepared in 1% BSA/PBS and 100 μl of antibody solution is used per well containing one piece of an epidermal or dermal sheet. The tissue is incubated for 1 h at

37 °C or overnight at 4 °C (*see* **Note 11**). The 96-well plates are covered with a lid or Parafilm during incubation to prevent any fluid evaporation. After incubation with antibody the sheets are washed three times for 10 min in 100 µl 1 % BSA/PBS in 96-well plates to remove unbound antibody. The sheets are carefully transferred from well to well with fine curved forceps. After washing steps, the sheets are embedded in VECTASHIELD® Antifade Mounting Medium on glass microscope slides and overlaid with slide coverslips.

Two- and Three-Step Staining Procedure/Indirect Staining

Besides using directly fluorochrome-coupled antibodies one has the option to use unconjugated primary antibodies, which are detected in a two or three step staining procedure. These staining techniques allow amplifying the fluorescent signal in case the detected molecule is only weakly expressed in the tissue. For the two-step staining procedure, sheets are incubated with the primary antibody followed by a fluorochrome-coupled secondary antibody directed against the host species of the primary antibody. For the three step staining a biotinylated secondary antibody against the host species of the primary antibody is used followed by a third amplification step with streptavidin, which binds to biotin, coupled to a fluorochrome (*see* **Note 12**). As described above stainings are performed in 100 µl antibody solution for 1 h at 37 °C. After each staining step the sheets are washed three times for 10 min in 100 µl 1% BSA/PBS in the 96 well plate, followed by embedding in VECTASHIELD® Antifade Mounting Medium on glass microscope slides.

Double Staining

Sometimes it is helpful to counterstain cells to simultaneously visualize two markers on the same cell, e.g., to visualize DC within the pool of $CD45^+$ leukocytes. In order to achieve this, both molecules can be stained concurrently with a mix of two fluorescently conjugated antibodies. When an indirect staining has to be performed, we advise to first stain the molecule that is indirectly labeled. It is important to block open binding sites of the secondary antibody with 10 % serum or 100 µg/ml Ig from the host species of the secondary antibody for 15 min at 37 °C (*see* **Note 13**). Then the counterstaining with another antibody can be performed. Species- or isotype-specific secondary antibodies can also be used to avoid cross-reactivity (*see* **Note 12**). An example for a Langerin and MHC-class II double staining is shown in Fig. 4.

3.4.2 Immunofluorescent Staining of Epidermal Sheets on Tape

Epidermal sheets are washed once in PBS and incubated in Glycine solution containing 0.1 % saponin and Fc-block for 5 min at room temperature. Meanwhile the antibody mix is prepared in 60 µl staining buffer per sheet (**Note 14**). A layer of Parafilm is placed at the bottom of a saturated humid chamber and a rectangle for each sheet is drawn on the Parafilm (leaving enough space between the rectangles). A drop of 50 µl staining solution is placed into each

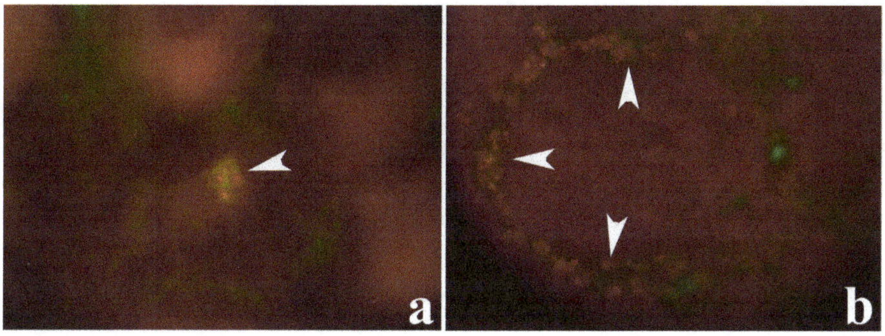

Fig. 4 Dermal sheets with lymphatic vessels containing migratory Langerin$^+$ skin DC. Dermal sheets from steady state skin (**a**) and inflammation induced by tape stripping (**b**) were stained with antibodies against Langerin (*red fluorescence*) and MHC-class II (*green fluorescence*). *Arrowheads* indicate lymphatic vessels filled with migratory skin DC. Double positive cells represent LC and Langerin$^+$ dermal DC, MHC-class II single positive cells represent Langerin^{neg} dermal DC and macrophages

rectangle and the sheet is placed carefully on top (tape facing upwards), avoiding air bubbles. The remaining 10 μl staining solution is used to fill up any blank area underneath the sheet if necessary. The epidermal sheets can be incubated for 1 h at room temperature or at 4 °C overnight, depending on the antibodies used (*see* **Notes 10** and **11**). After incubation the sheets are washed three times in PBS and placed on glass slides (tape facing downwards). The sheets are encircled with Pap-Pen and mounted with ProLong® Gold Antifade with DAPI. Slides can be stored like this for up to 2 years at 4 °C.

3.5 Monitoring of Skin DC—Preparation and Staining of Cryosections

3.5.1 Preparation of Cryosections

Mice are sacrificed and ears are cut off at their base. Tissue is embedded in colorless Neg50-Frozen-Section Medium and 8 μm skin sections are prepared from hardened tissue (−30 °C) in a freezing microtome at −27 °C. Cryosections are placed on poly-L-lysine coated microscopic slides, where they are dried for 1 h at room temperature. Afterwards the microscopic slides with sections can be either stored long-term at −20 °C or used instantly for immunofluorescence staining.

3.5.2 Staining of Cryosections

Frozen sections are taken out from the freezer and are placed in a humid chamber for 20 min at room temperature. The sections are fixed with acetone for 10 min at room temperature in glass cuvettes. Afterwards acetone needs to evaporate, so let the sections dry for another 10 min. Before staining draw a circle with a hydrophobic slide marker (Pap Pen) around each tissue sections to prevent spilling of antibody solution. The sections are stained by applying 100 μl of antibody solution onto the tissue, which is then incubated for 30 min at 37 °C or overnight at 4 °C (*see* **Note 11**). Antibody dilutions are prepared in 1% BSA/PBS. As described above for sheet staining, the cryosections can be stained with one or a mixture of primary antibodies in a one, two or three step staining procedure, depending on the expression levels of the molecule to be detected. Incubations should be performed in a closed humid chamber to avoid liquid evaporation. Following antibody incubation sections are washed three times for 5 min in 1 % BSA/PBS to remove unbound antibody. At the end of the staining process sections are embedded in VECTASHIELD® Antifade Mounting Medium on glass microscope slides and covered with slide coverslips. Stained sections can be stored at 4 °C for up to 1–2 years.

3.6 Analysis of Migratory Skin DC from Lymph Nodes by Flow Cytometry

3.6.1 Preparation of a Single Cell Suspension

After FITC painting cervical and, if FITC was also applied onto the back, inguinal lymph nodes are isolated and collected in 1.5 ml Eppendorf tubes. 200 μl of digestion mix are added to each tube and the lymph nodes are cut into very small pieces (clean scissors between samples to avoid cross-contamination). Another 800 μl of digestion mix are added and the samples are incubated for 45 min at 37 °C, shaking at ~1000 rpm. After incubation 20 μl 500 mM EDTA solution per 1 ml digestion mix (final concentration 10 mM) are added and the samples are incubated for additional 5 min at room temperature to separate T cell/ DC clusters. The cell suspension is passed over a 70 μm cell strainer and the strainer is rinsed with 10 ml PBS/ 2 mM EDTA. The cells are centrifuged for 5 min at 400×*g* at 4 °C and the supernatant is discarded. The cells are resuspended in an appropriate volume of PBS/2 mM EDTA and counted. The cell concentration is adjusted to 10^6 cells per 50 μl and 10^6 cells (50 μl) are taken per staining.

3.6.2 Flow Cytometric Analysis of Migratory DC in Skin-Draining Lymph Nodes After FITC Painting

10^6 cells are used per staining and are incubated with Fc-block for 10 min at room temperature. For the detection of migratory DC the cells are stained with an antibody cocktail including fixable Life/dead marker in AmCyan (eBioscience), CD103 in PE (clone 2E7), MHC-II in PerCP-Cy5.5 (clone M5/114.15.2), CD11b in PE-Cy7 (clone M1/70), Langerin in Alexa 647 (clone 929 F3.01, Dendritics), CD11c in APC-Cy7 (clone N418), and CD24 in Pacific blue (clone M1769) in FACS buffer. The cells are incubated with the antibody cocktail for 1 h at 4 °C in the dark. Following this incubation, the cells are washed with PBS/2 mM EDTA, resuspended in 100 μl FACS buffer and acquired immediately with a flow cytometer. An example for the FACS analysis of FITC positive migratory cells is provided in Fig. 5 (*see* **Note 15**).

4 Notes

1. Inflammation and emigration of LC from the epidermis can be induced in every inbred mouse strain; nevertheless, the degree of skin inflammation might vary between strains.
2. We recommend not mixing male and female mice in experimental groups. The development of skin inflammation can

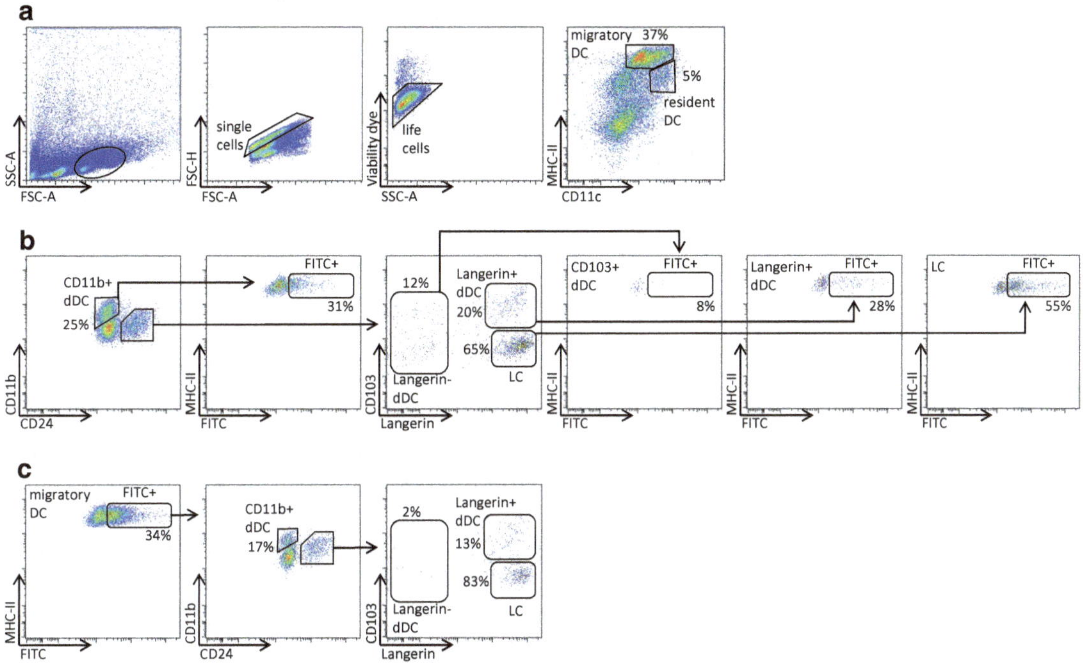

Fig. 5 Flow cytometric analysis of migratory skin DC in skin-draining lymph nodes after FITC painting. (**a**) To identify migratory DC a gate is drawn around mononuclear cells. Single cells are determined with the area and the height of the FSC. Dead cells are excluded by life/dead staining. Migratory DC are defined as MHC-$II^{high}CD11c^{int}$ cells and can be analyzed in two different ways: (**b**) By gating on DC subsets like $CD11b^+$ dermal DC, LC and $Langerin^+$ dermal DC first and then analyzing frequencies of $FITC^+$ cells or (**c**) by gating on $FITC^+$ cells within the migratory DC subset first and then dividing them into the respective skin DC subsets. While CD24 mirrors Langerin expression in the epidermis, this correlation is less pronounced in skin-draining lymph nodes [8]. The indicated percentages represent the frequencies of DC subsets of the respective parental gate

vary between the sexes due to differences in skin thickness and weight.

3. According to our experience Tesa tape crystal clear is the only tape that does not tarnish after contact with acetone or alcohol. Furthermore it does not impair fluorescence microscopy since it stays completely transparent.
4. In early experiments using tape stripping LC were physically extracted with help of the tape [21, 22]. Milder tape stripping induces inflammation followed by emigration of LC from the epidermis [19]. Tape stripping triggers the upregulation of mRNA for pro-inflammatory cytokines like IL-1α, IL-1β, and TNF-α in the skin [23], cytokines that are important for the migration of LC [24].
5. First signs of Langerhans cell emigration can be observed after 24 h, when the cells change their morphology to leave the epidermis (Fig. 2).
6. Epidermis should be easily removable from the dermis in one piece. If this is not the case the digestion might be incomplete,

then incubate the skin for another 5–10 min. Make sure that all epidermal pieces are peeled off from the dermis.

7. Epidermal and dermal sheets can be stored long-term at −20 °C without any loss of quality. Freshly prepared and frozen sheets show comparable staining results.
8. If the ears are still highly inflamed depilation can damage the delicate epidermis, in this case the depilation step should be skipped.
9. In case of strong tissue inflammation the skin will be oozing fluid, which prevents it from sticking to the tape properly. In this case the ears can be pre-fixed in ice-cold acetone for 20 min prior to splitting them into halves to dehydrate the tissue.
10. If high background fluorescence is an issue (e.g., after topical FITC painting), the sheets can be exposed to light for a minimum of 4 h prior to immunofluorescence staining. Alternatively, epidermal sheets can be incubated for 20 min in 0.1% Sudan black in 70% ethanol after immunofluorescence staining. This will result in a blackening of the tape, without interfering with the antibody staining.
11. The decision how long primary antibodies are incubated with the sheets depends on the expression levels of the molecules to be detected. We recommend shorter incubation of 1 h at 37 °C for strongly expressed molecules and longer incubation overnight at 4 °C for weakly expressed molecules.
12. Indirect staining in a two or three step procedure can result in unspecific background staining especially in dermal sheets. In order to quench this effect as well as antibody cross-reactivity between species, blocking with normal serum (5% v/v) from the host species of the secondary antibody can be performed before the staining procedure is started. In addition, secondary antibodies should be carefully titrated.
13. Alternatively, the secondary antibody can be replaced by a F(ab) fragment; a monovalent antibody molecule still binding to its antigen but lacking the Fc portion. Using a F(ab) fragment as secondary antibody can improve the staining results, because (1) it eliminates nonspecific binding between Fc portions of antibodies and Fc receptors on cells and (2) F(ab) fragments do not interfere with specific anti-Fc mediated secondary antibody detection.
14. In case of a weak staining result due to low expression of the target molecule, the signal intensity can be increased by replacing the staining solution with a so-called staining enhancer, such as the Thermo Scientific Pierce Immunostain Enhancer.
15. This basic protocol can be used to generally analyze migratory DC after the induction of skin inflammation, e.g., tape stripping, without the possibility to identify FITC$^+$ recent skin immigrants.

Acknowledgements

The authors would like to thank the members of the Clausen and the Stoitzner laboratories for their support and the members of the animal facilities of the University Medical Center Mainz and the Medical University of Innsbruck for responsible animal husbandry. J.L.O. is a fellow of the Fritz-Thyssen Foundation (10.15.1.02OMN), D.O. is supported by a scholarship from the Austrian Science Fund (FWF-T-007370), B.E.C. is supported by the DFG (CL 419/2-1) and the Research Center for Immunotherapy (FZI) Mainz, and P.S. is supported by grants form the Austrian Science Fund (P-27001-B13, ZFW011010-015).

References

1. Clausen BE, Stoitzner P (2015) Functional specialization of skin dendritic cell subsets in regulating T cell responses. Front Immunol 6:534
2. Romani N, Clausen BE, Stoitzner P (2010) Langerhans cells and more: langerin-expressing dendritic cell subsets in the skin. Immunol Rev 234:120–41
3. Jiang A, Bloom O, Ono S, Cui W, Unternaehrer J, Jiang S, Whitney JA, Connolly J, Banchereau J, Mellman I (2007) Disruption of E-cadherin-mediated adhesion induces a functionally distinct pathway of dendritic cell maturation. Immunity 27:610–24
4. Steinman RM, Hawiger D, Nussenzweig MC (2003) Tolerogenic dendritic cells. Annu Rev Immunol 21:685–711
5. Banchereau J, Steinman RM (1998) Dendritic cells and the control of immunity. Nature 392:245–52
6. Dalod M, Chelbi R, Malissen B, Lawrence T (2014) Dendritic cell maturation: functional specialization through signaling specificity and transcriptional programming. EMBO J 33:1104–16
7. Steinman RM, Banchereau J (2007) Taking dendritic cells into medicine. Nature 449:419–26
8. Henri S, Poulin LF, Tamoutounour S, Ardouin L, Guilliams M, de Bovis B, Devilard E, Viret C, Azukizawa H, Kissenpfennig A, Malissen B (2010) CD207+ CD103+ dermal dendritic cells cross-present keratinocyte-derived antigens irrespective of the presence of langerhans cells. J Exp Med 207:189–206
9. Tamoutounour S, Guilliams M, Montanana Sanchis F, Liu H, Terhorst D, Malosse C, Pollet E, Ardouin L, Luche H, Sanchez C, Dalod M, Malissen B, Henri S (2013) Origins and functional specialization of macrophages and of conventional and monocyte-derived dendritic cells in mouse skin. Immunity 39:925–38
10. Geissmann F, Manz MG, Jung S, Sieweke MH, Merad M, Ley K (2010) Development of monocytes, macrophages, and dendritic cells. Science 327:656–61
11. Malissen B, Tamoutounour S, Henri S (2014) The origins and functions of dendritic cells and macrophages in the skin. Nat Rev Immunol 14:417–28
12. Seré K, Baek JH, Ober-Blöbaum J, Müller-Newen G, Tacke F, Yokota Y, Zenke M, Hieronymus T (2012) Two distinct types of Langerhans cells populate the skin during steady state and inflammation. Immunity 37:905–16
13. Pulendran B, Tang H, Denning TL (2008) Division of labor, plasticity, and crosstalk between dendritic cell subsets. Curr Opin Immunol 20:61–7
14. Honda T, Nakajima S, Egawa G, Ogasawara K, Malissen B, Miyachi Y, Kabashima K (2010) Compensatory role of Langerhans cells and langerin-positive dermal dendritic cells in the sensitization phase of murine contact hypersensitivity. J Allergy Clin Immunol 125:1154–1156.e2
15. Noordegraaf M, Flacher V, Stoitzner P, Clausen BE (2010) Functional redundancy of Langerhans cells and Langerin+dermal dendritic cells in contact hypersensitivity. J Invest Dermatol 130:2752–9
16. Kautz-Neu K, Noordegraaf M, Dinges S, Bennett CL, John D, Clausen BE, von Stebut E (2011) Langerhans cells are negative regulators of the anti-Leishmania response. J Exp Med 208:885–91
17. Igyártó BZ, Haley K, Ortner D, Bobr A, Gerami-Nejad M, Edelson BT, Zurawski SM, Malissen B, Zurawski G, Berman J, Kaplan DH (2011) Skin-resident murine dendritic cell subsets promote

distinct and opposing antigen-specific T helper cell responses. Immunity 35:260–72

18. Flacher V, Tripp CH, Mairhofer DG, Steinman RM, Stoitzner P, Idoyaga J, Romani N (2014) Murine Langerin + dermal dendritic cells prime CD8+ T cells while Langerhans cells induce cross-tolerance. EMBO Mol Med 6:1191–204
19. Holzmann S, Tripp CH, Schmuth M, Janke K, Koch F, Saeland S, Stoitzner P, Romani N (2004) A model system using tape stripping for characterization of Langerhans cell-precursors in vivo. J Invest Dermatol 122:1165–74
20. Juhlin L, Shelley WB (1977) New staining techniques for the Langerhans cell. Acta Derm Venereol 57:289–96
21. Lessard RJ, Wolff K, Winkelmann RK (1968) The disappearance and regeneration of Langerhans cells following epidermal injury. J Invest Dermatol 50:171–9
22. Streilein JW, Lonsberry LW, Bergstresser PR (1982) Depletion of epidermal langerhans cells and Ia immunogenicity from tape-stripped mouse skin. J Exp Med 155:863–71
23. Wood LC, Jackson SM, Elias PM, Grunfeld C, Feingold KR (1992) Cutaneous barrier perturbation stimulates cytokine production in the epidermis of mice. J Clin Invest 90:482–7
24. Stoitzner P, Zanella M, Ortner U, Lukas M, Tagwerker A, Janke K, Lutz MB, Schuler G, Echtenacher B, Ryffel B, Koch F, Romani N (1999) Migration of langerhans cells and dermal dendritic cells in skin organ cultures: augmentation by TNF-alpha and IL-1beta. J Leukoc Biol 66:462–70

Chapter 4

Visualization of the T Cell Response in Contact Hypersensitivity

Gyohei Egawa and Kenji Kabashima

Abstract

Contact hypersensitivity (CHS) is the most basic murine model for type IV hypersensitivity. This dermatitis model is mediated by hapten-sensitized, skin-infiltrating T cells. Recent intravital imaging studies have demonstrated the dynamic migratory property of skin-infiltrating T cells and the orchestrated interaction of T cells with dermal dendritic cells. Multiphoton microscopy enables the direct, three-dimensional, and minimally invasive imaging of in vivo skin samples with high spatiotemporal resolution. Here, we describe a basic method for the intravital imaging of skin-infiltrating T cells in the DNFB-induced CHS response.

Key words Adoptive transfer, Contact hypersensitivity, Dendritic cell, Hapten, Imaging, Multiphoton microscopy, T cell

1 Introduction

Contact hypersensitivity (CHS) is a murine model for contact dermatitis, a prototypic T cell-mediated delayed-type (type IV) hypersensitivity response [1, 2]. The CHS response is induced by the penetration of small compounds called haptens through the skin barrier (Fig. 1). Haptens activate keratinocytes to produce various proinflammatory mediators such as tumor necrosis factor (TNF)-α and interleukin (IL)-1α/β, which promote the migration and maturation of skin dendritic cells (DCs) [3, 4]. Cutaneous DCs, including epidermal Langerhans cells, capture the haptens and carry them to the draining lymph nodes and present them to naïve T cells (sensitization phase). T cells that recognize the haptens are activated and proliferate and then circulate throughout the body. Upon rechallenge with the same hapten, hapten-specific T cells are promptly recruited to the lesional skin and induce skin inflammation (elicitation phase) [5]. Recently, using an intravital imaging technique, we visualized the cluster formation of skin-infiltrating T cells in the vicinity of dermal blood capillaries with dermal DCs and macrophages [6]. Hapten-specific T cells interact with dermal

Björn E. Clausen and Jon D. Laman (eds.), *Inflammation: Methods and Protocols*, Methods in Molecular Biology, vol. 1559, DOI 10.1007/978-1-4939-6786-5_4, © Springer Science+Business Media LLC 2017

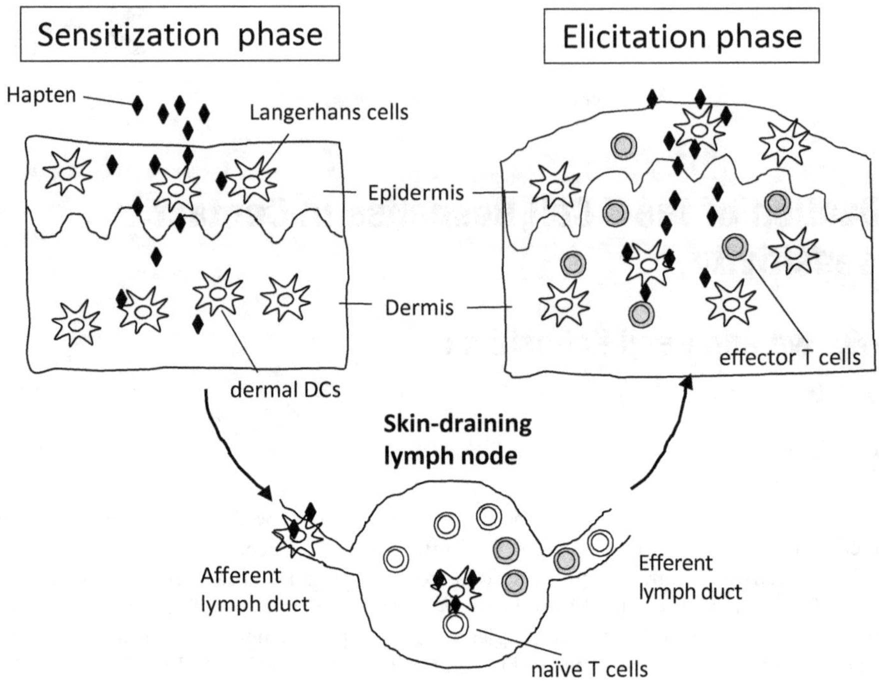

Fig. 1 Schematic representation of a CHS reaction. During the sensitization phase, hapten-bearing dendritic cells (DCs) migrate into draining lymph node and present antigens to naïve T cells. During the elicitation phase, activated-effector T cells infiltrate into the skin and interact with cutaneous DCs

DCs for hours and proliferate and produce interferon (IFN)-γ in situ.

Intravital imaging is an important technique to capture dynamic biological events such as immune responses. Multiphoton (MP) microscopy (also referred to as two-photon excitation microscopy) was first described by Denk et al. [7] and is now commonly used for intravital imaging. Compared with conventional single-photon excitation microscopy, two-photon excitation microscopy allows deeper tissue penetration with less photodamage, achieving high spatiotemporal resolution. MP can provide substantial information that is not available using traditional methods such as histological and flow cytometer-based analysis. Since noninvasive intravital imaging is easy with mouse ear skin, various kinds of cutaneous immune responses have been visualized thus far [8, 9].

Here we describe a basic method for the in vivo imaging of skin-infiltrating T cells in the CHS response. We provide a detailed description of the induction of the DNFB-mediated CHS response, T cell-labeling, the adoptive transfer of T cells, and how to investigate mouse ear skin with MP microscopy.

2 Materials

2.1 Animals

1. 6–8-week-old, sex- and weight-matched mice (*see* **Notes 1** and **2**).
2. CD11c-enhanced yellow fluorescent protein (EYFP) mice (available from Jax®: stock number 008829) (*see* **Note 3**).
3. Langerin-enhanced green fluorescent protein (EGFP) mice (available from Jax®: stock number 016939) (*see* **Note 4**).

2.2 Induction of the Contact Hypersensitivity Response

1. Electric shaver.
2. 2,4-dinitrofluorobenzene (DNFB) (*see* **Note 5**).
3. Olive oil.
4. Acetone.

2.3 Adoptive Transfer of Effector T Cells

1. Standard equipments to collect lymph nodes including cell culture dish, a 40-μm nylon cell strainer, 1 ml syringe, 15 ml centrifuge tube, and 1 ml microcentrifuge tube.
2. 30-gauge needle insulin syringe.
3. 2% RPMI: RPMI 1640 medium supplemented with 2% fetal calf serum.
4. 10% RPMI: RPMI 1640 medium supplemented with 10% fetal calf serum.
5. Phosphate buffered saline (PBS):1.37 M NaCl, 0.027 M KCl, 0.081 M Na_2HPO_4, 0.0147 M KH_2PO_4.
6. MACS buffer: PBS supplemented with 0.5% bovine serum albumin and 2 mM EDTA.
7. Pan T cell isolation KIT, mouse (Miltenyi Biotec, Bergisch Gladbach, Germany) (*see* **Note 6**).
8. Magnetic cell-sorting device (Miltenyi Biotec).
9. CellTrace CFSE dye (Thermo Fisher Scientific, Lafayette, CO, USA).
10. Cellracker Red CMTPX dye (Thermo Fisher Scientific).

2.4 Intravital Imaging of the Skin

1. Two-photon microscope with a tunable (690–1040 nm) Ti/sapphire laser (Mai Tai DeepSee, Spectra-Physics, Santa Clara, CA, USA) (*see* **Note 7**).
2. Inhalation anesthesia apparatus for small animals.
3. Cover glass (24 × 24/24 × 50 mm).
4. Hair removal cream (*see* **Note 8**).
5. Pentobarbital sodium: 10% (v/v) solution in PBS (*see* **Note 9**).
6. Isoflurane.
7. Grease.
8. Immersion oil.

3 Methods

3.1 Sensitize Mice with DNFB

Before sensitizing mice, keep mice calm in a cage for at least 24 h (*see* **Note 10**).

1. Prepare 0.5 % (w/v) DNFB solution (*see* **Notes 5** and **11**).
2. Shave the abdominal hair thoroughly using an electric shaver (*see* **Note 12**).
3. Grasp the mouse in one hand and paint 20 μl of 0.5 % DNFB solution on the shaved abdomen (Fig. 2) (*see* **Note 13**).
4. Air-dry the DNFB solution.
5. Sensitize at least 5 mice (*see* **Note 14**).
6. Keep the mice calm for 5 days (*see* **Note 15**).

3.2 Adoptive Transfer of Sensitized T Cells

3.2.1 Preparation of Single Cell Suspension of Lymph Node Cells

All buffers should be kept on ice (>10 °C).

1. Euthanize mice with the proper procedure.
2. Collect both sides of the axillary and inguinal lymph nodes (*see* **Note 16**). Put lymph nodes into 5 ml of 2 % RPMI in a 15 ml centrifuge tube and keep on ice.
3. Using a syringe plunger, mash the lymph nodes through a 40-μm cell strainer.
4. Centrifuge at 3000 × *g* for 3 min at 4 °C and discard supernatant.
5. Resuspend cells in 10 ml of MACS buffer.

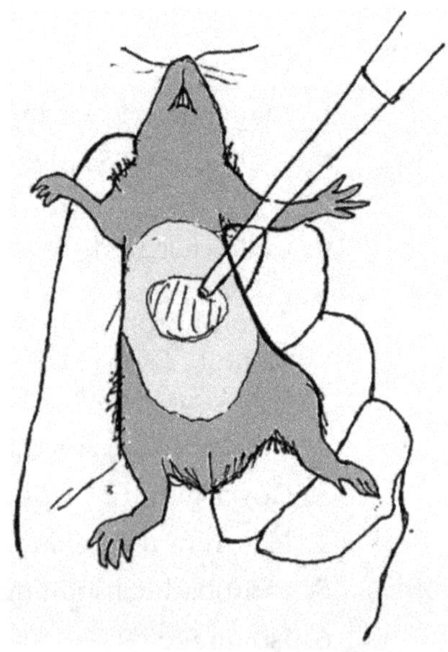

Fig. 2 Mouse sensitization. Hold a mouse in one hand and paint the hapten solution onto the shaved abdomen as shown

6. Count cells (*see* **Note 17**).
7. Centrifuge at 3000 ×g for 3 min at 4 °C and discard supernatant.

3.2.2 Isolation of T cells with Magnetic Cell Sorter

1. Resuspend cells in 40 μl of MACS buffer per 10^7 cells.
2. Add 10 μl of biotin-antibody cocktail per 10^7 cells.
3. Mix well and incubate for 5 min on ice.
4. Add 10 ml of MACS buffer.
5. Centrifuge at 3000 ×g for 3 min at 4 °C and discard supernatant.
6. Resuspend cells in 80 μl of MACS buffer per 10^7 cells.
7. Add 20 μl of anti-biotin microbeads per 10^7 cells.
8. Mix well and incubate for 10 min on ice.
9. Wash cells as in **steps 4** and **5**.
10. Resuspend cells in 1 ml MACS buffer.
11. To remove cell clumps, filter the cell suspension through a 40-μm cell strainer.
12. Isolate T cells with a magnetic cell sorter (*see* **Note 18**).
13. Count cells (*see* **Note 19**).
14. Centrifuge at 3000 ×g for 3 min at 4 °C and discard supernatant.

3.2.3 Cell Labeling with Fluorescent Dyes

1. Resuspend cells in 1 ml of PBS (*see* **Note 20**).
2. Prepare 1 ml of 10 μM fluorescent dye (CFSE or CMTPX) solution in PBS.
3. Mix cell solution with fluorescent dye solution (1:1).
4. Incubate for 10 min at 37 °C, inverting the tube every 3 min (*see* **Note 21**).
5. Add 10 ml of ice-cold 10% RPMI.
6. Centrifuge at 3000 ×g for 3 min at 4 °C and discard supernatant.
7. Wash cells as in **steps 5** and **6**.
8. Count cells.
9. Resuspend in 300 μl of 2% RPMI.

3.2.4 Adoptive Transfer of T cells via Tail Vein

1. Heat CD11c-EYFP mice with a heating lamp for 5 min (*see* **Note 22**).
2. Fix the mice using a mouse holder.
3. Inject 300 μl of T cell suspension into the tail vein with a 30-gauge insulin syringe.
4. Proceed to the elicitation of CHS within 2 days.

3.3 Intravital Imaging of CHS Response in the Ear Skin

3.3.1 Elicitation of CHS Response

1. Prepare 0.3% (w/v) DNFB solution (*see* **Notes 5** and **23**).
2. Anesthetize recipient mice by the intraperitoneal injection of 10% pentobarbital sodium solution (10 μl per g body weight) (*see* **Note 24**).
3. Grasp the mouse in one hand and paint 20 μl of 0.3% DNFB solution on the left ear skin (10 μl to the dorsal side and 10 μl to the ventral side).
4. Air-dry the DNFB solution.

3.3.2 Mouse Preparation for Intravital Imaging

1. Apply the hair removal cream to the ventral and dorsal side of the left ear skin. Three minutes later, remove the cream from the ear using wet cotton or running water (*see* **Note 25**).
2. Apply the grease to the dorsal side of the left ear using a cotton swab (*see* **Note 26**).
3. Attach the 24×24 mm cover glass to the dorsal side of the left ear.

3.3.3 Placing the Mouse onto the Microscope Stage

Place the mouse on a heating pad at 37 °C throughout the imaging procedure.

1. If necessary, place a single drop of immersion oil on the objective lens.
2. Cover the central hole of the microscope stage with 24×50 mm cover glass and fix it with tape (*see* **Note 27**).
3. Place a drop of immersion oil onto the cover glass just above the objective lens.
4. Place a mouse onto the stage. Sandwich the ear between two cover glasses (Fig. 3) (*see* **Note 28**).
5. Connect the mouse to the anesthetic apparatus. Flow 1% isoflurane at a rate of 1 L/min (*see* **Note 29**).
6. Stabilize the mouse using taping.

3.3.4 Start Imaging

1. Set the appropriate excitation laser wavelength. The ideal excitation wavelength is 940–960 nm for EYFP and EGFP and 780–800 nm for CFSE and CMTPX [10]. Collagen fibers in the dermis can be visualized by second harmonic generation (Fig. 4).
2. Commence imaging. We typically take stacks of 15–20 images, spaced 3.5 μm apart, every 1–5 min for 3–12 h (*see* **Note 30**).

4 Notes

1. The CHS response is influenced by the hair cycle. It is suppressed in the anagen (hair-growth) phase. To avoid this, the sensitization of CHS should be completed within the first telogen (resting) phase (6–8 weeks after birth).

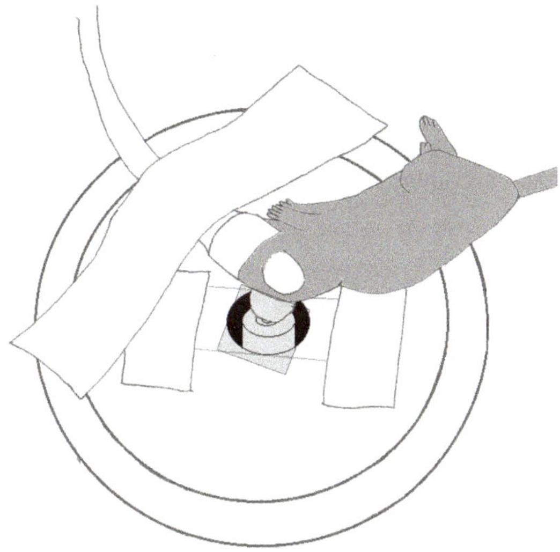

Fig. 3 Fix mouse on the stage. The ear lobe is sandwiched between two coverslips

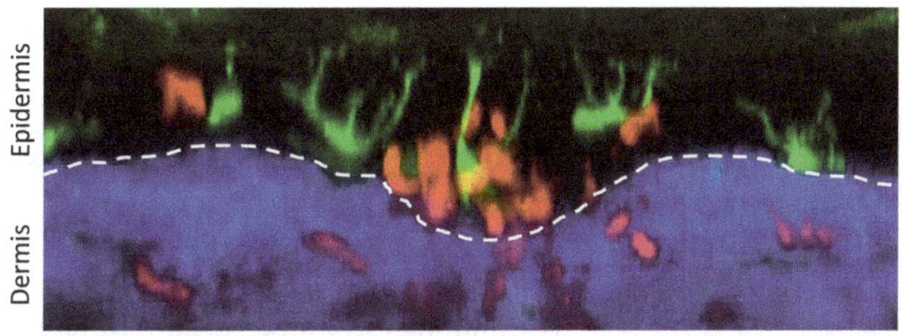

Fig. 4 Sample image. Skin-infiltrating T cells (*red*) interact with Langerhans cells (*green*). The *white-dashed line* represents the border between the epidermis and dermis. *Blue*: collagen fibers

2. The CHS response is influenced by mouse strain. In general, the CHS response is stronger in BALB/c mice than C57BL/6 mice.
3. CD11c, also known as integrin αX, is expressed in both epidermal Langerhans cells (LCs) and dermal DCs. CD11c expression is, however, sometimes weak in LCs. This strain is suitable for the observation of dermal DCs.
4. Langerin, a C-type lectin, is specifically and extensively expressed in LCs and dermal Langerin$^+$ DCs. This strain is suitable for the observation of LCs.
5. A variety of haptens are used for the induction of the CHS response. The standard hapten application chart is shown in Table 1.

Table 1
Standard hapten application for CHS response[a]

	Sensitization			Elicitation		
	Concentration (%)	Solvent	Dose (μl)	Concentration (%)	Solvent	Dose (μl)
DNFB	0.5	Acetone–olive oil (4:1)	25	0.3	Acetone–olive oil (4:1)	20
TNCB	7.0	Acetone–olive oil (4:1)	100	1.0	Acetone–olive oil (9:1)	20
Oxazolone	3.0	100% EtOH	150	1.0	100% EtOH	20
FITC	0.5	Acetone–dibutyl phthalate (1:1)	400	0.5	Acetone–dibutyl phthalate (1:1)	20

[a]*DNFB* 2,4-dinitrofluorobenzene, *TNCB* 2,4,6-trinitrochlorobenzene, *FITC* fluorescein isothiocyanate

6. $CD4^+$ T cell isolation kit, $CD8^+$ T cell isolation kit, and CD90.2 microbeads are also available.
7. An inverted microscope is better suited for observation of the skin than an upright microscope, because of the ease of fixing the ear.
8. Hair removal cream for humans is suitable.
9. The anesthesia is maintained for 1–1.5 h with intraperitoneal administration of pentobarbital sodium. Anesthetic gases such as isoflurane are suitable for longer anesthesia.
10. Immune responses, including the CHS response, may be suppressed in stressed mice. Mice should be accustomed to their housing before sensitization.
11. The specific gravity of DNFB is 1.482 g/cm^3. To prepare 6 ml of 0.5% DNFB solution, mix 20 μl of DNFB with 4.8 ml acetone and 1.2 ml olive oil.
12. Care should be taken not to damage the skin during shaving.
13. Paint DNFB solution on the center of the abdomen in a coin-sized area (Fig. 2).
14. We generally use five sensitized mice for transferring the sensitized T cells into one recipient mouse.
15. The number of DNFB-sensitized T cells in the draining lymph nodes reaches a peak at 5 or 6 days post-sensitization.
16. The draining lymph nodes of the abdominal skin are the axillary and inguinal lymph nodes. If mice are sensitized on the ear skin or the back skin, collect the auricular or brachial lymph nodes, respectively.

17. Approximately 10^8 cells can be harvested from the draining lymph nodes of five sensitized mice.
18. Separate T cells manually with MACS columns or automatically with an autoMACS pro separator.
19. Approximately $1.0–2.0 \times 10^7$ T cells are harvested from the draining lymph nodes of five sensitized mice. Note that not all T cells are DNFB-specific T cells. If necessary, keep a 50 μl aliquot for flow cytometry to ensure the purity of T cells.
20. Cells should be labeled in a medium without FCS. FCS significantly interferes with the linkage of fluorescent dye to the cells.
21. Do not exceed 10 min since the fluorescent dye solution is cell-toxic.
22. Use Langerin-EGFP mice if the interaction between T cells and epidermal Langerhans cells is the target of observation.
23. To prepare 5 ml of 0.3% DNFB solution, mix 10 μl of DNFB with 4 ml acetone and 1 ml olive oil.
24. The body temperature of the mouse will drop, particularly after the anesthesia. Keep the mouse on a heating pad and warm it sufficiently.
25. Ensure that the hair removal cream does not stay on the ear for more than 5 min. The cream is stimulative and may modify skin inflammation.
26. Handle the ear gently to prevent injuries arising from friction.
27. Avoid the formation of bubbles when immersion oil is placed between the objective lens and the cover glass.
28. Do not apply strong pressure to the ear as it may disturb blood and lymph circulation, which are important for intravital imaging studies.
29. The flow rate of isoflurane needs to be increased depending on the body weight of the mouse.
30. We observed that labeled effector T cells started to appear in the dermis within 6 h post-elicitation and formed clusters with $EYFP^+$ dermal dendritic cells. The clusters became larger and more evident after 24 h [6].

Acknowledgment

This work was supported by Grants-in-Aid for Scientific Research from the Ministry of Education, Culture, Sports, Science and Technology of Japan.

References

1. Kaplan DH, Igyártó BZ, Gaspari AA (2012) Early immune events in the induction of allergic contact dermatitis. Nat Rev Immunol 12(2):114–124
2. Honda T, Egawa G, Grabbe S, Kabashima K (2013) Update of immune events in the murine contact hypersensitivity model: toward the understanding of allergic contact dermatitis. J Invest Dermatol 133(2):303–315
3. Cumberbatch M, Kimber I (1995) Tumour necrosis factor-alpha is required for accumulation of dendritic cells in draining lymph nodes and for optimal contact sensitization. Immunology 84(1):31
4. Cumberbatch M, Dearman R, Kimber I (1997) Langerhans cells require signals from both tumour necrosis factor α and interleukin 1β for migration. In: Dendritic cells in fundamental and clinical immunology. Springer, pp. 125–128
5. Egawa G, Nakamizo S, Natsuaki Y, Doi H, Miyachi Y, Kabashima K (2013) Intravital analysis of vascular permeability in mice using two-photon microscopy. Sci Rep 3:1932
6. Natsuaki Y, Egawa G, Nakamizo S, Ono S, Hanakawa S, Okada T, Kusuba N, Otsuka A, Kitoh A, Honda T (2014) Perivascular leukocyte clusters are essential for efficient activation of effector T cells in the skin. Nat Immunol 15(11):1064–1069
7. Denk W, Strickler JH, Webb WW (1990) Two-photon laser scanning fluorescence microscopy. Science 248(4951):73–76
8. Li JL, Goh CC, Keeble JL, Qin JS, Roediger B, Jain R, Wang Y, Chew WK, Weninger W, Ng LG (2012) Intravital multiphoton imaging of immune responses in the mouse ear skin. Nat Protoc 7(2):221–234
9. Kabashima K, Egawa G (2014) Intravital multiphoton imaging of cutaneous immune responses. J Invest Dermatol 134(11):2680–2684
10. Cahalan MD, Parker I, Wei SH, Miller MJ (2002) Two-photon tissue imaging: seeing the immune system in a fresh light. Nat Rev Immunol 2(11):872–880

Chapter 5

Ultraviolet Radiation-Induced Immunosuppression: Induction of Regulatory T Cells

A. Bruhs and T. Schwarz

Abstract

Solar/ultraviolet (UV) radiation exerts a variety of biological effects, including suppression of the immune system. UV-induced immunosuppression is induced by suberythemogenic/physiological UV doses, and it affects primarily T-cell driven immune reactions. Another characteristic feature of UV-induced immunosuppression is its antigen-specificity. This is due to the induction of T cells with suppressive features, called regulatory T cells. Since UV-induced regulatory T cells may harbor therapeutic potential phenotypic and functional characterization of these cells is ongoing. Most of these studies have been performed in the murine model of contact hypersensitivity. In this protocol we describe a method for the UV-induced suppression of the induction of contact hypersensitivity and the adoptive transfer of immune response.

Key words Contact hypersensitivity, Immunosuppression, Regulatory T cells, Tolerance, Ultraviolet radiation

1 Introduction

It is well known for decades that ultraviolet (UV) radiation in particular the mid wave range (UVB, 290–320 nm) suppresses the immune system. UV-induced immunosuppression exerts unique features: (1) It is caused by low suberythemogenic doses. (2) It is antigen-specific and thus differs from immunosuppression caused by drugs. (3) Primarily T-cell-driven reactions are affected [1]. Most of the relevant studies have been performed in the model of contact hypersensitivity (CHS) in mice. Topical application of contact allergens (haptens) on the skin results in obligatory sensitization. Upon successful sensitization a specific ear swelling response can be induced by applying much lower concentrations of the same hapten on one ear (ear challenge; Fig. 1a). This concentration does not induce swelling in non-sensitized mice, thus excluding a toxic reaction. In addition, other unrelated haptens do not induce ear challenge in sensitized mice, indicating the antigen-specificity of this immune response.

Björn E. Clausen and Jon D. Laman (eds.), *Inflammation: Methods and Protocols*, Methods in Molecular Biology, vol. 1559, DOI 10.1007/978-1-4939-6786-5_5,

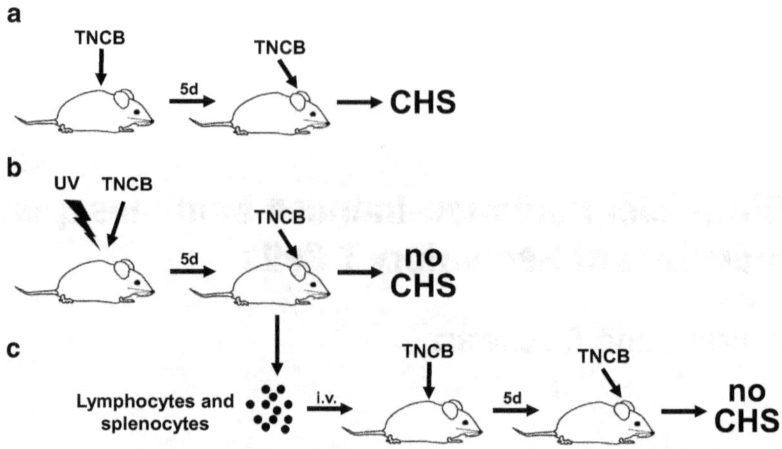

Fig. 1 UV radiation induces antigen-specific immunotolerance. (**a**) Epicutaneous application of a contact allergen (e.g., 2,4,6-trinitrochlorobenzene [TNCB]) on the back of the mice followed by a challenge 5 days later on the left ear results in contact hypersensitivity (CHS) indicated by an ear swelling response. (**b**) In contrast, application of the contact allergen onto UV-exposed skin does not result in CHS. (**c**) Lymphocytes and splenocytes obtained from UV-tolerized mice suppress sensitization against the same hapten in recipient mice after adoptive transfer

Application of haptens onto skin which has been exposed to suberythemogenic doses of UVB radiation does not result in sensitization [2]. Since irradiation and hapten application take place in the same area, this phenomenon is called local immunosuppression. More importantly, application of haptens onto UV-exposed skin results in long term immunosuppression since these mice cannot be resensitized at later time points even without being further UV exposed. However, all other immune responses are unaffected, indicating the antigen specificity of UVR-induced immunosuppression.

Antigen specificity is due to the induction of antigen-specific regulatory T cells (Treg) [3] Injection of T cells obtained from UV- and hapten-treated mice into naïve syngeneic mice renders the recipients resistant to sensitization (adoptive transfer; Fig. 1b). Again suppression after adoptive transfer is antigen-specific since all other immune responses against unrelated haptens are not affected in the recipient mice [3]. Utilizing adoptive transfer experiments it was shown that UV-induced Treg belong to the $CD4^{+}CD25^{+}$ subtype and express Foxp3, CTLA-4, GITR and neuropilin [4–7]. Upon antigen-specific stimulation UV-induced Treg release interleukin-10 which is crucially involved in UV-induced immunosuppression [5, 8].

Phototherapy is utilized for various inflammatory dermatoses which equally well respond to immunosuppressive drugs [9]. Hence, one relevant mode of action of phototherapy may be immunosuppression. In contrast to immunosuppressive drugs, phototherapy is not associated with the typical long term side effects including superinfections. This might be due to the antigen-specificity caused by Treg. Hence studies are ongoing to further characterize UV-induced Treg phenotypically and functionally with the ultimate aim to utilize these cells in a therapeutic setting but not only for dermatoses but also for other inflammatory and (auto)immune diseases.

2 Materials

2.1 UV-Irradiation of Mice

1. Adult female mice (6–7 weeks old) that have been bred and housed under specific and pathogen-free conditions (*see* **Note 1**).
2. Shaving device (e.g., Oster A-2).
3. UV-source (e.g., TL12 fluorescent lamps, Philips, Eindhoven, The Netherlands).
4. Stopwatch.

2.2 Induction of Contact Hypersensitivity

1. Adult female mice (6–7 weeks old) that have been bred and housed under specific and pathogen-free conditions.
2. 1% (w/v) 2,4,6-trinitrochlorobenzene (TNCB) in 4:1 acetone–olive oil (*see* **Note 2**).
3. 0.5% (w/v) TNCB in 4:1 acetone–olive oil (*see* **Note 2**).
4. Spring loaded micrometer.

2.3 Isolation of Lymphocytes and Splenocytes

1. 70% (v/v) ethanol.
2. Sterile surgical instruments including forceps and pairs of scissors (*see* **Note 3**).
3. Dissecting board and needles.
4. RPMI complete medium: RPMI 1640 supplemented with 10% FCS, 2 mM l-glutamine and 100 U/ml Penicillin/Streptomycin.
5. Tubes of appropriate size for lymph nodes and spleen.
6. Metal cell strainers (mesh size 100 μm).
7. 60 mm Petri dishes.
8. 5 ml syringes.
9. Disposable nylon cell strainers (mesh size 70 μm).
10. Erythrocyte lysing buffer: 150 mM NH_4Cl, 10 mM $KHCO_3$, 1 mM NaEDTA, pH 7.5 (*see* **Note 4**).
11. Hemocytometer.

2.3.1 Separation of CD4⁺CD25⁻ and CD4⁺CD25⁺ T Cells from Lymphocytes and Splenocytes

1. Magnetic cell sorter (e.g., autoMACS® Pro Separator, Miltenyi Biotec, or equivalent) including required equipment as columns and buffers for the separation procedure.
2. $CD4^+CD25^+$ Regulatory T Cell Isolation Kit, mouse (Miltenyi Biotec, or equivalent).
3. MACS running buffer: DPBS supplemented with 2 mM EDTA and 0.5 % (w/v) BSA.
4. Allophycocyanin (APC)-conjugated CD4 antibody for flow cytometry.
5. APC-conjugated Ig antibody for flow cytometry.
6. Phycoerythrin (PE)-conjugated Ig antibody for flow cytometry.
7. Sterile FACS staining buffer: DPBS supplemented with 1 % (w/v) BSA.
8. Sterile FACS blocking buffer: DPBS supplemented with 3 % (w/v) BSA.
9. Flow cytometer and appropriate analysis software.

2.4 Adoptive Transfer of Immune Response

1. 70 % (v/v) ethanol.
2. 0.9 % sodium chloride injection solution.
3. 1 ml syringes and needles (30G × ½ inch).
4. Red heat lamp.
5. Mouse restrainer usable for tail vein injection.
6. Adult female mice (6–7 weeks old) that have been bred and housed under specific and pathogen-free conditions as recipients.

3 Methods

3.1 UV-Induced Suppression of the Induction of CHS in Mice

The contact hypersensitivity (CHS) reaction is a common in vivo assay to study cell-mediated host immune responses to contact allergens. The vast majority of contact allergens used in this model are chemically reactive substances of low molecular weight which have to bind to proteins of the host to exert their antigenic properties. Thus, these substances are also called haptens. Topical application of haptens onto razor-shaved skin of mice results in sensitization in almost all animals treated (Fig. 1a). In contrast, if the hapten is painted on skin that was immediately before exposed to rather low doses of UVB radiation, CHS is not induced (Fig. 1b).

1. On the first day of UV-treatment a large area of the back of the animals is shaved thoroughly (*see* **Note 5**).
2. The shaved backs are exposed to UV radiation (*see* **Note 6**) delivered from a bank of four TL12 fluorescent lamps (Philips,

Eindhoven, The Netherlands), which emit most of their energy within the UVB range (290–320 nm) with an emission peak at 313 nm. Mice (*see* **Note 7**) are exposed to UV daily for 4 consecutive days (1000 J/m^2/exposure).

3. *Sensitization phase:* 24 h after the last UV exposure mice are sensitized by the epicutaneous application of 50 μl of 1% TNCB solution to the surface of the irradiated area.
4. *Elicitation phase:* 5 days after sensitization each side of the left ear is treated with 10 μl of 0.5% TNCB solution (20 μl total). The vehicle acetone–olive oil is applied to the right ear. Naïve mice that were not exposed to the sensitizing dose of TNCB (**step 3**) serve as negative controls to exclude nonspecific ear swelling induced by the irritating effects of the chemical.
5. After 24 h ear thickness is measured with a spring-loaded micrometer (*see* **Note 8**). CHS response is determined as the amount of swelling of the hapten-challenged ear compared with the thickness of the vehicle-treated ear in sensitized animals and is expressed as centimeters $\times 10^{-3}$ (mean ± SD).

3.2 Adoptive Transfer of Immune Response

UV-induced tolerance can be adoptively transferred into naïve recipients via injection of T cells. As described in several publications [10–12] lymphocytes and splenocytes obtained from UV- and hapten-treated mice are sufficient to suppress immune responses in recipient mice upon adoptive transfer (Fig. 1c). Isolation and injection of enriched $CD4^+CD25^+$ Treg from bulk cells will increase the suppressive efficacy in recipients (*see* **Note 9**).

3.2.1 Dissection of the Spleen and Lymph Nodes and Preparation of a Single-Cell Suspension

1. Mice are killed by cervical dislocation and placed with the left side up on a dissecting board.
2. Wet fur with 70% ethanol and cut away about 1 cm^2 of the skin, about half-way between the front and back legs (*see* **Note 10**). The spleen should now be visible under the peritoneum. The spleen is dissected and placed into RPMI complete medium.
3. The mouse is now extended on the back, with the limbs spread and fixed with needles in the four paws. Using forceps and a pair of scissors, the skin is cut along the ventral midline from the groin to the chin, being careful to only cut the skin and not the peritoneal wall. Four further incisions are made from the start of the first incision downward to the knees and elbows on both sides. Pull the skin back on the sides and fix the skin with needles.
4. The inguinal, the axillary and the brachial lymph nodes are dissected and placed into RPMI complete medium.
5. Spleens and lymph nodes can be pooled (*see* **Note 11**).
6. Spleens and lymph nodes are put into a sterile metal cell-strainer, the remaining medium is discarded. The strainer containing organs is placed into a 60 mm Petri dish and 4 ml of fresh RPMI complete medium are added.

7. Using the barrel of a 5 ml syringe, spleens and lymph nodes are pressed through the strainer until only fibrous tissue remains in the strainer. The strainer is washed with fresh RPMI complete medium.
8. The cells are resuspended using a serological pipette and sieved through a 70 μm nylon mesh cell strainer into a 50 ml conical tube. Cells are centrifuged at 300 × *g* for 5 min at 4 ° C and resuspended thoroughly in 0.5–3 ml erythrocytes lysis buffer (*see* **Note 12**) and incubated on ice for not more than 90 s (*see* **Note 13**).
9. The reaction is stopped by adding at least twice the volume of RPMI complete medium. To get rid of precipitates that may form after adding the medium, the cell suspension is sieved through a 70 μm nylon mesh cell strainer into a new 50 ml conical tube. Cells are washed with fresh medium and centrifuged at 300 × *g* for 5 min at 4 °C and resuspended in 10–20 ml RPMI complete medium, depending on cell density.
10. Using a hemocytometer cells are counted and the absolute cell number is calculated.

For adoptive transfer experiments we usually inject 5×10^7 lymphocytes in 200 μl of a 0.9 % sodium chloride injection solution per mouse. This amount is sufficient to suppress immune responses in recipient mice, but it can be scaled up to 1×10^8 lymphocytes. Alternatively pure Treg can be isolated as described in the following section.

For adoptive transfer of bulk lymphocytes directly proceed to Subheading 3.2.3.

3.2.2 Isolation of $CD4^+CD25^+$ Treg from a Single-Cell Suspension

The methodology described here is for using the Miltenyi MACS isolation and autoMACS Pro Separator usage. One could also use other magnetic separation techniques. Volumes for magnetic labeling given below are for an initial starting cell number of up to 10^7 lymphocytes. For larger initial cell numbers, scale up volumes accordingly.

1. The lymphocytes from Subheading 3.2.1 are counted and centrifuged at 300 × *g* for 10 min. The supernatant is aspirated completely and the cells are resuspended in 40 μl MACS Running Buffer.
2. 10 μl of Biotin-Antibody Cocktail (*see* **Note 14**) are added and the mixture is incubated for 10 min at 4–8 °C.
3. 30 μl MACS Running Buffer, 20 μl of Anti-Biotin MicroBeads, and 10 μl of CD25-PE antibody are added to the cells, mixed well and refrigerated for additional 15 min in the dark at 4–8 °C.
4. Cells are washed by adding 1–2 ml of MACS Running Buffer per 10^7 total cells and centrifuged at 300 × *g* for 10 min. The supernatant is removed completely and the cells are

resuspended in 500 μl MACS Running Buffer for up to 10^8 cells. For larger cell numbers the appropriate amounts of buffer have to be used.

5. After preparing and priming the autoMACS Pro Separator, the magnetically labeled cells are fractionated using the separation program "Depl025". During this procedure $CD4^+$ T cells are enriched by depletion of unwanted cells. Both fractions are collected and the CD4 positive cells are counted. CD4 negative cells are discarded (*see* **Note 15**).
6. $CD4^+$ T cells are centrifuged at 300 × *g* for 10 min and resuspended in 90 μl of MACS Running Buffer per 10^7 initially used lymphocytes.
7. 10 μl of Anti-PE MicroBeads are added to cells, mixed and the suspension is refrigerated for 15 min in the dark at 4–8 °C.
8. Cells are washed by adding 1–2 ml of MACS Running Buffer per 10^7 total cells and centrifuged at 300 × *g* for 10 min. The supernatant is removed completely and the cells are resuspended in 500 μl MACS Running Buffer for up to 10^8 cells. For larger cell numbers the appropriate amounts of buffer have to be used.
9. The magnetically labeled $CD4^+$ T cells are applied to the autoMACS Pro Separator and fractionated using the separation program "Possld2". Both fractions are collected: The negative fraction contains $CD4^+CD25^-$ T cells and the positive fraction is the enriched $CD4^+CD25^+$ Treg fraction.

For adoptive transfer experiments, we usually inject 5×10^5 enriched Treg in 200 μl of a 0.9% sodium chloride solution per mouse into the tail veins.

Flow Cytometry Analysis of Fractionated $CD4^+$ T-Cells

The enrichment of Treg is proved by double staining of CD4 and CD25 followed by FACS analysis. As T cells are already labeled with a CD25-PE antibody during the MACS isolation procedure (Subheading 3.2.2, **step 3**), cells have to be stained only with a fluorochrome conjugated anti-CD4 antibody.

1. About 2–5 × 10^5 cells in 100 μl of $CD4^+CD25^-$ and $CD4^+CD25^+$ T cells are prepared in a 96-well U-bottom microplate. One well of T cells for IgG control should be also included. Preparation of two wells with $CD4^+CD25^-$ Treg for single staining is recommended for proper compensation of the FACS device.
2. Cells are centrifuged at 300 × *g* for 5 min, resuspended in 100 μl FACS blocking buffer and incubated for 30 min at 4–8 °C.
3. Cells are centrifuged at 300 × *g* for 5 min and resuspended in 100 μl FACS staining buffer.
4. An appropriate amount of an APC-conjugated CD4 antibody or IgG antibody is added to the respective wells and cells are incubated for 60 min at 4–8 °C.

5. Cells are centrifuged at 300 × *g* for 5 min, washed once with FACS staining buffer, resuspended in 400 μl FACS staining buffer and subjected to FACS analysis (Fig. 2).

3.2.3 Intravenous Injection of Isolated Cells into Naïve Mice

For adoptive transfer experiments we usually inject 5×10^7 lymphocytes or 5×10^5 enriched Treg in 200 μl of a 0.9 % sodium chloride injection solution per mouse.

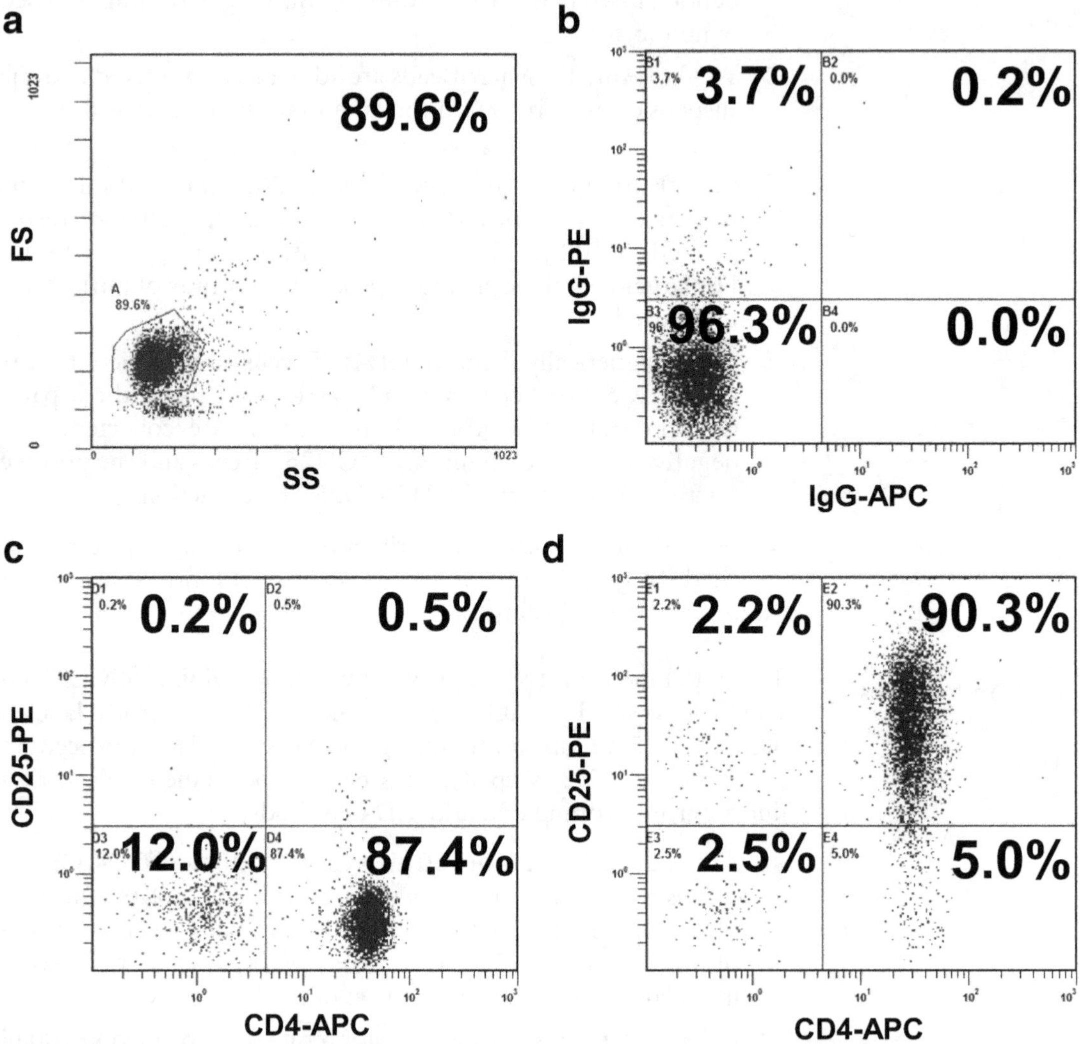

Fig. 2 Separation of CD4⁺CD25⁻ and CD4⁺CD25⁺ T cells from lymphocytes. Lymphocytes from UV-radiated donors were isolated, separated in CD4⁺CD25⁻ and CD4⁺CD25⁺ T cells by magnetobead separation, stained with CD4 and CD25 antibodies, and subjected to FACS analysis. (**a**) Gating strategy to identify lymphocytes. (**b**) CD4⁺CD25⁺ Treg stained with PE and APC-conjugated IgG antibodies. (**c**) CD4⁺CD25⁻ T cells stained with CD4-APC and CD25-PE antibodies. (**d**) CD4⁺CD25⁺ Treg stained with CD4-APC and CD25-PE antibodies

1. Cells are adjusted to the desired concentrations with 0.9% sodium chloride and taken up by a syringe. Air bubbles are completely removed.
2. Using a red heat lamp, the tail of the mouse is warmed up in order to dilate the veins (*see* **Note 16**).
3. The mouse is placed into a restraining device. The tail is grasped and gentle pressure is applied in order to stabilize the tail and raise the veins. The lateral veins are located superficially and can be visualized by slight rotation of the tail.
4. Alcohol is applied to the injection site. By maintaining the needle and the syringe parallel to the tail, the vein is punctured and the cells are injected by gentle pressure.
5. Once the cells are injected, the needle is removed and pressure applied with a clean gauze to the injection site to stop bleeding.
6. Continue with **step 3**, Subheading 3.1 for sensitization and challenging.

4 Notes

1. We prefer using female mice. But the model also works fine with male mice. An age of at least 6 weeks ensures a fully developed immune system [13].
2. Be careful when working with TNCB! Always wear safety glasses and gloves. As a potent sensitizer it is an irritant to eyes, skin, digestive tract, and respiratory tract and very toxic by inhalation, ingestion, and skin contact. There is also a potential fire and explosion hazard.
3. Use two sets of surgical instruments consisting of two forceps and one pair of scissors: one for making the incisions through the skin and a different one for the section of the inner part and dissection of the organs of the mouse. This lowers the risk of contamination.
4. Erythrocyte lysis buffer can be prepared as a 10× solution and stored in 1 ml aliquots at −20 ° C. Once thawed and diluted, the 1× solution is stored at 4 °C and used within 4 weeks.
5. Ensure no mice get hurt by shaving the back. Do not irradiate or sensitize mice with injured skin! You can also shave the mice one day prior to irradiation or sensitization. Potential irritations from shaving might disappear in the meantime.
6. Prior to radiation, the intensity (mW/cm^2) of the UV output has to be measured in a constant distance (we use 30 cm) using a UV-Meter. Based on this measurement, the time of UV exposure is calculated so that the UV dose of 1000 J/m^2/exposure

will be delivered to the mice placed in the same distance. You can use a mouse cage base placed in this distance from the fluorescent lamp to ensure delivery of the correct UV dose.

7. Up to three mice can be irradiated at the same time. It is not necessary to protect their eyes.
8. For experienced persons it is possible to measure ear thickness without anesthesia of the mice. The mouse has to be properly restrained with pressure behind the neck and immobilized on a tabletop. We prefer using an isofluran vaporizer for very short procedures like ear challenge and ear swelling measurements. The use of isofluran inhalant anesthesia for rodent procedures is recommended, due to its wide safety margin, reliability, ease of administration, and rapid return to consciousness for animals after end of exposure.
9. The $CD4^{+}CD25^{-}$ fraction can also be used in further experiments. The cells can be stimulated with various substances or molecules in vitro and injected in mice to test the suppressive capacity of in vitro stimulated $CD4^{+}CD25^{-}$ T cells in different models. We have shown this for example for the antimicrobial peptide mBD14 [14].
10. Do not cut away too much of the skin as it would impede or even preclude the subsequent dissection of the inguinal lymph node.
11. Spleens and lymph nodes from up to six mice can be pooled and processed at the same time.
12. The amount of lysis buffer used depends on the pellet size. You can approximately calculate 0.5 ml lysis buffer per mouse.
13. The erythrocyte lysis step can be skipped when the suspension is subjected to magnetic separation as in the first separation step the erythocytes will be depleted.
14. Non-$CD4^{+}$ cells are indirectly magnetically labeled with a cocktail of biotin-conjugated antibodies. The cocktail contains antibodies against CD8a, CD11b, CD45R, CD49b, and Ter-119.
15. $CD4^{+}$ T cells are pre-enriched by depletion of unwanted cells. The antibody cocktail described in **Note 14** labels all cells excluding CD4 positive cells. Keep in mind that when using the MACS program "Depl025" the so-called "positive fraction" contains the labeled, CD4 negative cells. The CD4 positive cells are unlabeled and thus collected in the so-called "negative fraction."
16. Warm up the tail for about 30–60 s using the red heat lamp. By holding mouse tail in front of the red heat lamp you prevent the mouse from over warming as your fingers also became warm.

References

1. Schwarz T (2010) The dark and the sunny sides of UVR-induced immunosuppression: photoimmunology revisited. J Invest Dermatol 130:49–54
2. Toews GB, Bergstresser PR, Streilein JW (1980) Epidermal Langerhans cell density determines whether contact hypersensitivity or unresponsiveness follows skin painting with DNFB. J Immunol 124:445–453
3. Elmets CA, Bergstresser PR, Tigelaar RE, Wood PJ, Streilein JW (1983) Analysis of the mechanism of unresponsiveness produced by haptens painted on skin exposed to low dose ultraviolet radiation. J Exp Med 158:781–794
4. Bruder D, Probst-Kepper M, Westendorf AM, Geffers R, Beissert S, Loser K et al (2004) Neuropilin-1: a surface marker of regulatory T cells. Eur J Immunol 34:623–630
5. Schwarz A, Beissert S, Grosse-Heitmeyer K, Gunzer M, Bluestone JA, Grabbe S et al (2000) Evidence for functional relevance of CTLA-4 in ultraviolet-radiation-induced tolerance. J Immunol 165:1824–1831
6. Schwarz A, Navid F, Sparwasser T, Clausen BE, Schwarz T (2011) In vivo reprogramming of UV radiation-induced regulatory T-cell migration to inhibit the elicitation of contact hypersensitivity. J Allergy Clin Immunol 128:826–833
7. Shimizu J, Yamazaki S, Takahashi T, Ishida Y, Sakaguchi S (2002) Stimulation of CD25(+) CD4(+) regulatory T cells through GITR breaks immunological self-tolerance. Nat Immunol 3:135–142
8. Shreedhar V, Giese T, Sung VW, Ullrich SE (1998) A cytokine cascade including prostaglandin E2, IL-4, and IL-10 is responsible for UV-induced systemic immune suppression. J Immunol 160:3783–3789
9. Weichenthal M, Schwarz T (2005) Phototherapy: how does UV work? Photodermatol Photoimmunol Photomed 21:260–266
10. Bruhs A, Haarmann-Stemmann T, Frauenstein K, Krutmann J, Schwarz T, Schwarz A (2014) Activation of the arylhydrocarbon receptor causes immunosuppression primarily by modulating dendritic cells. J Invest Dermatol 135(2):435–444
11. Navid F, Boniotto M, Walker C, Ahrens K, Proksch E, Sparwasser T et al (2012) Induction of regulatory T cells by a murine beta-defensin. J Immunol 188:735–743
12. Schwarz A, Navid F, Sparwasser T, Clausen BE, Schwarz T (2012) 1,25-dihydroxyvitamin D exerts similar immunosuppressive effects as UVR but is dispensable for local UVR-induced immunosuppression. J Invest Dermatol 132:2762–2769
13. Holsapple MP, West LJ, Landreth KS (2003) Species comparison of anatomical and functional immune system development. Birth Defects Res B Dev Reprod Toxicol 68:321–334
14. Bruhs A, Schwarz T, Schwarz A (2015) Prevention and mitigation of experimental autoimmune encephalomyelitis by murine beta-defensins via induction of regulatory T cells. J Invest Dermatol 136:173–181. doi:10.1038/jid.2015.405

Chapter 6

Surgical Denervation in the Imiquimod-Induced Psoriasiform Mouse Model

Armanda J. Onderdijk, Ineke M. Hekking-Weijma, Edwin F. Florencia, and Errol P. Prens

Abstract

Psoriasis is a chronic inflammatory skin disease with a prevalence of 2–3%. It appears to result from a combination of genetic and environmental factors, but the precise pathogenesis is still unknown. Neurogenic inflammation is involved in psoriasis pathogenesis as well, but the role of neurogenic factors is currently unclear. Molecular studies often involve material obtained from patients. However, many questions and especially experimental manipulations are not suited for study in humans. Imiquimod application on mouse skin leads to immune cell infiltration, inflammation with intense redness, epidermal thickening, and scaling that jointly greatly resembles human psoriasis. Here we describe the use of surgical denervation in the imiquimod-induced psoriasiform model, to study the role of skin innervation and neuropeptides in the pathogenesis of psoriasis.

Key words Imiquimod, Psoriasis, Mouse model, Denervation, Nerves, Neuropeptides, (γδ) T cells, IL-17, IL-23, TLR7

1 Introduction

Psoriasis affect millions of people worldwide, yet the precise pathogenesis is still unknown [1]. The most common form (approximately 90%) is plaque type psoriasis also called psoriasis vulgaris. This common disease is characterized by hyperproliferation of keratinocytes and immune cell infiltration including T cells, dendritic cells and neutrophils in the dermis and epidermis. Clinically patients suffer from red, indurated, scaly lesions that can cover the whole body. In the current view on psoriasis, genetically predisposed keratinocytes are triggered by environmental factors such as mechanical trauma or certain drugs. This results in the production of antimicrobial peptides including HBD2 (beta-defensin) and LL-37 (cathelicidin). LL-37 can form complexes with self DNA and RNA, which subsequently activate plasmacytoid dendritic cells that produce IFN-α, IL-1, IL-12, and IL-23. These cytokines lead to the activation of innate lymphoid cells and (γδ) T cells and cause the differentiation of Th1 and Th17

Björn E. Clausen and Jon D. Laman (eds.), *Inflammation: Methods and Protocols*, Methods in Molecular Biology, vol. 1559, DOI 10.1007/978-1-4939-6786-5_6, © Springer Science+Business Media LLC 2017

cells and LL-37 specific effector T cells that migrate to the skin. These T cells and their cytokines lead to a vicious cycle of inflammation that cannot be hampered by the regulatory system [2]. Several observations point to a role for nerves and neuropeptides in psoriasis, including: clearance of psoriatic lesions after inadvertent denervation, symmetry of psoriasis lesions, exacerbation of disease by psychological stress, and an increase in nerves and neuropeptides in lesional psoriatic skin [3]. Molecular studies often involve material obtained from patients. However, many questions and especially experimental manipulations are not suited for study in humans. Animal studies are required to further define the role of neurogenic inflammation in this complex disease. Imiquimod is a TLR7 agonist that signals via the receptor on macrophages, dermal dendritic cells (DC) and plasmacytoid DC via MyD-88 dependent signaling pathways [4]. Signaling via this route activates a.o. the transcription factor Nf-κB. In humans imiquimod is used for the treatment of genital warts, actinic keratosis and superficial basal cell carcinoma. In patients treated with imiquimod, psoriatic skin lesions can be induced and preexisting psoriasis can be exacerbated [5–10]. These clinical findings led us to develop the imiquimod-induced psoriasiform mouse model [11] which is now used worldwide [12]. Repeated imiquimod application on mouse skin leads to immune cell infiltration, inflammation with intense redness, epidermal thickening, and scaling that jointly greatly resembles human psoriasis. The imiquimod-mouse model is dependent on the IL-17/IL-23 axis and largely resembles the initation phase of human psoriatic lesions [11]. The cutaneous gene expression profiles associated with the imiquimod-induced psoriasiform phenotype exhibited statistically significant similarity to the expression profile of psoriasis in humans [13]. A great advantage of this model that it is very quick and robust, in which clinical psoriasis lesions can be obtained by the consecutive application of Aldara™ for 5 days or more on the shaved back of mice. The model is especially suitable for studying the acute phase of psoriasis and greatly facilitates research on the mechanism of action that drives psoriasis inflammation. Many groups have studied components of the skin inflammation in psoriasis by using this model [14–17]. We have used the model to better understand the involvement of nerves and neuropeptides in psoriasis (unpublished data). In this chapter we describe in detail the use of the imiquimod-induced psoriasiform mouse model and the method of surgical denervation.

2 Materials

2.1 Surgical Denervation in the Imiquimod-Induced Psoriasiform Mouse Model

1. Anesthesia: isoflurane: 2% in O_2 1 L/min.
2. Shaving device: use a special small animal clipper to avoid damage to the skin.
3. Surgical microscope: magnification range 2 to 12×.

4. Surgical instruments: needle holder, scissors, forceps, microsurgical scissors, microsurgical forceps.
5. Suture material: vicryl 6/0, FS-3 needle.

2.2 Imiquimod Induced Psoriasiform Skin Inflam mation

1. Imiquimod 5% cream (Aldara™, Meda Pharma). Additives: isostearic acid, benzyl alcohol, cetyl alcohol, stearyl alcohol, white soft paraffin, polysorbate 60, sorbitan stearate, glycerol, methyl hydroxybenzoate, propyl hydroxybenzoate, xanthan gum, purified water.
2. Control vehicle cream: Aldara base cream without imiquimod when available, or a comparable compounded neutral cream.
3. Female C57BL/6 mice 6–11 weeks of age, weight matched, approximately 23 g. Housing under standard animal facility conditions: controlled temperature, humidity, food and water ad lib. In principle, any wild type or transgenic mouse can be used.
4. Balance to assess animal weight.
5. Protective gloves.
6. Murine Psoriasis Area and Severity Index (PASI) score table.
7. Absolute digimatic micrometer.

3 Methods

3.1 Surgical Denervation in the Imiquimod-Induced Psoriasiform Mouse Model

1. Carry out the surgery under clean but not necessarily sterile circumstances, using surgical gloves and thoroughly cleaned instruments.
2. Bring the animal under deep anesthesia using isoflurane 2% in O_2 1 L/min (*see* **Note 1**).
3. Shave the back of the animal and both flanks thoroughly (*see* **Note 2**).
4. *Denervation operation procedure* (*see* **Note 3**): adjust the microscope, use 4× magnification to open the skin and fascia. Make a 2 cm longitudinal incision along the midline of the back starting at lumbar 2 over the thoracic curvature up to thoracic 10. Divide the underlying fascia carefully over almost the complete length of the skin incision. Only the nerves of the right side of the dorsal skin are transected (Fig. 1). Separate the fascia of the right lateral side from the underlying muscles by blunt dissection and retract the fascia along with the skin (*see* **Note 4**). Adjust the microscope to a 6 to 8× magnification. Identify the 12th rib and find the 12th thoracic nerve parallel to the rib. Expose and mobilize the branch for a distance of about 5–8 mm distal from the intervertebral foramen. Locate six more nerve branches distal from the 12th thoracic nerve, expose and mobilize them in the same way. When all seven branches are located

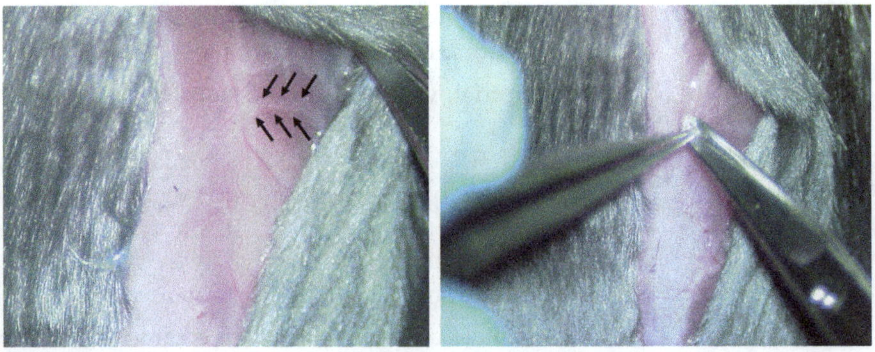

Fig. 1 Surgical denervation procedure. Microscopic image before transection of the nerves. *Arrows* point to nerve branches

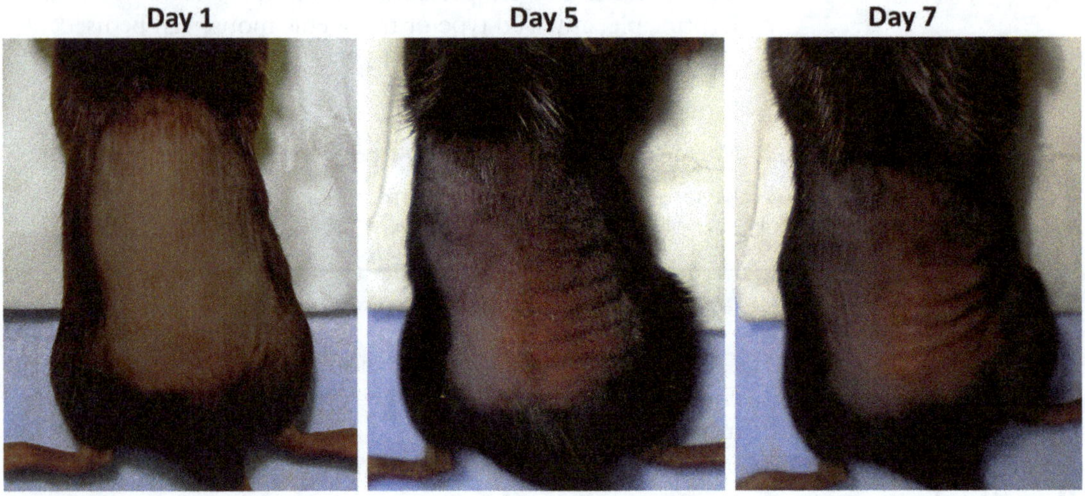

Fig. 2 Imiquimod-induced psoriasiform skin inflammation. Clinical result of daily topical application of 62.5 mg of commercially available Aldara™ cream on the shaved right back area (before application (baseline), day 5 and day 7)

and exposed, cut the branches one by one as close to the skin as possible starting at the thoracic side (*see* **Note 5**). Bring the skin carefully back into its original position. Close the skin with 5–6 interrupted stitches using 6/0 vicryl on a FS-3 needle (Ethicon). *Sham operation procedure*: operate the mice in exactly the same way without cutting the nerves after exposure and mobilization of the nerve branches (*see* **Note 6**).

3.2 Induction of Psoriasiform Dermatitis by Imiquimod Treatment

1. The day previous to the induction of psoriasiform dermatitis (*see* **Note 2**), the back side area of the animals (*see* **Note 7**) is cautiously shaved clearing the area for imiquimod treatment and concurrently preventing lesions and possible cutaneous irritation (Fig. 2). The baseline weight is determined using a balance.

2. The animals are weighed daily (*see* **Note 8**) and receive a daily topical administration of 62.5 mg of commercially available Aldara™ cream on their shaved right back and when applicable on the right ear for the experimentally defined consecutive days (typically 6–8) (*see* **Note 9**). The mice of the control group receive a daily topical administration of control cream (*see* **Note 10**). The untreated left back area is the internal experimental control. The application of Aldara™ represents a daily dose of 3.125 mg of imiquimod.
3. Assessment of local modified PASI of psoriasiform skin inflammation: from the onset of the experiment, the PASI score assessment is used to monitor the progress of the psoriatic inflammation in the animals (Fig. 2). The PASI-score erythema (redness, Fig. 3a) and desquamation (scaling, Fig. 3b) are clinically determined using the scoring table. The induration (thickness) is further determined by micrometer measurements.
4. The cutaneous induration is measured by lifting up the skin and spanning the fixed targeted area with gloves covered index fingers and thumbs. Duplo measurements of the induration are acquired at the mid-section of the spanned skin using an absolute digimatic micrometer.

4 Notes

1. During the surgical procedure it is important to prevent dehydration of the eyes of the mice by application of ointment to the eyes.
2. Shave the skin of the mice carefully to avoid damage to the skin. The reaction of the skin upon shaving can interfere with the results of the experiment, therefore the application of imiquimod starts after1 day.
3. In addition to biomedical training and IACUC-permission, one needs basic anatomical knowledge and basic surgical skills to perform this procedure (making an incision, transecting the nerves and closing the skin with stitches).
4. Handle the skin with great care. Underlying nerves can easily be damaged.
5. Be sure the nerves are clearly visible before they are cut, this will avoid incomplete disconnection.
6. Per animal it takes 30 min initially for the total surgical denervation procedure (including shaving). When one is experienced the average time spent per animal will be 20 min. In principle all animals survive the procedure when performed carefully.

a **Back skin scoring for redness**

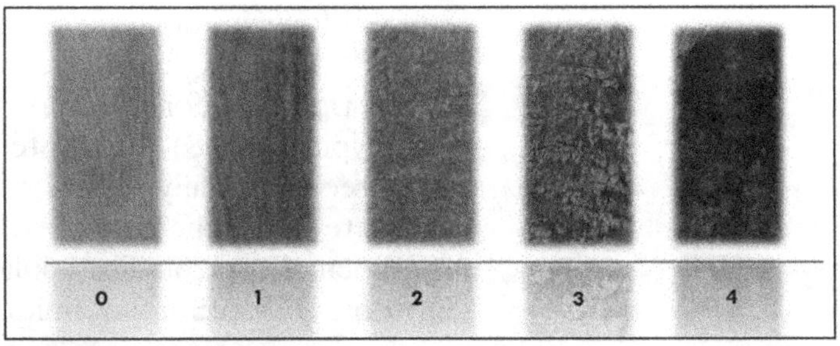

Redness	Score
None	0
Light red	1
Red not dark	2
Dark red	3
Extremely red	4

b **Back skin scoring for scaling**

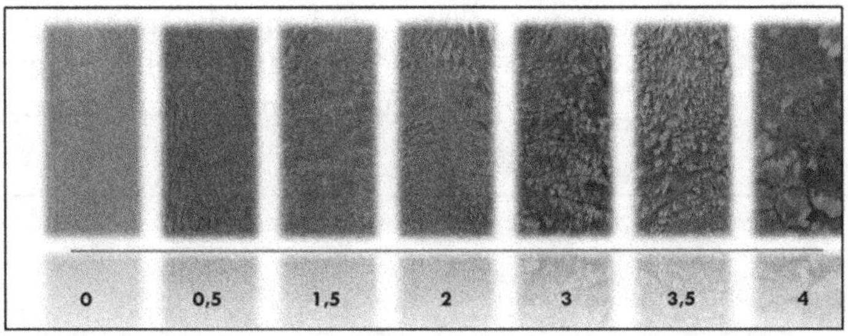

Scaling	Score
None	0
Thin scales, limited surface area	1
Thicker (mild) scales, modest surface area	2
Thick scales, rough, larger surface area	3
Very robust scales, vast surface area	4

Fig. 3 Modified Psoriasis Area and Severity Index (PASI). Clinical scoring based on a modified Psoriasis Area and Severity (PASI) to score psoriasiform skin inflammation in mice; redness (erythema) score (**a**) and scaling score (**b**)

7. Psoriasiform skin inflammation can be induced by imiquimod in every inbred mouse strain. The scoring of redness in white vs. brown/black mice is essentially equal, but in Balb/C mice the skin inflammation is easier assessable compared to C57Bl/6 mice, because of the skin pigmentation. However, due to availability of the various transgenic and knockout mice, we generally use the C57Bl/6 strains in experiments. In addition, because of a more pronounced skin inflammation, we routinely use females.

8. If the weight loss of the mice is more than 15 % from baseline, 300 μL of phosphate buffered saline (PBS) has to be injected intraperitoneally. Usually a single injection suffices. This weight loss occurs more frequently in C57Bl/6 mice, probably because their response to imiquimod is more Th1-driven, whereby more IL-1 and IL-6 is produced, leading to a fever response and dehydration.
9. Ten days after denervation nerves regenerate into the murine back skin, this limitates the time frame that can be studied.
10. Note that the additives in vehicle cream may induce alterations that are TLR-7 independent including activation of the NRLP1 inflammasome by isostearic acid [18].

References

1. Nestle FO, Kaplan DH, Barker J (2009) Psoriasis. N Engl J Med 361:496–509
2. Perera GK, Di Meglio P, Nestle FO (2012) Psoriasis. Annu Rev Pathol 7:385–422
3. Saraceno R, Kleyn CE, Terenghi G et al (2006) The role of neuropeptides in psioriasis. Br J Dermatol 155(5):876–882
4. Hemmi H, Kaisho T, Takeuchi O et al (2002) Small anti-viral compounds activate immune cells via the TLR7 MyD88-dependent signaling pathway. Nat Immunol 3(2):196–200
5. Smith WA, Siegel D, Lyon VB et al (2013) Psoriasiform eruption and oral ulcerations as adverse effects of topical 5% imiquimod treatment in children: a report of four cases. Pediatr Dermatol 30(6):e157–e160
6. Patel U, Mark NM, Machler BC et al (2011) Imiquimod 5% cream induced psoriasis: a case report, summary of the literature and mechanism. Br J Dermatol 164(3):670–672
7. Fanti PA, Dika E, Vaccari S et al (2006) Generalized psoriasis induced by topical treatment of actinic keratosis with imiquimod. Int J Dermatol 45:1464–1465
8. Rajan N, Langtry JA (2006) Generalized exacerbation of psoriasis associated with imiquimod cream treatment of superficial basal cell carcinoma's. Clin Exp Dermatol 31:140–141
9. Gilliet M, Conrad C, Geiges M et al (2004) Psoriasis triggered by toll-like receptor 7 agonist imiquimod in the presence of dermal plasmacytoid dendritic cell precursors. Arch Dermatol 140(12):1490–1495
10. Wu JK, Siller G, Strutton G (2004) Psoriasis induced by topical imiquimod. Australas J Dermatol 45:47–50
11. van der Fits L, Mourits S, Voerman JSA et al (2009) Imiquimod-induced psoriasis-like skin inflammation in mice is mediated via the IL-23/IL-17 axis. J Immunol 182:5836–5845
12. Flutter B, Nestle FO (2013) TLRs to cytokines: mechanistic insights from the imiquimod mouse model of psoriasis. Eur J Immunol 43:3138–3146
13. Swindell WR, Johnston A, Carbajal S et al (2011) Genome-wide expression profiling of five mouse models identifies similarities and differences with human psoriasis. PLoS One 6:e18266
14. Yoshiki R, Kabashima K, Honda T et al (2014) IL-23 from Langerhans cells is required for the development of imiquimod-induced psoriasis-like dermatitis by induction of IL-17A- producing gammadelta T cells. J Invest Dermatol 134:1912–1921
15. Wohn C, Ober-Blöbaum JL, Haak S et al (2013) Langerin(neg) conventional dendritic cells produce IL-23 to drive psoriatic plaque formation in mice. Proc Natl Acad Sci U S A 110(26):10723–10728. doi:10.1073/1307569110
16. Works MG, Yin F, Yin CC et al (2014) Inhibition of Tyk2 and JAK1 ameliorates imiquimod-induced psoriasis-like dermatitis by inhibiting IL-22 and the IL-23/IL-17 axis. J Immunol 193:3278–3287
17. Hoste E, Denecker G, Gilbert B et al (2013) Caspase-14-deficient mice are more prone to the development of parakeratosis. J Invest Dermatol 133:742–750
18. Walter A, Schäfer M, Cecconi V et al (2013) Aldara activates TLR-7 independent immune defense. Nat Commun 4:1560

Chapter 7

Xenotransplantation Model of Psoriasis

Jeremy Di Domizio, Curdin Conrad, and Michel Gilliet

Abstract

Psoriasis is a chronic autoimmune skin disease affecting approximately 2% of the population with a major psychosocial and socioeconomic impact. A causal therapy leading to permanent cure is not available, and current treatments only lead to limited amelioration, and therefore new therapeutic targets need to be identified. Recent works demonstrated a predominant role of T_H17 cells in the pathogenesis of psoriasis; yet the underlying molecular mechanisms driving the development of the disease are still largely elusive. Several mouse models of psoriasis including drug-induced models (topical application of imiquimod to the skin) and genetically engineered mice (constitutive activation of epidermal STAT3, epidermal deletion of JunB/c-Jun, and epidermal overexpression of Tie2) have been used to study the pathophysiology of the disease; however such models cannot fully recapitulate all molecular and cellular pathways occurring in human psoriasis. Xenotransplantation of human pre-psoriatic skin onto immunodeficient mice and triggering its conversion into a psoriatic plaque is the best model to dissect the mechanisms occurring during the development of human psoriasis. One model is based on the transplantation of human pre-psoriatic skin onto SCID mice followed by the transfer of activated autologous T cells. The ex vivo activation of T cells required to induce the psoriatic conversion of the graft limits the study of early events in the pathogenesis of psoriasis. Another model is based on transplantation of human pre-psoriatic skin onto AGR129 mice. In this model, the skin grafting is sufficient to activate human cells contained in the graft and trigger the conversion of the graft into a psoriatic skin, without the need of transferring activated T cells. Here we review the methodological aspects of this model and illustrate how this model can be used to dissect early events of psoriasis pathogenesis.

Key words Preclinical model, Psoriasis, Xenotransplant

1 Introduction

Psoriasis is a chronic-relapsing inflammatory skin disease characterized by the formation of erythematous scaly plaques due to aberrant hyperproliferation and altered differentiation of keratinocytes leading to epidermal hyperplasia. Psoriatic skin inflammation is also characterized by immune cell infiltrates among which T cells are the main components. The IL-23/IL-17 axis has now been extensively demonstrated to be required for the formation of psoriasis through the generation of T_H17 cells [1, 2]. T_H17 cells have been shown to drive autoimmune inflammation in predisposed individuals [1, 3].

Björn E. Clausen and Jon D. Laman (eds.), *Inflammation: Methods and Protocols*, Methods in Molecular Biology, vol. 1559, DOI 10.1007/978-1-4939-6786-5_7, © Springer Science+Business Media LLC 2017

They mainly produce IL-17A, IL-17F, IL-21, IL-22, and IL-26 [4–7]. IL-17A, and IL-17F can induce chemokine production by epithelial cells leading to innate immune cell infiltration [8]. IL-22 induces proliferation of epithelial cells and is involved in epidermal acanthosis [9, 10]. Furthermore, IL-22 and IL-17 both induce epithelial cell activation and production of antimicrobial peptides [9]. IL-21 does not have a direct inflammatory role but amplifies and stabilizes the development of T_H17 cells [11]. Although the role of T_H17 cells has been well defined in sustaining skin inflammation, early events driving the autoimmune T cell cascade and the development of psoriasis have remained unclear.

Mouse models offer an experimental system that allows investigation of these events. Several mouse models of psoriasis have been developed including the imiquimod-induced model (topical application of a TLR7 agonist to the skin), the K5-Stat3C model (expression of a constitutively active mutant STAT3 in basal keratinocytes), the K5-Tie2 model (overexpression of the endothelial specific tyrosine kinase in basal keratinocytes), the JunB/c-Jun model (keratinocyte-specific deletion of JunB and c-Jun in adult mice). Despite the many disparities between mice and human skin such as the denser distribution of hair follicles, thinner epidermis, and the presence of an underlying muscle layer in mouse skin, these mouse models recapitulate some aspects of human psoriasis including the epidermal hyperproliferation, thickening and altered differentiation of the epidermis, an inflammatory infiltrate that includes T cells, altered vascularization and responsiveness to current anti-psoriatic therapies. However, it is also clear that these models do not represent all aspects of human psoriasis, which has been nicely confirmed on the transcriptomics level [12].

Xenotransplantation models in which human uninvolved skin of a psoriasis patient is grafted onto immunodeficient mice and converted into a human psoriatic plaque appear to be the most reliable model of psoriasis development. One model is based on the transplantation of uninvolved (pre-psoriatic) skin of a psoriasis patient onto SCID mice, which are deficient in T- and B cells and therefore do not reject the human skin xenograft. In this model, the graft converts into a psoriatic plaque upon intradermal injection of autologous $CD4^+$ T cells activated by IL-2 and bacterial-derived superantigen (SEB/SEC2) [13]. The requirement of implanting ex vivo activated T cells limits the use of this model to investigate early innate events in the development of psoriasis, in particular the events preceeding T cell activation.

Another xenotransplantation model is the AGR129 mouse model of psoriasis. In addition to not having T and B cells, AGR129 mice also lack type I and type II IFN receptors, which reduces NK cell activity leading to improved acceptance of human skin grafts. In the AGR129 mouse model, the pre-psoriatic graft spontaneously converts into a fully fledged psoriatic lesion within 35 days [14, 15]. The conversion is triggered by the transplantation procedure itself (a Koebner phenomenon) and involves the activation of human immune cells present in the engrafted skin. The development of the psoriatic lesion is characterized by the expansion of skin-resident T cells that produce pro-inflammatory cytokines and accumulate in both the dermis and epidermis and precedes the hyperproliferation of keratinocytes [14, 16]. This expansion step relies on the proliferation of T resident memory cells as human T cell recirculation to the mouse lymphoid organs has not been observed [14, 16] and is in line with findings demonstrating that some antigen-experienced memory T cells remain permanently embedded within the tissues [17].

Several major advances in the understanding of psoriasis pathogenesis have been made using this model:

1. Plasmacytoid dendritic cells (pDC) infiltrating pre-psoriatic skin are activated to produce type I IFN leading to the subsequent activation of Th17 cells by conventional dendritic cells [15].
2. Conventional dendritic cells in psoriatic skin produce IL-23 and blocking IL-23 inhibits the Th17-mediated development of psoriasis [18].
3. T cells activated in the dermis migrate into the epidermis via VLA-1 to induce the epidermal psoriatic phenotype [16].
4. Intraepidermal CD8 T cells produce the majority of Th17 cytokines and trigger the development of the epidermal psoriatic phenotype [19].

In this chapter, we describe the establishment of the xenotransplantation model and how it can be used to dissect the initial events occurring during the development of psoriasis.

2 Materials

2.1 Harvesting Human Pre-psoriatic Skin

1. Chronic plaque-type psoriasis patient.
2. Surgical scissors.
3. Gauze compresses.

2.2 Engraftment of Pre-psoriatic Skin Onto Immunodeficient Mice

1. 7–8-week-old, sex- and weight-matched AGR129 mice (B6.129S2-Rag2tm1.1Cgn-Ifnar1tm1Agt-Ifngr1tm1Agt/J).
2. Inhalation narcosis device.
3. Shaving razor.
4. Hair removal cream.
5. Surgical scissors.

6. 3M™ Vetbond™ Tissue adhesive.
7. Non-adhesive, stretchable, air-permeable bandage.
8. Analgesics (Buprenorphin, Acetaminophen).
9. Antibiotics (Amoxicilline).

2.3 Histological Analysis of the Newly Developed Psoriatic Skin Lesion

1. Scissors and tweezers.
2. Histology molds.
3. Tissue freezing embedding medium (O.C.T.).
4. Cryostat.

2.4 Flow Cytometry Analysis of the Dermal Infiltrate

1. Enzyme cocktail (RPMI 1640 medium supplemented with 1% penicillin/streptomycin, 1 mg/ml Dispase, 1 mg/ml collagenase, and 0.1% DNase).
2. FACS buffer (PBS supplemented with 2% fetal calf serum and 2 mM EDTA).
3. Fluorescently labeled antibodies and DAPI.
4. Flow cytometer.

3 Methods

3.1 Harvesting Human Pre-psoriatic Skin

1. Around 4 cm wide keratome skin biopsies in the pre-lesional area (normal-appearing skin at a distance of around 1–2 cm from the lesion) are taken from the buttocks or upper thigh of patients with confirmed plaque-type psoriasis (*see* **Note 1**).
2. Skin samples are trimmed, kept in PBS-immersed gauze compresses to avoid dryness, and rapidly grafted onto mice (within 3 h).
3. Keratome skin samples are cut into smaller pieces (around 0.5×0.5 cm in size) for grafting onto mice.

3.2 Engraftment of Pre-psoriatic Skin Onto Immunodeficient Mice

1. AGR129 mice are anesthetized during the whole procedure (15 min) by inhalation narcosis with Isofluran (dosage 2.5% and induction at 5%).
2. Mice backs are shaved (electrical razor) and depilated (hair removal cream).
3. A piece of skin of around 6 mm is removed from the back of mice and a piece of human skin obtained from keratome biopsies will be adapted into the wound and sealed by 3M™ Vetbond™ Tissue adhesive.
4. A non-adhesive dressing and a strechable, air-permeable bandage is applied to guarantee optimal healing of the graft without substantially hindering the mice in mobility and food/water intake. A 2.5 cm wide bandage is wrapped around the belly and the back between the hind and forelegs and thus does

not perturbate the moving of mice (*see* **Note 2**). The dressing and the healing of the graft must be checked twice daily for 48 h, daily for the next 3 days, and every other day for up to 28 days. The dressing bandage can be removed 7 days after engraftment (*see* **Note 3**).

5. Analgesia is given to mice as subcutaneous injection of 0.1 mg/kg buprenorphin right after and 12 h after surgery (*see* **Notes 4** and **5**).

3.3 Blocking the Activity of Potentially Involved Factors

1. The development of a fully psoriatic lesion requires the sequential involvement of activated pDC in the dermis that produce type I IFN and expansion of T cells into the epidermis that produce IL-17 (Fig. 1).
2. To assess the role of a given cytokine or cell type in the development of psoriasis, 10 μg of isotype control or blocking antibodies targeting the desired candidate are injected subcutaneously, intraveneously, or intraperitoneally at day 1 (*see* **Note 6**). The solution is injected as 50 μl containing 10 μg of antibody, which corresponds to a 0.2 mg/ml solution.
3. The antibody solution is injected every third day until 35 days (or less according to the kind of antibody) to maintain the blockade during the development of the psoriatic lesion.

3.4 Histological Analysis of the Newly Developed Psoriatic Skin Lesion

1. To determine whether the human xenograft develops into a psoriatic skin, grafted skins are excised at day 35 and frozen in OCT-embedded molds in liquid nitrogen, and stored at −80 °C until use.
2. 6-μm skin sections are cut with a cryostat.

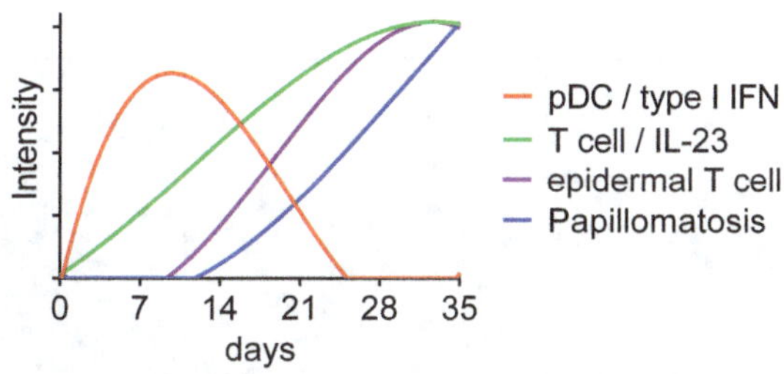

Fig. 1 Sequential events occurring during the development of psoriasis. Schematic representation of the different immunological events preceding the formation of psoriasis skin lesions. Within the first week following engraftment of nonpsoriatic skin onto AGR129 mice, pDC present in the dermis are activated to produce type I IFN (*red line*). This type I IFN production drives the induction of IL-23, the expansion of T cells, and their differentiation into T_H17 cells in the following weeks (*green line*). Activated T cells further infiltrate the epidermis and produce IL-17 and IL-22 (*purple line*) that induce hyperproliferation of keratinocytes, epidermal acanthosis, and changes characteristic of a psoriatic skin lesion (*blue line*)

3. Sections are stained with hematoxylin and eosin according to standard protocols for histological analysis. A psoriatic skin will show typical hallmarks of psoriasis such as acanthosis, parakeratosis, focal loss of granular layer, and dermal immune cell infiltration mainly composed of T cells (Fig. 2).
4. To determine whether abnormal keratinocyte proliferation and differentiation exists, sections are stained with fluorescently labeled anti-Ki67 and anti-involucrin respectively. Intense Ki67 positive keratinocytes with a broader expression of involucrin within the epidermal layers are found in psoriatic lesions.

3.5 Flow Cytometry Analysis of the Dermal Infiltrate

1. To determine the nature of the immune cell infiltrate in the newly developed psoriatic lesion, grafted skins are excised at day 35 (or at earlier time points in the case of a kinetics analysis), dermal sheets are separated from epidermal sheets, minced and digested with 1 mg/ml Dispase and 1 mg/ml collagenase for 30 min at 37 °C to yield single cell suspensions.
2. Cell suspensions are filtered through a 70 μm cell strainer onto a 50-ml centrifuge tube and washed with 50 ml of PBS at 500 × *g* for 5 min.
3. Cells are resuspended in 200 μl of FACS buffer containing the desired fluorescently labeled antibodies (Table 1) and DAPI to exclude dead cells, and stained for 15 min at 4 °C.
4. Cells are then washed with 5 ml of PBS at 500 × *g* for 5 min, resuspended in 200 μl of FACS buffer and immediately acquired on a flow cytometer.

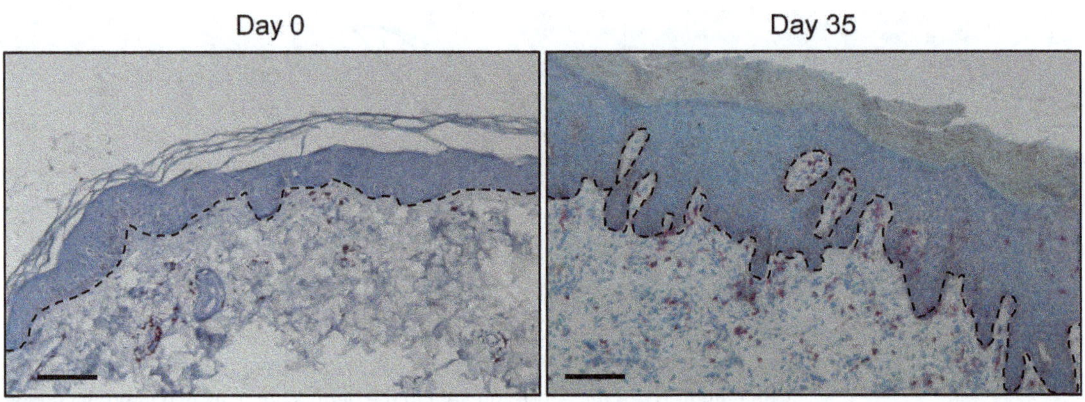

Fig. 2 Expansion of dermal T cells during the development of psoriasis. Pictures of cryosections stained for CD3 (*red*) and hematoxylin (*blue*) of nonpsoriatic skin on the day of transplantation onto AGR129 mice (Day 0), and after development of fully fledged psoriasis on day 35. Histological analysis demonstrates the expansion of $CD3^+$ T cells in the dermis and their infiltration into the epidermis after 35 days. Scale bars, 20 μm

Table 1
List of antibodies used for flow cytometry analysis

Antigen	Cell expression	Clone	Supplier/dilution
CD3	T cells	HIT3a	BD Pharmingen™/1/10
CD4	T cell subset, mono, macro, pDC	SK3	BD Pharmingen™/1/10
CD8	T cell subset, NK	SK1	BD Pharmingen™/1/10
CD11c	DC, myeloid cells, B cells, T cell subset	S-HCL-3	BD Pharmingen™/1/100
CD45RA	Naive and effector T cells	HI100	BD Pharmingen™/1/10
CD45RO	Central and effector memory T cells	UCHL1	BD Pharmingen™/1/10
CD123	pDC, basophils, macro, DC	AC145	Miltenyi Biotec/1/20
HLA-DR	Macro, B cells, DC	G46-6	BD Pharmingen™/1/10
BDCA-2	pDC	AC144	Miltenyi Biotec/1/20
TNF	TNF-producing cells	MAb11	BD Pharmingen™/1/5
IFN-α_2	IFN-α_2-producing cells	225.C	Chromaprobe, Inc./1/5
IFN-γ	IFN-γ-producing cells	B27	BD Pharmingen™/1/5

4 Notes

1. Patients do not receive topical or systemic therapy for at least 4 weeks before the study.
2. The bandage is rather tight and is held in place well. Mice rarely remove the bandage within these first 7 days before removal (clearly less than 5%). The dressing is verified every day after surgery and must be redone in case a loose bandage is observed.
3. We cut open the bandage above the belly, afterwards it more or less falls off by itself. The bandage sticks more to itself than on the mouse hairs when put around the belly. It will therefore not strip mouse hair when removed.
4. Usage of NSAID is not feasible in our model as the inflammatory reaction plays an essential role in the development of psoriasis.
5. Mice weight must be monitored daily for the first 7 days, and every other day for up to 35 days. If weight loss exceeds 10%, mice must be euthanized and the experiment terminated.
6. The route of injection and the dosage depends on the nature of the antibody. For therapeutic antibodies already used in the clinic, refer to its precise dosage and administration route.

References

1. Gaffen SL, Jain R, Garg AV, Cua DJ (2014) The IL-23-IL-17 immune axis: from mechanisms to therapeutic testing. Nat Rev Immunol 14(9):585–600
2. van der Fits L, Mourits S, Voerman JS, Kant M, Boon L, Laman JD et al (2009) Imiquimod-induced psoriasis-like skin inflammation in mice is mediated via the IL-23/IL-17 axis. J Immunol 182(9):5836–5845
3. Langrish CL, Chen Y, Blumenschein WM, Mattson J, Basham B, Sedgwick JD et al (2005) IL-23 drives a pathogenic T cell population that induces autoimmune inflammation. J Exp Med 201(2):233–240
4. Wilson NJ, Boniface K, Chan JR, McKenzie BS, Blumenschein WM, Mattson JD et al (2007) Development, cytokine profile and function of human interleukin 17-producing helper T cells. Nat Immunol 8(9):950–957
5. Manel N, Unutmaz D, Littman DR (2008) The differentiation of human T(H)-17 cells requires transforming growth factor-beta and induction of the nuclear receptor RORgammat. Nat Immunol 9(6):641–649
6. Bettelli E, Korn T, Oukka M, Kuchroo VK (2008) Induction and effector functions of T(H)17 cells. Nature 453(7198):1051–1057
7. Donnelly RP, Sheikh F, Dickensheets H, Savan R, Young HA, Walter MR (2010) Interleukin-26: an IL-10-related cytokine produced by Th17 cells. Cytokine Growth Factor Rev 21(5):393–401
8. Ye P, Rodriguez FH, Kanaly S, Stocking KL, Schurr J, Schwarzenberger P et al (2001) Requirement of interleukin 17 receptor signaling for lung CXC chemokine and granulocyte colony-stimulating factor expression, neutrophil recruitment, and host defense. J Exp Med 194(4):519–527
9. Wolk K, Witte E, Witte K, Warszawska K, Sabat R (2010) Biology of interleukin-22. Semin Immunopathol 32(1):17–31
10. Ma HL, Liang S, Li J, Napierata L, Brown T, Benoit S et al (2008) IL-22 is required for Th17 cell-mediated pathology in a mouse model of psoriasis-like skin inflammation. J Clin Invest 118(2):597–607
11. Nurieva R, Yang XO, Martinez G, Zhang Y, Panopoulos AD, Ma L et al (2007) Essential autocrine regulation by IL-21 in the generation of inflammatory T cells. Nature 448(7152):480–483
12. Swindell WR, Johnston A, Carbajal S, Han G, Wohn C, Lu J et al (2011) Genome-wide expression profiling of five mouse models identifies similarities and differences with human psoriasis. PLoS One 6(4):e18266
13. Nickoloff BJ, Wrone-Smith T (1999) Injection of pre-psoriatic skin with CD4+ T cells induces psoriasis. Am J Pathol 155(1):145–158
14. Boyman O, Hefti HP, Conrad C, Nickoloff BJ, Suter M, Nestle FO (2004) Spontaneous development of psoriasis in a new animal model shows an essential role for resident T cells and tumor necrosis factor-alpha. J Exp Med 199(5):731–736
15. Nestle FO, Conrad C, Tun-Kyi A, Homey B, Gombert M, Boyman O et al (2005) Plasmacytoid predendritic cells initiate psoriasis through interferon-alpha production. J Exp Med 202(1):135–143
16. Conrad C, Boyman O, Tonel G, Tun-Kyi A, Laggner U, de Fougerolles A et al (2007) Alpha1beta1 integrin is crucial for accumulation of epidermal T cells and the development of psoriasis. Nat Med 13(7):836–842
17. Gaide O, Emerson RO, Jiang X, Gulati N, Nizza S, Desmarais C et al (2015) Common clonal origin of central and resident memory T cells following skin immunization. Nat Med 21(6):647–653
18. Tonel G, Conrad C, Laggner U, Di Meglio P, Grys K, McClanahan TK et al (2010) Cutting edge: a critical functional role for IL-23 in psoriasis. J Immunol 185(10):5688–5691
19. Di Meglio P, Villanova F, Navarini AA, Mylonas A, Tosi I, Nestle FO, Conrad C (2016) Targeting CD8(+) T cells prevents psoriasis development. J Allergy Clin Immunol 138(1):274–276.e6

Chapter 8

A Mouse Model for Atopic Dermatitis Using Topical Application of Vitamin D3 or of Its Analog MC903

Verena Moosbrugger-Martinz, Matthias Schmuth, and Sandrine Dubrac

Abstract

Atopic dermatitis (AD) is a chronic relapsing inflammatory skin disease with pruritus and high prevalence. Indeed, 15–30% of children and 2–10% of adults from industrialized countries are affected. Acute AD lesions are characterized by epidermal hyperplasia associated with a dominant Th2/Th17 immune response and dermal inflammatory infiltrates. Moreover, the expression of alarmins such as TSLP, IL-33, and IL-25 is upregulated in acute AD lesions. Topical application of vitamin D3 or of its low-calcemic analog MC903 induces changes in skin morphology and inflammation resembling immune perturbations observed in acute lesions of patients with AD. Mice treated with MC903 or vitamin D3 additionally display increased serum IgE levels, as observed in patients with extrinsic AD. Interestingly, these symptoms are not dependent on mouse gender or on genetic background. Thus, the easiness of this mouse model renders it very attractive to study immunologic abnormalities involved in AD development or maintenance. Furthermore, this model might be useful for preclinical studies aiming at unraveling new therapeutic strategies to treat AD. In this chapter, we describe the induction and major features of MC903 and vitamin D3-induced AD-like inflammation in mice.

Key words Atopic dermatitis, MC903, Mouse model, Thymic stromal lymphopoietin (TSLP), Skin, Type 2 T helper cells (Th2), Vitamin D3

1 Introduction

Atopic dermatitis (AD) is a chronic relapsing non-contagious inflammatory skin disease accompanied by pruritus. Its onset occurs early in life, most commonly between 6 weeks and 6 months of age. Its incidence culminates around the age of 2 years and then slowly diminishes. In 50–70% of cases, the disease progressively regresses and disappears during adolescence. Atypically, AD can develop with a late onset (<18 years old). Worldwide, the prevalence of AD is relatively high by affecting 15–30% of children and 2–10% of adults. Noticeably, AD prevalence underwent a marked increase during the past 30 years, potentially resulting from increased pollution [1]. In atopic children, regression of

Björn E. Clausen and Jon D. Laman (eds.), *Inflammation: Methods and Protocols*, Methods in Molecular Biology, vol. 1559, DOI 10.1007/978-1-4939-6786-5_8, © Springer Science+Business Media LLC 2017

eczema can coincide with the development of asthma or allergic rhinitis, whose incidence starts increasing at the age of 2 and 5 years, respectively. However, incidence of asthma peaks around an age of 5 years and then slowly decreases to reach its minimal incidence at 15 years. Incidence of allergic rhinitis remains stable throughout life [2].

The pattern of AD skin lesions is related to patients' age. In the perinatal period, erythematous and papulovesicular eruptions with oozing and crusting are often observed on the face, scalp, and flexures. Later, in childhood, AD is characterized by generalized dry skin and persistent lichenified flexural lesions on arms and legs. When AD persists or appears in adults, the disease is mostly localized on extremities (feet and hands) and flexures (elbows, knees, and neck). It can also manifest as an atopic red face, as chronic lichenified eczema on the trunk, or as subacute or psoriasiform [3]. The course of AD varies in individuals according to psychologic state and environment. The physical and environmental factors involved in adults differ from those in children and this may be responsible for the different patterns of skin involvement and for the atypical morphologies [3].

Primary genetic defects affecting keratinocytes and compromising the skin barrier are believed to substantially contribute to AD development. The defective epidermal barrier permeability has long been assumed to be a consequence of the immunological abnormalities observed in AD ("inside-to-outside" paradigm). Later, skin barrier dysfunction was proposed as the "driving force" of AD pathogenesis ("outside-to-inside" paradigm). Nowadays, an "outside-to-inside, back-to-outside" paradigm predominates. In this pathogenic model, initial skin barrier impairment favors allergen/hapten/chemical ingress in the stratum corneum, which are taken up by Langerhans cells (LCs) [4]. Activated LCs then migrate to regional lymph nodes to prime naïve $CD4^+$ T-lymphocytes into Type 2 T helper (Th2)/allergic cells or locally activate memory Th2 cells [5–7]. Th2 cytokines such as IL-4 and IL-13, produced not only by skin T cells but also by innate lymphoid cells type 2 (ILCs2), then downregulate genes important to skin barrier function such as filaggrin (FLG), involucrin or loricrin, further increasing skin permeability to allergens/haptens/chemicals [8–10]. This vicious cycle might be amplified by the hyper-proliferation of LCs which has previously been reported in AD skin [11]. The "outside-to-inside, back-to-outside" paradigm is strengthened by recent work showing that increased transepidermal water loss (TEWL) in newborns precedes overt AD symptoms [12].

Primary skin barrier disturbances observed in AD are, in part, driven by loss-of-function mutations in the gene encoding the epidermal protein filaggrin (FLG) [13]. However, other genes important for skin barrier function are potentially involved. Meta-analysis of genome-wide association studies identified other risk loci linked to AD and involved in epidermal proliferation and differentiation [14, 15]. However, to date, only FLG mutations were found to predict dose-dependent alterations in the permeability of epidermal barrier [16–18]. In patients with AD, the epidermal barrier defect is also provoked by abnormal lipid composition and organization of the straum corneum and by an altered epidermal lipid metabolism [9, 19–22]. These cutaneous lipid abnormalities can result from upstream genetic alterations in lipid-related genes but also in genes related to keratinocyte differentiation [16].

During flares, two skin states, i.e., nonlesional vs. lesional coexist in AD patients. Nonlesional skin, despite a normal appearance, shows epidermal hyperplasia, increased TEWL, and is associated with deregulated keratinocyte differentiation, a less acidic skin surface pH and subclinical signs of inflammation [23]. Increased numbers of $Ki67^+$ keratinocytes and upregulation of keratin 16 expression demonstrate a stimulation of keratinocyte proliferation in nonlesional skin. This keratinocyte hyper-proliferation is not counteracted by increased apoptosis [24]. Moreover, $CD3^+$ and $CD11c^+$ cells are more abundant in nonlesional AD than in healthy skin [23]. Furthermore, the transcription of genes involved in both epidermal homeostasis and immune response is largely altered in nonlesional AD when compared to healthy skin. The expression of genes encoding for major terminal differentiation proteins, including loricrin, FLG, involucrine, corneodesmosine, late cornified envelope and small proline rich proteins is downregulated [23]. Interestingly, protein levels of Claudin 4, a protein essential for tight junctions, are enhanced in nonlesional AD when compared to healthy and lesional skin [25]. The expression of the T-cell trafficking chemokines, CCL17, CCL5, CCL11, CCL18 and the expression of IL-13 considered as Th2 mediators are markedly increased whereas expression of genes involved in Th1/IFNγ signaling is moderately triggered in nonlesional AD [23]. Furthermore, expression of IL-23/p19 and p40 is increased, suggesting a partial upregulation of the Th17 immune response [23]. A Th22 immune response is not induced in nonlesional skin with expression of IL-22 similar in nonlesional AD and healthy skin [26, 27]. Thus, nonlesional skin mainly displays a Th2/Th17 immune response. Expression of antimicrobial peptides such as hBD-2 and LL-37 [28, 29] and neutrophil numbers [30] are unaltered in nonlesional skin when compared to healthy skin and it remains unknown whether nonlesional AD skin is infiltrated by increased numbers of ILCs2. Thus, the contribution of innate immunity to nonlesional AD might rather be minor.

Lesional AD skin exhibits major epidermal hyperplasia, spongiosis, lichenification, overt inflammation, possibly bacterial as well as viral superinfection. Moreover, lesional AD is characterized by severe skin barrier impairment associated with dramatic increase of TEWL and strong downregulation of keratinocyte differentiation.

Skin lesions of AD patients are infiltrated with various immune cells, such as eosinophils, basophiles, mast cells, dendritic cells (DCs), $CD8^+$ T cells, $CD4^+$ T cells, and ILCs2 [31]. Recent work has shown that neutrophils and neutrophil-related molecule such as DEFB4 and CXCL1 are increased in skin lesions of AD patients when compared to nonlesional skin, thus changing the classical view on the contribution of neutrophils to AD [30]. Moreover, higher levels of neutrophils in lesional AD are associated with *Staphylococcus aureus* infection and *Staphylococcal* coagulase-induced supraepidermal crust formation [30]. Others reported lower numbers of polymorphonuclear leukocytes, NK cells and plasmacytoid DCs (pDCs) in AD lesions, potentially explaining microbial superinfection [32]. Thus, both abnormal adaptive and innate immunity contribute to lesional AD [32].

Lesional AD skin develops in two phases, i.e., the acute phase which lasts only a few hours followed by the chronic phase. Acute lesions are characterized by a Th2 dominant immune response and epidermal hyperplasia, very similar to nonlesional AD. However, acute lesions additionally exhibit increased expression of alarmins such as IL-25, IL-33, and thymic stromal lymphopoietin (TSLP) which are produced by damaged epidermal cells, mostly keratinocytes [33]. These alarmins are believed to promote Th2 immune response, thus perpetuating immune abnormalities [33]. Because the acute phase of lesional AD only lasts a few hours, the literature mostly reports data on the chronic phase of lesional AD. Immune abnormalities observed in chronic AD lesions are more complex than in acute lesions because Th1, Th17, Th22, and Th2 immune responses coexist [26, 27, 34]. Acute and chronic AD lesions can be distinguished by differential expression pattern of various molecules (Table 1) [35, 36]. Most of AD skin lesions are colonized with microbes [37]. Microbial superinfection triggers receptors such as the protease-activated receptors (PARs), the Toll-like receptors (TLRs), the C-type lectins (CLRs), and inflammasomes which, in turn, induce NF-κB activation, reactive oxygen species (ROS) production, and the release of innate pro-Th2 cell cytokines including alarmins and granulocyte-macrophage colony-stimulating factor (GM-CSF) by epidermal cells [33, 37]. Subsequently, ILCs2 are recruited to AD skin lesions by TSLP, IL-25, IL-33 but also by prostaglandin D2 [31–33, 38, 39]. Thus, in chronic AD lesions, microbial superinfection sustains inflammation by triggering innate immunity via keratinocyte activation.

Various mouse models have been developed in order to better understand the pathogenesis of AD or to evaluate efficacy of potential therapies. However, there are no perfect mouse models for AD because genetically- or chemically-induced AD in mice only recapitulates part of the features observed in AD patients but never all [7, 40]. The choice of a mouse model to study AD should be tailored to the question asked. The mouse model using vitamin D3

Table 1
Cytokine expression profile in acute versus chronic AD lesions

	Acute lesions	Chronic lesions
IL-4	↑	~↑
IL-5	=	↑
IL-10	↑	↑
IL-13	~↑	↑
IL-31	↑	↑
CCL18	~↑	↑
CCL5	~↑	↑
CCL13	=	↑
CCL11	↑	↑
TSLP	↑	↑
TSLPR	~↑	↑
OX40L	=	=
IL-9	~↑	~↑
IL-22	↑	↑
S100A7	↑	↑
S100A8	↑	↑
S100A9	↑	↑
S100A12	↑	↑
IL-32	↑	↑
IFN-γ	=	↑
IL-8	~↑	~↑
IL-1β	~↑	~↑
IFN-α	=	~↑
CXCL9	=	↑
CXCL10	=	↑
CXCL11	=	↑
IL-17A	~↑	~↑
IL-23p19	~↑	=
IL-23p40	~↑	~↑
CCL20	↑	↑
Foxp3	=	↑

Expression compared to nonlesional AD [35, 36], = unchanged expression, ~↑ non significantly increased, ↑ significantly increased or its low-calcemic analog, MC903 has been developed by Li et al. in 2006 [41]. In this model, vitamin D3 or MC903 induces overexpression of TSLP by keratinocytes leading to the development of AD-like inflammation [41, 42] and of asthma [43, 44]. Mice treated with MC903 or vitamin D3 exhibit epidermal hyperplasia associated with increased dermal inflammatory infiltrates consisting of eosinophils and $CD3^+$, $CD4^+$, $CD11c^+$, $GR\text{-}1^+$, and mast cells [41]. Skin treated with MC903 shows increased levels of TSLP, IL-4, IL-5, IL-13, IL-31, IL-10, IL-8, IFN-γ, and TNF-β [5, 41]. Thus, in this model, a mixed Th2/Th1 immune response is triggered by MC903/vitamin D3 treatment. However, it remains unknown whether MC903 or vitamin D3 enhances a Th17 or a Th22 immune response in mouse skin. Moreover, vitamin D3- or MC903-treated mice display increased serum IgE [5, 41], as observed in extrinsic AD. The induction of AD-like symptoms by vitamin D3 or MC903 requires both adaptive and innate immunity. Indeed, this model has been used to demonstrate the pathogenic role of LCs in the development of AD [5] and their hyper-proliferation in AD skin [11]. Furthermore, topical applications of MC903 and TSLPR deficient mice have been employed to demonstrate that TSLP signaling in $CD4^+$ T cells is required for memory formation of Th2 cells [45]. Recently, this model has been utilized to show a TSLP-dependent, IL-33-independent recruitment of ILCs2 to AD skin [39] and that AD-like inflammation is improved by microRNA-146a through suppression of innate immune responses in keratinocytes [46]. Finally, $RAG1^{-/-}$ mice treated with MC903 display epidermal hyperplasia, increased skin expression of TSLP, IL-4, IL-6, IL-10, and IFN-γ, and increased skin infiltration with ILCs2, eosinophils, mast cells, and $CD11c^+$ cells [39, 41].

Thus, the MC903- or vitamin D3-based AD mouse model nicely recapitulates important hallmarks of lesional AD. Therefore, it can be used to address still unanswered questions related to the complex immune interplay that characterizes lesional AD. Furthermore, this model might help in deciphering abnormal adaptive and innate immune responses in AD. The epidermal barrier function has not yet been investigated in this model, which could be useful to detail the effects of cutaneous immunity on stratum corneum and tight junction barriers. Moreover, this mouse model could be used to evaluate the relation between AD and asthma.

To conclude, the big advantage of this model is its easiness. Indeed, it suffices to topically apply vitamin D3 or MC903 to mouse skin for several days to obtain AD-like inflammation recapitulating major AD features [41]. This model does not require tape stripping which can be tricky, application of occlusive patches onto mouse back that are sometimes not easy to manage, topical application of hazardous agents such as oxazolone or 2,4-dinitrofluorobenzene (DNFB), or complex genetic manipulations that take months or years to be established. In this chapter, we will provide all technical details for topically applying vitamin D3 or MC903 to mouse skin in order to obtain AD-like inflammation.

2 Materials

1. 8–10-week-old, sex- and weight-matched mice (*see* **Note 1**).
2. Ethanol 99 % grade pure.
3. A high precision balance.
4. Safe-lock 1.5 ml black Eppendorf tubes (light safe).
5. Eventually a shaving devise and a depilatory cream.
6. MC903 (also called calcipotriol, >98 %, Tocris). The working concentration for MC903 is 45 μM. It can be prepared with an initial concentration of 450 μM as follows: Dissolve 1 mg MC903 (MM = 412.6 g/mol) in 5.386 ml ethanol. Further dilute this stock solution ten times in ethanol to reach the working concentration of 45 μM. Prepare 1 ml aliquots in small sterile black Eppendorf tubes (safe-lock, light safe) and store at −20 °C. Aliquots should not repeatedly be thawed and frozen because of subsequent ethanol evaporation, which will concentrate the chemical (*see* **Notes 2–4**). Argon can be applied to the Eppendorf tubes to avoid oxidation of MC903 for long-term storage (*see* **Note 5**).
7. Vitamin D3 (also called 1α,25-dihydroxyvitamin D3 or cholecalciferol, >98 % HPLC, Sigma-Aldrich). Dissolve vitamin D3 in ethanol to a working concentration of 50 μM. It can be prepared as an initial solution of 500 μM as follows: Dissolve 1 mg vitamin D3 (MM = 384.339 g/mol) in 5.204 ml ethanol. Dilute this solution ten times with ethanol to reach the working concentration of 50 μM. Use the same storage conditions as described for MC903 (*see* **Notes 2–5**).

3 Methods

Compounds can be topically applied to mouse ears under short anesthesia with ketamine or isoflurane. Because MC903 is a low-calcemic vitamin D3 analog, it can be applied to mouse skin at higher concentrations and for a longer time than vitamin D3. Therefore, MC903 can be applied not only to mouse ears but also to mouse back skin after hair removal (please see below). Vitamin D3 should only be applied to mouse ears because of it adverse effects on systemic calcium metabolism.

3.1 Induction of AD-Like Skin Inflammation

3.1.1 Topical Application of MC903

1. When MC903 is applied to mouse back skin, hair should be removed 3 days before starting the topical applications (*see* **Note 6**).
2. To induce AD-like inflammation with MC903, compound should topically be applied once daily as follows for (1) mouse ears (12.5 μl on dorsal and ventral ear side for a total volume of 25 μl per ear) or (2) back skin (25 μl for a skin area the size of a quarter). Altogether, 1.125 nmol MC903 will be applied per ear or per back skin area every day (*see* **Note 1**).
3. The sequence of treatment will be the following: 5 days treatment, 2 days interruption, 5 days treatment, 2 days interruption, 1 or 2 days treatment (for a 15–16 day-treatment period). Control animals are treated in parallel with ethanol only (Fig. 1).

3.1.2 Topical Application of Vitamin D3

1. When vitamin D3 is used, only one ear should be treated because of adverse effects on systemic calcium metabolism (*see* **Notes 1** and **2**).
2. To induce AD-like inflammation with vitamin D3, the compound should topically be applied to one mouse ear (10 μl on dorsal and ventral ear side for a total volume of 20 μl per ear) once daily. Altogether, 0.4 nmol vitamin D3 will be applied per ear and per day according to the following treatment sequence: 4 days treatment, 3 days interruption, 4 days treatment (for a 11 day-treatment period) (*see* **Notes 1** and **2**). Control animals are treated in parallel with ethanol only (see diagram below).

3.2 Evaluation of Atopic Inflammation

The time course of inflammation can be monitored by measuring ear thickness with a caliper under light anesthesia (Fig. 2a). Upon treatment, inflammation develops as skin hyper-vascularization and subsequent skin redness becomes visible (Fig. 2b). Auricular lymph nodes are also enlarged after treatment (Fig. 2c) (*see* **Note 7**).

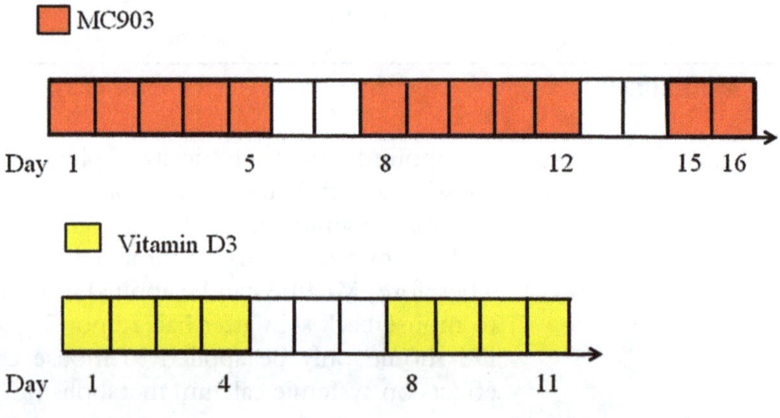

Fig. 1 Diagrams showing the daily treatment scheme for MC903 (in *red*) and for vitamin D3 (in *yellow*)

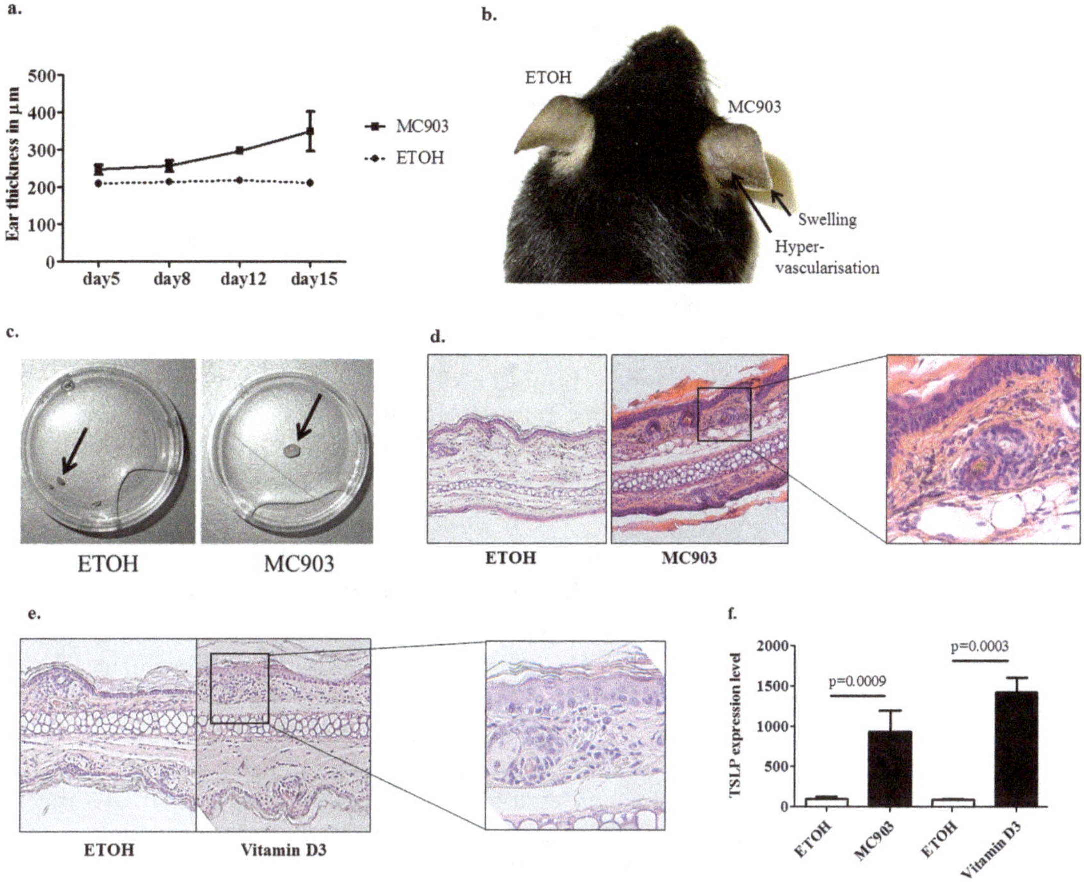

Fig. 2 MC903 induces atopic dermatitis-like inflammation in mice. C57BL/6 mice were topically treated with MC903 on right ear or with ethanol on left ear for 15 days as follow: 5 days topical treatment, 2 days interruption, 5 days treatment, 2 days interruption, 1 day topical treatment. (**a**) Time course of ear thickness. Days on *x*-axis refer to days after start of the treatment. (**b**) Pictures of a representative mouse on day 15 showing ear thickening and hyper-vascularization (*arrows*) for the ear side treated with MC903. (**c**) Pictures of representative auricular lymph nodes from a mouse treated for 15 days with MC903 or ethanol (ETOH). Pictures of representative H&E staining from mouse ears after topical treatment with ethanol or MC903 (**d**) or vitamin D3 according to the 11-day protocol (**e**). Magnification ×100 (*left panel*) or ×400 (*right panel*). (**f**) Histogram showing expression of TSLP, measured by quantitative PCR, in mouse ears treated with ethanol, or MC903 or vitamin D3. Results are expressed as % of controls and shown as Mean ± SEM. Statistical significance was determined by a Student-*t*-test

Histological analysis of mouse skin shows epidermal hyperplasia and dermal inflammatory infiltrates mostly consisting of lymphocytes, macrophages, eosinophils and neutrophils (Fig. 2d) (*see* **Note 8**). The vitamin D3-related symptoms are attenuated due to shorter treatment time and lower dose of the compound used (Fig. 2e). However, this protocol is sufficient to induce a robust TSLP overexpression in mouse skin (Fig. 2f) (*see* **Note 9**).

4 Notes

1. This model works in mice regardless of sex and genetic background (Balb/c versus C57BL/6).
2. Mice treated with vitamin D3 will lose weight over time during the experiment due to interactions between vitamin D3 and calcium metabolism. Therefore, MC903 should be preferred to vitamin D3. In case, MC903 is not available, a careful follow up of the mice should be done; only mice weighting more than 25 g should be used for the experiment.
3. Compounds should be stored at −20 °C protected from light and in aliquots. If possible, remove oxygen in tubes with argon prior storage (*see* **Note 5**). Tubes should have a safe lock and be additionally sealed with Parafilm to avoid ethanol evaporation.
4. Aliquots of working solution should be prepared to be only used once. Otherwise, air can induce compound oxidation and ethanol evaporation.
5. Argon is sold as a bottle of gas. The bottle output is usually connected to flexible plastic tubing at the end of which a glass Pasteur pipette or a pipette tip is inserted. After opening of the bottle to release the gas, apply the Pasteur pipette in the Eppendorf tubes for 30 s at least. It takes a bit of time to eliminate all oxygen. The duration of argon diffusion depends on the volume of liquid in the tube.
6. It is important to remove hair 3 days prior to topical treatment. These 3 days are required for skin recovery after hair removal which inflicts skin traumas. Mice are anesthetized and shaved on a large back skin area with a shaving device. Then, a thick layer of depilatory cream is applied onto skin for 4–7 min and washed away with water only. Cream should be entirely removed and mice carefully dried using handkerchiefs. To help mice to recover from anesthesia and hair removal, they can be placed on a warming table at 35 °C. If no warming table is available, mice can be placed in between two latex gloves filled with warm water. This recovery procedure should not exceed 20 min.
7. Auricular lymph nodes can be further used for flow cytometry analyses or for cell cultures as follows: place auricular lymph node(s) in a 6 well-plate containing 2 ml Hank's buffer without calcium and magnesium and 2% FCS. Then, dislocate lymph nodes with curved pincers and pipet the bulk into a 50 ml Falcon tube. Wash the well that has contained lymph nodes with 2 ml Hank's buffer and 2% FCS and add to Falcon tube. Auricular lymph nodes are then digested with collagenase D (120 μl of a 40 mg/ml solution) for 25 min at 37 °C under shaking. Stop the digestion by adding EDTA (80 μl of a 0.5 M solution) for 5 min at 37 °C under shaking. Single cell

suspension is obtained by filtering cells through a 40 μm cell strainer, washed with cold PBS and centrifuged. Finally, dissolve the pellet in cold PBS or R10 medium, count cells in a hemocytometer.

8. To perform H&E staining on mouse ears, disinfect tissue with 70% ethanol, remove and fix it overnight at 4 °C in 1 ml of a 4% formalin solution. Then, embed ½ ear in paraffin and cut in 3 μm sections with a microtome. Hematoxylin and eosin staining is then done as follows: after deparaffinization with successive xylene and ethanol baths, sections are first stained with haematoxylin (3×5 min), washed with 1% acid alcohol for 2 min and then further stained with eosin for 2 min. After extensive washings, sections are mounted and examined under a light microscope.
9. To measure expression of TSLP in mouse ears, the following protocol can be utilized: RNAse-free tubes and solutions should be used throughout all RNA preparation and RNA Zap® (Ambion) should be used to clean up instruments. First disinfect ears with 70% ethanol, remove and immediately shock freeze it in liquid nitrogen. Ears can be stored at −80 °C for a few days or used on the same day to prepare RNA. Skin contains RNases; therefore it is always better to prepare RNA from skin as soon as possible after removal because the storage can induce RNA degradation. RNA is then prepared as follows (adapted from TRIzol data sheet): add 1 ml TRIzol to ½ mouse ear and homogenize with a homogenizer. Incubate samples for at least 5 min at room temperature. Then, add 200 μl chloroform and mix tubes by inverting for 15 s. Incubate samples at room temperature for at least 2 min and centrifuge at 12,000×*g* for 15 min at 4 °C. Pipet the aquous phase (the upper color-less phase) and transfer into a clean tube. Add 500 μl isopropanol and mix by inverting 5–10 times. Let RNA precipitation at −20 °C overnight. Then, centrifuge samples at 12,000×*g* for 10 min at 4 °C. A white pellet should be visible at the bottom of the tube. To ensure visualization of a pellet, GlycoBlue™ (Thermofisher) (1:1000) can be added to the mixure prior overnight precipitation. After centrifugation, remove supernatant, add 1 ml 75% ethanol and centrifuge samples at 7500×*g* for 10 min at 4 °C. Carefully remove ethanol and let the tube drying by inverting on a clean tissue for 5–10 min at room temperature. Clean swabs can alternatively serve at drying residual ethanol on tube walls. When the pellet is dried up, add 50 μl TE buffer and vortex well. Samples can be further incubated at 55–60 °C for 10 min to inactivate proteins (Table 2). Then, genomic DNA can be removed from samples by DNase treatment according to manufacturer's instructions (Ambion, Austin, TX). The removal of genomic

Table 2
Summary for RNA and cDNA preparation from mouse ears

RNA preparation 50 μl		**cDNA preparation 100 μl**	
Step 1: Homogenization	½ ear + 1 ml TRIzol	*Step 1*: Denaturation step	1 μg RNA + 4 μl Hexamer (*see* **Note 11**) + 10 μl 10 mM dNTP + (qsp 54 μl RNase-free water) Incubate for 5 min at 65 °C
Step 2: Dissociation of nucleoprotein complex	Incubation for 5 min at room temperature	*Step 2*: To bring all reagents at room temperature	20 μl 5× buffer + 10 μl 0.5 M DTT Incubate for 10 min at 25 °C
Step 3: Isolation of nucleic acids	+200 μl chloroform Mix Centrifuge at 12,000 × *g* for 15 min at 4 °C Transfer color-less phase into a fresh tube	*Step 3*: cDNA synthesis	2 μl Superscript II (200 U/ml) Incubate for 50 min at 42 °C
Step 4: Precipitation of nucleic acids	+500 μl isopropanol Mix Precipitate overnight at −20 °C	*Step 4*: Enzyme inactivation	Incubate for 5 min at 96 °C
Step 5: Isolation of nucleic acids	Centrifuge at 12,000 × *g* for 10 min at 4 °C	*Step 5*: Storage	cDNA can be stored at 4 °C for short term and at −20/−80 °C for longer storage
Step 6: Wash	+1 ml 75% ethanol Centrifuge at 7500 × *g* for 10 min at 4 °C		
Step 7: RNA solution	Dry pellet + TE buffer		
Step 8: Inactivation of proteins	10 min at 55–60 °C		
Step 9: RNA concentration	Dilute 1:100 RNA in RNAse-free distilled water and measure absorbance at 260 vs. 280 nm		

DNA allows a more sensitive detection of changes in gene expression. Ultimately, prepare random primed cDNA from total RNA (Superscript II RNase H-reverse transcriptase; Life Technologies) (Table 2). Real-time PCR (Real-time PCR detection system CFX96; Biorad) is performed using the Brilliant III Ultra-Fast Quantitative PCR Kit from Agilent technologies according to manufacturer's instructions. Taqman primer and probe mix are used with this kit and increase PCR specificity. Sequences for probes and primers specific for mouse TATA binding protein (*see* **Note 10**) and for mouse TSLP mRNA molecules are synthesized by Microsynth (Balgach, Switzerland): TSLP forward primer 5′CCT TCA CTC CCC GAC AAA AC3′, TSLP reverse primer 5′GCC TGG GCA GTG GTC ATT3′ and TSLP Taqman probe FAM-5′TTG CCC GGA GAA CAA GAG AAG CCC T3′-TAMRA; TATA binding protein forward primer 5′ACTTCGTGCAAGA AATGCTGAA3′, TATA binding protein reverse primer 5′TGTCCGTGGCTCTCTTATTCTCA3′ and TATA binding protein Taqman probe FAM-5′TCCCAAGCGATTTGC TGCAGTCATC3′-TAMRA. Aleternatively, pre-made primer and probe mix are commercially available (Applied Biosystems). RT-PCR is performed with a first cycle at 95 °C for 3 min and then 39 cycles as follows: 5 s at 95 °C, 10 s at 60 °C with the current kit.

10. TATA binding protein is a good housekeeping gene for skin. Alternatively, cyclophilin can be used. These two housekeeping genes are best for the skin. Other housekeeping genes such as 36B4 and beta-2-microglobulin work also satisfyingly.
11. Hexamers are synthesized by Microsynth (Balgach, Switzerland) and prepared as a 100 μM stock solution in RNase-free distilled water. Dissolve hexamers in distilled water, vortex, incubate for 5 min at 55 °C, vortex, further incubate for 3 min at 55 °C, cool down on ice and store at −20 °C.

References

1. Miller RL, Peden DB (2014) Environmental effects on immune responses in patients with atopy and asthma. J Allergy Clin Immunol 134:1001–1008
2. Barnetson RS, Rogers M (2002) Childhood atopic eczema. BMJ 324:1376–1379
3. Correale CE, Walker C, Murphy L, Craig TJ (1999) Atopic dermatitis: a review of diagnosis and treatment. Am Fam Physician 60:1191–1198
4. Yoshida K, Kubo A, Fujita H, Yokouchi M, Ishii K, Kawasaki H, Nomura T, Shimizu H, Kouyama K, Ebihara T, Nagao K, Amagai M (2014) Distinct behavior of human Langerhans cells and inflammatory dendritic epidermal cells at tight junctions in patients with atopic dermatitis. J Allergy Clin Immunol 134:856–864
5. Elentner A, Finke D, Schmuth M, Chappaz S, Ebner S, Malissen B, Kissenpfennig A, Romani N, Dubrac S (2009) Langerhans cells are critical in the development of atopic dermatitis-like inflammation and symptoms in mice. J Cell Mol Med 13:2658–2672
6. Nakajima S, Igyártó BZ, Honda T, Egawa G, Otsuka A, Hara-Chikuma M, Watanabe N, Ziegler SF, Tomura M, Inaba K, Miyachi Y, Kaplan DH, Kabashima K (2012) Langerhans cells are critical in epicutaneous sensitization with protein antigen via thymic stromal lymphopoietin receptor signaling. J Allergy Clin Immunol 129:1048–1055.e1046
7. Dubrac S, Schmuth M, Ebner S (2010) Atopic dermatitis: the role of Langerhans cells in disease pathogenesis. Immunol Cell Biol 88:400–409
8. Howell MD, Kim BE, Gao P, Grant AV, Boguniewicz M, DeBenedetto A, Schneider L, Beck LA, Barnes KC, Leung DY (2009) Cytokine modulation of atopic dermatitis filaggrin skin expression. J Allergy Clin Immunol 124:R7–R12

9. Elias PM, Schmuth M (2009) Abnormal skin barrier in the etiopathogenesis of atopic dermatitis. Curr Opin Allergy Clin Immunol 9:437–446
10. Elias PM, Feingold KR (2001) Does the tail wag the dog? Role of the barrier in the pathogenesis of inflammatory dermatoses and therapeutic implications. Arch Dermatol 137:1079–1081
11. Chorro L, Sarde A, Li M, Woollard KJ, Chambon P, Malissen B, Kissenpfennig A, Barbaroux JB, Groves R, Geissmann F (2009) Langerhans cell (LC) proliferation mediates neonatal development, homeostasis, and inflammation-associated expansion of the epidermal LC network. J Exp Med 206:3089–3100
12. Kelleher M, Dunn-Galvin A, Hourihane JO, Murray D, Campbell LE, McLean WH, Irvine AD (2015) Skin barrier dysfunction measured by transepidermal water loss at 2 days and 2 months predates and predicts atopic dermatitis at 1 year. J Allergy Clin Immunol 135:930–935.e931
13. Palmer CN, Irvine AD, Terron-Kwiatkowski A, Zhao Y, Liao H, Lee SP, Goudie DR, Sandilands A, Campbell LE, Smith FJ, O'Regan GM, Watson RM, Cecil JE, Bale SJ, Compton JG, DiGiovanna JJ, Fleckman P, Lewis-Jones S, Arseculeratne G, Sergeant A, Munro CS, El Houate B, McElreavey K, Halkjaer LB, Bisgaard H, Mukhopadhyay S, McLean WH (2006) Common loss-of-function variants of the epidermal barrier protein filaggrin are a major predisposing factor for atopic dermatitis. Nat Genet 38:441–446
14. Paternoster L, Standl M, Chen CM, Ramasamy A, Bønnelykke K, Duijts L, Ferreira MA, Alves AC, Thyssen JP, Albrecht E, Baurecht H, Feenstra B, Sleiman PM, Hysi P, Warrington NM, Curjuric I, Myhre R, Curtin JA, Groen-Blokhuis MM, Kerkhof M, Sääf A, Franke A, Ellinghaus D, Fölster-Holst R, Dermitzakis E, Montgomery SB, Prokisch H, Heim K, Hartikainen AL, Pouta A, Pekkanen J, Blakemore AI, Buxton JL, Kaakinen M, Duffy DL, Madden PA, Heath AC, Montgomery GW, Thompson PJ, Matheson MC, Le Souëf P, Australian Asthma Genetics Consortium (AAGC), St. Pourcain B, Smith GD, Henderson J, Kemp JP, Timpson NJ, Deloukas P, Ring SM, Wichmann HE, Müller-Nurasyid M, Novak N, Klopp N, Rodríguez E, McArdle W, Linneberg A, Menné T, Nohr EA, Hofman A, Uitterlinden AG, van Duijn CM, Rivadeneira F, de Jongste JC, van der Valk RJ, Wjst M, Jogi R, Geller F, Boyd HA, Murray JC, Kim C, Mentch F, March M, Mangino M, Spector TD, Bataille V, Pennell CE, Holt PG, Sly P, Tiesler CM, Thiering E, Illig T, Imboden M, Nystad W, Simpson A, Hottenga JJ, Postma D, Koppelman GH, Smit HA, Söderhäll C, Chawes B, Kreiner-Møller E, Bisgaard H, Melén E, Boomsma DI, Custovic A, Jacobsson B, Probst-Hensch NM, Palmer LJ, Glass D, Hakonarson H, Melbye M (2012) Meta-analysis of genome-wide association studies identifies three new risk loci for atopic dermatitis. Nat Genet 44:187–192
15. Weidinger S, Willis-Owen SA, Kamatani Y, Baurecht H, Morar N, Liang L, Edser P, Street T, Rodriguez E, O'Regan GM, Beattie P, Fölster-Holst R, Franke A, Novak N, Fahy CM, Winge MC, Kabesch M, Illig T, Heath S, Söderhäll C, Melén E, Pershagen G, Kere J, Bradley M, Lieden A, Nordenskjold M, Harper JI, McLean WH, Brown SJ, Cookson WO, Lathrop GM, Irvine AD, Moffatt MF (2013) A genome-wide association study of atopic dermatitis identifies loci with overlapping effects on asthma and psoriasis. Hum Mol Genet 22:4841–4856
16. Gruber R, Elias PM, Crumrine D, Lin TK, Brandner JM, Hachem JP, Presland RB, Fleckman P, Janecke AR, Sandilands A, McLean WH, Fritsch PO, Mildner M, Tschachler E, Schmuth M (2011) Filaggrin genotype in ichthyosis vulgaris predicts abnormalities in epidermal structure and function. Am J Pathol 178:2252–2263
17. Kezic S, O'Regan GM, Yau N, Sandilands A, Chen H, Campbell LE, Kroboth K, Watson R, Rowland M, McLean WH, Irvine AD (2011) Levels of filaggrin degradation products are influenced by both filaggrin genotype and atopic dermatitis severity. Allergy 66:934–940
18. Brown SJ, Kroboth K, Sandilands A, Campbell LE, Pohler E, Kezic S, Cordell HJ, McLean WH, Irvine AD (2012) Intragenic copy number variation within filaggrin contributes to the risk of atopic dermatitis with a dose-dependent effect. J Invest Dermatol 132:98–104
19. Dahten A, Mergemeier S, Worm M (2007) PPARgamma expression profile and its cytokine driven regulation in atopic dermatitis. Allergy 62:926–933
20. Koro O, Furutani K, Hide M, Yamada S, Yamamoto S (1999) Chemical mediators in atopic dermatitis: involvement of leukotriene B4 released by a type I allergic reaction in the pathogenesis of atopic dermatitis. J Allergy Clin Immunol 103:663–670
21. Janssens M, van Smeden J, Gooris GS, Bras W, Portale G, Caspers PJ, Vreeken RJ, Hankemeier T, Kezic S, Wolterbeek R, Lavrijsen AP, Bouwstra JA (2012) Increase in short-chain ceramides correlates with an altered lipid organization and

decreased barrier function in atopic eczema patients. J Lipid Res 53:2755–2766

22. van Smeden J, Janssens M, Kaye EC, Caspers PJ, Lavrijsen AP, Vreeken RJ, Bouwstra JA (2014) The importance of free fatty acid chain length for the skin barrier function in atopic eczema patients. Exp Dermatol 23:45–52
23. Suárez-Fariñas M, Tintle SJ, Shemer A, Chiricozzi A, Nograles K, Cardinale I, Duan S, Bowcock AM, Krueger JG, Guttman-Yassky E (2011) Nonlesional atopic dermatitis skin is characterized by broad terminal differentiation defects and variable immune abnormalities. J Allergy Clin Immunol 127:954–964. e951–954
24. Rebane A, Zimmermann M, Aab A, Baurecht H, Koreck A, Karelson M, Abram K, Metsalu T, Pihlap M, Meyer N, Fölster-Holst R, Nagy N, Kemeny L, Kingo K, Vilo J, Illig T, Akdis M, Franke A, Novak N, Weidinger S, Akdis CA (2012) Mechanisms of IFN-γ-induced apoptosis of human skin keratinocytes in patients with atopic dermatitis. J Allergy Clin Immunol 129:1297–1306
25. Gruber R, Börnchen C, Rose K, Daubmann A, Volksdorf T, Wladykowski E, Vidal-Y-Sy S, Peters EM, Danso M, Bouwstra JA, Hennies HC, Moll I, Schmuth M, Brandner JM (2015) Diverse regulation of Claudin-1 and Claudin-4 in atopic dermatitis. Am J Pathol 185(10):2777–2789
26. Mansouri Y, Guttman-Yassky E (2015) Immune pathways in atopic dermatitis, and definition of biomarkers through broad and targeted therapeutics. J Clin Med 4(5):858–873
27. Eyerich K, Novak N (2013) Immunology of atopic eczema: overcoming the Th1/Th2 paradigm. Allergy 68:974–982
28. Clausen ML, Jungersted JM, Andersen PS, Slotved HC, Krogfelt KA, Agner T (2013) Human β-defensin-2 as a marker for disease severity and skin barrier properties in atopic dermatitis. Br J Dermatol 169:587–593
29. Goo J, Ji JH, Jeon H, Kim MJ, Jeon SY, Cho MY, Lee SH, Choi EH (2010) Expression of antimicrobial peptides such as LL-37 and hBD-2 in nonlesional skin of atopic individuals. Pediatr Dermatol 27:341–348
30. Dhingra N, Suárez-Fariñas M, Fuentes-Duculan J, Gittler JK, Shemer A, Raz A, Fischetti VA, Krueger JG, Guttman-Yassky E (2013) Attenuated neutrophil axis in atopic dermatitis compared to psoriasis reflects TH17 pathway differences between these diseases. J Allergy Clin Immunol 132:498–501.e493
31. Kim BS (2015) Innate lymphoid cells in the skin. J Invest Dermatol 135:673–678
32. Maintz L, Novak N (2011) Modifications of the innate immune system in atopic dermatitis. J Innate Immun 3:131–141
33. Hammad H, Lambrecht BN (2015) Barrier epithelial cells and the control of type 2 immunity. Immunity 43:29–40
34. Tintle S, Shemer A, Suárez-Fariñas M, Fujita H, Gilleaudeau P, Sullivan-Whalen M, Johnson-Huang L, Chiricozzi A, Cardinale I, Duan S, Bowcock A, Krueger JG, Guttman-Yassky E (2011) Reversal of atopic dermatitis with narrow-band UVB phototherapy and biomarkers for therapeutic response. J Allergy Clin Immunol 128:583–593.e581–584
35. Gittler JK, Shemer A, Suárez-Fariñas M, Fuentes-Duculan J, Gulewicz KJ, Wang CQ, Mitsui H, Cardinale I, de Guzman Strong C, Krueger JG, Guttman-Yassky E (2012) Progressive activation of T(H)2/T(H)22 cytokines and selective epidermal proteins characterizes acute and chronic atopic dermatitis. J Allergy Clin Immunol 130:1344–1354
36. Soumelis V, Reche PA, Kanzler H, Yuan W, Edward G, Homey B, Gilliet M, Ho S, Antonenko S, Lauerma A, Smith K, Gorman D, Zurawski S, Abrams J, Menon S, McClanahan T, de Waal-Malefyt RR, Bazan F, Kastelein RA, Liu YJ (2002) Human epithelial cells trigger dendritic cell mediated allergic inflammation by producing TSLP. Nat Immunol 3:673–680
37. Baker BS (2006) The role of microorganisms in atopic dermatitis. Clin Exp Immunol 144:1–9
38. Salimi M, Barlow JL, Saunders SP, Xue L, Gutowska-Owsiak D, Wang X, Huang LC, Johnson D, Scanlon ST, McKenzie AN, Fallon PG, Ogg GS (2013) A role for IL-25 and IL-33-driven type-2 innate lymphoid cells in atopic dermatitis. J Exp Med 210:2939–2950
39. Kim BS, Siracusa MC, Saenz SA, Noti M, Monticelli LA, Sonnenberg GF, Hepworth MR, Van Voorhees AS, Comeau MR, Artis D (2013) TSLP elicits IL-33-independent innate lymphoid cell responses to promote skin inflammation. Sci Transl Med 5:170ra116
40. Jin H, He R, Oyoshi M, Geha RS (2009) Animal models of atopic dermatitis. J Invest Dermatol 129:31–40
41. Li M, Hener P, Zhang Z, Kato S, Metzger D, Chambon P (2006) Topical vitamin D3 and low-calcemic analogs induce thymic stromal lymphopoietin in mouse keratinocytes and trigger an atopic dermatitis. Proc Natl Acad Sci U S A 103:11736–11741
42. Li M, Hener P, Zhang Z, Ganti KP, Metzger D, Chambon P (2009) Induction of thymic stromal lymphopoietin expression in keratinocytes is necessary for generating an atopic dermatitis

upon application of the active vitamin D3 analogue MC903 on mouse skin. J Invest Dermatol 129:498–502

43. Leyva-Castillo JM, Hener P, Jiang H, Li M (2013) TSLP produced by keratinocytes promotes allergen sensitization through skin and thereby triggers atopic march in mice. J Invest Dermatol 133:154–163
44. Zhang Z, Hener P, Frossard N, Kato S, Metzger D, Li M, Chambon P (2009) Thymic stromal lymphopoietin overproduced by keratinocytes in mouse skin aggravates experimental asthma. Proc Natl Acad Sci U S A 106:1536–1541
45. Wang Q, Du J, Zhu J, Yang X, Zhou B (2015) Thymic stromal lymphopoietin signaling in CD4(+) T cells is required for TH2 memory. J Allergy Clin Immunol 135:781–791.e783
46. Rebane A, Runnel T, Aab A, Maslovskaja J, Rückert B, Zimmermann M, Plaas M, Kärner J, Treis A, Pihlap M, Haljasorg U, Hermann H, Nagy N, Kemeny L, Erm T, Kingo K, Li M, Boldin MP, Akdis CA (2014) MicroRNA-146a alleviates chronic skin inflammation in atopic dermatitis through suppression of innate immune responses in keratinocytes. J Allergy Clin Immunol 134:836–847.e811

Chapter 9

Particle Bombardment of Ex Vivo Skin to Deliver DNA and Express Proteins

Ena Sokol, Miranda Nijenhuis, Klaas A. Sjollema, Marcel F. Jonkman, Hendri H. Pas, and Ben N.G. Giepmans

Abstract

Particle bombardment of gold microparticles coated with plasmids, which are accelerated to high velocity, is used for transfection of cells within tissue. Using this method, cDNA encoding proteins of interest introduced into ex vivo living human skin enables studying of proteins of interest in real time. Here, technical aspects of particle bombardment of ex vivo skin are described using green fluorescent protein (GFP) as readout for efficiency. This method can be applied on numerous tissues, including in living model animals.

Key words Particle bombardment, Exogenous proteins, Green fluorescent protein, Helios gene gun, Ex vivo living human skin, Blistering diseases, Live imaging

1 Introduction

Particle bombardment is used as a physical method of cell transfection in which high density subcellular-sized particles coated with DNA are accelerated to high velocity to enter cells [1]. The gene gun was introduced in the 1980s to deliver DNA with brute force into plant cells to overcome the hard physical cell wall [2, 3]. Subsequently, the method was applied to mammalian cells, live mice, and intact brain slices [1, 4–6]. To date, gene delivery by particle bombardment has found its way to target cancer cells for therapy [7], and in several studies in rodents models to study vaccination [8], aiming to reduce the effects of inflammation [6], and to decolorize pigmented skin [4].

We use gene gun-mediated delivery of plasmids encoding green fluorescent protein (GFP) and/or chimeras to study pemphigus, an autoimmune blistering disease leading to loss of cell–cell adhesion in the skin and/or mucosa [9–11]. The autoantibodies target desmogleins (Dsg1–4) [12], building blocks of cell–cell adhesion structures (desmosomes) that provide strength to the tissue [13, 14].

Björn E. Clausen and Jon D. Laman (eds.), *Inflammation: Methods and Protocols*, Methods in Molecular Biology, vol. 1559, DOI 10.1007/978-1-4939-6786-5_9, © Springer Science+Business Media LLC 2017

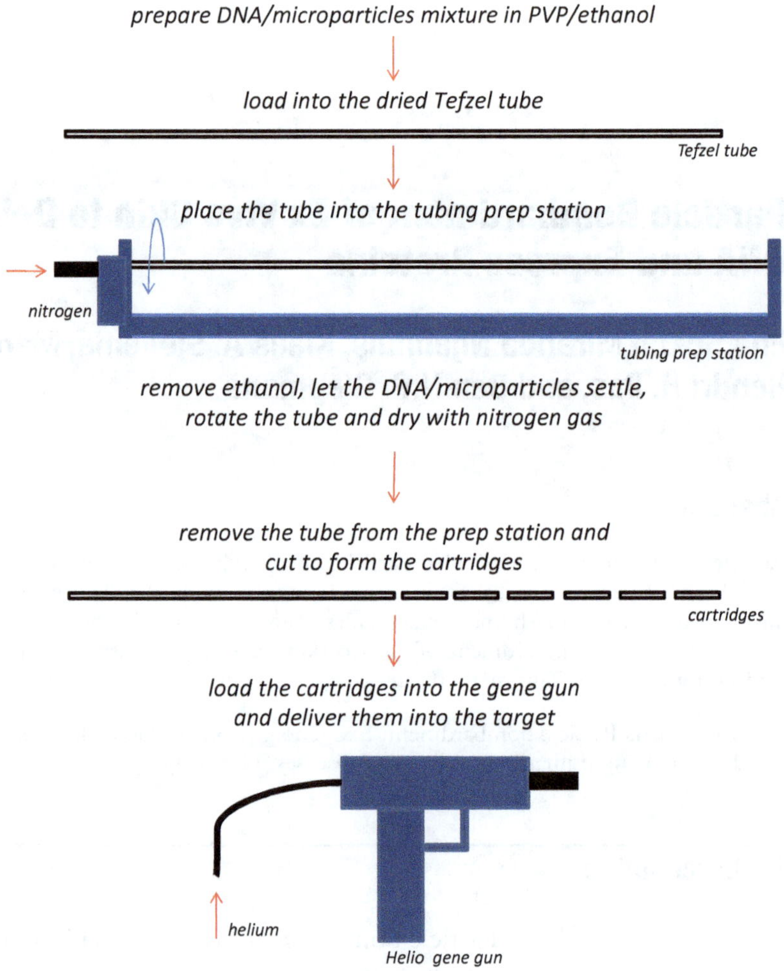

Fig. 1 Workflow of DNA–microparticles preparation

In search for the pemphigus pathomechanisms, several models are used: monolayers of cultured keratinocytes, skin 3D rafts, passive transfer mouse models, and ex vivo living human skin [15]. In cultured cell monolayers, autoantibodies (IgG) from a subtype of pemphigus patients cause internalization of Dsg3 followed by clustering of non-internalized Dsg3 proteins that form 'linear array' structures [16]. It is unknown if such a mechanism also occurs in patients, but auto-antibody-targeted desmogleins are relocalized and clustered in human skin. Loss of cell–cell adhesion can be induced in our cultured skin model within 24 h [17].

To follow the fate of IgG and desmoglein in tissue, we implement particle bombardment with a gene gun to deliver exogenous DNA encoding a chimeric of a desmosomal protein and a fluorescent protein in ex vivo living human skin. These can be imaged in real time using live fluorescence microscopy, thus

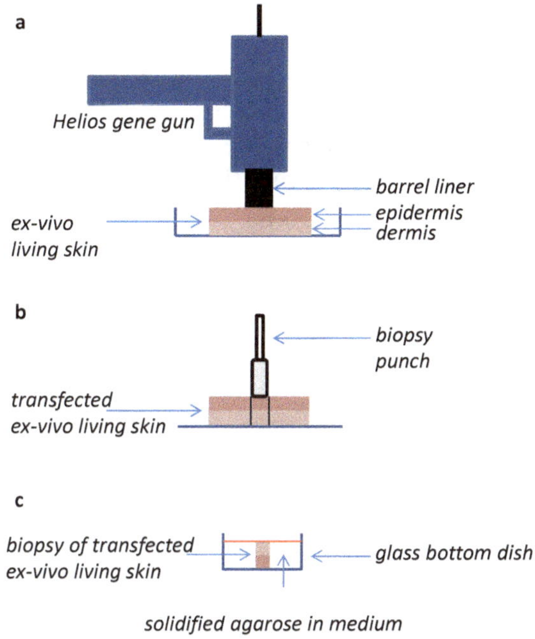

Fig. 2 Delivery of DNA–microparticles into the skin and preparation for live imaging. (**a**) DNA coated on the microparticles is delivered into the ex vivo living human skin using the Helios gene gun. The barrel liner is placed on the epidermal surface. (**b**) A punch biopsy is taken from the transfected skin ideally while the skin is placed on a silicone mold and stretched (not shown). (**c**) The transfected skin biopsy is placed into the glass bottom dish and stabilized using low melting point agarose in medium. Note that the epidermis is placed down because we use an inverted microscope. The level of medium is indicated with a *red line*. Check **Note 12** when using an upright microscope

bypassing the need for fixation and permeabilization or physical sectioning [18]. Here, the protocol for delivery of DNA and analysis of the expression in ex vivo skin is described. The protocol can be applied or used as a starting point to introduce cDNA encoding proteins of interest in skin of animals models.

The general bombardment workflow (Fig. 1) is as follows: preparation of (1) DNA–microparticles mixture; (2) the cartridges; (3) the tissue; followed by (4) DNA delivery into the tissue and finally (5) analysis by fluorescence microscopy. First, a suspension of DNA and microparticles is made which is injected into a tubing system and equally redistributed on the tubing prep station. The tube with DNA–microparticles is cut into the smaller pieces: the bullets. These are loaded into the Helios gene gun. Under pressure of helium, DNA–microparticles suspension coated on the inner side of the cartridges is propelled into the target tissue (Fig. 2). The fluorescent protein will be expressed and is typically analyzed after 1 day using live imaging, but can also be examined in cryosections.

2 Materials

2.1 Materials for Preparation of DNA–Microparticles Mixture

1. Gold microparticles.
2. Polyvinylpyrrolidone (PVP), a stock of 20 mg/ml in ethanol, store up to 1 month at −20 °C.
3. 0.5 M spermidine. Prepare 1 ml of 0.5 M spermidine in 100% ethanol.
4. Purified plasmid DNA (1 mg/ml) in distilled water.
5. 1 M calcium chloride.
6. Vortex device.
7. Ultrasonic cleaner.
8. 15 ml tubes.
9. 1.5 ml microfuge tubes.
10. 100% ethanol.
11. Analytical balance.

2.2 Materials for Loading the DNA–Microparticles

1. Gene gun tubing prep station.
2. Tetzel tubing.
3. Tank with regulator with compressed nitrogen of grade 4.5 (99.995%) or more.
4. Nitrogen hose.
5. Adaptor tubing.
6. 10 ml syringe.
7. Tubing cutter.
8. Scissors.
9. Marking pen.

2.3 Materials for Delivery of the DNA–Microparticles into the Target

1. Helios gene gun.
2. Tank with regulator with compressed helium of grade 4.5 (99.995%) or more.
3. Barrel liners washed in 70% ethanol.
4. Cartridge holder washed in 70% ethanol.
5. Helium hose.
6. Ear protection.
7. Gloves.
8. Flow hood.

2.4 Target Tissue

1. Redundant human skin or animal skin.
2. Cell medium, like Dulbecco's Modified Eagle Medium (DMEM) with 10% fetal bovine serum (FBS).

3. Hank's balanced salt solution (HBSS).
4. Sterile surgical scissors.
5. Sterile surgical tweezers.
6. Sterile 6-well plates.
7. Gloves.
8. Flow hood.

2.5 Examination of Transfection

1. Fluorescence microscope.
2. 6 mm sterile biopsy punch.
3. Sterile silicone mold.
4. Sterile needles of 0.5×16 mm.
5. Cell medium, like DMEM without phenol red, supplemented with 10% FBS.

2.6 Preparation for Imaging of Transfected Tissue

1. Fluorescence microscope.
2. Low melting point agarose.
3. Cell medium, like DMEM without phenol red, supplemented with 10% FBS.
4. Sterile 35 mm glass bottom dishes.
5. Sterile tweezers.

2.7 Material for Tissue Sectioning and Examination

1. Liquid nitrogen.
2. Liquid nitrogen tank.
3. Small metal cans for biopsies.
4. Cryostat.
5. Hair dryer.
6. Microscopic glass.
7. Fluorescence microscope.
8. Nuclear stain.
9. Mounting medium.

3 Methods

3.1 DNA–Microparticles Mixture

Purified plasmid DNA is precipitated on the microparticles and loaded in the Tefzel tube to prepare the cartridges. The DNA–microparticles will be propelled into the target tissue by helium pressure.

It is important to optimize the ratio between the amount of DNA and microparticles and the amount of microparticles delivered per target, the concentration of PVP and to define the optimal helium pressure that will lead to the most efficient protein expression (*see* **Note 1**). Here we use parameters that are optimal for delivery of DNA encoding GFP to the epidermis of ex vivo living human skin. The 1 ml DNA–microparticles mixture will create 17 cartridges (*see* **Note 2**).

1. Prepare PVP in 100% ethanol with a concentration of 0.1 mg/ml.
2. Weigh 8.33 μg of 1.0 μm gold microparticles in a 1.5 ml microfuge tube. For other sized microparticles *see* **Note 3**.
3. Add 100 μl of 0.5 M spermidine to the gold microparticles.
4. Vortex for 5 s, then sonicate in the ultrasonic cleaner for 5 s.
5. Add 16.6 μg of plasmid DNA. If using more than one plasmid with different tags, all of them should be added at this step.
6. Vortex for 5 s.
7. Sonicate for 5 s.
8. Add 100 μl of 1 M $CaCl_2$ in a dropwise manner.
9. Leave for 10 min at room temperature to precipitate.
10. Spin 15 s and discard the supernatant, which should be clear.
11. Resuspend the pellet and wash 3× with 1 ml ethanol discarding the supernatants.
12. Add PVP–ethanol (0.1 mg/ml) to the pellet to reach a final volume of 1 ml. For larger volumes *see* **Note 4**.
13. The suspension can be directly used or stored at −20 °C up to 2 months.

3.2 DNA–Microparticles Cartridges

Cartridges are prepared by loading the DNA–microparticles suspension into the prep station provided by the Helios gene gun system (Fig. 1). The suspension is evenly loaded and microparticles with DNA are settled inside the Tetzel tube and evenly distributed by rotations, while ethanol is removed and the tube is dried by nitrogen gas. The cartridges are made by cutting the Tetzel tube with the DNA–microparticles coated inside and can be inspected under the light microscope to determine the presence of microparticles and their density. Follow the manufacturer's protocol to set up the tube preparation station.

1. Insert uncut Tefzel tube into the tubing prep station connected to the nitrogen source.
2. Adjust the nitrogen flow on the prep station to 0.3–0.4 l per minute (LPM).
3. Dry the tube with nitrogen for 15 min prior the loading of the DNA–microparticles mixture.
4. Turn off the nitrogen flow.
5. Remove the dried Tefzel tube from the prep station and cut 75 cm of the tube (*see* **Note 5**).

6. Vortex the DNA–microparticles suspension, so that all the clumps are removed.
7. Connect a 10 ml syringe with a support tube to the Tefzel tube.
8. Bring the DNA–microparticles suspension with a syringe into the Tefzel tube and bring back the tube to the horizontal position to the prep station.
9. Allow the DNA–microparticles to settle for 5 min.
10. Using the connected syringe move the liquid back by constant speed (*see* **Note 6**) leaving the settled microparticles in.
11. Discard the liquid and disconnect the syringe.
12. Turn the rotator on.
13. Open the nitrogen gas, adjust the flow to 0.4 LPM and leave for 5 min while rotating.
14. Turn off the rotator and the nitrogen flow.
15. Inspect under the light microscope the presence of gold microparticles and mark with a pen the beginning and the end of the Tefzel tube with microparticles.
16. Cut the empty pieces of the Tefzel tube with scissors.
17. Cut the Tefzel tube with microparticles using the cutting device to create cartridges.
18. The cartridges can be directly inserted in the Helios gen gun to deliver DNA to the target tissue or can be stored at 4 °C. It is recommended not to store them longer than 1 month.
19. Prior to delivery into the skin it is recommended to test the cartridges (*see* **Note 7**).

3.3 Manipulation of the Target Tissue

We use live human skin taken immediately after surgery (*see* **Note 8**) [19]. Prior to receiving the skin prepare the hood and all the necessary materials and always work with gloves.

1. Upon receiving the skin, transfer it into a sterile plastic tube.
2. Wash the skin in HBSS and inspect the pieces of the skin (*see* **Notes 9** and **10**).
3. If subdermal tissue is present, remove it using sterile scissors.
4. With sterile scissors cut pieces more than 1 × 1 cm that will fit the barrel of the gene gun.
5. Place the pieces into the 6-well dishes with appropriate medium, so that the epidermis is in contact with the air. Do not submerge the skin completely in the medium!

3.4 Delivery of the DNA–Microparticles into Tissue

Cartridges with DNA–microparticles are loaded into the Helios gene gun and under helium pressure propelled into the tissue. We use helium pressure of 300 lb per square inch (psi) for the delivery.

See **Note 1** for the optimization and **Note 11** for testing the Helios gene gun. The Helios gene gun should be set according to the manufacturer's protocol.

1. Load the cartridges into the cartridge holder starting from number 1.
2. Place the holder into the Helios gene gun.
3. Place the linear barrel into the Helios gene gun.
4. Connect the Helios gene gun with the helium tank and set to 300 psi.
5. Place the battery into the Helios gene gun.
6. Place ear protection.
7. Remove the medium from a well with the targeted tissue.
8. Place the linear barrel vertical to the skin touching the epidermal side.
9. Activate the safety interlock and press the trigger button to deliver the DNA–microparticles.
10. Add new medium into the well with the transfected skin leaving the epidermis in the air.
11. Repeat the DNA delivery depending on the number of cartridges and samples. Before discharging the next cartridge change its position in the cartridge holder in the Helios gene gun in order to propelle the appropriate cartridge.
12. Leave the skin in the incubator of 37 °C with 5% CO_2 overnight.

3.5 Examination of Transfection

The transfected tissue can be examined for protein expression 24 h after transfection. It can be examined in the uncut version (the whole piece of skin) or in form of biopsies (Fig. 3).

1. If using an inverted microscope, skin can be examined in ocular mode to detect the fluorescent signal (GFP) in 6 well dishes from the **steps 3** and **4**.
2. If the fluorescent signal is positive proceed with **step 3**.
3. In the flow hood, stretch the skin on a silicone mold using sterile needles.
4. Cut 6-mm biopsies from the transfected piece of skin on the mold.
5. Place the biopsies in glass bottom dishes.
6. Add an appropriate amount of medium.
7. Examine fluorescence: We use the Lambda mode of a Zeiss 780 microscope (Fig. 4) to check emission spectra. Note that skin auto-fluoresces and therefore it is essential to perform this step.

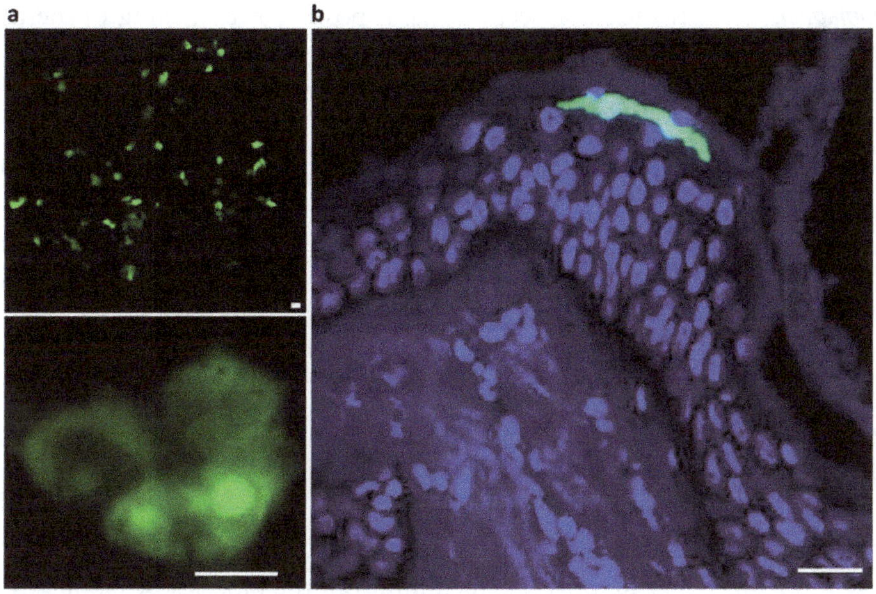

Fig. 3 Analysis of GFP in transfected living skin. (**a**) Skin after delivery of DNA encoding GFP in full thickness and imaged from the epidermal side. *Top*: Around 60 GFP positive cells. *Bottom*: enlarged region showing two transfected cells. (**b**) Cross section of transfected skin showing localization of the transfected cell (*green*) in relation to the epidermal layers (nuclei have been counterstained; *blue*). Bars: 20 μm

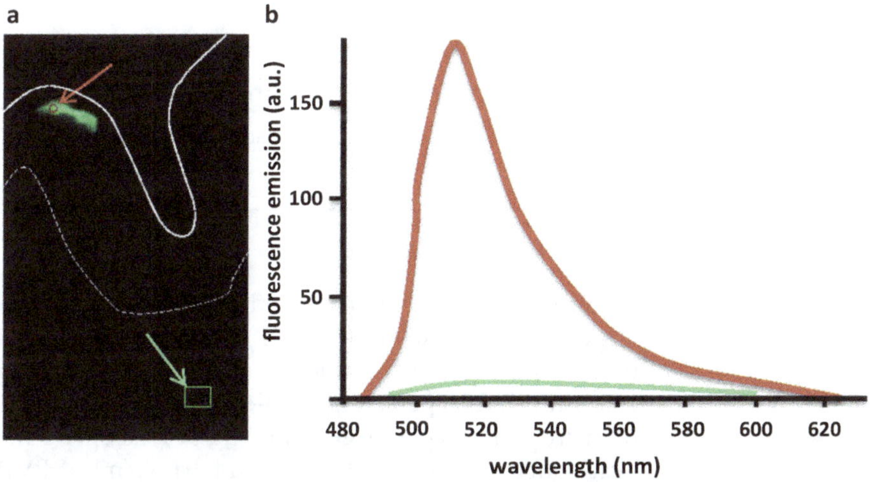

Fig. 4 GFP emission from transfected ex vivo living human skin. (**a**) Section of skin after gene-delivery imaged in lambda mode with 488 nm excitation. (**b**) Emission from areas indicated with *arrows*. The colors of the regions of interest match the colors used in the spectra. Note that the emission of the *red area* corresponds to the known GFP emission spectra. *a.u.* arbitrary units

3.6 Live Imaging of Transfected Tissue

If the fluorescent signal is positive live imaging of the transfected tissue can be performed. To keep the biopsy stable, these are incubated in low melting point agarose mixed with medium, which solidifies at room temperature.

1. Prepare low melting point agarose (0.4 % together in medium) and keep at 37 °C.
2. Place skin biopsy (*see* **Note 12**) in a 35 mm glass bottom dish.
3. Pour the low melting point agarose in the dish with the biopsy.
4. Leave at room temperature to solidify.
5. Place into the microscope and perform live imaging.

3.7 Cyrosectioning of Transfected Tissue

If the fluorescent signal is positive, it is optional to examine which epidermal/dermal layer is transfected. This can be done by cryosectioning the tissue biopsies (Figs. 3 and 4). The sections can be further stained for other molecules or features of interest.

1. Remove the medium from the biopsies by tapping these a few times on tissue paper.
2. Place the biopsy in the cap of the metal can.
3. Place the metal can with the biopsy in it in the liquid nitrogen.
4. Store at −80 °C or proceed directly with sectioning.
5. Cut 4 μm sections in the cryostat and place sections on the microscopic glass.
6. Dry with the hair dryer for 15 min.
7. Optionally perform nuclear staining or immunolabeling.
8. Examine the sections for fluorescence (Fig. 2b).

4 Notes

1. Optimize the parameters for efficient DNA delivery into the target in the following order: (1) helium pressure, (2) concentration of PVP, (3) the amount of gold per target and (4) the amount of DNA per 1 mg of microparticles. Start with 0.5 mg of microparticles per target and 2 μg of DNA per 1 mg of gold. Test concentrations of 0, 0.05, and 1 mg/ml of PVP and test helium pressure of 50, 100, 200, and 400 psi.
2. 1 ml DNA–microparticles suspension can fill 21.5 cm of the Tefzel tube, of which around 17 cartridges can be made. In order to fill the complete Tefzel tube of 76.2 cm that can fit into the tube prep station 3 ml of suspension should be made which can fill off approximately 63.5 cm leaving free ends.

3. The sizes of microparticles are 0.6, 1.0, and 1.6 μm gold. It is recommended to test which are the most suitable for the desired target tissue.
4. If a larger volume of DNA–mircoparticles solution is used, add 200 μl of PVP–ethanol in appropriate concentration, resuspend and transfer to a 15 ml tube (**step 12**). Next, add the PVP–ethanol to generate the appropriate final volume.
5. The entire 75 cm Tefzel tube should be used, even if the solution only partially fills the tube.
6. Load the DNA–microparticles suspension into the Tefzel tube with a constant speed. It is recommended to practice by loading ethanol and removing ethanol at a rate of 1.27–2.54 cm/s. If a peristaltic pump is available it should be calibrated and used.
7. Validate the DNA–microparticles by transfecting an easier target, such as cell lines, prior to delivery to skin. Remember to use lower helium pressure for cell lines and primary cells. We recommend 100 psi.
8. Keep the time to transfer the skin from the clinic to the lab to a minimum (<30 min). We have noticed changes in the ultrastructure of the human skin if the time is prolonged.
9. Size and shape of the human skin pieces depends on the surgery type. Chose the operation type were it is possible to have bigger skin pieces with less of subdermal tissue.
10. Never pick up the skin by the dermal side, it is very sticky to the tweezers and hard to manipulate. Always try to hold the skin at the epidermal side.
11. Test the Helios gene gun before the delivery of the DNA–microparticles using an empty cartridge holder.
12. When using an inverted microscope, the epidermis should be in contact with the glass bottom of the dish and the whole biopsy should be merged in medium/low melting point agarose. If an upright microscope is used, the epidermis is up and in contact with air.

Acknowledgment

We thank Oscar Stassen and Elly Hol (Free University Amsterdam, now Utrecht University) for training. Part of the work has been performed in the UMCG Microscopy and Imaging Center (UMIC). Funding for these studies was provided by the Netherlands Organization for Scientific Research (*NWO 175-010-2009-023*) and the Gratama Foundation.

References

1. Uchida M, Li XW, Mertens P et al (2009) Transfection by particle bombardment: delivery of plasmid DNA into mammalian cells using gene gun. Biochim Biophys Acta 1790(8):754–764
2. Klein TM, Fromm M, Weissinger A et al (1988) Transfer of foreign genes into intact maize cells with high-velocity microprojectiles. Proc Natl Acad Sci U S A 85(12):4305–4309
3. Klein TM, Arentzen R, Lewis PA et al (1992) Transformation of microbes, plants and animals by particle bombardment. Biotechnology (N Y) 10(3):286–291
4. Yang CH, Shen SC, Lee JC et al (2004) Seeing the gene therapy: application of gene gun technique to transfect and decolour pigmented rat skin with human agouti signalling protein cDNA. Gene Ther 11(13):1033–1039
5. Lo DC, McAllister AK, Katz LC (1994) Neuronal transfection in brain slices using particle-mediated gene transfer. Neuron 13(6):1263–1268
6. Lu B, Scott G, Goldsmith LA (1996) A model for keratinocyte gene therapy: preclinical and therapeutic considerations. Proc Assoc Am Physicians 108(2):165–172
7. Zilony N, Tzur-Balter A, Segal E et al (2013) Bombarding cancer: biolistic delivery of therapeutics using porous Si carriers. Sci Rep 3:2499
8. Chen CH, Ji H, Suh KW et al (1999) Gene gun-mediated DNA vaccination induces antitumor immunity against human papillomavirus type 16 E7-expressing murine tumor metastases in the liver and lungs. Gene Ther 6(12):1972–1981
9. Stanley JR, Amagai M (2006) Pemphigus, bullous impetigo, and the staphylococcal scalded-skin syndrome. N Engl J Med 355(17):1800–1810
10. Ioannides D, Lazaridou E, Rigopoulos D (2008) Pemphigus. J Eur Acad Dermatol Venereol 22(12):1478–1496
11. Sokol E, Kramer D, Diercks GF et al (2015) Large-scale electron microscopy maps of patient skin and mucosa provide insight into pathogenesis of blistering diseases. J Invest Dermatol 135(7):1763–1770
12. Garrod DR, Merritt AJ, Nie Z (2002) Desmosomal cadherins. Curr Opin Cell Biol 14(5):537–545
13. Amagai M, Stanley JR (2012) Desmoglein as a target in skin disease and beyond. J Invest Dermatol 132(3 Pt 2):776–784
14. Waschke J (2008) The desmosome and pemphigus. Histochem Cell Biol 130(1):21–54
15. van der Wier G, Pas HH, Jonkman MF (2010) Experimental human cell and tissue models of pemphigus. Dermatol Res Pract 2010:143871
16. Jennings JM, Tucker DK, Kottke MD et al (2011) Desmosome disassembly in response to pemphigus vulgaris IgG occurs in distinct phases and can be reversed by expression of exogenous Dsg3. J Invest Dermatol 131(3):706–718
17. Oktarina DA, van der Wier G, Diercks GF et al (2011) IgG-induced clustering of desmogleins 1 and 3 in skin of patients with pemphigus fits with the desmoglein nonassembly depletion hypothesis. Br J Dermatol 165(3):552–562
18. Schnell U, Dijk F, Sjollema KA et al (2012) Immunolabeling artifacts and the need for live-cell imaging. Nat Methods 9(2):152–158
19. Oktarina DA, Poot AM, Kramer D et al (2012) The IgG "lupus-band" deposition pattern of pemphigus erythematosus: association with the desmoglein 1 ectodomain as revealed by 3 cases. Arch Dermatol 148(10):1173–1178

Part II

Inflammation of the Lung

Chapter 10

Murine Models of Allergic Asthma

Eline Haspeslagh, Nincy Debeuf, Hamida Hammad, and Bart N. Lambrecht

Abstract

Allergic asthma is a heterogeneous inflammatory lung disease affecting millions of people worldwide and with a steadily increasing incidence. Mouse models have been of utmost importance in uncovering key inflammatory cell types, cytokines, and pathways in the development and maintenance of allergic asthma. Historically, the mainstay in experimental asthma research was sensitizing rodents to the model protein antigen ovalbumin (OVA) with the pro-Th2 adjuvant aluminum hydroxide, followed by repetitive OVA exposures to the airways to initiate a Th2-skewed adaptive immune response leading to eosinophilic airway inflammation and airway hyperreactivity (AHR). In the last 5 years, OVA is often replaced by naturally occurring allergens such as house dust mite (HDM) or cockroach extracts, but the principle of first sensitizing and then repetitively challenging mice with the same antigen is unchanged. Here, we describe an often used and relevant HDM-based protocol to establish acute allergic asthma, and the methods we have developed to rapidly analyze inflammatory cell infiltration in the bronchalveolar lavage fluid by flow cytometry. Moreover, we explain the methods to restimulate T cells from lung-draining mediastinal lymph nodes with HDM to allow the measurement of cytokine secretion profiles of allergen reactive T cells.

Key words Acute allergic asthma, Bronchoalveolar lavage, Eosinophilia, Flow cytometry, House dust mite (HDM), Mediastinal lymph nodes, Murine model, Ovalbumin (OVA)

1 Introduction

Worldwide, more than 300 million people suffer from asthma and its incidence is continuously increasing. Asthma is a chronic airway disorder characterized by lung inflammation, airway hyperreactivity (AHR) to nonspecific stimuli and recurring episodes of airway obstruction, sometimes leading to permanent airway remodeling and impaired airway function. Allergic asthma, which accounts for about 80% of asthma cases, is often described as a Th2-driven disease characterized by IL-5 dependent lung eosinophilia, IL-4 dependent elevated IgE serum levels and IL-13 dependent AHR and goblet cell metaplasia (GCM) [1, 2]. Not surprisingly, high levels of Th2 cytokines can be detected in lung tissue and bronchoalveolar lavage (BAL) fluid. Current treatments for asthma

Björn E. Clausen and Jon D. Laman (eds.), *Inflammation: Methods and Protocols*, Methods in Molecular Biology, vol. 1559, DOI 10.1007/978-1-4939-6786-5_10, © Springer Science+Business Media LLC 2017

mainly consist of inhaled corticosteroids and long acting bronchodilators, and act in reducing the symptoms without curing the disease. Although these treatments are effective in most patients, they can be unsuccessful in some patients and may have side effects [3]. Thus, there is a continuous search for better targeted treatment strategies that are based on mechanistic insights into disease development and progression.

Mouse models have been of invaluable importance in elucidating key cytokines, cellular networks and pathways in both the development and effector phases of allergic asthma. Recently several new drugs that were discovered in mouse models (such as neutralizing IL-5 antibodies in eosinophil-rich asthma) have been approved by the Food and Drug Administration. Until a decade ago, the model antigen ovalbumin (OVA) was the mainstay in murine asthma models. In these protocols, mice were first immunized systemically once or twice with OVA via intraperitoneal (i.p.), intradermal or subcutaneous injection, typically together with the adjuvant aluminium hydroxide (alum) to skew the resulting immune response towards a Th2-driven response. This was followed by repetitive intratracheal (i.t.), intranasal (i.n.), or aerosolized OVA-challenges, resulting in an acute and robust influx of eosinophils in the lungs and the establishment of AHR [4]. OVA-models are rather cheap and are easy to use considering the tools available. For example, the TCR transgenic OT-I and OT-II mice, that possess OVA-specific CD8+ and CD4+ T cells, respectively, are commercially available. Moreover, OVA-based models have proven extremely valuable in uncovering critical steps in the induction and maintenance of Th2-mediated asthma. For example, it has been shown that the observed eosinophilia and AHR are independent of IgE or B cells, but require the activation of CD4+ T lymphocytes via IL-4 mediated activation of the STAT6 pathway [5, 6]. The resulting Th2 cells secrete amongst others IL-5 and IL-13, which play a prominent role in eosinophil activation, and airway remodeling and mucus hyperplasia, respectively [7, 8]. The critical role of dendritic cells (DCs) in the OVA asthma model has been studied in models where DCs were depleted during either sensitization or challenge to OVA and in studies in which the i.p. sensitization of OVA/alum was shown to be completely dependent on monocyte derived DCs [9–11].

However, newly developed drugs targeting the identified key players and showing efficacy in the murine OVA-model often did not prove successful in clinical trials [12–14]. Differences in the underlying mechanisms of disease between OVA-mice and human patients may account for the failures in clinical translation. Repetitive OVA sensitization via the lung only leads to a very weak response after OVA-challenges. In the absence of TLR agonists, the outcome of OVA inhalation can even be immunological tolerance. Robust sensitization via the pulmonary route requires the concomitant administration of the TLR4 agonist LPS [15]. In this scenario of pulmonary sensitization, TLR activation by LPS and/or other immunostimulating pathogen associated molecular patterns (PAMPs) is necessary for the maturation and activation of antigen presenting cells (APCs), like DCs. Moreover, the LPS dose can influence the resulting immune response; whereas OVA administered together with high LPS doses induces a Th1-like response, low doses of concomitant LPS lead to a Th2-like immune response. The use of alum bypasses the requirement for PAMPs, but might therefore also bypass innate signals and pathways that naturally occur in human sensitization and can modify the resulting immediate and effector immune responses to allergens.

Recently, new acute models of allergic asthma have been validated that make use of naturally occurring allergens, such as extracts of house dust mite, cockroach or *Alternaria alternata*. In these models, sensitization is carried out via the pulmonary route, without any need for adjuvant, and triggers a vast immediate innate immune response next to the initiation of adaptive immunity [16]. These models mimic human disease more closely and aid in unraveling important aspects of allergic sensitization that were not significant in the OVA-induced model, such as the necessity of epithelial expressed TLR4 for efficient sensitization to HDM [17].

It should be taken into account that also these models show caveats worth mentioning. Whereas human asthma is a chronic condition, inflammation and AHR typically resolve in acute murine models when challenges are stopped [18]. Next, it is now appreciated that asthma is a very heterogeneous disease with multiple phenotypes and endotypes. For example, one subset of patients has very high levels of neutrophils and Th17-associated cytokines in BAL, which is not reflected in the standard HDM-induced asthma model [19]. Depending on the research question, chronic model or models of neutrophilic asthma can be used to bypass these issues. Still, to resolve questions about the eosinophil-rich, steroid-sensitive endotype of human asthma, which is present in about half of the patients, the HDM-induced asthma model proved to be a valid model.

In this protocol, we explain how to establish HDM-induced or OVA-induced acute allergic asthma in mice and how to analyze the influx of inflammatory cells in BAL fluid by flow cytometry. Moreover, we describe how to restimulate the T cells from mediastinal lymph nodes (MLNs) with HDM to study their capacity to secrete Th2 and other cytokines. These are two main read-outs informative for the strength and the nature of the adaptive immune response.

2 Materials

2.1 Establishment of a Mouse Model of HDM-Induced Acute Allergic Asthma

1. 6–8 week old C57Bl/6 mice, ideally specified-pathogen free (*see* **Notes 1** and **2**).

2. Small animal anesthesia device compatible with isoflurane and a connected induction chamber.
3. Vertical restraining device for intratracheal installation (*see* Fig. 1).
4. Non-sharp forceps.
5. Isoflurane.
6. House dust mite (HDM) extract from Greer Laboratories, diluted in sterile phosphate buffered saline (PBS) to a concentration of 5 mg protein content/mL (*see* **Notes 3** and **4**).

2.2 Establishment of a Mouse Model of OVA-Induced Acute Allergic Asthma

1. Standard laboratory equipment including a shaker, a balance, ethanol 70% (v/v), syringes, and 26 gauge needles.
2. Small animal aerosol inhalation chamber with nebulizer.
3. OVA grade V and grade III from Sigma Aldrich.
4. Sterile aluminum hydroxide ($Al(OH_3)$).
5. Sterile PBS.

2.3 Analysis of the Infiltration of Inflammatory Cells in BAL Fluid

1. Standard laboratory equipment including syringes, needles (23 and 26 gauge), a centrifuge, an aspirator, a round bottom 96-well plate, and fluorescence-activated cell sorting (FACS) tubes.
2. Dissection material including forceps and scissors.
3. A three laser flow cytometer.
4. A light microscope, Bürker chamber, and trypan blue for manual cell counting.
5. Cannulas, made of 23 Gauge needles with a small piece of polyethylene tubing around the sharp needle points.
6. Small strings.

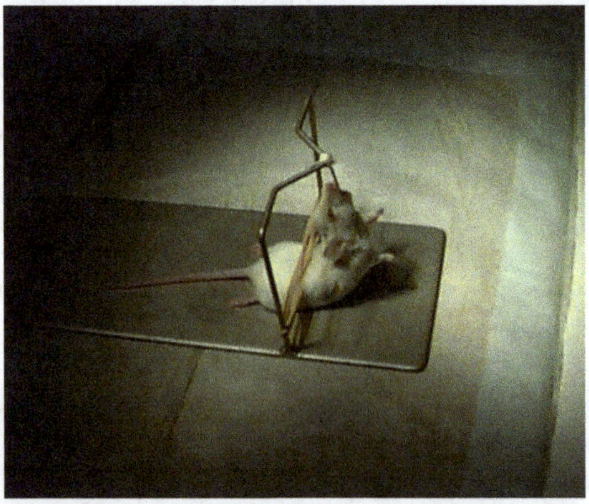

Fig. 1 Vertical mouse restraining device for intratracheal instillation

7. Pentobarbital or another anesthetic.
8. PBS containing 0.5 mM EDTA for taking BAL fluid.
9. FACS buffer consisting of PBS containing 0.25 % BSA, 0.5 mM EDTA, and 0.05 % NaN_3 (*see* **Note 5**).
10. (Optional) osmotic lysis buffer: ddH_2O containing 0.83 % NH_4Cl, 0.1 % $KHCO_3$, and 0.1 M EDTA at a pH between 7.1 and 7.4 (adjusted with HEPES).
11. Staining mix comprised of antibodies in Table 1, diluted in FACS buffer (*see* **Notes 5** and **6**).

2.4 Restimulation of MLN Cells with HDM

1. Standard laboratory equipment including a 24-well plate, 100 or 70 μm meshes, small petri dishes, and syringes (all sterile).
2. Dissection material including forceps and scissors.
3. A CO_2 incubator.
4. A sterile 96-well culture plate.
5. A light microscope, Bürker chamber, and trypan blue for manual cell counting.
6. House dust mite (HDM) extract (Greer Laboratories), diluted in sterile PBS to a concentration of 5 mg protein content/mL.
7. Tissue culture medium (TCM), consisting of $RPMI^-$ 1640 medium with GlutaMAX-1 (diluted according to manufactur-

Table 1
Antibody composition of the flow cytometry staining mix for analysis of BAL fluid (*see* also Notes 5 and 6)

Specificity	Clone	Fluorochrome	Excitation laser	Species	Isotype	Supplier	Dilution
Siglec-F	E50-2440	PE	488 or 561 nm	Rat	IgG2a	BD Pharmingen	1/1000
CD3e	145-2C11	PE-Cy5	488 or 561 nm	Armenian Hamster	IgG	Tonbo Biosciences	1/200
CD19	eBio1D3	PE-Cy5	488 or 561 nm	Rat	IgG2a	eBioscience	1/400
CD11c	N418	PE-Cy7	488 or 561 nm	Armenian Hamster	IgG	eBioscience	1/800
CD11b	M1/70	BD Horizon V450	405 nm	Rat	IgG2b	BD Pharmingen	1/800
Ly-6G	1A8	AF700	633 nm	Rat	IgG2a	BD Pharmingen	1/500
MHC-II	M5/114.15.2	APC-eFluor780	633 nm	Rat	IgG2b	eBioscience	1/1000
CD16/CD32 (Fc-block)		Unlabeled					1/400

er's instructions), 5% fetal calf serum, gentamycin (diluted according to manufacturer's instructions) and 5×10^{-5} M β-mercaptoethanol.

3 Methods

3.1 Establishment of a Mouse Model of HDM-Induced Acute Allergic Asthma

1. Dilute the HDM stock (5 mg/mL) to 12.5 μg/mL in sterile PBS (1 μg in 80 μL/mouse) under sterile conditions (*see* **Note** 7).
2. Intratracheal instillation: on day 0, anesthetize mice with 2–2.5% isoflurane in air or O_2, then place them on the restraining device in a vertical head-up position with the hind legs on the bench, and by fixing the two front teeth in a loop of string (*see* Fig. 1). Gently pull the tongue out with non-sharp forceps to prevent any swallowing. Pipet 80 μL of diluted HDM extract, or 80 μL PBS as a control, into the mouth and keep mice in this position until all the fluid is inhaled (*see* **Notes 8** and **9**).
3. Dilute the HDM stock (5 mg/mL) to 250 μg/mL in sterile PBS (10 μg in 40 μL/mouse) under sterile conditions (*see* **Note** 7).
4. From days 7 to 11, challenge the mice daily intranasally by pipetting 40 μL of diluted HDM extract directly into the nostrils of isoflurane (2%)-sedated mice (*see* **Note 10**).

3.2 Establishment of a Mouse Model of OVA-Induced Acute Allergic Asthma

1. Prepare an OVA/alum solution of 500 μL sterile PBS per mouse containing 20 μg/mL OVA grade V and 2 mg/mL Alum. Just before use, rotate for 30 min at room temperature.
2. Intraperitoneal (i.p.) injection: on days 0 and 7, disinfect and clean the belly of the mice by spraying 70% ethanol (v/v) and inject 500 μL OVA/alum solution, or 500 μL PBS as a control in the left lower quadrant just beneath the nipple with a 26 G needle. Hold the mice with their head downwards to make sure organs are not pricked (*see* **Note 11**).
3. From days 14 to 20, daily challenge mice in an inhalation chamber by aerosolizing about 10 mL of 1% OVA grade III in sterile PBS with a nebulizer (*see* **Note 12**).

3.3 Collection and Analysis of Bronchoalveolar Lavage (BAL) Fluid

1. Three or four days after the last challenge, euthanize mice by giving them an overdose of pentobarbital (100 μL i.p. with 26 G needle).
2. Cut the chest wall open up to the chin and remove fat, salivary glands and the surrounding tegument to expose the trachea. Make a small incision in the trachea between the first and second cartilage ring, bring in a cannula and retain it by knotting

a string around the cannula and trachea. Collect BAL fluid in a 15 mL tube by flushing the lungs three times with 1 mL of PBS containing 0.5 mM EDTA via a 1 mL syringe inserted in the cannula (*see* **Notes 13** and **14**). Repeat this step two times to reach a volume of 3 mL.

3. Centrifuge the BAL fluid for 7 min at $400\times g$ and 4 °C. Discard the supernatant, resuspend the pellet containing the cells in 200 μL FACS buffer, and transfer to a 96-well round bottom plate. Centrifuge the plate for 3 min at $400\times g$ and 4 °C, remove supernatant and again resuspend in 200 μL FACS buffer (*see* **Notes 15** and **16**).
4. Take a small sample (10 or 20 μL) and manually count cells.
5. Take some cells from every sample, pool and redistribute in seven wells for single stains and an unstained control. For one single stain, 50,000 cells are sufficient.
6. Centrifuge the plate for 3 min at $400\times g$ and 4 °C, discard supernatant and stain a maximum of 5×10^6 cells in 100 μL staining mix, consisting of Fc-block, SiglecF-PE, CD3-PE-Cy5, CD19-PE-Cy5, CD11c-PE-Cy7, CD11b-V450, Ly6G-AF700, and MHC-II-APC-eFluor780 in FACS buffer. Incubate for 30 min at 4 °C in the dark (*see* **Notes 5** and **6**).
7. Add 100 μL FACS buffer and centrifuge the plate ($400\times g$, 4 °C, 3 min). Remove supernatant, resuspend in 200 μL FACS buffer and transfer to FACS tubes for acquisition with a flow cytometer.

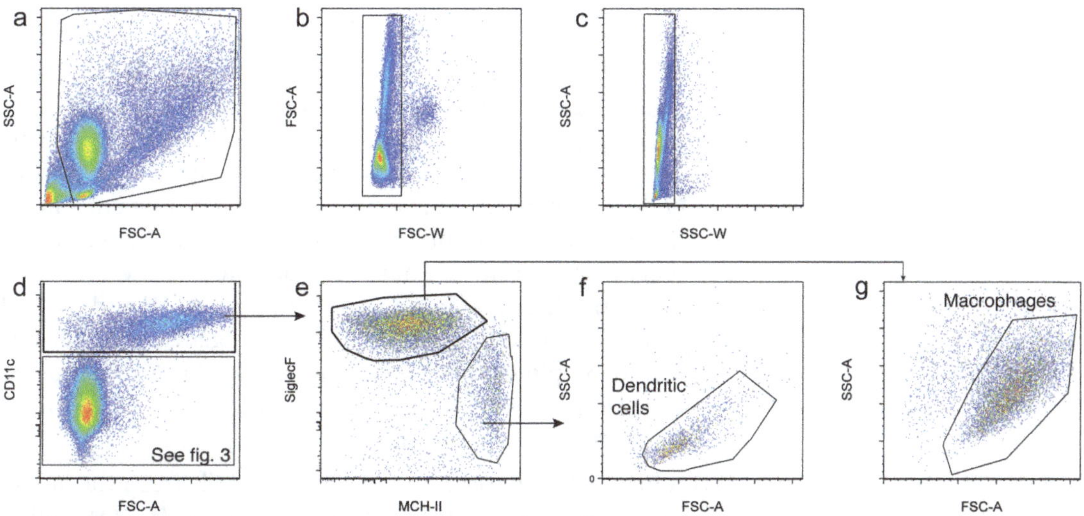

Fig. 2 Flow cytometry gating strategy for inflammatory cell populations in BAL fluid. Hierarchical gating of non-debris, single cells, CD11c^{hi} cells, and DCs and macrophages. See text for details

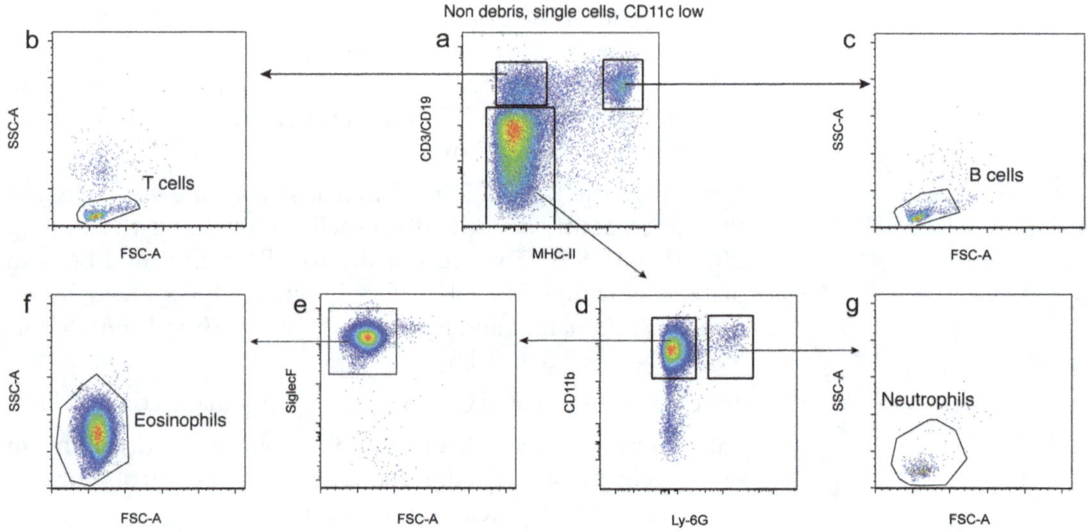

Fig. 3 Flow cytometry gating strategy for inflammatory cell populations in BAL fluid. Hierarchical subdivision of CD11c^{low} cells (*see* Fig. 1) in T cells, B cells, neutrophils, and eosinophils. See text for details

8. Several gating strategies are possible, but we propose a straightforward and validated strategy depicted in Figs. 2 and 3 that is consistently used in our lab (*see* **Note 17**).
   (a) Plot forward scatter-area (FSC-A) against side scatter-A (SSC-A) and exclude the debris that can be recognized as events with a very low signal for one or both parameters, in the lower left corner and at the edges of this plot (Fig. 2a). FSC-A and SSC-A are dependent on the size and the complexity of the cell, respectively. Events with very low FSC-A or SSC-A are too small to be cells and should therefore not be analyzed further.
   (b) Discriminate the doublets from the analysis. When a cell doublet passes the laser, the width (W), which is the time necessary for the doublet to pass the laser beam, will be higher than the W of a singlet. In contrast, the height (H), which is the maximum signal of the event and is dependent on the pulse voltage, is similar between singlets and doublets. Therefore, doublets show a disproportion when comparing the parameters W and H and can be excluded by plotting FSC-W against FSC-H, followed by plotting SSC-W against SSC-H. Similarly, one can also plot FSC-W against FSC-A ($A = W \times H$) followed by plotting SSC-W against SSC-A (Fig. 2b, c).
   (c) (Optional) If desirable, exclude dead cells from the analysis (*see* **Note 5**). Plot the fixable Live/Dead (L/D) marker against FSC-A. Gate out the dead cells that are L/D^{high} and small (low FSC-A). Cells with an intermediate to high

L/D signal and a high FSC-A tend to be big autofluorescent cells such as macrophages and are considered alive.

(d) Separate the remaining alive single cells in two populations based on CD11c expression (Fig. 2d). $CD11c^{high (hi)}$ cells comprise both dendritic cells (DCs) and macrophages, whereas all other cell populations are $CD11c^{low}$.

(e) In the $CD11c^{hi}$ gate, macrophages and DCs can be distinguished from each other based on SiglecF and MHC-II signal (Fig. 2e). Alveolar macrophages express high levels of SiglecF whereas DCs are negative for SiglecF. Both cell populations express MHC-II, but macrophages at intermediate (int) levels and DCs at high levels. Check whether the $SiglecF^{hi}MHC\text{-}II^{int}$ cells delineated as macrophages have high FSC-A and SSC-A values, which is expected for the big and complex alveolar macrophages of the lungs (Fig. 2g). $SiglecF^{-}MHC\text{-}II^{hi}$ cells that range from $FSC\text{-}A^{low}$ $SSC\text{-}A^{low}$ to $FSC\text{-}A^{int}$ $SSC\text{-}A^{int}$ are defined as DCs (Fig. 2f).

(f) In the $CD11c^{low}$ gate, lymphocytes can be distinguished as cells expressing either CD3 (T cells) or CD19 (B cells). In this gating strategy, antibodies to both CD3 and CD19 are coupled to the same fluorochrome (PE-Cy5), therefore T and B cells are to be discriminated from each other based on the MHC-II expression on B cells that is not present on T cells (Fig. 3a). Both $CD11c^{low}CD3/CD19^{+}MCH\text{-}II^{-}$ T cells and $CD11c^{low}CD3/CD19^{+}MCH\text{-}II^{+}$ B cells are small and not complex cells with a low FSC-A and SSC-A (Fig. 3b, c).

(g) Cells that are both low for CD11c, CD3 and CD19 and high for CD11b are either eosinophils or neutrophils (Fig. 3d). Neutrophils are $CD11b^{hi}Ly\text{-}6G^{+}$ cells that have a similar FSC-A as lymphocytes but a slightly higher SSC-A (Fig. 3g). $CD11b^{hi}Ly\text{-}6G^{-}$ cells, that moreover highly express SiglecF, are denoted as eosinophils (Fig. 3e). The small but very complex eosinophils occupy a notable area in the FSC-A-SSC-A plot, consisting of the $FSC\text{-}A^{low}$ $SSC\text{-}A^{hi}$ events (Fig. 3f).

9. For every cell population, absolute numbers can be calculated by multiplying percentages obtained from the FACS software with total cell counts from manual counting, and dividing the result by 100. A representative result is shown in Fig. 4 (*see* **Note 18**).

3.4 Restimulation of Mediastinal Lymph Node (MLN) Cells with HDM

1. After taking the BAL from mice, cut the rib cage open, move the lungs upwards or sidewards and collect mediastinal lymph nodes (MLNs) in a 24-well plate in a sterile, rich buffer (HBSS or RPMI) on ice. MLNs are located underneath the right lung

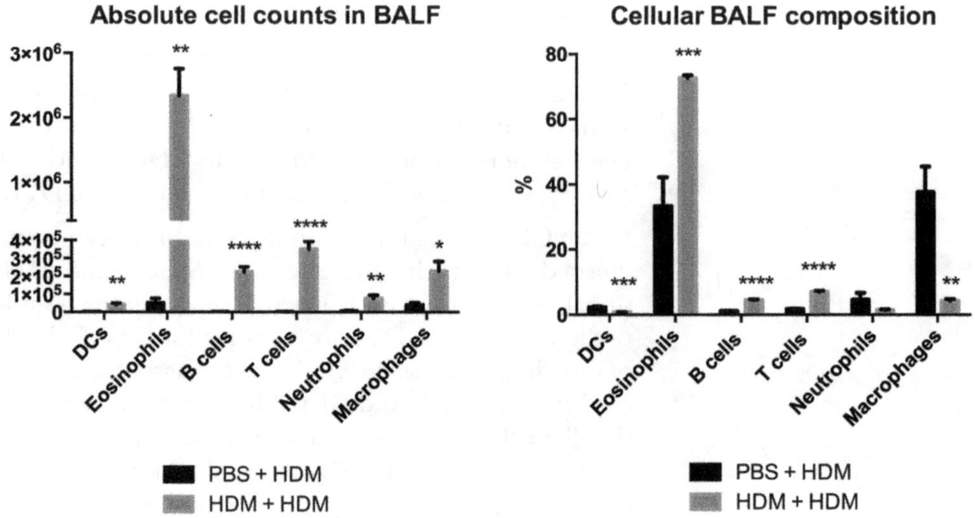

Fig. 4 Representative inflammatory cell infiltration in the BAL fluid (BALF) for a standard HDM-induced asthma protocol. Mice are sensitized intratracheally with 1 μg HDM extract or mock-sensitized with PBS, followed by five consecutive HDM-challenges (10 μg intranasally) 1 week later. Four days after the last challenge, eosinophil counts in BAL fluid are expected to be around two million. *$p<0.05$; **$p<0.01$; ***$p<0.001$; ****$p<0.0001$

lobes next to the right lateral border of the trachea and just below the thymus (*see* **Note 19**).

2. Homogenize the MLNs under sterile conditions with the tamping bar of a syringe, through a 70 or 100 μm mesh, in a small petri dish in 2 × 500 μL TCM. Pipet the cell suspension from the petri dish into a 15 mL tube.
3. Manually count cells and bring samples to a concentration of two million cells/mL by adding TCM, or by centrifuging and resuspending in the appropriate volume of TCM.
4. For every sample, seed 6 wells of a round bottom 96-well culture plate with 200,000 cells in 100 μL TCM per well.
5. Dilute the HDM stock (5 mg/mL) to 30 μg/mL in TCM (6 × 100 μL per MLN) and add 100 μL of diluted HDM extract to every well.
6. Incubate for 3–4 days in a CO_2 incubator at 37 °C and 5 % CO_2.
7. Spin cells down (400 × *g*, 3 min, 4 °C).
8. For every sample, pool supernatant of the 6 wells into 1 well of a 24-well plate and freeze at −20 °C for subsequent analysis of cytokines by ELISA. A representative result is shown in Fig. 5.

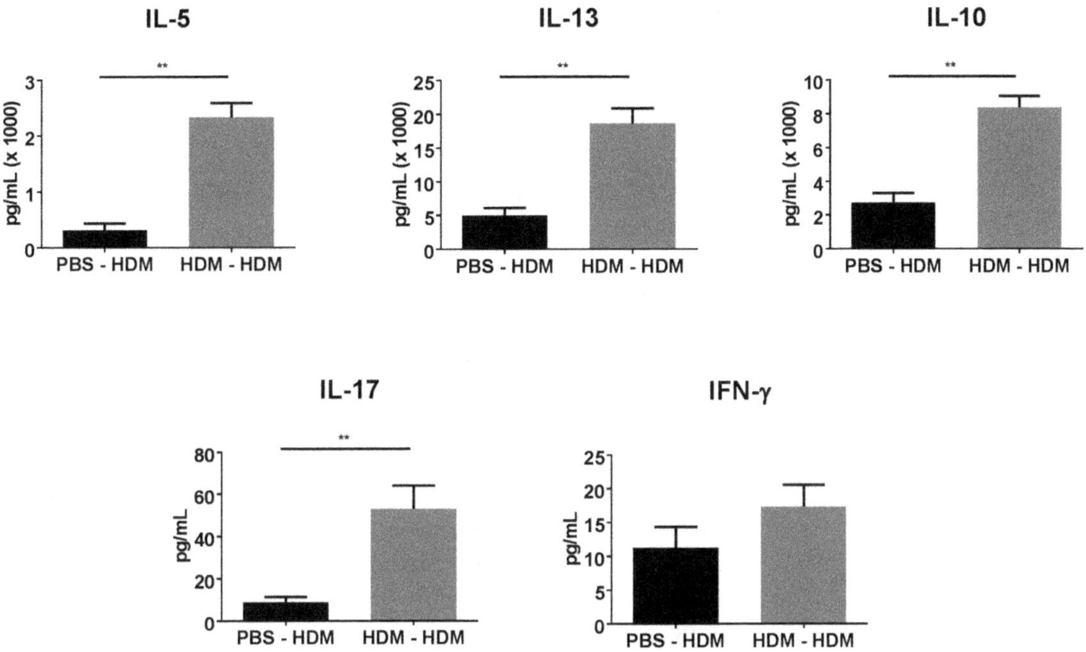

Fig. 5 Representative cytokine secretion levels in supernatants of HDM-restimulated MLN cell cultures for a standard HDM-induced asthma protocol. Mice are sensitized intratracheally with 1 μg HDM extract or mock-sensitized with PBS, followed by five consecutive HDM-challenges (10 μg intranasally) 1 week later. Four days after the last challenge, MLNs are collected, homogenized to single cell suspensions and restimulated in vitro with HDM for 3 days. MLN cells from HDM-sensitized and -challenged mice secrete significantly more Th2, Th17 and Treg cytokines in their culture supernatants. $^{**}p<0.01$

4 Notes

1. 6–8 mice per group are usually enough to obtain statistically significant results. For control groups, in which variation tends to be lower, three or four animals may suffice.
2. The strength and nature of responses to OVA, HDM, Der p 1 (a major HDM allergen), and other aeroallergens differ between mouse strains. Generally, in models of acute asthma, pulmonary eosinophilia and Th2 cytokine levels in BAL are significantly higher in C57Bl/6 mice than in BALB/c mice, whereas they exhibit a less pronounced AHR [20–22]. Mouse strains might also differ in the underlying pathophysiological mechanisms leading to the hallmarks of allergic airway disease. For example, eosinophils are necessary for AHR induction in C57Bl/6 mice, a requirement not observed in BALB/c mice [6, 23, 24]. Furthermore, A/J mice exhibit intrinsic AHR without any allergen exposure and that is independent of T and B cells and IL-4 signaling [25]. For this reason, carefully select the mouse strain best fit for your research question.

3. On a bottle of HDM extract, two concentrations are depicted: use the protein content and NOT the dry weight (wt) to make your dilution.
4. HDM batches, even when bought from the same company, are not standardized and may therefore vary in composition (e.g., LPS, β-glucan and chitin content, protease activity). Recently it has been shown in an HDM-based model of allergic asthma that adding LPS and β-glucans to the HDM leads to a strong pulmonary infiltration of neutrophils on top of eosinophils [26]. Also other experiments showed that LPS can vastly influence the asthmatic response, and that the precise effect is dependent on the dose and the timing of administration [17, 27]. Thus, HDM batches varying in these components can profoundly affect Th-skewing properties. When using a new HDM batch for the first time, it is very useful to first characterize the response induced by your particular batch by doing some standard read-outs of interest. Great care should be taken when you switch to a new batch within the same project, and results from the two batches should carefully be compared.
5. BAL fluid contains very little dead cells, however, some scientists still prefer to add a Fixable Live/Dead stain to the antibody mix, for example L/D-eFluor506. In this case, use PBS instead of FACS buffer for all steps.
6. Several panel designs targeting the same cell surface markers are possible. If another panel is designed, or if antibodies are bought from different suppliers, it is most safe to choose for the same antibody clones. New antibodies should first be validated and checked for their optimal dilution and staining conditions before using them in the complete staining mix.
7. In our lab, a standard sensitization dose of 1 μg HDM extract is used, followed by a standard challenge dose of 10 μg for five times (the "1/10" protocol). This can be adapted to lower doses if there is a suspicion that mild effects are masked by the robust response after sensitization and challenge, or to higher doses when the read-out(s) of interest are hard to detect. Always keep in mind that changing the doses of sensitization or challenges might change the mechanisms behind the observed responses. For example, $Flt3l^{-/-}$ mice, lacking CD103+ cDCs and CD11b+ cDCs, show a significantly reduced influx of eosinophils when using the standard "1/10"protocol. This suggests that monocyte-derived DCs (moDCs), the only remaining lung DC population, are not capable of inducing asthma in this setting. However, when sensitization and challenge doses are increased to 100 μg, asthma is induced in $Flt3l^{-/-}$ mice, demonstrating that moDCs do sensitize mice for HDM when the sensitization dose is high [28]. Similar dose dependent effects have also been described

in a cockroach model of asthma [29] and in OVA-protocols, for example in AHR induction, which is mast cell-dependent in low challenge frequency/dose protocols, but mast cell-independent in protocols with higher frequency and dose of challenges [30].

8. It may take some practice to identify when the mice are sedated enough (to have adequate time to carry out the i.t. installation) but not too much to avoid them breathing in little shocks. This depends on the device but typically, we wait until the respiratory rate is slow and restful, then wait another 10–20 s before removing the mice from the isoflurance device for instillation.
9. C57Bl/6 and BALB/c mice show a very different behavior when being exposed to isoflurane. When using BALB/c mice, the timeframe during which the mice are optimally sedated for i.t. and i.n. instillation (enough but not too much) is shorter.
10. The exact timing when an i.n. challenge is given is critical and it may take practice to recognize when the mice should be removed from the isoflurane device. Typically, the percentage of administered isoflurane is slightly lower than for i.t. instillation (2 versus 2.5 %) and the mice can be challenged from the moment the breathing is slow and restful without additional waiting. When carried out correctly, it takes less than a minute for the mice to wake up.
11. Always gently mix the OVA/alum solution by inverting the tube (or syringe) a few times to make sure that OVA and alum are homogenously distributed in the tube (or syringe) and that all the mice are injected with the same amounts of OVA/alum.
12. 1 % OVA dilutions in sterile PBS can be made beforehand and stored in the −20 °C freezer for a couple of months.
13. Pay attention not to put the cannula too deep into the trachea; it should not reach the bifurcation of the bronchi.
14. Sometimes, it can be hard to recover the BAL fluid from the lungs because a vacuum is created; in this case, the vacuum can be disrupted by carefully moving the cannula a bit less deep in the trachea. Watch out not to pull it out completely.
15. We use this two-step redilution scheme because after aspiration of the supernatant from the 15 mL tube, a little bit of fluid is always left at the edges of the tube and consequently cells may not be resuspended in exactly the same volume after the addition of FACS buffer. This is important since the absolute cell counts is one of the main read-outs of this protocol.
16. Usually, the cell suspensions contain very little red blood cells (RBCs). However, if some cell pellets stain red, you may facilitate the manual cell counting by lysing the RBCs. After the

first centrifugation round, discard the supernatant and add 300 μL osmotic lysis buffer directly to the 15 mL tubes at room temperature. After 3 min, neutralize with an excess of PBS (or FACS buffer), centrifuge and resuspend the samples in 200 μL FACS buffer for transfer to the 96-well plate.

17. Eosinophils and neutrophils are the most significant inflammatory cell populations in the BALF. By making use of a hierarchical gating in which both cell types are only identified in the end, possible contaminations of these gates with other cell types are minimized.
18. As a rule of thumb, eosinophil percentages above 50% indicate successful sensitization and challenging.
19. In PBS controls, MLNs can be extremely small and hard to see. It helps to carefully push with a forceps on the surrounding fat and tissue to move the MLNs upwards and out of their surroundings. If MLNs are really big, pay attention not to break them. It may be useful to first detach the MLNs from their surroundings by gently pulling at the strings keeping them in place. Do not confuse the MLNs with the thymus just above them, which is larger and stiffer.

Acknowledgments

Eline Haspeslagh is supported by the Research Foundation Flanders (FWO).

References

1. Robinson DS, Qutayba H, Ying S, Tsicopoulos A, Barkans J, Bentley AM, Corrigan C, Durham SR, Kay B (1992) Predominant Th2-like bronchoalveolar T-lymphocyte population in atopic asthma. N Engl J Med 326(5):298–304
2. Holgate ST, Polosa R (2008) Treatment strategies for allergy and asthma. Nat Rev Immunol 8:218–230. doi:10.1038/nri2262
3. Barnes PJ (2011) Glucocorticosteroids: current and future directions. Br J Pharmacol 163:29–43. doi:10.1111/j.1476-5381.2010.01199.x
4. Kumar RK, Herbert C, Foster PS (2008) The "classical" ovalbumin challenge model of asthma in mice. Curr Drug Targets 9:485–494. doi:10.2174/138945008784533561
5. Corry DB, Grünig G, Hadeiba H, Kurup VP, Warnock ML, Sheppard D, Rennick DM, Locksley RM (1998) Requirements for allergen-induced airway hyperreactivity in T and B cell-deficient mice. Mol Med 4:344–355
6. Corry DB, Folkesson HG, Warnock ML, Erle DJ, Matthay MA, Wiener-Kronish JP, Locksley RM (1996) Interleukin 4, but not interleukin 5 or eosinophils, is required in a murine model of acute airway hyperreactivity. J Exp Med 183:109–117. doi:10.1084/jem.183.1.109
7. Mould AW, Ramsay AJ, Matthaei KI, Young IG, Rothenberg ME, Foster PS (2000) The effect of IL-5 and eotaxin expression in the lung on eosinophil trafficking and degranulation and the induction of bronchial hyperreactivity. J Immunol 164:2142–2150, ji_v164n4p2142 [pii]
8. Ingram JL, Kraft M (2012) IL-13 in asthma and allergic disease: asthma phenotypes and targeted therapies. J Allergy Clin Immunol 130:829–842. doi:10.1016/j.jaci.2012.06.034
9. Lambrecht BN, Salomon B, Klatzmann D, Pauwels RA (1998) Dendritic cells are required for the development of chronic eosin-

ophilic airway inflammation in response to inhaled antigen in sensitized mice. J Immunol 160:4090–4097

10. Lambrecht BN, Peleman RA, Bullock GR, Pauwels RA (2000) Sensitization to inhaled antigen by intratracheal instillation of dendritic cells. Clin Exp Allergy 30:214–224, cea818 [pii]
11. Kool M, Soullié T, van Nimwegen M, Willart MAM, Muskens F, Jung S, Hoogsteden HC, Hammad H, Lambrecht BN (2008) Alum adjuvant boosts adaptive immunity by inducing uric acid and activating inflammatory dendritic cells. J Exp Med 205:869–882. doi:10.1084/jem.20071087
12. Borish LC, Nelson HS, Lanz MJ, Claussen L, Whitmore JB, Agosti JM, Garrison L (1999) Interleukin-4 receptor in moderate atopic asthma. A phase I/II randomized, placebo-controlled trial. Am J Respir Crit Care Med 160:1816–1823
13. Kips JC, O'Connor BJ, Langley SJ, Woodcock A, Kerstjens HAM, Postma DS, Danzig M, Cuss F, Pauwels RA (2003) Effect of SCH55700, a humanized anti-human interleukin-5 antibody, in severe persistent asthma: a pilot study. Am J Respir Crit Care Med 167:1655–1659. doi:10.1164/rccm.200206-525OC
14. Leckie MJ, Ten Brinke A, Khan J, Diamant Z, O'Connor BJ, Walls CM, Mathur AK, Cowley HC, Chung KF, Djukanovic R, Hansel TT, Holgate ST, Sterk PJ, Barnes PJ (2000) Effects of an interleukin-5 blocking monoclonal antibody on eosinophils, airway hyperresponsiveness, and the late asthmatic response. Lancet 356:2144–2148. doi:10.1016/S0140-6736(00)03496-6
15. Eisenbarth SC, Piggott DA, Huleatt JW, Visintin I, Herrick CA, Bottomly K (2002) Lipopolysaccharide-enhanced, toll-like receptor 4-dependent T helper cell type 2 responses to inhaled antigen. J Exp Med 196:1645–1651. doi:10.1084/jem.20021340
16. Jacquet A (2011) The role of innate immunity activation in house dust mite allergy. Trends Mol Med 17:604–611. doi:10.1016/j.molmed.2011.05.014
17. Hammad H, Chieppa M, Perros F, Willart MA, Germain RN, Lambrecht BN (2009) House dust mite allergen induces asthma via Toll-like receptor 4 triggering of airway structural cells. Nat Med 15:410–416. doi:10.1038/nm.1946
18. McMillan SJ, Lloyd CM (2004) Prolonged allergen challenge in mice leads to persistent airway remodelling. Clin Exp Allergy 34:497–507. doi:10.1111/j.1365-2222.2004.01895.x
19. Martin RA, Hodgkins SR, Dixon AE, Poynter ME (2014) Aligning mouse models of asthma to human endotypes of disease. Respirology 19:823–833. doi:10.1111/resp.12315
20. Kelada SNP, Wilson MS, Tavarez U, Kubalanza K, Borate B, Whitehead GS, Maruoka S, Roy MG, Olive M, Carpenter DE, Brass DM, Wynn TA, Cook DN, Evans CM, Schwartz DA, Collins FS (2011) Strain-dependent genomic factors affect allergen-induced airway hyperresponsiveness in mice. Am J Respir Cell Mol Biol 45:817–824. doi:10.1165/rcmb.2010-0315OC
21. Morokata T, Ishikawa J, Ida K, Yamada T (1999) C57BL/6 mice are more susceptible to antigen-induced pulmonary eosinophilia than BALB/c mice, irrespective of systemic T helper 1/T helper 2 responses. Immunology 98:345–351. doi:10.1046/j.1365-2567.1999.00890.x
22. Van Hove CL, Maes T, Cataldo DD, Guéders MM, Palmans E, Joos GF, Tournoy KG (2009) Comparison of acute inflammatory and chronic structural asthma-like responses between C57BL/6 and BALB/c Mice. Int Arch Allergy Immunol 149:195–207. doi:10.1159/000199715
23. Lee JJ, Dimina D, Macias MP, Ochkur SI, McGarry MP, O'Neill KR, Protheroe C, Pero R, Nguyen T, Cormier SA, Lenkiewicz E, Colbert D, Rinaldi L, Ackerman SJ, Irvin CG, Lee NA (2004) Defining a link with asthma in mice congenitally deficient in eosinophils. Science 305:1773–1776. doi:10.1126/science.1099472
24. Humbles AA, Lloyd CM, McMillan SJ, Friend DS, Xanthou G, McKenna EE, Ghiran S, Gerard NP, Yu C, Orkin SH, Gerard C (2004) A critical role for eosinophils in allergic airways remodeling. Science 305:1776–1779. doi:10.1126/science.1100283
25. Hadeiba H, Corry DB, Locksley RM (2000) Baseline airway hyperreactivity in A/J mice is not mediated by cells of the adaptive immune system. J Immunol 164:4933–4940, ji_v164n9p4933 [pii]
26. Hadebe S, Kirstein F, Fierens K, Chen K, Drummond RA, Vautier S, Sajaniemi S, Murray G, Williams DL, Redelinghuys P, Reinhart TA, Fallert Junecko BA, Kolls JK, Lambrecht BN, Brombacher F, Brown GD (2015) Microbial ligand costimulation drives neutrophilic steroid-refractory asthma. PLoS One 10:e0134219. doi:10.1371/journal.pone.0134219
27. Schuijs MJ, Willart MA, Vergote K, Grad D, Deswarte K, Ege MJ, Madeira FB, Beyaert R (2015) Farm dust and endotoxin protect against allergy through A20 induction in lung epithelial cells. Science 349:1907–1911

28. Plantinga M, Guilliams M, Vanheerswynghels M, Deswarte K, Branco-Madeira F, Toussaint W, Vanhoutte L, Neyt K, Killeen N, Malissen B, Hammad H, Lambrecht BN (2013) Conventional and monocyte-derived CD11b+dendritic cells initiate and maintain T helper 2 cell-mediated immunity to house dust mite allergen. Immunity 38:322–335. doi:10.1016/j.immuni.2012.10.016
29. Walzer T, Brawand P, Swart D, Tocker J, De Smedt T (2005) No defect in T-cell priming, secondary response, or tolerance induction in response to inhaled antigens in Fms-like tyrosine kinase 3 ligand-deficient mice. J Allergy Clin Immunol 115:192–199. doi:10.1016/j.jaci.2004.08.046
30. Kobayashi T, Miura T, Haba T, Sato M, Serizawa I, Nagai H, Ishizaka K (2000) An essential role of mast cells in the development of airway hyperresponsiveness in a murine asthma model. J Immunol 164:3855–3861. doi:10.4049/jimmunol.164.7.3855

Chapter 11

Subcutaneous and Sublingual Immunotherapy in a Mouse Model of Allergic Asthma

Laura Hesse and Martijn C. Nawijn

Abstract

Allergic asthma, caused by inhaled allergens such as house dust mite or grass pollen, is characterized by reversible airway obstruction, associated with an eosinophilic inflammation of the airways, as well as airway hyper responsiveness and remodeling. The inhaled allergens trigger a type-2 inflammatory response with involvement of innate lymphoid cells (ILC2) and Th2 cells, resulting in high production of immunoglobulin E (IgE) antibodies. Consequently, renewed allergen exposure results in a classic allergic response with a distinct early and late phase, both resulting in bronchoconstriction and shortness of breath. Allergen specific immunotherapy (AIT) is the only treatment that is capable of modifying the immunological process underlying allergic responses including allergic asthma and both subcutaneous AIT (SCIT) as well as sublingual AIT (SLIT) have proven clinical efficacy in long term suppression of the allergic response. Although these treatments are very successful for rhinitis, application of AIT in asthma is hampered by variable efficacy, long duration of treatment, and the risk of severe side-effects. A more profound understanding of the mechanisms by which AIT achieves tolerance to allergens in sensitized individuals is needed to improve its efficacy. Mouse models have been very valuable as a preclinical model to characterize the mechanisms of desensitization in AIT and to evaluate novel approaches for improved efficacy. Here, we present a rapid and reproducible mouse model for allergen-specific immunotherapy. In this model, mice are sensitized with two injections of allergen absorbed to aluminum hydroxide to induce allergic sensitization, followed by subcutaneous injections (SCIT) or sublingual administrations (SLIT) of the allergen as immunotherapy treatment. Finally, mice are challenged by three intranasal allergen administrations. We will describe the protocols as well as the most important read-out parameters including measurement of invasive lung function measurements, serum immunoglobulin levels, isolation of broncho-alveolar lavage fluid (BALF), and preparation of cytospins. Moreover, we describe how to restimulate lung single cell suspensions, perform flow cytometry measurements to identify populations of relevant immune cells, and perform ELISAs and Luminex assays to measure the cytokine concentrations in BALF and lung tissue.

Key words Allergic asthma, Subcutaneous immunotherapy (SCIT), Sublingual immunotherapy (SLIT), Mouse model, Grass pollen (GP), House dust mite (HDM), FlexiVent, Flow cytometry, Bronchoalveolar lavage, Eosinophilia

1 Introduction

Asthma is the result of a complex interaction between genetic susceptibility and environmental factors that lead to the inception of the disease only in the susceptible individual. The most common

Björn E. Clausen and Jon D. Laman (eds.), *Inflammation: Methods and Protocols*, Methods in Molecular Biology, vol. 1559,
DOI 10.1007/978-1-4939-6786-5_11, © Springer Science+Business Media LLC 2017

asthma phenotype is allergic asthma, which is caused by inhaled allergens such as grass pollen (GP), ragweed, cat and dog allergens, and house dust mites (HDM) [1, 2]. Patients suffering from allergic asthma have reversible airway obstruction, associated with an eosinophilic inflammation, hyper responsiveness and remodeling of the airways. The worldwide prevalence of allergic asthma has dramatically increased over the last 25 years, currently affecting over 330 million people.

The inflammatory response in allergic asthma is characterized by the presence of high levels of cytokines such as IL-4, IL-5, and IL-13, produced by both innate lymphoid cells (ILCs) and T helper 2 (Th2) cells [3]. These cytokines contribute to the pathological changes of the airways observed in allergic asthma such as the influx of eosinophils, mucus hypersecretion, airway hyper responsiveness and airway wall remodeling. In addition, the Th2 dominated adaptive response to the inhaled allergens result in the presence of allergen-specific IgE. Allergen-induced cross-linking of IgE bound to the cell surface of mast cells and basophils through the high affinity IgE receptor will induce degranulation of these cells resulting in the acute allergic response, leading to bronchoconstriction and vasodilation. The subsequent influx of inflammatory cells including Th2 cells will result in activation of these cells upon local antigen presentation of the causative allergen, inducing the late-phase response. Upon recurrent exposure to the allergen, a chronic and poorly resolving inflammation around the small airways results in permanent changes to the airway wall.

Currently available asthma therapies are focused on controlling the ongoing inflammatory process, mainly with inhaled corticosteroids (ICS), in combination with long acting beta agonists (LABA) or leukotriene receptor antagonists (LTRA) [4]. Notwithstanding the clinical success in achieving asthma control, current asthma treatment regimens fail to cure the disease, as evidenced by ongoing airway wall remodeling even in well-controlled asthma patients and an unaltered risk for asthma attacks either upon daily ICS use compared to intermittent ICS use or upon cessation of ICS treatment [5, 6]. Moreover, a subset of patients with severe asthma exists that does not respond to steroid treatment [7, 8]. These shortcomings of current mainstream asthma therapy indicate the failure of this therapeutic approach to address the underlying, causative immunological mechanisms, resulting in a transient suppression of symptoms of asthma in most patients.

The only treatment known to date that is capable of modifying the immunological process underlying allergic asthma is allergen-specific immunotherapy (AIT) [9]. Unlike standard asthma treatment, AIT has been shown to provide a long-term protection against asthma attacks that is maintained upon cessation of therapy and to reduce medication use in allergic asthma. AIT involves the administration of gradually increasing amounts of allergen extracts for a period of 3–5 years with the aim of achieving a state of immunological tolerance and subsequently a reduction of clinical manifestations in the allergic patients [10]. A Cochrane systematic review on the application of subcutaneous AIT (SCIT) in asthma reported an overall efficacy in suppression of symptom score, medication use and both allergen-specific and nonspecific bronchial hyperresponsiveness [11]. Sublingual AIT (SLIT) treatment for house dust mite allergy reduced the use of ICS (relative mean reduction of 50%) while maintaining asthma control [12]. In addition to suppressing asthma symptoms and achieving reduced medication use, grass pollen AIT has also been found to prevent progression to asthma in children with seasonal allergic rhinoconjunctivitis [10]. Also AIT treatment has been shown to prevent progression to asthma in a subset of children [13].

Although the mechanism behind successful immunotherapy remains, at least in part, unknown, the beneficial effects of AIT are ascribed to a shift from the Th2 profile seen in allergic asthma towards a protective T regulatory (Treg) profile that suppresses allergen specific responses [14]. Clinical improvement after AIT is associated with increased levels of neutralizing antibodies, production of IL-10 and TGF-β, and increased $CD4^{+}FoxP3^{+}$ Treg numbers and resolution of Th2 inflammation [15–18]. For instance, GP SCIT treatment has been shown to induce regulatory T cell numbers in nasal tissue, associated with reduced tissue Th2 and eosinophil cell numbers [17]. Moreover, PBMCs from AIT treated patients cultured in the presence of allergens produce increased levels of IL-10 and TGF-β, reflecting an increased presence or activity of regulatory T cells [18]. In addition, a recent study employing tetramer technology to track individual Th cell clones in GP allergic patients elegantly showed that successful GP SCIT was associated with a selective loss of those allergen-specific Th2 clones that were found to be increased in number in GP allergic patients compared to non-allergic control subjects [16]. Furthermore, blocking IgGs has been suggested to contribute to successful AIT, since increased levels of IgGs in serum of AIT-treated patients has been associated with the alleviation of allergic symptoms [19–21]. The blocking IgG hypothesis states that blocking antibodies produced by B cells upon tolerance induction contribute to successful AIT in two ways. First, by binding to the allergen directly and thereby competing with specific IgE preventing cross-linking and subsequent mast cell and basophil degranulation as well as preventing IgE facilitated antigen presentation. Second, the specific IgG antibodies can bind to FcγRIIB expressed by B cells, mast cells, and basophils, which can, upon allergen-mediated IgG cross-linking, provide a negative intracellular signal and prevent activation, even upon co-aggregation with FcεRI.

While SCIT and SLIT have been widely accepted as effective therapeutic alternatives for allergic rhinoconjuncivitis, application in asthma is hampered by the long duration of treatment required to achieve long-lasting relieve of symptoms, the variable efficacy in allergic asthma and concerns regarding the safety of treatment. SCIT injections of allergen extracts have a potential risk of anaphylactic reactions, with an incidence of severe anaphylactic responses reported to be at around one in a million injections [22]. Therefore, outpatient clinic visits are required for the administration and monitoring of the therapy [23]. In developing more convenient alternatives, SLIT has been developed as a less invasive alternative with proven clinical effects for patients suffering from allergic rhinitis [24]. Herein, uptake of the allergen takes place in the oral mucosa, where mucosal Langerhans cells in humans and oral macrophage-like cells in mice have been implicated [25]. Although the mechanism of action remains to be elucidated, advantages include the absence of the involvement of the clinic, ease of use (droplets or fast dissolving tablets), and relative costs. Understanding the mechanisms by which AIT suppresses the allergen-induced asthma symptoms is needed to redesign AIT for better efficacy and optimal safety, in particular in asthmatic patients.

Previously, animal models have proven to be valuable as a preclinical model to improve AIT and to unravel the mechanisms of desensitization involved. The development of a predictive and reproducible AIT protocol was initially based on a mouse model of allergic asthma using the standard model antigen ovalbumin (OVA) [26]. Herein, mice were sensitized with OVA without the use of an adjuvant in seven intraperitoneal injections, followed after 2 weeks by SCIT treatment using three injections of OVA (1 mg), and after another 2 weeks challenged by OVA (2 mg/ml) inhalation once a day (5 min) for 8 consecutive days. The outcome parameters of SCIT treatment were OVA-specific immunoglobulin (Ig) levels: sp-IgE, -IgG1 and IgG2a, airway eosinophilia, airway hyperresponsiveness (AHR), and proinflammatory cytokine production by antigen specific T cells (Th2 mediated response), such as interleukin 4 (IL-4), IL-5, and IL-13. In the initial studies, no adverse events were recorded in the BALB/c strain of mice, while the experimental SCIT treatment effectively reduced airway inflammation and AHR and induced spIgG1 and spIgG2a serum levels. In addition, spIgE levels were also increased, in accordance with the initial rise of spIgE in human subjects treated with SCIT. Importantly however, SCIT treatment in the OVA mouse model prevented the increase of spIgE levels after allergen challenge, which is readily observed in control treated mice [27]. After several improvements, the protocol was reduced to two intraperitoneal injections containing OVA accompanied by a sensitizing adjuvant, Alum (mixture of aluminum hydroxide and magnesium hydroxide) and three intranasal challenges containing high dose aerosolized OVA. In addition, OVA SCIT treatment was also found to be effective in sensitized mice that were challenged by

OVA inhalation prior to SCIT treatment, indicating the ability of the experimental treatment to suppress an established allergic airway inflammatory response [28]. Throughout the years, this mouse model for SCIT has been used to improve our understanding of the mechanisms of desensitization [26, 29–31]. Examples include the requirement on neutralizing antibody responses [28], the crucial role of IL-10 in the induction of tolerance, the essential contribution of $CD4^{+}FoxP3^{+}$ T regulatory cells (Treg). Aside from studies on the involvement of B and T lymphocytes, the crucial role of the antigen presenting cells, mostly DCs, have been investigated extensively. DCs play a key role in the generation of adaptive T cell subsets and, depending on their maturation state, DCs can respond either immunogenic, in a sensitizing fashion, or tolerogenic [32]. Tolerogenic DCs have a semi-mature or immature phenotype, characterized by increased expression of major histocompatibility complex class II (MHC-II) and B7-2, low expression of CD40, and no production of proinflammatory cytokines (IL-6 and TNFα). Studies have shown that incubation of immature DCs with $CD4^{+}$T cells induce antigen specific Tregs [33, 34], postulating that immature DCs play a critical role in Treg cell generation and peripheral tolerance. Based on these findings, AIT can be improved when allergen administration is accompanied by inhibition of DC maturation or prevention of DC dependent costimulation. One approach explored to this end is the use of $1,25(OH)_2$vitamin D_3, the active metabolite of vitamin D, since it inhibits NF-κB signaling via the RelB protein, which is essential for DC differentiation and maturation. Indeed, using the OVA-SCIT mouse model, co-administration of $1,25(OH)_2VitD_3$ has been shown to potentiate the suppressive effects of AIT [29]. In addition, CTLA4-Ig (Abatacept) was found to enhance efficacy of SCIT in the OVA mouse model [35].

Although using this mouse model of immunotherapy has provided a much more detailed insight in the immunological mechanisms, it should not be forgotten that it is merely an experimental preclinical model using a purified protein (OVA) that lacks the properties of natural allergens, and which in fact is able to induce tolerance when inhaled by naïve mice [36]. Therefore, the classical model allergen OVA was replaced with a natural allergen extract that is also used in human SCIT, such as GP and HDM, and the GP and HDM SCIT protocols for allergic asthma have been optimized regarding administered allergen doses (*unpublished data*). Second, other administrative routes were optimized, based on a SLIT mouse model of allergic rhinitis [37]. Both administrative routes have been validated and standardized allowing a head-to-head comparison. This model allows in-depth characterization of the mechanisms of SCIT and SLIT treatment for allergic asthma, as well as their optimization using novel approaches including peptide SCIT treatment or use of alternative formulations and adjuvantia.

In this protocol, we explain how subcutaneous and sublingual routes of allergen-specific immunotherapy can be applied in a mouse model of allergic asthma using natural allergen extracts. We provide an overview of the most important outcome parameters for translational studies, including invasive lung function measurements for AHR, specific IgE and IgG levels in serum, ear swelling tests for the early phase response and measurement of lung tissue and airway inflammation. Moreover, we describe how to restimulate lung single cell suspensions, perform flow cytometry measurements to identify populations of relevant immune cells, and perform ELISAs and Luminex assays to measure the cytokine concentrations in BALF and lung tissue.

2 Materials

2.1 Subcutaneous and Sublingual Immunotherapy in a Mouse Model of Allergic Asthma

1. 7–9-week-old BALB/cByJ mice (females) housed in individually ventilated cages (IVC).
2. Syringes (1 ml) and 25 G needles.
3. 20 μl pipet and tips.
4. 15 ml tubes.
5. Sterile phosphate buffered saline (PBS).
6. Rough extract grass pollen (GP, *Phleum pratense*; *Phl p*) **or** crude extract house dust mite (HDM, *Dermatophagoides pteronyssinus*; *Der p*), resuspended according to **Note 1**.
7. Sterile aluminum hydroxide ($Al(OH_3)$), 20% (Imject® Alum).

2.2 Ear Swelling Test and Blood Withdrawal via Orbital Puncture

1. Small animal anesthesia device compatible with isoflurane and a connected induction chamber.
2. Isoflurane (2-chloro-2-(difluoromethoxy)-1,1,1-trifluoroethane, 4.5 %, halocarbon, isoflurane USP, liquid for inhalation).
3. Oxygen (1.5 ml/min O_2).
4. Sterile phosphate buffered saline (PBS).
5. Rough extract grass pollen (GP, *Phleum pratense*; *Phl p*) **or** crude extract house dust mite (HDM, *Dermatophagoides pteronyssinus*; *Der p*).
6. 30 G Insulin syringes (0.3 ml 0.30 mm × 8 mm).
7. 1 ml MiniCollect® serum tubes (Greiner Bio-One).
8. Glass microcapillary tubes: micro hematocrit tubes (Na-Heparinized 80 IU/ml).
9. 1.5 ml tubes and a centrifuge.
10. Digimatic pressure-limited micrometer.
11. Regular hand tissues, hand gloves, and sterile tissues.

2.3 Lung Function Measurement and Section

1. Ligatures (6/0 and 3/0), silicon tubing (0.28 mm and OD: 0.61 mm), syringes (1 and 5 ml), and 25 G needles.
2. 20 G intravenous cannula for tracheal cannulation and calibration (pink, 20GA 1.16IN 1.1 × 30 mm BD Insyte-W™).
3. 1.5 ml tubes, 15 ml tubes, 24-well cell culture plates, MiniCollect® serum tubes, and 2 ml cryogen vials.
4. Sterile PBS, PBS supplemented with bovine serum albumin (BSA, 5 %, heat shock fraction, protease free, low endotoxin, suitable for cell culture, pH 7, ≥98 %) and a complete protease inhibitor cocktail tablet (cOmplete Mini), and sterile RPMI1640.
5. Ketamine (100 mg/ml), Domitor (1 mg/kg), Rocuronium bromide (10 μg/ml), sterile methacholine.
6. Chirurgical microscope (40×) and basic micro-chirurgical instrument set.
7. FlexiVent (SCIREQ), computers, and FlexiWare Software.
8. Weighing scale (precision > 0.1 g).
9. Manometer with syringe and closing valves.
10. Micro pulse-oxymeter for small animals.
11. Heating mats for small animals.

2.4 Analysis of the Infiltration of Inflammatory Cells in BAL Fluid

1. Microscope slides (76 × 26 mm), Shandon filter cards and 70 % ethanol.
2. Cytospin cuvette and metal cytospin slide holder and its driver.
3. Pipet-man® with associated pipettes and tips.
4. Cyto-centrifuge (Shandon, cytospin 3), regular centrifuge and aspirator.
5. Cell counter machine, 10 ml Coulter counter cups, Isoton II, and Lyzerglobin.
6. Sterile PBS, bovine serum albumin (BSA, 5 %, heat shock fraction, protease free, low endotoxin, suitable for cell culture, pH 7, ≥98 %).
7. Sterile lysis buffer containing 155 mmol/l NH_4Cl, 10 mmol/l $KHCO_3$, and 0.1 mmol/l EDTA.
8. Medion Diagnostics Diff-Quick staining set.
9. A light microscope with 20×, 40×, and 100× magnification lenses, immersion oil, and a differential cell counter.

2.5 Preparation of Single Cell Suspensions of Lung Tissue, Spleen, and Draining Lymph Nodes

1. Standard laboratory equipment including ice, 24-well plates, petri dishes, sterile scalpels, pipets, Pipet-man with associated pipets, 50 ml tubes, 70 μm nylon cell strainers and the plunger of a 5 ml syringe.
2. Safety cabinet (down-flow cabinet) with a closed suction system, and a standard centrifuge.

3. Sterile RPMI1640, and sterile 500 ml RPMI1640 supplemented with: 10% (50 ml) fetal calf serum (FCS, complement inactivated), L-glutamine (200 mM in 0.85% NaCl solution),

   5 ml of 10,000 U/ml penicillin with 10,000 μg/ml streptomycin (PenStrep), (*optional*) 3% bovine serum albumin (BSA, heat shock fraction, protease free, low endotoxin, suitable for cell culture, pH 7, ≥98%), (*optional*) 5 ml MEM vitamin solution (100×).
4. 4 mg/ml collagenase A and 0.1 mg/ml DNAse I.
5. Cell counter machine, 10 ml Coulter counter cups, Isoton II, and Lyzerglobin.
6. Cryogen vials, a Stratagene box, −80 °C freezer, and liquid nitrogen storage.
7. Storage medium for cells in liquid nitrogen: 50% HBSS, 40% FCS, and 10% DMSO.

2.6 Restimulation of Lung Cells and Draining Lymph Node (DLN) Cells

1. Safety cabinet (down-flow cabinet) with a closed suction system, standard centrifuge, and a CO_2 incubator.
2. Petri dishes, sterile scalpels, pipets, and Pipet-man® with associated pipets.
3. Supplemented RPMI1640 and a single cell suspension resulted from Subheading 2.5.
4. A sterile U-bottom 96-well cell culture plate.
5. Rough extract grass pollen (GP, *Phleum pratense*; *Phl p*) **or** crude extract house dust mite (HDM, *Dermatophagoides pteronyssinus*; *Der p*).

2.7 Homogenization of Lung Tissue for Total Protein and Cytokine Analysis

1. Homogenizer, 1.5 ml tubes, 96-well flat bottom ELISA plates, cryogen vials, and ELISA plate reader.
2. BCA protein assay kit.
3. Demi water, Tween 20, and 70% ethanol.
4. Luminex buffer containing 50 mM Tris–HCl, 150 mM NaCl, 0.002% Tween, pH 7.5, and (*optional*) one tablet complete protease inhibitor cocktail tablet/100 ml buffer (cOmplete Mini), and (*optional*) one tablet PhosSTOP phosphatase inhibitor cocktail tablet/100 ml buffer. Luminex buffer can be aliquoted and stored at −20 °C.

2.8 Analysis of Immunoglobulin Levels in Serum and Cytokine Levels in BAL Fluid, Supernatant of Restimulated Single Cell Suspensions, and Lung Tissue Homogenates

1. ELISAs for immunoglobulins: total IgE, -IgA, -IgG1, and -IgG2a, as well as specific (sp)IgE, spIgG1, and spIgG2a.
2. ELISAs for cytokines of interest like, IL-4, IL-5, IL-10, IL-13, and IFNγ.
3. Luminex assay for mouse cytokines, choose your cytokines of interest and combine them in a single Mouse Magnetic Luminex Screening Assay [LXSAMSM].
4. For an overview of all antibodies included in the immunoglobulin-ELISAs, we would like to refer to Table 1. For the allergen specific IgE ELISA, we use a "home-made" biotinylated allergen as a second antibody (*see* **Note 13**). To include a reference line in all specific Ig-ELISAs we use a collection of pooled sera from asthmatic mice (positive controls). As an example, we include here the total Immunoglobulin E levels in serum:
   (a) NUNC Maxisorp 96-well flat bottom ELISA plates, multichannel pipet and associated tips, ELISA plate-washer, -shaker, -and reader.
   (b) ELISA buffer containing: 6.06 g/l Tris (50 mM), 8 g/l NaCl (136.9 mM), 0.05% Tween 20, 0.744 g/l EDTA (2 mM), pH 7.2, and freshly add 5 g/l BSA.
   (c) Wash buffer containing PBS and 0.05% Tween 20.
   (d) Coat: purified rat anti-mouse IgE, clone R35-72 (*see* Table 1).
   (e) Standard: purified mouse IgE κ isotype control, clone C38-2.
   (f) Samples: mouse serum collected on different time points.
   (g) Second antibody: biotin rat anti-mouse IgE, clone R35-118.
   (h) Avidin horseradish peroxidase (HRP), OPD peroxidase substrate, and 4 M H_2SO_4.

2.9 Quantification of DCs, T Cell Populations and Innate Lymphoid Cells in Lung Single Cell Suspensions Using Flow Cytometry

1. FACS tubes (polystyrene) for samples and singles during staining, 30 μm filter top FACS tubes, standard centrifuge, three laser flow cytometer (FacsVerse).
2. FACS buffer containing: 1% BSA in PBS.
3. Block buffer containing: 2% normal rat serum (NRS) and 5% FcBlock (purified and unlabeled CD16/32 antibody) in FACS buffer. For intracellular blocking, use 2% NRS and 5% FcBlock in PERM buffer (*see* Subheading 2.9, **item 6**).
4. Staining antibodies diluted in FACS buffer according to manufacturers' protocol (*see* Tables 2 and 3). In some cases, the dilution of every antibody can be adjusted depending on the intensity of the fluorescent signal.

Table 1
Overview of immunoglobulin ELISA antibodies

ELISA	Layer	Antibody	Stock	Dilution	Supplier
Total IgE	Capture	Purified Rat Anti-Mouse IgE (R35-72)	0.5 mg/ml	1:500	BD Bioscience
	Block	ELISA buffer containing 1% BSA	Pure	300 μl	Lab EXPIRE
	Sample	Mice Sera samples (Pre- and Post-sera)	Pure	Pre 1:30, Post 1:60	Animal Centre
	Standard	Purified Mouse IgE κ Isotype Control (C38-2)	0.5 mg/ml	Start 2500 ng/ml, twofold dilution steps	BD Bioscience
	Detection	Biotin Rat Anti-Mouse IgE (R35-118)	0.5 mg/ml	1:500	BD Bioscience
Total IgG1	Capture	Purified Rat Anti-Mouse IgG1 (A85-3)	0.5 mg/ml	1:200	BD Bioscience
	Block	ELISA buffer containing 1% BSA	Pure	300 μl	Lab EXPIRE
	Sample	Mice Sera samples (Pre- and Post-sera)	Pure	1:300,000	Animal Centre
	Standard	Purified Mouse IgG1, κ Isotype Control (MOPC-31C)	0.5 mg/ml	Start 750 ng/ml, threefold dilution steps	BD Bioscience
	Detection	Biotin Rat Anti-Mouse IgG1 (A85-1)	0.5 mg/ml	1:500	BD Bioscience
Total IgG2a	Capture	Purified Rat Anti-Mouse IgG2a (R11-89)	0.5 mg/ml	1:200	BD Bioscience
	Block	ELISA buffer containing 1% BSA	Pure	300 μl	Lab EXPIRE
	Sample	Mice Sera samples (Pre- and Post-sera)	Pure	1:50	Animal Centre
	Standard	Purified Mouse IgG2a κ Isotype Control (G155-178)	0.5 mg/ml	Start 500 ng/ml, twofold dilution steps	BD Bioscience
	Detection	Biotin Rat Anti-Mouse IgG2a (R19-15)	0.5 mg/ml	1:500	BD Bioscience
Total IgA	Capture	Purified anti-mouse IgA Antibody (RMA-1)	0.5 mg/ml	1:100	BioLegend
	Block	ELISA buffer containing 1% BSA	Pure	300 μl	Lab EXPIRE
	Sample	Mice Sera samples (Post-sera)	Pure	Post 1:50	Animal Centre
	Standard	Purified mouse IgA	1000 ng	Start 1000 ng/ml, threefold dilution steps	Bethyl Laboratories
	Detection	Biotin Rat Anti-Mouse IgA (C10-1)	0.5 mg/ml	1:250	BD Bioscience

spIgE	Capture	Purified Rat Anti-Mouse IgE (R35-72)	0.5 mg/ml	1:500	BD Bioscience
	Block	ELISA buffer containing 3% powdered milk (ELK)	Pure	300 μl	Campina
	Sample	Mice Sera samples (Pre- and Post-sera)	Pure	Pre 1:30, Post 1:60	Animal Centre
	Standard	Pooled reference serum positive	Pure	Start 1:2, twofold dilution steps	Animal Centre
	Detection	Biotinylated allergen (*see* **Note 13**)	3.9 mg/ml	1:150	Lab EXPIRE
spIgG1	Capture	Crude or rough extract Allergen (*see* **Note 1**)	1 mg/ml	1:100	ALK Abello/ Citeq Biologics
	Block	ELISA buffer containing 1% BSA	Pure	300 μl	Lab EXPIRE
	Sample	Mice Sera samples (Pre- and Post-sera)	Pure	1:300,000	Animal Centre
	Standard	Pooled reference serum positive	Pure	Start 1:50,000, twofold dilution steps	Animal Centre
	Detection	Biotin Rat Anti-Mouse IgG1 (A85-1)	0.5 mg/ml	1:500	BD Bioscience
spIgG2a	Capture	Crude or rough extract Allergen (*see* **Note 1**)	1 mg/ml	1:100	ALK Abello/ Citeq Biologics
	Block	ELISA buffer containing 1% BSA	Pure	300 μl	Lab EXPIRE
	Sample	Mice Sera samples (Pre- and Post-sera)	Pure	1:50	Animal Centre
	Standard	Pooled reference serum positive	Pure	Start 1:25, twofold dilution steps	Animal Centre
	Detection	Biotin Rat Anti-Mouse IgG2a (R19-15)	0.5 mg/ml	1:500	BD Bioscience

Table 2
Antibodies used for FACS analysis of innate lymphocytes

Specificity	Clone	Isotype	Staining	Supplier
Brilliant Violet 605™ anti-mouse Ly-6A/E (Sca-1) Antibody	D7	Rat IgG2a, κ	Extracellular	BioLegend
PerCP/Cy5.5 anti-mouse/ human KLRG1 (MAFA) Antibody	2F1/KLRG1	Syrian hamster IgG	Extracellular	BioLegend
Anti-Mouse CD3e PE	145-2C11	Armenian Hamster IgG	Extracellular	eBioscience
Anti-Mouse CD5 PE	53-7.3	Rat IgG2a, κ	Extracellular	eBioscience
Anti-Mouse CD19 PE	eBio1D3 (1D3)	Rat IgG2a, κ	Extracellular	eBioscience
Anti-Mouse NK1.1 PE	PK136	Mouse IgG2a, κ	Extracellular	eBioscience
Anti-Mouse Fc epsilon Receptor I alpha (FceR1) PE	MAR-1	Armenian Hamster IgG	Extracellular	eBioscience
Anti-Mouse CD11b PE	M1/70	Rat IgG2b, κ	Extracellular	eBioscience
Anti-Mouse CD11c PE	N418	Armenian Hamster IgG	Extracellular	eBioscience
Anti-Mouse Ly-6G (Gr-1) PE	RB6-8C5	Rat IgG2b, κ	Extracellular	eBioscience
Anti-Mouse TER-119 PE	TER-199	Rat IgG2b, κ	Extracellular	eBioscience
T1/ST2 (IL-33R) Monoclonal Antibody, FITC	DJ8	IgG1	Extra- and Intracellular	mdbiosciences
Anti-Mouse CD45 APC	30-F11	Rat IgG2b, κ	Extracellular	eBioscience
Anti-Mouse CD127 APC-eFluor® 780	A7R34	Rat IgG2a, κ	Extracellular	eBioscience
Anti-Human/Mouse Gata-3 PE-Cyanine7	TWAJ	Rat IgG2b, κ	Intracellular	eBioscience

Table 3
Antibodies used for FACS analysis of T cells and DCs

Specificity	Clone	Isotype	Staining	Supplier
Brilliant Violet 605™ anti-mouse CD4 Antibody	GK1.5	Rat IgG2b, κ	Extracellular	BioLegend
Anti-Mouse CD103 (Integrin alpha E) FITC	2E7	Armenian Hamster IgG	Extracellular	eBioscience
Anti-Mouse CD11b APC	M1/70	Rat IgG2b, κ	Extracellular	eBioscience
Anti-Mouse CD11c APC-eFluor® 780	N418	Armenian Hamster IgG	Extracellular	eBioscience
Anti-Mouse F4/80 Antigen PE-Cyanine7	BM8	Rat IgG2a, κ	Extracellular	eBioscience
Anti-Human/Mouse Gata-3 PerCP-eFluor® 710	TWAJ	Rat IgG2b, κ	Intracellular	eBioscience
Anti-Mouse/Rat Foxp3 PE	FJK-16s	Rat IgG2a, κ	Intracellular	eBioscience

5. Fixable live/dead (L/D) cell stain: 1/1000 dilution in PBS (V450 dye).
6. Foxp3/transcription factor staining buffer set containing: fixation/permeabilization concentrate (00-5123), fixation/permeabilization diluent (00-5223), and permeabilization buffer (10×, 00-8333, eBioscience). Dilute the concentrate (1 part) with the diluent (3 parts) prior to use (is called FIX). Dilute the buffer 10× in demi water (PERM buffer).

3 Methods

3.1 Subcutaneous and Sublingual Immunotherapy in a Mouse Model of Allergic Asthma

1. **Sensitization**

   Mice are injected intraperitoneally on days 1 and 14, with GP or HDM allergen extract absorbed to alum dissolved in PBS (total volume 100 μl, *see* Fig. 1 and **Note 2**). For GP sensitization, a rough extract of grass pollen (GP, *Phleum pratense*; *Phl p*) containing 8 μg *Phl p5a* total protein dissolved in 80 μl PBS (*see* **Note 1**, for GP stock solutions) is added to 20 μl Imject alum for each mouse that needs to be sensitized. For sensitization against HDM, (*Dermatophagoides pteronyssinus*; *Der p*) 5 μg HDM extract in 80 μl PBS is added to 20 μl Imject alum for each mouse (*see* **Note 1** for HDM stock solutions).

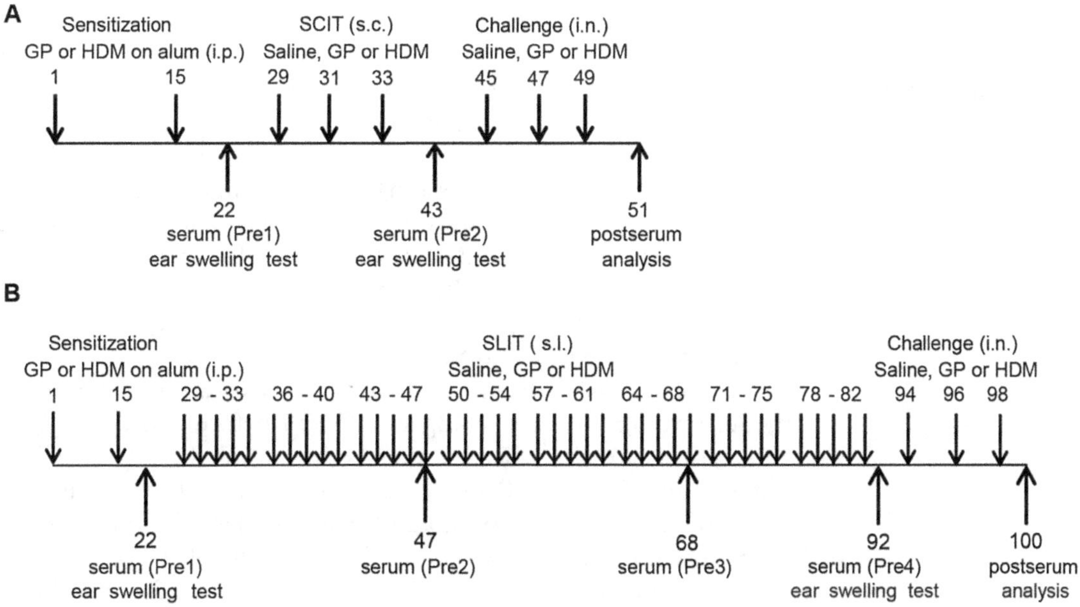

Fig. 1 Overview of AIT-treatment protocols in BALBcByJ mice. (**a**) Outline of the SCIT protocol. (**b**) Outline of the SLIT protocol. Serum is taken before SCIT (Pre1), before challenge (Pre2 in case of SCIT and Pre4 in case of SLIT), and after challenges (Post). In case of SLIT, we include two extra serum-time points (Pre2 and Pre3) during SLIT. Ear swelling tests (EST) are performed before AIT (to confirm sensitization) as well as after AIT (to confirm effect of AIT)

2. **SCIT treatment**

   Mice are SCIT treated on days 29, 31, and 33, by subcutaneous injections (*see* **Note 3**) of the allergen dissolved in PBS (total volume of 100 μl, Fig. 1a). For GP-SCIT (*Phleum pratense*; *Phl p*), dissolve 500 μg *Phl p* protein in 100 μl PBS per injection per mouse. For HDM-SCIT (*Dermatophagoides pteronyssinus*; *Der p*) use 250 μg HDM in 100 μl PBS per injection per mouse.

3. **SLIT treatment**

   Mice are SLIT treated for 5 days a week for 8 consecutive weeks (from day 29 until day 82), by sublingual administration (*see* **Note 4**) of the allergen dissolved in PBS (total volume of 5 μl, Fig. 1b). For GP-SLIT (*Phleum pratense*; *Phl p*), use 500 μg *Phl p* in 5 μl PBS per administration per mouse. For HDM-SLIT (*Dermatophagoides pteronyssinus*; *Der p*), use 250 μg HDM protein in 5 μl PBS per administration per mouse.

4. **Allergen Challenges**

   SCIT treated mice are challenged on days 45, 47, 49, while SLIT treated mice are challenged on days 94, 96, 98, by intranasal administration (*see* **Note 5**) of the allergen dissolved in PBS (total volume of 25 μl, Fig. 1). For GP challenges, use 40 μg *Phl p* protein in 25 μl PBS per administration per mouse. For HDM challenges, use 25 μg HDM in 25 μl PBS per administration per mouse.

3.2 Ear Swelling Test and Blood Withdrawal via Orbital Puncture

After sensitization, during SLIT and after SCIT (*see* Fig. 1), all mice receive a retro-orbital puncture to collect blood (*see* **Note 6**, Pre1-serum; max. 8 ml/kg in 14 days), while under anesthesia (4.5%, 1.5 ml isoflurane/min O_2). Per sample ten small drops are collected in miniCollect tubes and centrifuged in the lab for 11 min at 18,000 ×*g*, after which serum is collected in 100 ml aliquots in 1.5 ml Eppendorf tubes and stored at −80 °C for analysis of immunoglobulins and cytokines. In combination with these procedures, the ear swelling tests (EST) are performed (*see* Figs. 1 and 2), before and after SCIT and SLIT.

The early phase response to allergen provocation is measured by performing an ear swelling test (EST) before and after SCIT and SLIT treatment. Mice are anesthetized using 4.5%, 1.5 ml isoflurane/min O_2 and 10 μl of PBS containing a low amount of allergen (either 1 μg GP or 0.5 μg HDM) is injected intradermal in the right ear of the mouse (*see* Fig. 2). As a control, 10 μl of PBS is injected intradermally in the mouse's left. After 1 or 2 h, ear thickness of both ears is measured using a digimatic pressure limited force-micrometer at 0.5 N (±0.15 N, *see* **Note 7**). The net thickness (Δ, in mm) can be calculated by subtracting the thickness of the left ear from the right ear (*see* Fig. 3a).

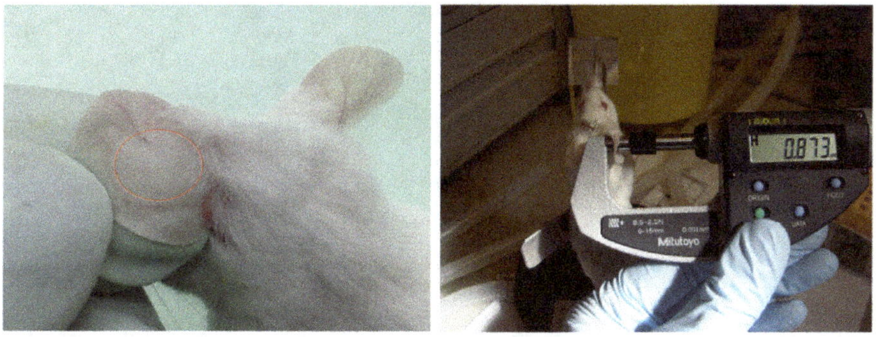

Fig. 2 Photos representing the ear swelling test. *Left*: Anesthetized mice are intradermally injected with 10 μl of PBS in the left ear as a control using a small insulin syringe. A small swelling will be visible just below the skin. *Right*: after 2 h, ear thickness of both ears is measured using a digimatic force-micrometer. It is important to keep the micrometer in a horizontal position

3.3 Lung Function Measurement and Section

Here, the methods and protocols described are based on the FlexiVent version 5.3 (Factory assigned IP address: 192.168.1.200). While we routinely use intravenous administration of methacholine and flexible cannulas for tracheal intubation, alternative approaches including methacholine inhalation and the use of rigid cannulas for tracheal intubation have been described as well [38]. In case immunohistochemical analyses of lung tissue, airway wall remodeling or inflammation is required, this is best performed on a separate group of mice as the forced oscillation technique of invasive airway resistance measurements can be disruptive of local tissue architecture.

1. **Calibration of FlexiVent** should be performed according to the manufacturer's instructions. Briefly, both airway and cylinder pressure need to be calibrated per mouse (weight adjusted) using a 1 ml syringe, a manometer, and a closed and open cannula. For the airway pressure, the first pressure point is zero, the second is the pressure after putting in 1 ml of air. For the cylinder pressure, a dynamic tubing calibration is required using the open and closed cannula according to the manufacturer's instructions.
2. Two days after the final challenge, mice were **weighed and anesthetized** with a mixture of 75 mg/kg ketamine (100 mg/ml) and 1 mg/kg domitor (0.5 mg/ml, *see* **Note 8**) by intraperitoneal injection (10 μl mix per gram bodyweight). Repeat this injection with 25 % of the initial dose every 20 min. Be aware that during the entire procedure the mice should be kept warm. Furthermore, heart rate, blood pressure and O_2 saturation should be monitored using a pulse-oximeter and recorded.
3. All anesthetized mice were cannulated with a 20 G **trachea cannula** and a jugular vein cannula, then placed on a computer-controlled small-animal ventilator (FlexiVent, SCIREQ).

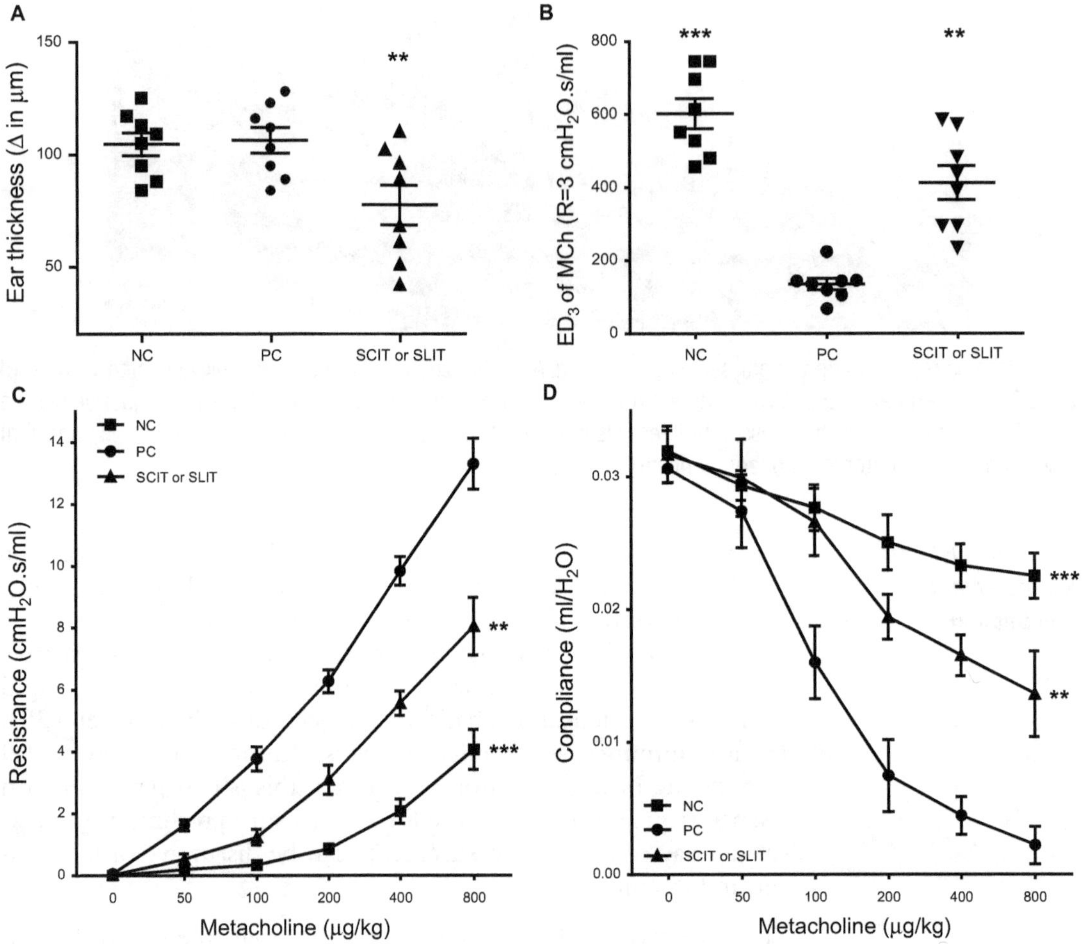

Fig. 3 Clinical manifestations after AIT. (**a**) IgE dependent allergic response plotted as net ear thickness (mm) 2 h after GP injection (1 kSQ) in the right ear and PBS in the left ear as a control, performed after AIT. Placebo-treated mice (NC and PC) provide similar swelling since both have been placebo treated and are not challenged yet. (**b**) Effective Dose (ED) of methacholine, when the airway resistance reaches 3 cmH_2O s/ml. (**c**) Airway hyperactivity (AHR) was measured by FlexiVent and plotted as airway resistance (*R* in cmH_2O s/ml) and as (**d**) Airway compliance (*C* in ml/cmH_2O). Absolute values are expressed as mean ± SEM ($n=8$). $^*P<0.05$, $^{**}P<0.01$, and $^{***}P<0.005$ compared to positive control. NC: negative control, PBS challenged; PC: positive control, GP challenged; SCIT or SLIT treated mice (300 kSQ), GP challenged

Tracheal cannulation: First, make an incision in the middle of the neck and tear the underlying tissue carefully with two sharp pair of tweezers till you see the muscle where the trachea is lying in. Be careful not to touch the gland around the trachea, to prevent increased mucus production. Then, tear the muscle open carefully, completely free the trachea from underlying tissue and place two ligatures, one at the top of the trachea and one at the bottom. Third, cut a hole in the trachea between the trachea rings and place the cannula in the trachea and close both ligatures. Attach the upper ligature to the cannula with a tight knot. Finally, attach the mice to the FlexiVent machine and set the program to standard breathing (script running on basic breathing, *see* **Note 9**).

Jugular vein cannulation: Make an imaginary line from the right armpit to the left foreleg and from the right armpit to the middle of the jaw, then make a 1.5 cm vertical incision (downwards) on the crossing. Similar as with the trachea cannula, tear the underlying tissue carefully with two sharp pairs of tweezers until you can see the jugular vein and clear it of any fat or surrounding connective tissue, allowing a curved surgical tweezer to maneuver underneath the jugular vein. Then, place a ligature (6/0) around the upper part of the jugular vein, close it and attach this ligature with some tape to the operating table to put some tension on it. Now, place a second ligature (6/0) 0.5 cm down, but do not close the knot completely. Place a bulldog clamp on the lower ligature to increase the tension and cut a hole in the vein between the two ligatures. Place the cannula through the hole in the jugular vein and close the bottom ligature. Test whether the cannula is in place by carefully pulling the plunger of the syringe. A properly cannulated jugular vein will allow blood to be present in the cannula. Fix the cannula with both ligatures. Now, several dosages of methacholine can be given through this cannula according to the FlexiVent's protocol (*see* **Notes 9** and **10**).

4. Before starting the **FlexiVent measurements**, all mice receive a muscle relaxant, 1 μl/g mouse rocuronium bromide (diluted to 0.125 mg/ml), which is repeated after the methacholine dosage of 100 μg/kg. When starting the protocol, make sure the positive end-expiratory pressure (PEEP) is set at 20 mm H_2O. According to the weight table (*see* **Note 11**), methacholine is administered intravenously in doses 0, 50, 100, 200, 400, and 800 μg/kg, and airway responsiveness is measured by obtaining airway resistance (R in cmH_2O s/ml), the Newtonian resistance (the resistance of the central or conducting airways, Rn in cmH_2O s/ml), and compliance (C in ml/H_2O). Immediately after each methacholine dose flush the tubing with 30 μl saline to make sure that all methacholine enters the body.
5. Immediately after this procedure, all mice were **sacrificed** under continued anesthesia by collecting blood through a vena cava puncture (post-serum) in a miniCollect tube. To start, the abdomen of the mouse is opened and the bowels are repositioned so that the vena cava is clearly visible. After fat removal, the vena cava can be punctured using a 25 G needle on a 1 ml syringe and take out approximately 1 ml of total blood volume.

6. Prepare the body for **Broncho-alveolar lavage** by opening the diaphragm so the lungs can fully collapse, but make sure not to damage the lungs by puncturing. Using a syringe containing 1 ml supplemented PBS (10 ml PBS + 1 protease cocktail inhibitor tablet and 3 % BSA on room temperature) on the trachea cannula, the lungs can be flushed gently. During drawback of this first ml of supplemented PBS, it is normal that a small amount remains in the lungs. Store the first ml in a 1.5 ml tube. Repeat this lavage for four times using regular PBS (non-supplemented, on room temperature) and collect this in a 15 ml tube. Store the first ml lavage on ice as BALF and the remaining 4 ml on ice to collect extra cells.
7. Hereafter, individual lung lobes and all other necessary organs can be collected and placed in RPMI1640 medium (~1 ml at 4 °C) and kept on ice. Also, individual lung lobes can be stored separately in cryogen-vials, and snap-frozen immediately after isolation in liquid nitrogen and stored at −80 °C for future analysis. Make sure that the empty cryovials have been weighed prior to dissection to allow measurement of the net weight of the lung lobe retrieved during section.
8. Finally, export all FlexiVent data to Excel files and store them according at the appropriate locations (backed-up network drive), for analysis of resistance and compliance values (*see* **Note 12**). After analysis of the data, resistance and compliance values can be plotted in a graph against the doses of MCh (*see* Fig. 3c, d). Furthermore, in analyzing the resistance data, one could calculate the effective dose (ED) of MCh necessary to increase AHR to an R of 3 cmH_2O s/ml (ED3) (*see* Fig. 3b). Appropriate statistical evaluation includes ANOVA, or in case of missing values a GEE analysis [39].

3.4 Analysis of the Infiltration of Inflammatory Cells in BAL Fluid

Inflammatory cell composition of BAL and lung tissue can be analyzed by manual counting of cytospin preparations or by flow cytometric analysis. While the latter allows for a far more detailed analysis, the former does require minimal time investment on the section day of the experiment.

1. First, all **cytospin slides** need to be numbered and coated. Open the slide holder by its driver, insert a clean slide with appropriate label in the slide holder, place a clean Shandon filter card on the slide in the holder, insert a clean cuvette in the holder above the filter card, and put the holder containing slide—filter card—cuvette in the cyto-centrifuge. Add 20 μl PBS containing 1 % BSA in the whole of cuvette and run the centrifuge at 550 × *g* for 1 min.
2. Centrifuge the first ml of the **BAL** cell suspension at 590 × *g*, 4 °C for 5 min and store the supernatant in 100 μl aliquots at

−80 °C. Do the same for the 15 ml tube containing the additional BAL cells, only discard the supernatant. Now, resuspend the pellet of the 15 ml tube in 500 μl lysis buffer and add this to the pellet of the first ml and incubate for 1 min at room temperature. Then, centrifuge the cells at 590 × *g*, 4 °C for 5 min, discard the supernatant and resuspend the pellet in 200 μl PBS containing 1 % BSA.

3. To **count** the cells, use an appropriately calibrated method for cell counting (resulting in a BALF **total cell count** (*T*)) and adjust the number of cells to 1×10^6 cells/ml (*see* Fig. 4a).
4. Prepare **cytospins** by adding 100 μl of the cell suspension (1×10^5 cells) to the cuvette of the coated slides and centrifuge at 550 × *g* at room temperature for 5 min. Carefully release the slides from the holder using the driver and let the slides air dry for 10 min at room temperature. Clean the cuvettes using demi-water and 70 % ethanol solution overnight.
5. Cytospin preparations are stained with a Diff-Quick staining set (manufacturer's protocol) and 300 cells per cytospin were evaluated using the differential cell counter and differentiated by an observer blinded to the experimental groups into **mononuclear cells** (M), **neutrophils** (N), and **eosinophils** (E) by standard morphology using a light microscope with 100× magnification in immersion oil (*see* Fig. 4b).

3.5 Preparation of Single Cell Suspensions of Lung Tissue, Spleen, and Draining Lymph Nodes

1. In preparing a **single cell suspension** from **mouse lung**, the left lung lobe (largest) of every mouse is transferred into a petri dish in the flow cabinet. Using a scalpel, the lobe is cut into a homogenous paste, dissolved in 2 ml RPMI1640 medium including 4 mg/ml collagenase A, 0.1 mg/ml DNase I, and 1 % BSA, and incubated for 1.5 h at 37 °C. A single cell suspension is generated by flushing the lung digest through a 70 μm cell strainer into a 50 ml tube. Cell strainers are washed with 2–5 ml of RPMI (at room temperature) in order to flush out remaining cells. The collection tubes are centrifuged at 350 × *g* for 5 min at 4 °C and the supernatant can be discarded. Pellets are resuspended in 1 ml lysis buffer and incubated for 3 min at room temperature. Cells are then centrifuged again at 350 × *g* for 5 min at 4 °C and supernatant is discarded. The cells are counted using a Coulter counter and used for cytospin (*see* Subheading 2.4 BAL Fluid) and restimulation (*see* Subheading 2.6).
2. **Single cell suspensions** of **spleen cells** are obtained in a similar fashion, although enzymatic digestion is only required in case of DC subset analyses. Single cell suspensions are generated by flushing the spleen tissue suspension through a 70 μm cell strainer and rinsing the strainer with 5 ml sterile RPMI1640,

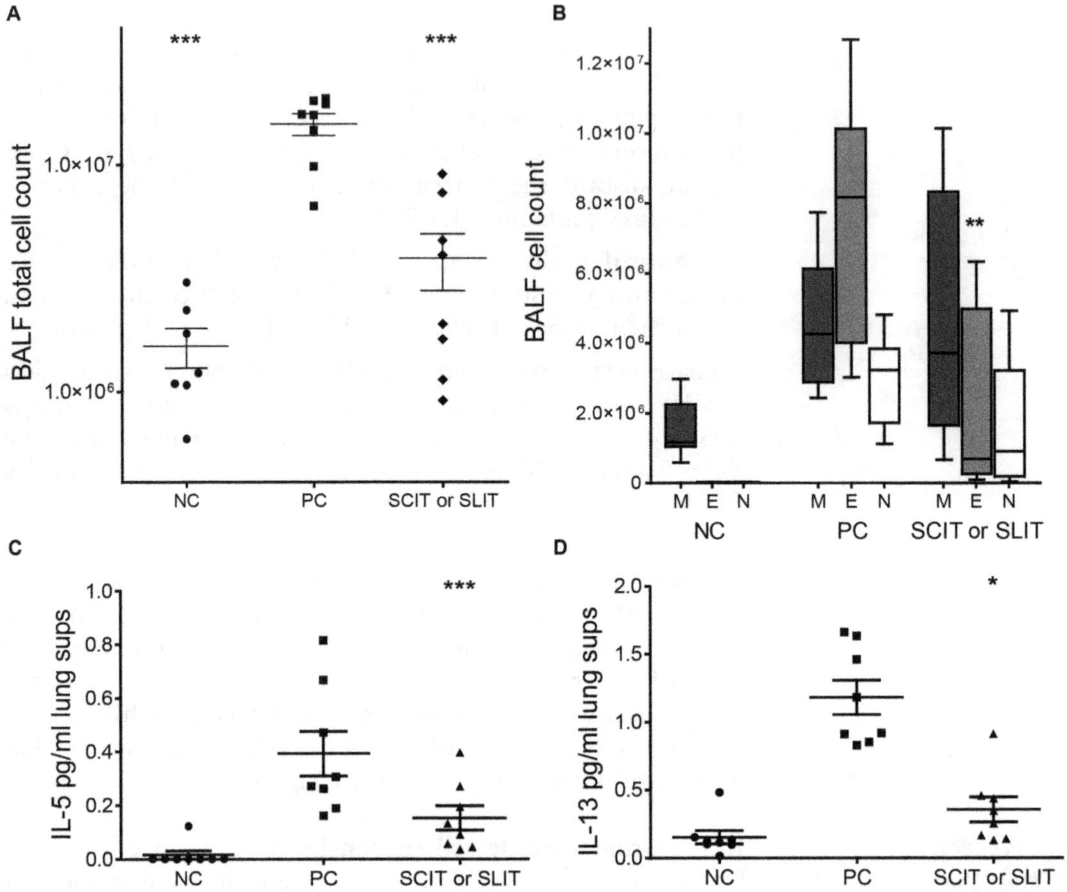

Fig. 4 The eosinophilic and proinflammatory cytokine response after AIT. (**a**) Total cell counts in broncho-alveolar lavage fluid (BALF). (**b**) Differential cytospin cell counts in BALF. *M* mononuclear cells, *E* eosinophils, *N* neutrophils. Absolute numbers are plotted as median and 10–90 interquartile. (**c** and **d**) Concentrations of IL-5 and IL-13 measured in restimulated single cell suspensions of lung cells. Concentrations were calculated as the concentration after 5 day-restimulation minus unstimulated control (PBS) and expressed as mean ± SEM ($n = 8$). $^{*}P < 0.05$, $^{**}P < 0.01$, and $^{***}P < 0.005$ compared to positive control

before centrifuging the spleen cells at 550 × *g* for 5 min. Discard the supernatant, add 1 ml lysis buffer and incubate for 10 min at room temperature. Wash the cells with 1 ml RMPI1640 twice and cells are ready for further use. For storage of the cells in liquid nitrogen, resuspend the cell pellet in 50 % HBSS, 40 % FCS, and add slowly 10 % DMSO, then divide the suspension over both cryogen vials, and place them in a Stratagene® box in the −80 °C overnight. The day after, transfer the vials into the liquid nitrogen.

3. Cells originating from the (lung) **draining lymph nodes** (DLN) can be processed in a similar fashion as the lung tissue cells.

3.6 Restimulation of Lung Cells and Draining Lymph Node (DLN) Cells

1. To evaluate the T cell responses in **lung tissue single cell suspensions**, 200,000 cells/well are restimulated in 250 μl RPMI1640 (supplemented with 10% FCS, pen/strep; 50 μM beta-ME) with either 0 or 30 μg of GP or HDM extract *in triplo* in 96-well plates (U-bottom). Lung cell cultures are incubated for 5 days at 37 °C and 5% CO_2. The supernatant of all wells are pooled per mouse, aliquoted *in triplo* and stored in −80 °C, for analysis of cytokines.
2. Cell suspensions from draining **lymph nodes** can be restimulated in a similar way as described above. Using a round-bottom 96-well plate, 200,000 cells/well can be restimulated with GP or HDM extracts (30 μg/well). Since lymph node-cell suspensions usually do not contain as much cells as the lung suspensions, here measurements can be done *in duplo*.

3.7 Homogenization of Lung Tissue for Total Protein and Cytokine Analysis

To measure levels of specific cytokines, chemokines or other mediators in lung tissue, individual lung lobes are used either freshly at the day of section, or at a later stage using lung lobes snap-frozen on the day of section and retrieved from −80 °C for analysis. Use the identical lung lobe for all mice in the experimental and control groups. Keep the lung lobes on ice at all times.

1. Weigh the cryogen vials containing the lung lobe and correct for the empty cryogen vial weight to obtain the net lung lobe weight (mg lung tissue).
2. Add Luminex buffer in a ratio of 1:5 weight/volume of each lung (1 mg lung + 4 μl buffer).
3. Homogenize the lung with the homogenizer (on ice!) for at least 1 min, until no more large pieces are visible. Then, clean the homogenizer (dismantle the crusher) with tab water (once) and ethanol (once) in between samples. Clean and dry the homogenizer.
4. Centrifuge the crushed lung samples at 12,000 × *g* for 20 min at 4 °C.
5. Collect supernatants, store them in 100 μl aliquots at −80 °C until further analysis, and discard the pellets.
6. When evaluating cytokine responses between experimental groups, it is important to measure cytokine-levels (ELISA) and plot them relative to protein content instead of per ml lung tissue homogenate. Protein concentrations retrieved from homogenization of lung lobes vary between individual mice, so this needs to be corrected for. Therefore, a BCA analysis can be performed to quantitate protein content of the lung tissue homogenates according to the manufacturer's protocol (Thermo Scientific, Waltham, MA, USA).

3.8 Analysis of Immunoglobulin Levels in Serum and Cytokine Levels in BAL Fluid, Supernatant of Restimulated Single Cell Suspensions and Lung Tissue Homogenates

1. ELISA measurements can be performed to determine the **immunoglobulin levels in serum** of total as well as GP- or HDM-spIgG1, GP- or HDM-spIgG2a, GP- or HDM-spIgE in serum taken at three different time points (pre1-, pre2-, and post-serum, stored at −80 °C).
2. Cytokine measurements in BAL fluid, supernatant of restimulated single cell suspensions and lung tissue homogenates can be performed by ELISA or multiplex analysis (a wide range of commercial suppliers available). For accurate quantification of cytokine levels by ELISA, samples should be stored at −80 °C until measurement, and, as a rule of thumb, samples should be processed within 3 months from isolation.
3. Protocol for Ig-ELISA measurements in sera: coat a high affinity binding 96-well flat bottom ELISA plate with 100 μl purified rat anti-mouse IgE/G1/G2a (*see* Table 1) in PBS overnight at 4 °C. Wash the plate five times using 300 μl wash buffer (PBS containing 0.05 % Tween 20) either with a ELISA plate washer or by hand. Block the plate using 300 μl ELISA buffer with 1 % BSA at room temperature for 1 h. Empty the plate, wash once with wash buffer, make sure the wells are emptied and add the samples and standard (both *in duplo*) in a total volume of 100 μl and incubate for 2 h at room temperature on the shaker 300 rpm. For concentration of the reference curve and the appropriate dilution of the serum samples please refer to Table 1. Usually, pre-sera samples will be diluted 1:30 and post-sera samples 1:60 in ELISA buffer; however several dilutions can be tested for optimal results. Wash the plate five times using 300 μl wash buffer. Add detection Ab diluted in ELISA buffer (*see* Table 1 and **Note 13**) to the plate in 100 μl and incubate for 1.5 h at room temperature on the shaker at 300 rpm. Wash the plate five times using wash buffer. Add 100 μl horseradish peroxidase (HRP) diluted 1:200 in ELISA buffer and incubate for 1 h at room temperature on the shaker 300 rpm. Wash the plate again and add 100 μl OPD peroxidase substrate (according to manufacturers' instructions) and incubate for 10 min in the dark until the coloring reaction is complete. Stop the reaction by adding 75 μl 4 M H_2SO_4 to each well. Read the optical density at 490 nm on the ELISA plate reader. Calculate the concentrations using of the sera samples based on the reference curve a four parameter model. The fit of the standard curve should be at least 0.95 (r^2). When performing multiple 96-well plates in one measurement, each plate should contain a standard curve as well as a few reference samples that are included on all plates for plate–plate comparison.

3.9 Quantification of DCs, T Cell Populations, and Innate Lymphoid Cells in Lung Single Cell Suspensions Using Flow Cytometry

Divide all lung single cell suspensions in the FACS tubes per mouse per mixture and use a small amount of cells for the single staining (two donors per single). Start with a wash using 300 μl FACS Buffer, centrifuge the cells at 590 × *g* for 5 min and remove supernatant. Then, resuspend in 100 μl FACS buffer, add an extracellular block using 100 μl Block buffer (2% NRS, 5% FcBlock in FACS buffer) and incubate for 10 min on room temperature. Centrifuge, remove supernatant and resuspend in 100 μl FACS buffer, add 100 μl extra-cellular staining, and incubate for 30 min on room temperature in the dark (*see* Tables 2 and 3 for the mixtures). Centrifuge and wash in 1000 μl FACS buffer then wash again in 1000 μl regular PBS. Resuspend in 100 μl PBS, add 75 μl fixable live dead V450 (1:1000 diluted in PBS) incubate for 15 min on room temperature in the dark. Wash once in 1000 μl regular PBS and resuspend in 1000 μl FIX, incubate for 30 min on room temperature in the dark. Without washing add 1000 μl PERM buffer. Centrifuge and remove supernatant and then resuspend in 100 μl PERM buffer containing 2% NRS and 5% FcBlock for intracellular blocking. After 10 min incubation, centrifuge, remove supernatant, and resuspend in 100 μl PERM buffer. Then add 100 μl intracellular staining (antibodies diluted in PERM buffer), and incubate for 30 min on room temperature in the dark (*see* Tables 2 and 3 for the mixtures). Without washing add 1000 μl PERM buffer, centrifuge and remove supernatant. Wash once more in 1000 μl FACS buffer and remove supernatant. Finally, resuspend 200 μl FACS buffer and transfer the cells to the 35 μm cell strainer FACS tube. Measure all singles and samples using a three laser flow cytometer (eight fluorochromes).

In analyzing the FCS files derived from the measurements, always start by setting the compensation settings using the single stained cells, depending on the program used. Once, these are corrected throughout the entire experiment, start the analysis by excluding all dead cells as well as doublets. The first can be done by plotting the area of the forward scatter (FSC-A) against the fixable live dead marker and exclude the dead cells (*see* Fig. 5a). Second, all doublets can be excluded using a small selection gate when plotting the area of the side scatter (SSC-A) against the width of the side scatter (SSC-W, *see* Fig. 5b). Then, depending on the mix gating strategies can be adjusted depending on which cell type needs to be identified and or quantified. Here, as an example, the gating strategy for ILC2s can be plotted as Lineage negative cells versus CD45 positive cells (*see* Table 2 and Fig. 5c). Subclassification can be done using GATA3 and CD127, markers that are both expressed by ILC2s (Fig. 5d).

For the identification of other cell types, CD4 and GATA3 can be used to identify Th2 cells, CD4 and FoxP3 can be used to identify

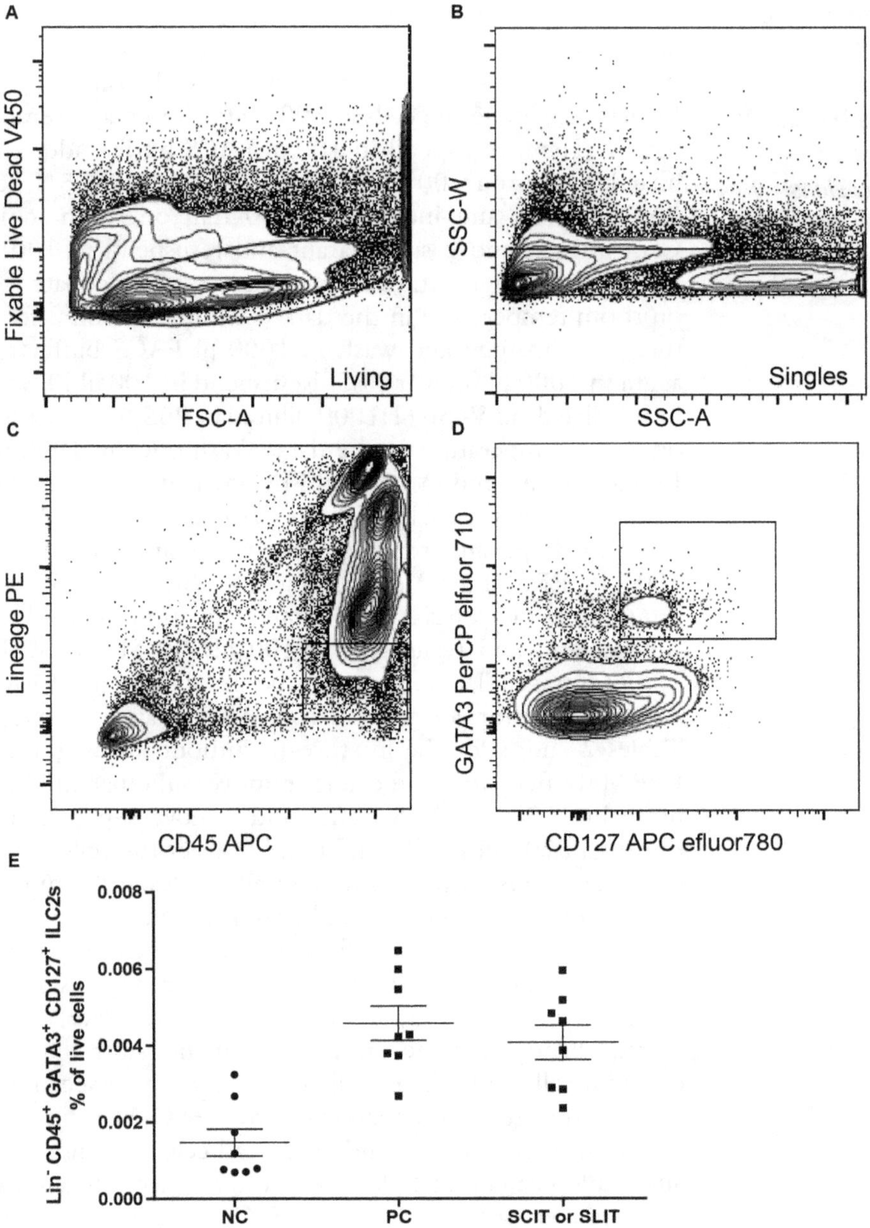

Fig. 5 Gating strategy for the identification of innate lymphoid cells type 2 (ILC2s) in the lung. (**a**) Gating of live cells. (**b**) Doublet cell exclusion. (**c**) Gating out the lineage negative cells and including the CD45 positive cells. (**d**) Gating for only the GATA3 and CD127 double positive cells. (**e**) ILC2s plotted as $Lineage^{-}CD45^{+}GATA3^{+}$ and $CD127^{+}$ % of live cells

Treg cells, and CD11b and CD103 can be used to identify subpopulations of different types of conventional DCs (*see* Table 3). The gating strategy starts similar as mentioned before, with the exclusion of dead cells and doublets.

4 Notes

1. **Stocks of GP**: dissolve the 204 mg dry matter of *Phleum pratense*, 225 (MP225PHLpra, 1006674 or 1031225) in 2.125 ml sterile PBS to get a solution containing 60 kSQ/μl (~96 μg/μl). Aliquot this stock in small 100 μl portions and store at −20 °C. **Stocks of HDM**: dissolve 25.0 mg DP extract FD 12C27 in 500 μl sterile PBS to get a solution containing 50 μg/μl HDM and aliquot this stock in 25 μl portions and store at −20 °C.
2. Performing **intraperitoneal injections**: the non-anesthetized animal is restrained manually (one-handed) and tilted head down at 35–40° angle so that the intestines fall away from the injection site. The needle is inserted into the lower right quadrant of the abdomen slightly off the midline anterior to the bladder. Slight negative pressure is applied to the syringe. To avoid the likelihood of puncturing or lacerating abdominal organs, a ½ inch, 27 G needle or insulin syringe is recommended. This route of administration allows for a volume of up to 1 ml be given safely to a mouse.
3. **Subcutaneous injections** can be used for administration of the allergen extracts. The non-anesthetized animal is held using a standard single handed restraint technique and a 25 G needle is inserted at the base of a skin tent created by the thumb and forefinger. A slight negative pressure is applied to the syringe to ensure proper placement is subcutaneous and not having accidently damaged a local vein. A total of 100 μl is injected.
4. For **sublingual administration**, the non-anesthetized animal is restrained manually (one-handed) and the head is tilted up at full vertical position. Tightly fix the fir between thumb and index finger, until the mice slightly stick out their tongue. Using a P20 pipet, 5 μl of allergen solution can be placed under the tongue, while ensuring that it stays there for 30 s minimum. It is of paramount importance that the mice do not swallow the allergen during the administration. After administration, maintain the restrained animal for 30 s up-straight to prevent swallowing until the mouse can be placed back in the individual ventilated cage (IVC).
5. The **intranasal challenges** are performed with the mouse lightly and quickly anesthetized using 4.5 % isoflurane in combination with 1 ml/min O_2. Mice are taken out of the anesthesia as soon as their breathing starts to slow down a bit. The mouse is manually restrained and the tail anchored between the small finger and the palm. The mouse is held in a supine position with the head elevated. Right before the mouse wakes

up (should be within 1 min), the end of a micropipette is placed at or in the external nares and then the solution is poured in. Pipet 25 μl of the allergen extract dissolved in PBS, quickly on each of the nares as the mouse wakes up and inhales into the lungs. Check visually whether the allergen solution has been inhaled by the mouse.

6. **Retro-orbital bleeding** targets the venous sinus located behind the eye. When correctly performed on these long-anesthetized mice using 4.5 % isoflurane in combination with 1 ml/min O_2, the eyes and health of the animal remain unaffected. Hold the anesthetized mouse on a flat surface and gently press it against the flat surface, to force blood from the thorax to the head. The forefinger of the same hand is used to pull the dorsal eyelid back producing slight exophthalmos (bulging of the eye). Then, use a glass microcapillary tube to penetrate the orbital conjunctiva at the medial or lateral canthus of the eye. As soon as blood accumulates in the capillary lift up the mouse and hold it above the MiniCollect tube and let ten drops of blood fall in. Be aware, the speed of which the blood drops in the tube can vary significantly! When punctured just right, you have to act quickly.
7. In using the **digimatic pressure-limited micrometer**, it is really important to keep it perfectly horizontal when measuring ear thickness. Therefore, all mice need to remain in the same horizontal position during the measurement. Mice receiving a light anesthesia, using 4.5 % isoflurane in combination with 1 ml/min O_2, can be placed on a small bridge/cup to make sure the ears are in the same horizontal position every time.
8. Mice can be anesthetized for invasive lung function measurement using the following dilution schedule:

	Solution	Administration	Dose
Ketamine	100 mg/ml	75 mg/ml	0.75 μl/g mouse
Domitor	0.5 mg/ml	1 mg/ml	1 μl/g mouse
Dilution scheme (100 mg/ml)			
	1 ml	5 ml	10 ml
Domitor	200 μl	1000 μl	2000 μl
Ketamine	75 μl	375 μl	750 μl
Saline	725 μl	3625 μl	7250 μl

9. A standard script is available within the FlexiWare software, which can be adjusted to the following format:

```
FlexiVent      script       ================
Script:   MCh IV DRC Author:   LH Date:   15-
02-2012 Changes:     LH: 8-6-2016 Adapted to
```

```
new software and doses Adapted to new doses and comments of Scireq crew 1. Added snapshot after TLC (for quality control) 2. Quick prime 3 instead of quick prime 2 (+ reduction of number of perturbations) 3. In template adaptation: addition of constant phase model for the quick prime perturbations (c) SCIREQ Inc. 2001-04
// Start of command section // ------------------------ Start Script, Format = 3.0; Title = MCh DRC with TLC; //Start DEFAULT ventilation (Depending on Template) 0:00 Ventilation DEFAULT; // Perform TLC maneuver immediately after attaching the animal 0:02 Prompt MESSAGE=Attach the animal, then click OK to perform two TLC maneuvers.; 0:00 Marker TEXT=Performing two TLC maneuvers at start of the experiment.; 0:00 Ventilation MODE=CFlow; F=10 br/min; Vt=40 ml/kg; IER=1; Pmax=30 cmH2O; 0:05 Ventilation DEFAULT; 0:15 Ventilation MODE=CFlow; F=10 br/min; Vt=40 ml/kg; IER=1; Pmax=30 cmH2O; 0:05 Ventilation DEFAULT; //Do a snapshot for quality control (check for leakage) 0:05 Perturbation NAME=Snapshot-240; // Log the substance 0:05 Marker TEXT=Start of MCh Dose response measurement.; // Start loop for Baseline 0:02 Loop Begin // Log next dose 0:00 Marker TEXT=Next dose: Baseline ; // Prepare to inject the mice 0:00 Prompt BEEP ; 0:00 Prompt MESSAGE=Press OK to start baseline measurement. ; 0:02 Marker TEXT=Mouse is being injected : Baseline; // Take 6 measurements directly after each other 0:00 Loop Begin 0:00 Perturbation NAME=QPrime3; 0:00 Loop Return MAXCOUNT=6; // Take 4 measurement for 4 times 0:00 Loop Begin 0:00 Perturbation NAME=QPrime3; 0:40 Loop Return MAXCOUNT=4 // Prompt user for next dose 0:20 Query MESSAGE=Continue with next dose? (No to restart previous dose); 0:00 Loop Return REPLY=NO ; // Start loop for 0 µg/kg 0:02 Loop Begin // Log next dose 0:00 Marker TEXT=Next dose: 0 ; // Prepare to inject the mice 0:00 Prompt BEEP ; 0:00 Prompt MESSAGE=Press OK when ready to inject mouse (0 µg/kg), and inject immediately thereafter. ; 0:02 Marker TEXT=Mouse is being injected:0 µg/kg; // Take
```

`6 measurements directly after each other 0:00 Loop Begin 0:00 Perturbation NAME=QPrime3; 0:00 Loop Return MAXCOUNT=6; // Take 4 measurement for 4 times 0:00 Loop Begin 0:00 Perturbation NAME=QPrime3; 0:40 Loop Return MAXCOUNT=4; // Prompt user for next dose 0:20 Query MESSAGE=Continue with next dose? (No to restart previous dose); 0:00 Loop Return REPLY=NO ; // Start loop for 50 µg/ kg →` **`repeat for the dosages`** `100, 200, 400 and 800 µg/ kg // End of script`

10. Before putting a new syringe on the IV-line, make sure there is no air remaining in the syringe and cannula (use 5 ml syringe with saline to fill the 1 ml syringe).
11. IV injection of several doses of methacholine: see dilution table and weights:

Dose (µg/kg)	Dose (mg/ml)
0	0
50	0.01562
100	0.03125
200	0.0625
400	0.125
800	0.25

Weight (g)	Injection volume (µl)
20	64
21	67
22	70
23	74
24	77
25	80
26	83
27	86
28	90
29	93
30	96
31	99
32	102
33	106

Weight (g)	Injection volume (μl)
34	109
35	112
36	115
37	118
38	122
39	129
40	128

12. Analysis of resistance and compliance data can be performed using the exported files. Herein, a clear stepwise report is made for every subject. When interested in the resistance and compliance values, simply highlight those, together with the COD values, the PEEP (and optional the Newtonian resistance R_N). Every dose of MCh gives a peak value in resistance (cmH_2O s/ml) and a bottom value in compliance (ml/H_2O). Highlight those for every dose of MCh and for every subject, and plot them. To ensure high quality data use the coefficient of determination (COD)-value with a cutoff of 8. This is a quality control parameter measuring the quality of the single compartment model fit. Alternatively, all values that are measured with sufficient technical quality (use COD value as a cutoff) can be plotted to calculate an area under the curve for each individual methacholine dose. Check whether the PEEP was registered as ~20 mm H_2O or ~2 cm H_2O.
13. Biotinylation of grass pollen and house dust mites is performed using the "Thermo Scientific EZ-Link Sulfo-NHS-LC-Biotin," an intermediate-length, water-soluble biotinylation reagent for labeling proteins (Thermo Scientific, 21327). According to the manufacturers' protocol, we can adjust the molar ratio of Sulfo-NHS-LC-Biotin to protein to obtain the level of incorporation desired (~4–6 biotin groups per allergen-particle). Calculate millimoles of biotin reagent to add to the reaction for a 20-fold molar excess: **mmol biotin** = ml protein × (mg protein/ml protein) × (mmol protein/mg protein) × (20 mmol biotin/mmol protein). Then, calculate microliters of 10 mM biotin reagent solution (stock) to add to the reaction: **μl biotin** = mmol biotin × (1,000,000 μl/l) × (l/10 mmol). Since, the rough extracts contain a mixture of proteins with a lot of different molecular weights, we make an estimate based on SDS-PAGE results. For the rough extract of GP, we calculated using an average molecular weight of 10,000 Da. An example: 1000 μl GP × (3.9 mg GP/1 ml GP) × (1 mmol GP/10,000 mg GP) × (5 mmol biotin/1 mmol GP) = 1.95×10^{-3} mmol biotin. Second, 1.95×10^{-3} mmol biotin × (1×10^{6} μl/l) × (l/10 mmol) = 195 μl

biotin. For the biotinylation reaction take the following steps: add 180 μl of ultrapure water to the 1 mg microtube to prepare a 10 mM solution of the biotin reagent (stock) and take out the calculated volume of biotin to add to your protein solution. Incubate for 2 h on ice or for 30 min on room temperature. For optimal performance and stability, we purify the labeled proteins using a Slide-A-Lyzer™ G2 Dialysis Cassettes, 3.5K MWCO, 0.5 ml according to the manufacturers' protocol (Thermo Scientific, 87722). In short, after hydrating the membrane in PBS for 2 min, using a 1 ml syringe with 18 G needle, slowly fill the cassette with your biotin–allergen mixture and withdraw any remaining air. Next, perform a typical dialysis procedure: 2 h at room temperature in 2 l PBS; then change the PBS and dialyze for another 2 h; change the buffer again and dialyze overnight at 4 °C. The next day, you can remove the purified sample and store aliquoted in the −20 °C freezer.

Acknowledgments

Laura Hesse is supported by the Dutch Lung Foundation (NAF10.060).

References

1. Kim HY, DeKruyff RH, Umetsu DT (2010) The many paths to asthma: phenotype shaped by innate and adaptive immunity. Nat Immunol 11:577–584. doi:10.1038/ni.1892
2. Weiss ST, Litonjua AA, Lange C, Lazarus R, Liggett SB, Bleecker ER, Tantisira KG (2006) Overview of the pharmacogenetics of asthma treatment. Pharmacogenomics J 6:311–326. doi:10.1038/sj.tpj.6500387
3. Lambrecht BN, Hammad H (2014) The immunology of asthma. Nat Immunol 16:45–56. doi:10.1038/ni.3049
4. Holgate ST, Polosa R (2008) Treatment strategies for allergy and asthma. Nat Rev Immunol 8:218–230. doi:10.1038/nri2262
5. Matte-Martyn A, Diaz-Granados N, Al-Saidi F, Cooper AB, Guest CB, Mazer CD, Mehta S, Stewart TE, Barr A, Cook D, Slutsky AS, Canadian Critical Care Trials Group (2011) Long-term inhaled corticosteroids in preschool children at high risk for asthma. N Engl J Med 354:683–693.doi:10.1056/NEJMoa1207363
6. Zeiger RS, Mauger D, Bacharier LB, Guilbert TW, Martinez FD, Lemanske RF, Strunk RC, Covar R, Szefler SJ, Boehmer S, Jackson DJ, Sorkness CA, Gern JE, Kelly HW, Friedman NJ, Mellon MH, Schatz M, Morgan WJ, Chinchilli VM, Raissy HH, Bade E, Malka-Rais J, Beigelman A, Taussig LM (2011) Daily or intermittent budesonide in preschool children with recurrent wheezing. N Engl J Med 365:1999–2001. doi:10.1056/NEJMoa1104647
7. Hancox RJ, Cowan JO, Flannery EM, Herbison GP, McLachlan CR, Taylor DR (2000) Bronchodilator tolerance and rebound bronchoconstriction during regular inhaled beta-agonist treatment. Respir Med 94:767–771. doi:10.1053/rmed.2000.0820, S0954-6111(00)90820-5 [pii]
8. Yim RP, Koumbourlis AC (2013) Tolerance & resistance to β2-agonist bronchodilators. Paediatr Respir Rev 14:195–198. doi:10.1016/j.prrv.2012.11.002
9. Jutel M (2014) Allergen-specific immunotherapy in asthma. Curr Treat Options Allergy 1:213–219. doi:10.1007/s40521-014-0013-1
10. Jacobsen L, Niggemann B, Dreborg S, Ferdousi H, Halken S, Høst A, Koivikko A, Norberg LA, Valovirta E, Wahn U, Möller C (2007) Specific immunotherapy has long-term preventive effect of seasonal and perennial asthma: 10-year follow-up on the PAT study. Allergy 62:943–948. doi:10.1111/j.1398-9995.2007.01451.x

11. Abramson MJ, Puy RM, Weiner JM (2010) Injection allergen immunotherapy for asthma. Cochrane Database Syst Rev (8):CD001186. doi:10.1002/14651858.CD001186.pub2
12. Mosbech H, Deckelmann R, De Blay F, Pastorello EA, Trebas-Pietras E, Andres LP, Malcus I, Ljørring C, Canonica GW (2014) Standardized quality (SQ) house dust mite sublingual immunotherapy tablet (ALK) reduces inhaled corticosteroid use while maintaining asthma control: a randomized, double-blind, placebo-controlled trial. J Allergy Clin Immunol. doi:10.1016/j.jaci.2014.03.019
13. Novembre E, Galli E, Landi F, Caffarelli C, Pifferi M, De Marco E, Burastero SE, Calori G, Benetti L, Bonazza P, Puccinelli P, Parmiani S, Bernardini R, Vierucci A (2004) Coseasonal sublingual immunotherapy reduces the development of asthma in children with allergic rhinoconjunctivitis. J Allergy Clin Immunol 114:851–857. doi:10.1016/j.jaci.2004.07.012
14. Passalacqua G (2014) Specific immunotherapy in asthma: a comprehensive review. J Asthma 51:29–33. doi:10.3109/02770903.2013.853082
15. Soyka MB, Van De Veen W, Holzmann D, Akdis M, Akdis CA (2014) Scientific foundations of allergen-specific immunotherapy for allergic disease. Chest 146:1347–1357. doi:10.1378/chest.14-0049
16. Wambre E, Delong JH, James EA, Torres-Chinn N, Pfützner W, Möbs C, Durham SR, Till SJ, Robinson D, Kwok WW (2014) Specific immunotherapy modifies allergen-specific CD4+ T-cell responses in an epitope-dependent manner. J Allergy Clin Immunol 133:872–879. doi:10.1016/j.jaci.2013.10.054
17. Radulovic S, Jacobson MR, Durham SR, Nouri-Aria KT (2008) Grass pollen immunotherapy induces Foxp3-expressing CD4+ CD25+ cells in the nasal mucosa. J Allergy Clin Immunol 121:1467–1472, 1472.e1. doi:10.1016/j.jaci.2008.03.013
18. Akdis CA, Akdis M (2015) Advances in allergen immunotherapy : aiming for complete tolerance to allergens. Sci Transl Med 7:1–6. doi:10.1126/scitranslmed.aaa7390
19. Nouri-Aria KT, Wachholz PA, Francis JN, Jacobson MR, Walker SM, Wilcock LK, Staple SQ, Aalberse RC, Till SJ, Durham SR (2004) Grass pollen immunotherapy induces mucosal and peripheral IL-10 responses and blocking IgG activity. J Immunol 172:3252–3259. doi:10.4049/jimmunol.172.5.3252
20. Francis JN, James LK, Paraskevopoulos G, Wong C, Calderon MA, Durham SR, Till SJ (2008) Grass pollen immunotherapy: IL-10 induction and suppression of late responses precedes IgG4 inhibitory antibody activity. J Allergy Clin Immunol 121:1120–1125.e2. doi:10.1016/j.jaci.2008.01.072
21. Akdis CA, Blesken T, Akdis M, Wüthrich B, Blaser K (1998) Role of interleukin 10 in specific immunotherapy. J Clin Invest 102:98–106. doi:10.1172/JCI2250
22. Epstein TG, Liss GM, Murphy-Berendts K, Bernstein DI (2014) AAAAI/ACAAI surveillance study of subcutaneous immunotherapy, years 2008–2012: an update on fatal and nonfatal systemic allergic reactions. J Allergy Clin Immunol Pract 2:161–167.e3. doi:10.1016/j.jaip.2014.01.004
23. Jacobsen L, Wahn U, Bilo MB (2012) Allergen-specific immunotherapy provides immediate, long-term and preventive clinical effects in children and adults: the effects of immunotherapy can be categorised by level of benefit—the centenary of allergen specific subcutaneous immunotherapy. Clin Transl Allergy 2:8. doi:10.1186/2045-7022-2-8
24. Durham SR, Emminger W, Kapp A, de Monchy JGR, Rak S, Scadding GK, Wurtzen PA, Andersen JS, Tholstrup B, Riis B, Dahl R (2012) SQ-standardized sublingual grass immunotherapy: confirmation of disease modification 2 years after 3 years of treatment in a randomized trial. J Allergy Clin Immunol 129:717–725.e5. doi:10.1016/j.jaci.2011.12.973
25. Didier A, Worm M, Horak F, Sussman G, de Beaumont O, Le Gall M, Melac M, Malling H-J (2011) Sustained 3-year efficacy of pre- and coseasonal 5-grass-pollen sublingual immunotherapy tablets in patients with grass pollen-induced rhinoconjunctivitis. J Allergy Clin Immunol 128:559–566. doi:10.1016/j.jaci.2011.06.022
26. Janssen EM, van Oosterhout AJ, Nijkamp FP, van Eden W, Wauben MH (2000) The efficacy of immunotherapy in an experimental murine model of allergic asthma is related to the strength and site of T cell activation during immunotherapy. J Immunol 165:7207–7214. doi:10.4049/jimmunol.165.12.7207
27. Janssen EM, Wauben MHM, Jonker EH, Hofman G, Van Eden W, Nijkamp FP, Van Oosterhout AJM (1999) Opposite effects of immunotherapy with ovalbumin and the immunodominant T-cell epitope on airway eosinophilia and hyperresponsiveness in a murine model of allergic asthma. Am J Respir Cell Mol Biol 21:21–29
28. Shirinbak S, Taher YA, Maazi H, Gras R, van Esch BC, Henricks PA, Samsom JN, Verbeek JS, Lambrecht BN, van Oosterhout AJM,

Nawijn MC (2010) Suppression of Th2-driven airway inflammation by allergen immunotherapy is independent of B cell and Ig responses in mice. J Immunol 185:3857–3865. doi:10.4049/jimmunol.0903909

29. Taher YA, van Esch BC, Hofman GA, Henricks PAJ, van Oosterhout AJM (2008) 1,25-Dihydroxyvitamin D3 potentiates the beneficial effects of allergen immunotherapy in a mouse model of allergic asthma: role for IL-10 and TGF-β. J Immunol 180:5211–5221. doi:10.4049/jimmunol.180.8.5211
30. Maazi H, Shirinbak S, Willart M, Hammad HM, Cabanski M, Boon L, Ganesh V, Baru AM, Hansen G, Lambrecht BN, Sparwasser T, Nawijn MC, van Oosterhout AJM (2012) Contribution of regulatory T cells to alleviation of experimental allergic asthma after specific immunotherapy. Clin Exp Allergy 42:1519–1528. doi:10.1111/j.1365-2222.2012.04064.x
31. Vissers JLM, van Esch BC, Hofman GA, van Oosterhout AJM (2005) Macrophages induce an allergen-specific and long-term suppression in a mouse asthma model. Eur Respir J 26:1040–1046. doi:10.1183/09031936.05.00089304
32. Kapsenberg ML (2003) Dendritic-cell control of pathogen-driven T-cell polarization. Nat Rev Immunol 3:984–993. doi:10.1038/nri1246
33. Jonuleit BH, Schmitt E, Schuler G, Knop J, Enk AH (2000) Induction of interleukin 10-producing, nonproliferating CD4+ T cells with regulatory properties by repetitive stimulation with allogeneic immature human dendritic cells. J Exp Med 192:1213–1222
34. Weiner HL (2001) The mucosal milieu creates tolerogenic dendritic cells and TRl and TH3 regulatory cells. Nat Immunol 2:671–672
35. Maazi H, Shirinbak S, den Boef LE, Fallarino F, Volpi C, Nawijn MC, van Oosterhout AJ (2013) Cytotoxic T lymphocyte antigen 4-immunoglobulin G is a potent adjuvant for experimental allergen immunotherapy. Clin Exp Immunol 172:113–120. doi:10.1111/cei.12041
36. Tan AM, Chen H-C, Pochard P, Eisenbarth SC, Herrick CA, Bottomly HK (2010) TLR4 signaling in stromal cells is critical for the initiation of allergic Th2 responses to inhaled antigen. J Immunol 184:3535–3544. doi:10.4049/jimmunol.0900340
37. Brimnes J, Kildsgaard J, Jacobi H, Lund K (2007) Sublingual immunotherapy reduces allergic symptoms in a mouse model of rhinitis. Clin Exp Allergy 37:488–497. doi:10.1111/j.1365-2222.2006.02624.x
38. Robichaud A, Fereydoonzad L, Urovitch IB, Brunet J-D (2015) Comparative study of three flexiVent system configurations using mechanical test loads. Exp Lung Res 41:84–92. doi:10.3109/01902148.2014.971921
39. Twisk JWR (2004) Longitudinal data analysis. A comparison between generalized estimating equations and random coefficient analysis. Eur J Epidemiol 19:769–776

Chapter 12

Characterization of Group 2 Innate Lymphoid Cells in Allergic Airway Inflammation Models in the Mouse

Bobby W.S. Li, Dior M.J.M. Beerens, Maarten D. Brem, and Rudi W. Hendriks

Abstract

Allergic asthma is a chronic inflammatory lung disease mediated by type 2 cytokines produced by T helper 2 (Th2) cells as well as the recently discovered group 2 innate lymphoid cells (ILC2). Due to a lack of unique markers, the accurate phenotypic characterization and quantification of ILC2 requires a comprehensive panel of fluorescently labeled antibodies. The markers that are currently used to characterize ILC2 have not been standardized and often vary between research groups, which poses significant challenges when comparing data. Intranasal administration of the pro-inflammatory cytokine IL-33 in mice is associated with strong, Th2 cell-independent ILC2 activation. ILC2 are also activated in mouse models of allergic asthma based on the physiologically relevant house dust mite (HDM) allergen, which parallel eosinophilic airway inflammation observed in asthma patients. Here, we describe the analysis of ILC2 by flow cytometry in these two commonly used allergic airway inflammation models in the mouse.

Key words Allergy and asthma, Group 2 innate lymphoid cells (ILC2), House dust mite, Interleukin-33, Murine airway inflammation model

1 Introduction

Asthma is a disease of the airways involving chronic inflammation and remodeling and is characterized by episodes of coughing, wheezing, and shortness of breath. Patients can be clustered into several endotypes based on symptoms, disease mechanisms and immunological profile, the most common being allergic asthma [1]. The T helper 2 (Th2) cell is classically placed in the center of the pathophysiology of allergic asthma. The Th2 signature cytokines IL-4, IL-5, and IL-13 are key orchestrators of the hallmarks of asthma. These include persistent inflammation, smooth muscle cell hyperplasia, mucous cell metaplasia, and airway hyperresponsiveness and remodeling [2]. Recently, innate counterparts of Th2 cells referred to as group 2 innate lymphoid

Björn E. Clausen and Jon D. Laman (eds.), *Inflammation: Methods and Protocols*, Methods in Molecular Biology, vol. 1559, DOI 10.1007/978-1-4939-6786-5_12,

cells (ILC2) have been identified as an innate source of type 2 cytokines and have been hypothesized to contribute to the pathogenesis of allergic asthma [3, 4].

Observations that a non-B/non-T cell population was capable of producing IL-5 and IL-13 in response to IL-25 were first made by Fort et al. in 2001 [5]. It was reported some years later that this IL-25-dependent population is an important source of type 2 cytokines and that these cells are critically involved in helminth expulsion [6]. In 2010, several independent research groups characterized this novel non-B/non-T lymphocyte population in fat associated lymphoid clusters, mesenteric lymph nodes, spleen, and liver and found them to be highly responsive to both IL-25 and IL-33, although different names were assigned to the cells at the time [7–9]. Cells with a similar phenotype and cytokine profile were also discovered in the lung in the context of influenza infection [10, 11]. A universal nomenclature was proposed and it is now generally accepted that in the mouse ILC2 are negative for classic hematopoietic lineage markers, express Sca-1, CD117 (c-kit), CD25 (IL-2Rα), CD127 (IL-7Rα), and T1/ST2 (IL-33R) on their cell surface, and are dependent on the transcription factor GATA3 [7–9, 12–15].

IL-25/IL-33-responsive ILC2 have also been found in human lungs and are enriched in the nasal polyps of patients suffering from chronic rhinosinusitis, a typical type 2 inflammatory disease [16]. These human ILC2 are defined by the expression of the seven-transmembrane prostaglandin D2 receptor CRTH2/CD294 and the natural killer marker CD161 and also require GATA3 [16, 17]. More recently, studies in asthmatic patients revealed increased numbers of ILC2 in peripheral blood and sputum, compared with healthy controls [18–20]. Moreover, this population appeared to be steroid insensitive, which is in agreement with in vitro studies showing that TSLP is a major determining factor in steroid sensitivity of ILC2 [20].

To explore the role of ILC2 in the complex inflammatory processes of allergic asthma, a number of mouse models have been developed that mimic allergy and asthmatic responses to physiological allergens. Intranasal administration of the protease allergen papain leads to activation of ILC2 and induces eosinophilic airway inflammation in wild-type as well as T and B cell-deficient *Rag1−/−* mice. However, *Rag2−/−Il2rg−/−* mice that additionally lack ILC2 do not mount an inflammatory response to papain and adoptive transfer of wild-type ILC2 into these mice restored inflammation [21]. In addition, ILC2-derived IL-13 promotes migration of activated lung dendritic cells towards the lymph nodes where subsequent T cell priming occurs, further suggesting a central role for ILC2 as early initiators of inflammation [22]. Experimental asthma models using the fungal allergen

Alternaria alternata have led to similar results, showing an IL-33-mediated inflammatory response orchestrated by activated ILC2 rather than Th2 cells [23, 24]. Together with data showing that ILC2 are capable of enhancing Th2 cell differentiation and function, these findings support a model in which ILC2 can become rapidly activated to provide an early source of type 2 cytokines and bridges the gap between innate and adaptive immunity [25, 26]. In contrast, *Rag1−/−* mice exposed to *Aspergillus fumigatus*, another fungal allergen, fail to develop airway inflammation and hyperresponsiveness. Moreover, ovalbumin-driven airway inflammation is attenuated upon depletion of $CD4^+$ T cells [27, 28]. In house dust mite (HDM)-induced allergic airway inflammation, blockade of CD28 signaling strongly diminishes airway hyperresponsiveness and pulmonary infiltrates of inflammatory cells in the lung [29]. Interestingly, chronic exposure to a cocktail of *Alternaria*, *Aspergillus*, and HDM synergistically induces airway inflammation, hyperresponsiveness, and remodeling that is dependent on adaptive immunity [30]. Taken together, these models instead indicate a critical role for T cells in mediating and maintaining allergic airway inflammation. Therefore, the contribution of ILC2 in the induction of allergic inflammation appears highly dependent on the allergen model.

Here, we describe in detail a T cell-independent and a T cell-dependent murine model for airway inflammation via intranasal administration of IL-33 or HDM, respectively. The alarmin cytokine IL-33 is constitutively expressed in the nucleus of airway epithelial cells and is released upon cellular stress or injury that occurs during exposure to a number of different environmental allergens [31]. IL-33 is a potent stimulator of ILC2 proliferation and cytokine production and intranasal administration of IL-33 leads to eosinophilic airway inflammation reminiscent of allergic asthma, which provides a unique tool to specifically investigate ILC2 function during inflammation [32–34]. A more physiologically relevant mouse model for allergic asthma employs HDM extract. Intranasal sensitization followed by provocation challenge with HDM produces eosinophilic infiltrates in the lung and airway hyperresponsiveness that closely resembles clinical observations in patients with allergic asthma [2]. Although there is abundant literature on mouse ILC2 in a variety of inflammatory diseases, the markers used to characterize ILC2 have not been standardized, which poses difficulties when comparing data from various publications. In this report, we provide a detailed insight into the induction of airway inflammation in mouse models based on exposure to IL-33 and HDM, focusing on the characterization of the ILC2 phenotype in bronchoalveolar lavage (BAL) fluid, lungs, and mediastinal lymph nodes (MLN) using flow cytometry.

2 Materials

Standard laboratory equipment including plates, tubes, syringes, pipettes, and centrifuges is not listed.

2.1 Induction of IL-33 and HDM-Induced Airway Inflammation

1. 8–16-week-old C57BL/6 mice housed in a specific-pathogen-free facility, fed ad libitum, and age- and gender-matched (*see* **Note 1**).
2. Recombinant mouse IL-33 (BioLegend, USA; 0.5 μg/40 μL; *see* **Note 2**).
3. HDM extract from *Dermatophagoides pteronyssinus* (Greer, USA; 1 μg/40 μL for sensitization and 10 μg/40 μL for challenge; *see* **Note 3**).
4. PBS.
5. Isoflurane anesthesia device.

2.2 Collection of BAL Fluid, Lungs, and MLN

1. Anesthetic and tools suitable for sacrificing mice (*see* **Note 4**).
2. Cannula: 23-gauge × 1¼ in. needle with the tip sheathed by ~10 mm of polyethylene tubing (inner diameter 0.58 mm/0.023 in.) to prevent puncturing of the airways (Fig. 1a).
3. Suture thread.
4. PBS containing 0.5 mM ethylenediaminetetraacetic acid (EDTA).
5. Hank's balanced salt solution (HBSS).

2.3 Preparation of Single-Cell Suspension

1. PBS containing 0.5 mM EDTA supplemented with 0.5% bovine serum albumin (BSA).
2. Osmotic lysis buffer: 8.3% NH_4Cl, 1% $KHCO_3$, and 0.04% Na_2EDTA in Milli-Q.
3. 100 μm nylon cell strainers.
4. RPMI 1640 Cell culture medium containing 10% fetal bovine serum (FBS).

2.4 Flow Cytometry

1. FACS-buffer containing 0.25% BSA, 0.5 mM EDTA, and 0.05% NaN_3 in PBS with a final pH of 7.2.
2. For intracellular transcription factor detection: eBioscience FoxP3/transcription factor staining kit containing (1) fixation and permeabilization concentrate and (2) diluent and (3) 10× wash buffer to be diluted in Milli-Q.
3. For intracellular cytokine detection: phorbol myristate acetate (PMA), ionomycin, and GolgiStop (BD Biosciences, USA). 4%

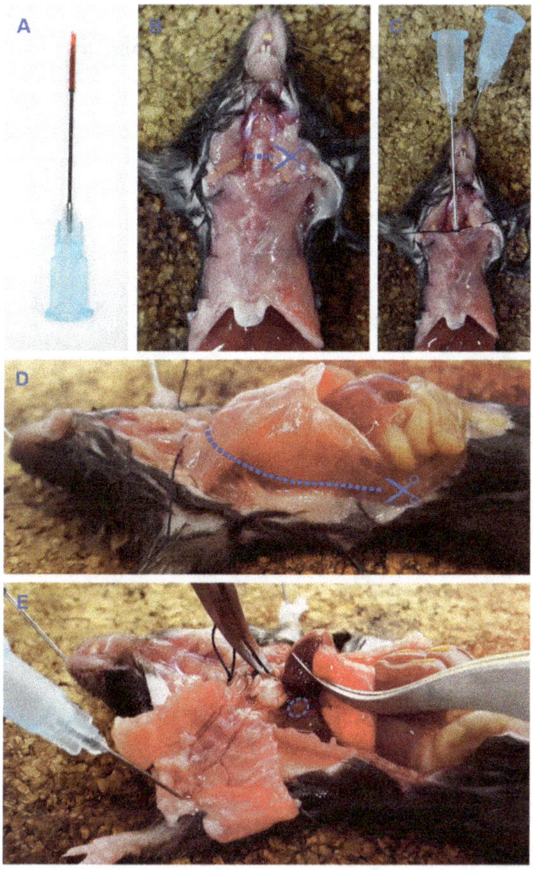

Fig. 1 Stepwise procedure for the collection of BAL fluid, lungs, and MLN. (**a**) A cannula used for the collection of BAL fluid. The polyethylene sheath prevents puncturing of the airways and is colored red to indicate its placement. (**b**) Preparation of the trachea for cannula insertion. The connective tissue is removed and a small incision is made between the tracheal cartilage along the *dotted blue line*. (**c**) Inserted cannula secured by suture thread. (**d**) The thoracic cavity can be opened by removing the diaphragm and cutting the ribs on both sides along the *dotted blue line*. (**e**) MLN can be exposed by lifting the right lung lobes and is situated below a blood vessel

paraformaldehyde (PFA) in PBS as stock solution, diluted 1:2 in PBS to a 2% working solution. Permeabilization and wash buffer of 0.5% saponin (Sigma-Aldrich, USA) in FACS-buffer.

4. Purified and unlabeled CD16/CD32 antibody (Fc-block, clone 2.4G2).
5. Fixable live/dead cell stain (Fixable Viability Dye eFluor® 506, eBioscience, USA).
6. Antibodies used for flow cytometry, listed in Table 1.
7. Data acquisition is performed using an LSR II flow cytometer (Beckton Dickinson, USA) equipped with three lasers and FACSDiva™ software (Beckton Dickinson, USA) and analyzed by FlowJo v10 (Tree Star Inc., USA) software.

Table 1
Antibodies used for flow cytometric analysis of ILC2, eosinophils, and neutrophils

Antibody	Conjugate	Clone	Company
ILC2 lineage mix			
B220	PE	RA3-6B2	eBioscience
CD3e	PE	145-2c11	eBioscience
CD4	PE	GK1.5	eBioscience
CD5	PE	53-7.3	eBioscience
CD11b	PE	M1/70	eBioscience
CD11c	PE	N418	eBioscience
CD19	PE	1D3	BD Biosciences
CD8a	PE	53-6.7	eBioscience
FcεRIα	PE	MAR-1	eBioscience
Gr-1	PE	RB6-8C5	BD Biosciences
NK1.1	PE	PK136	eBiosciences
TER-119	PE	TER-119	eBioscience
ILC2 surface markers			
CD45	PE-CF594	I3/2.3	Abcam
ICOS	APC	C398.4A	eBioscience
KLRG1	Biotin	2F1/KLRG1	BioLegend
MHCII	Brilliant Violet 650	M5/114.15.2	BD Biosciences
Sca-1	Brilliant Violet 786	D7	BD Biosciences
T1/ST2	Biotin	DJ8	MD Bioproducts
T1/ST2	FITC	DJ8	MD Bioproducts
Streptavidin	APC-eFluor 780		eBioscience
CD25	PerCP-Cy5.5	PC61.5	eBioscience
CD127	PE-Cy7	A7R34	eBioscience
CD127	eFluor450	A7R34	eBioscience
ILC2 transcription factors			
GATA3	eFluor 660	TWAJ-14	eBioscience
ILC2 cytokines			
Amphiregulin	Biotin	Polyclonal	R&D Systems
IL-4	Brilliant Violet 711	11B11	BD Biosciences
IL-5	APC	TRFK-5	BD Biosciences
IL-13	eFluor 450	eBio13A	eBioscience
Eosinophil and neutrophil surface markers			
Gr-1	APC-eFluor 780	RB6-8C5	eBioscience
Siglec-F	PE	E50-2440	BD Biosciences

3 Methods

3.1 Intranasal Injection

1. Mice are placed in a small gas chamber and are exposed to 2.5 % isoflurane anesthesia with an oxygen airflow of 1 L/min (VerEquip).
2. When the breathing rate has dropped to approximately two breaths per second, hold the mouse by the scruff of the neck with the abdomen facing you and tilt the body to a 45° angle.
3. Carefully place a drop of liquid on the tip of the nose using a pipette and wait for the mouse to inhale (*see* **Note 5**).
4. Once the droplet has been successfully inhaled and the breathing rate of the mouse starts to increase, place it on its back in the cage.

3.2 IL-33-Induced Airway Inflammation

1. Mice are administered 0.5 μg recombinant IL-33 in 40 μL PBS via intranasal injection under isoflurane anesthesia, as described above, three times with 1 day of rest between each injection.
2. Organs of interest are harvested 1 day after the final injection.
3. Control mice are treated with PBS.

3.3 HDM-Induced Airway Inflammation

1. Mice are sensitized with 1 μg HDM extract dissolved in 40 μL PBS via intranasal injection under isoflurane anesthesia as described above.
2. After a resting period of 7 days, mice are challenged daily to 10 μg HDM extract dissolved in 40 μL PBS by intranasal injection for 5 consecutive days.
3. Organs of interest are harvested 1 day after the final challenge.
4. Control mice are sensitized with PBS and are challenged with HDM.

3.4 Collection of BAL Fluid, Lungs, and MLN

1. Mice are sacrificed, using 75 mg/kg ketamine combined with 1 mg/kg medetomidine intraperitoneally (i.p.).
2. A midline incision is made to retract the skin and the connective tissue surrounding the trachea is carefully removed.
3. A suture thread is placed underneath the trachea by carefully lifting it with tweezers. This will be used to secure the cannula in the next step.
4. A small incision between the tracheal cartilage is made to insert a cannula, be careful not to sever the entire trachea (Fig. 1b). The cannula is secured in place using the suture thread in **step 3** by tying a knot around the portion of the trachea housing the cannula (Fig. 1c).

5. A syringe containing 1 mL PBS supplemented with 0.5 mM EDTA is attached to the cannula. The lungs are subsequently washed by gently flushing. Afterwards, the syringe is uncoupled and the aspirated BAL fluid is collected in a tube.
6. **Step 5** is repeated two more times for a total of ~3 mL BAL fluid.
7. The thoracic cavity is then opened by removing the diaphragm and cutting the ribs on both sides along the dorsal plane. The connective tissue between the thymus and the ribcage is removed and a transversal cut is made above the heart to completely expose the lungs (Fig. 1d).
8. The MLN is situated underneath the right lung lobes below a blood vessel and can be carefully extracted using tweezers and placed in HBSS for further processing (Fig. 1e).
9. Lungs lobes are separated from the bronchi and placed in HBSS for further processing.

3.5 Preparation of Single-Cell Suspensions

Lung and MLN tissue are mechanically disrupted on a 100 μm cell strainer using the plunger of a syringe. The strainers are flushed with 5 mL PBS containing 0.5 mM EDTA and 0.5 % BSA to extract an optimal amount of cells.

1. BAL fluid, lung, and MLN cell suspensions are centrifuged at 4 °C 400 × g for 7 min and the supernatant from the BAL fluid may be collected for the detection of cytokine levels by ELISA (not discussed here). Lung and MLN supernatants are discarded.
2. BAL and MLN cell pellets are resuspended in an appropriate volume of cell culture medium for cell counting and are ready for flow cytometric applications.
3. The cell pellet from the lung is resuspended in 1 mL osmotic lysis buffer and incubated at room temperature for 2 min. Lysis is stopped by adding 10 mL cold PBS and the suspension is centrifuged at 4 °C 400 × g for 7 min and the supernatant is removed.
4. Cells are resuspended in cold cell culture medium and after a sample is taken to determine absolute cell numbers, they are ready for flow cytometric applications.

3.6 Flow Cytometry

3.6.1 Intracellular Flow Cytometry Staining Protocol for ILC2 Detection

1. To detect cytokine production, one million cells per well in a 96-well plate are stimulated with PMA (50 ng/mL; diluted from a 1000× stock solution) and ionomycin (300 ng/mL diluted from a 1000× stock solution), and GolgiStop (1:1500) diluted in cell culture medium for 4 h at 37 °C prior to antibody staining.
2. For surface marker staining, one million cells are placed in each well of a 96-well plate and are incubated with 40 μL primary antibody mix in FACS buffer containing Fc-block for 30 min at 4 °C.

3. The samples are then washed once with FACS buffer and once with PBS.
4. Following this, the cells are incubated with fixable live/dead stain with 40 μL secondary antibody mix in PBS and incubated for 15 min at 4 °C.
5. For intracellular transcription factor detection: cells are washed in PBS, fixed and permeabilized using eBioscience fixation and permeabilization buffer for 30 min at 4 °C, followed by two washing steps using eBioscience wash buffer. Next, the pellet is incubated with 40 μL tertiary antibody mix in wash buffer for 60 min at 4 °C. Finally, the samples are washed, once with wash buffer and once with FACS buffer, before being resuspended in FACS buffer and measured by a flow cytometer within 1 day (*see* **Note 6**).
6. For intracellular cytokine detection: cells are washed in PBS and fixed using 2% PFA for 15 min at 4 °C followed by two washes with PBS. After fixation, the cells are permeabilized with permeabilization and wash buffer containing 0.5% saponin for 15 min at 4 °C. Next, the cell pellet is incubated with 40 μL tertiary antibody mix in perm/wash buffer for 60 min at 4 °C. Finally, the samples are washed once with perm/wash buffer and once with FACS buffer before being resuspended in FACS buffer and acquired within 1 day (*see* **Note 6**).

3.6.2 Analysis of Allergic Airway Inflammation by Flow Cytometry

The number of eosinophils present in the BAL fluid can be used as an indicator for the severity of allergic inflammation. Successful induction of airway inflammation yields large numbers of granulocytes, characterized by high side scatter (SSC) and relative low forward scatter (FSC) values, of which 90% or more consist of Siglec-F^+ eosinophils (Fig. 2a). These percentages generally translate to between ~0.5 and ~1.0 million eosinophils in the BAL fluid. Cellular infiltrates can also be seen in the lungs and typically accumulate around the bronchioles and blood vessels. In addition, thickened alveolar septa are also observed (Fig. 2b).

3.6.3 Analysis of ILC2 by Flow Cytometry

To quantify ILC2 in the BAL fluid, living cells that are negative for the live/dead stain are selected. However, it should be kept in mind that macrophages are autofluorescent and therefore positive in the live/dead staining, irrespective of their viability, and are therefore also excluded. Furthermore, it is possible to remove any debris in this step that may interfere with subsequent gating. ILC2 are relatively small cells and fall within the general lymphocyte gate in the FSC/SSC plot. CD45 expression is used to exclude all nonleukocyte populations and the lineage markers are compiled in a "dump" channel to readily exclude major hematopoietic cell populations. ILC2 do not express lineage markers and express high levels of surface Sca-1. Furthermore, they also express the IL-33R

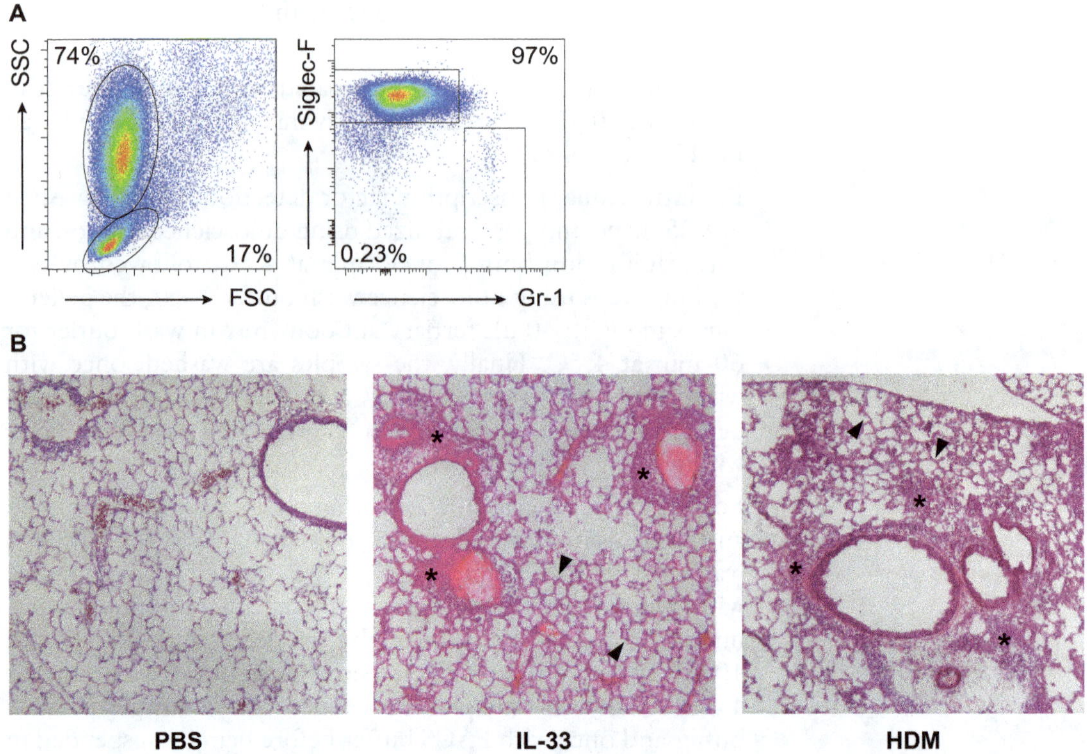

Fig. 2 Extent of eosinophilic inflammation in BAL fluid and lungs after IL-33 or HDM treatment. (**a**) Flow cytometric identification of eosinophils and neutrophils in the BAL fluid of IL-33-treated mice. Granulocytes are gated on the basis of high SSC and low FSC values and discriminated as eosinophils or neutrophils using Siglec-F and Gr-1, respectively. (**b**) Hematoxylin and eosin (H&E) staining of lung sections from PBS, IL-33, and HDM-treated mice, showing perivascular infiltrates (indicated by *asterisks*) and thickening of alveolar walls (indicated by *arrow heads*)

component T1/ST2 and intracellular GATA3 (Fig. 3a). Because GATA3, T1/ST2 and Sca-1 are also expressed by Th2 cells, it is critically important to optimize the lineage mix and to conservatively gate for lineage-negative cells to ensure no T cells are included within the ILC2 gate. The level of GATA3 expression within the ILC2 population is variable between different tissues (Fig. 3b). This likely reflects the activation state, as we observed that GATA3 levels increase when ILC2 are activated by IL-33 stimulation.

Although GATA3 is a consistent marker for ILC2, it is a nuclear protein that requires fixation and permeabilization steps for its detection. For applications where this is not desirable, such as live cell sorting, surface CD127 may be used as a replacement in conjunction with Sca-1 and T1/ST2. Although CD25 is also frequently associated with ILC2, its expression is variable (Fig. 3c). The observed differential expression on ILC2, depending on the type of stimulus applied, precludes the usage of CD25 as a surface

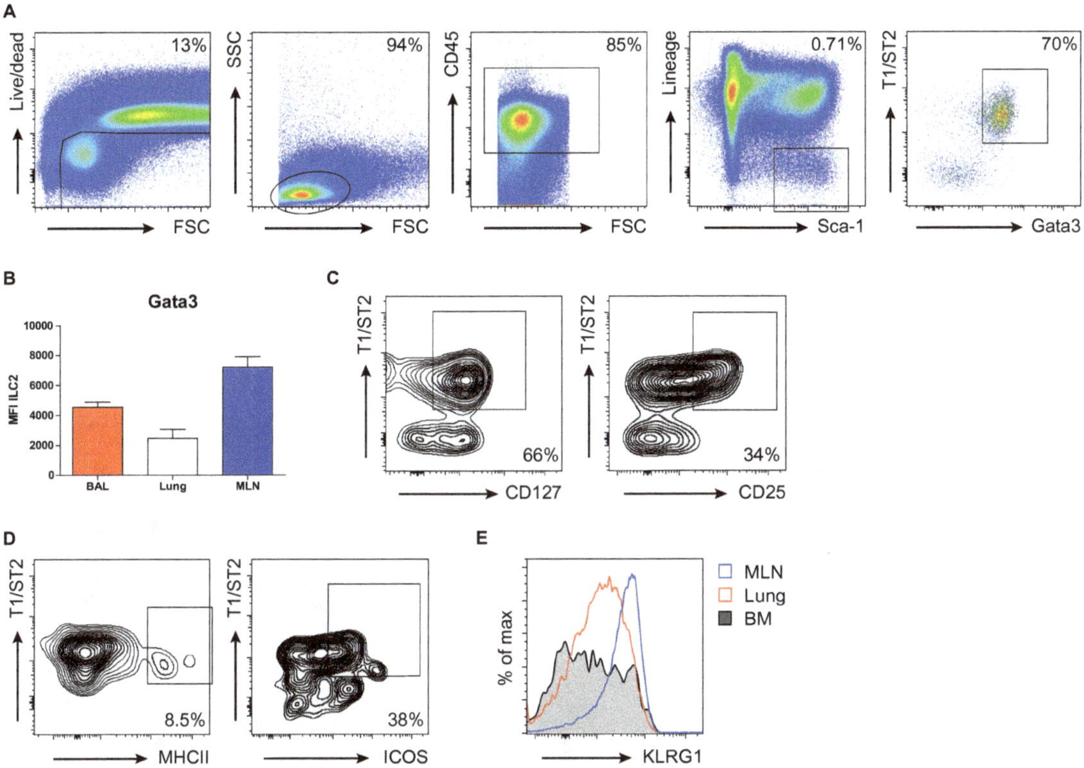

Fig. 3 Gating strategy for the identification of ILC2 in BAL fluid of HDM-treated mice. (**a**) After exclusion of dead cells and debris and gating for CD45+ lymphocytes, ILC2 are lineage-negative and express high levels of Sca-1, T1/ST2, and intracellular GATA3. (**b**) GATA3 expression level by ILC2 is variable between tissues, as shown by mean fluorescence intensity (MFI) values. (**c**) Alternative gating strategy for ILC2 from Lineage– Sca-1+ cells without intracellular staining, using CD127 as an additional marker. CD25 expression is variable within this population. (**d**) Analysis of MHCII and ICOS expression in ILC2. (**e**) Comparative analysis of KLRG1 expression in ILC2 derived from bone marrow (BM), lung, and MLN. Data are shown as mean ± SEM of $n = 5$ mice per group. All flow cytometry panels are pooled data from >4 mice

marker for accurate quantification of ILC2 numbers. A fraction of ILC2 express MHCII and ICOS (Fig. 3d) and have sparked investigations into the interaction of ILC2 with other immune cells [25, 35]. Expression of the co-inhibitory killer-cell lectin like receptor G1 (KLRG1) has been proposed as a marker acquired by mature ILC2 under inflammatory conditions [15, 36] and is differentially expressed between tissues (Fig. 3e).

ILC2 produce IL-5 and IL-13 in steady state and rapidly expand and upregulate their cytokine production upon stimulation. Amphiregulin production is low in resting ILC2 and is significantly upregulated when exposed to IL-33 or HDM (Fig. 4a). CD25 is expressed by ~50% of ILC2 in the lung in steady state. Administration of IL-33 results in a homogeneous ILC2 population that consistently expresses high levels of CD25. However, HDM stimulation leads to the expansion of $CD25^{lo/-}$ ILC2 that still possess the same cytokine profile as 'classical' CD25⁺ ILC2 (Fig. 4b, c). Additionally, these CD25$^{lo/-}$ ILC2 are present in higher numbers in this model and significantly contribute to the total population of type 2 cytokine producing cells (Fig. 4d). It is conceivable that the CD25$^{lo/-}$ILC2 population is also prominent in other allergen-based mouse models of lung inflammation. We therefore suggest the use of this marker as a method to discriminate between subpopulations of ILC2 rather than a characteristic to quantify ILC2 numbers.

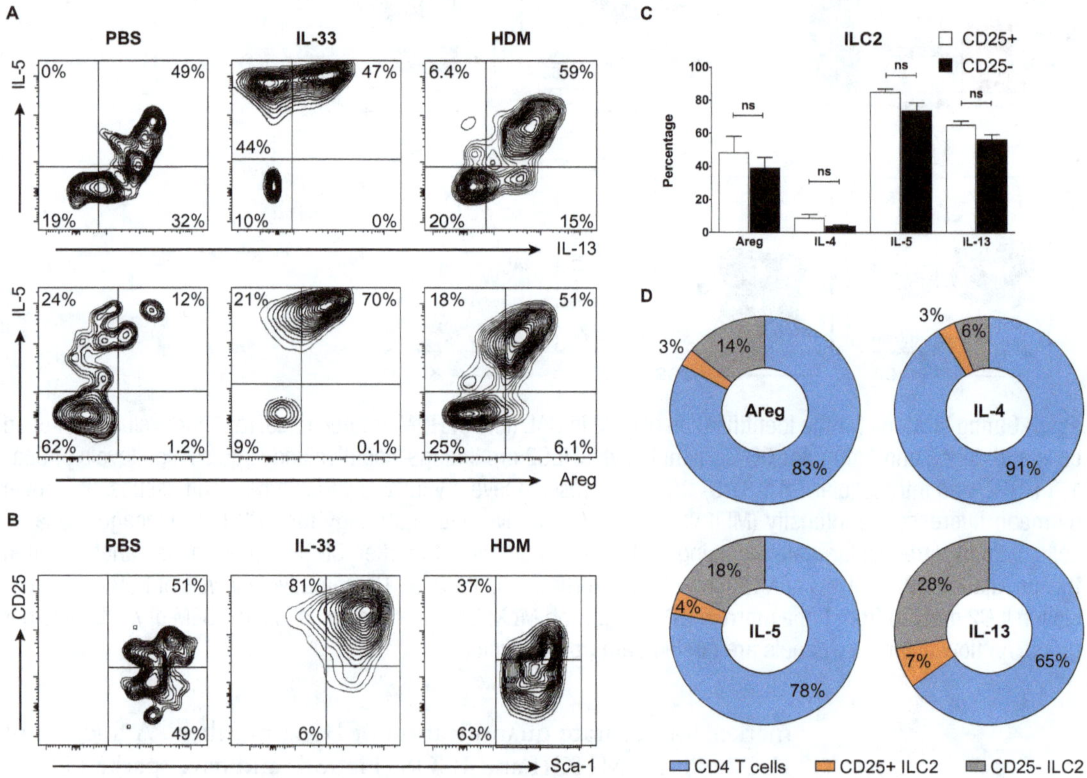

Fig. 4 CD25⁻ and CD25⁺ ILC2 secrete similar amounts of cytokines in HDM-treated mice. (**a**) Flow cytometric analysis of intracellular cytokine production of BAL fluid ILC2 in PBS, IL-33, or HDM-treated mice after stimulation of single-cell suspensions with PMA/ionomycin and GolgiStop for 4 h. (**b**) Expression of CD25 in BAL fluid derived ILC2 is dependent on the type of stimulation used. (**c**) Analysis of cytokine profiles of CD25⁻ and CD25⁺ ILC2 from BAL fluid of HDM-treated mice. (**d**) Relative contribution of various cell populations to amphiregulin (Areg), IL-4, IL-5, and IL-13 producing cells in BAL fluid of HDM-treated mice. Single-cell suspensions were stimulated with PMA/ionomycin in the presence of GolgiStop for 4 h and intracellular cytokine expression was quantified. Proportions of cytokine producing cells (expressed as percentages of the total number of cytokine-producing cells) were determined by flow cytometry in ILC2 and CD4 T cells. Data are shown as mean ± SEM of $n = 4–6$ mice per group. All flow cytometry panels are pooled data from >4 four mice. A Mann–Whitney U test was used to determine statistical significance between CD25⁻ and CD25⁺ ILC2 in HDM-treated mice

4 Notes

1. Our observation is that female C57BL/6 mice tend to develop more severe eosinophilic lung inflammation than male mice and therefore it is crucial to gender match between experimental groups. Difference in the severity of inflammation also exists between various mouse strains.
2. The potency of recombinant mouse IL-33 diminishes over time and has an effective shelf life of 3 months if stored at −80 °C and 1 week if stored at 4 °C. Avoid repeated freeze–thaw cycles.
3. HDM extract is a natural product and has a variable composition between batches. It is important to note the endotoxin content of each batch and to compare the immune response generated between new and old batches in order to ensure similar levels of inflammation. If necessary, perform titrations of different amounts of HDM during challenge.
4. Cervical dislocation is not a viable option due to a high chance of tearing the trachea, thus preventing the placement of a cannula for BAL fluid extraction. Euthanasia by inhalation of CO_2 gas potentially damages the immune cells in the lungs, and thus we recommend methods employing intraperitoneal overdose of anesthetic agents like ketamine/medetomidine.
5. If the mice are placed in the isoflurane chamber for extended periods of time (>1 min), they may become too deeply anesthetized and have trouble adequately inhaling the droplet. This is characterized by an extremely slow breathing rate of less than once per second. To avoid this, do not anesthetize more than four mice simultaneously to ensure optimal anesthesia. Additionally, it is normal for some mouse strains such as the C57BL/6 mice to hold their breath for a short amount of time during intranasal administration. We recommend not to exceed a volume of 80 μL for intranasal injections.
6. It is possible to leave the cells in the fixation step overnight at 4 °C and continue the FACS stain the next day if time is an issue.

Acknowledgments

The authors thank Dr. A. KleinJan (Erasmus MC) for critical reading of the manuscript and Dr. O. Corneth (Erasmus MC) for providing photographs of mouse dissections. This work was partly supported by the Lung Foundation Netherlands (Grant 3.2.12.67).

References

1. Lotvall J, Akdis CA, Bacharier LB, Bjermer L, Casale TB, Custovic A, Lemanske RF Jr, Wardlaw AJ, Wenzel SE, Greenberger PA (2011) Asthma endotypes: a new approach to classification of disease entities within the asthma syndrome. J Allergy Clin Immunol 127:355–360
2. Lambrecht BN, Hammad H (2015) The immunology of asthma. Nat Immunol 16:45–56
3. Eberl G, Colonna M, Di Santo JP, McKenzie AN (2015) Innate lymphoid cells. Innate lymphoid cells: a new paradigm in immunology. Science 348:aaa6566
4. Li BW, Hendriks RW (2013) Group 2 innate lymphoid cells in lung inflammation. Immunology 140:281–287
5. Fort MM, Cheung J, Yen D, Li J, Zurawski SM, Lo S, Menon S, Clifford T, Hunte B, Lesley R, Muchamuel T, Hurst SD, Zurawski G, Leach MW, Gorman DM, Rennick DM (2001) IL-25 induces IL-4, IL-5, and IL-13 and Th2-associated pathologies in vivo. Immunity 15:985–995
6. Fallon PG, Ballantyne SJ, Mangan NE, Barlow JL, Dasvarma A, Hewett DR, McIlgorm A, Jolin HE, McKenzie AN (2006) Identification of an interleukin (IL)-25-dependent cell population that provides IL-4, IL-5, and IL-13 at the onset of helminth expulsion. J Exp Med 203:1105–1116
7. Moro K, Yamada T, Tanabe M, Takeuchi T, Ikawa T, Kawamoto H, Furusawa J, Ohtani M, Fujii H, Koyasu S (2010) Innate production of T(H)2 cytokines by adipose tissue-associated c-Kit(+)Sca-1(+) lymphoid cells. Nature 463:540–544
8. Neill DR, Wong SH, Bellosi A, Flynn RJ, Daly M, Langford TK, Bucks C, Kane CM, Fallon PG, Pannell R, Jolin HE, McKenzie AN (2010) Nuocytes represent a new innate effector leukocyte that mediates type-2 immunity. Nature 464:1367–1370
9. Price AE, Liang HE, Sullivan BM, Reinhardt RL, Eisley CJ, Erle DJ, Locksley RM (2010) Systemically dispersed innate IL-13-expressing cells in type 2 immunity. Proc Natl Acad Sci U S A 107:11489–11494
10. Chang YJ, Kim HY, Albacker LA, Baumgarth N, McKenzie AN, Smith DE, Dekruyff RH, Umetsu DT (2011) Innate lymphoid cells mediate influenza-induced airway hyperreactivity independently of adaptive immunity. Nat Immunol 12:631–638
11. Monticelli LA, Sonnenberg GF, Abt MC, Alenghat T, Ziegler CG, Doering TA, Angelosanto JM, Laidlaw BJ, Yang CY, Sathaliyawala T, Kubota M, Turner D, Diamond JM, Goldrath AW, Farber DL, Collman RG, Wherry EJ, Artis D (2011) Innate lymphoid cells promote lung-tissue homeostasis after infection with influenza virus. Nat Immunol 12:1045–1054
12. Spits H, Artis D, Colonna M, Diefenbach A, Di Santo JP, Eberl G, Koyasu S, Locksley RM, McKenzie AN, Mebius RE, Powrie F, Vivier E (2013) Innate lymphoid cells—a proposal for uniform nomenclature. Nat Rev Immunol 13:145–149
13. Saenz SA, Siracusa MC, Perrigoue JG, Spencer SP, Urban JF Jr, Tocker JE, Budelsky AL, Kleinschek MA, Kastelein RA, Kambayashi T, Bhandoola A, Artis D (2010) IL25 elicits a multipotent progenitor cell population that promotes T(H)2 cytokine responses. Nature 464:1362–1366
14. Klein Wolterink RG, Serafini N, van Nimwegen M, Vosshenrich CA, de Bruijn MJ, Fonseca Pereira D, Veiga Fernandes H, Hendriks RW, Di Santo JP (2013) Essential, dose-dependent role for the transcription factor Gata3 in the development of IL-5+ and IL-13+ type 2 innate lymphoid cells. Proc Natl Acad Sci U S A 110:10240–10245
15. Hoyler T, Klose CS, Souabni A, Turqueti-Neves A, Pfeifer D, Rawlins EL, Voehringer D, Busslinger M, Diefenbach A (2012) The transcription factor GATA-3 controls cell fate and maintenance of type 2 innate lymphoid cells. Immunity 37:634–648
16. Mjosberg JM, Trifari S, Crellin NK, Peters CP, van Drunen CM, Piet B, Fokkens WJ, Cupedo T, Spits H (2011) Human IL-25- and IL-33-responsive type 2 innate lymphoid cells are defined by expression of CRTH2 and CD161. Nat Immunol 12:1055–1062
17. Mjosberg J, Bernink J, Golebski K, Karrich JJ, Peters CP, Blom B, te Velde AA, Fokkens WJ, van Drunen CM, Spits H (2012) The transcription factor GATA3 is essential for the function of human type 2 innate lymphoid cells. Immunity 37:649–659
18. Bartemes KR, Kephart GM, Fox SJ, Kita H (2014) Enhanced innate type 2 immune response in peripheral blood from patients with asthma. J Allergy Clin Immunol 134:671–678.e4
19. Smith SG, Chen R, Kjarsgaard M, Huang C, Oliveria JP, O'Byrne PM, Gauvreau GM, Boulet LP, Lemiere C, Martin J, Nair P, Sehmi R (2016) Increased numbers of activated group 2 innate lymphoid cells in the airways of patients with severe asthma and persistent airway eosinophilia. J Allergy Clin Immunol 137(1):75–86.e8

20. Kabata H, Moro K, Fukunaga K, Suzuki Y, Miyata J, Masaki K, Betsuyaku T, Koyasu S, Asano K (2013) Thymic stromal lymphopoietin induces corticosteroid resistance in natural helper cells during airway inflammation. Nat Commun 4:2675
21. Halim TY, Krauss RH, Sun AC, Takei F (2012) Lung natural helper cells are a critical source of Th2 cell-type cytokines in protease allergen-induced airway inflammation. Immunity 36:451–463
22. Halim TY, Steer CA, Matha L, Gold MJ, Martinez-Gonzalez I, McNagny KM, McKenzie AN, Takei F (2014) Group 2 innate lymphoid cells are critical for the initiation of adaptive T helper 2 cell-mediated allergic lung inflammation. Immunity 40:425–435
23. Doherty TA, Khorram N, Sugimoto K, Sheppard D, Rosenthal P, Cho JY, Pham A, Miller M, Croft M, Broide DH (2012) Alternaria induces STAT6-dependent acute airway eosinophilia and epithelial FIZZ1 expression that promotes airway fibrosis and epithelial thickness. J Immunol 188:2622–2629
24. Doherty TA, Khorram N, Chang JE, Kim HK, Rosenthal P, Croft M, Broide DH (2012) STAT6 regulates natural helper cell proliferation during lung inflammation initiated by Alternaria. Am J Physiol Lung Cell Mol Physiol 303:L577–L588
25. Mirchandani AS, Besnard AG, Yip E, Scott C, Bain CC, Cerovic V, Salmond RJ, Liew FY (2014) Type 2 innate lymphoid cells drive CD4+ Th2 cell responses. J Immunol 192:2442–2448
26. Drake LY, Iijima K, Kita H (2014) Group 2 innate lymphoid cells and CD4 T cells cooperate to mediate type 2 immune response in mice. Allergy 69(10):1300–1307
27. Corry DB, Grunig G, Hadeiba H, Kurup VP, Warnock ML, Sheppard D, Rennick DM, Locksley RM (1998) Requirements for allergen-induced airway hyperreactivity in T and B cell-deficient mice. Mol Med 4:344–355
28. Doherty TA, Soroosh P, Broide DH, Croft M (2009) CD4+ cells are required for chronic eosinophilic lung inflammation but not airway remodeling. Am J Physiol Lung Cell Mol Physiol 296:L229–L235
29. Gogishvili T, Luhder F, Kirstein F, Nieuwenhuizen NE, Goebbels S, Beer-Hammer S, Pfeffer K, Reuter S, Taube C, Brombacher F, Hunig T (2012) Interruption of CD28-mediated costimulation during allergen challenge protects mice from allergic airway disease. J Allergy Clin Immunol 130:1394–1403.e4
30. Iijima K, Kobayashi T, Hara K, Kephart GM, Ziegler SF, McKenzie AN, Kita H (2014) IL-33 and thymic stromal lymphopoietin mediate immune pathology in response to chronic airborne allergen exposure. J Immunol 193:1549–1559
31. Cayrol C, Girard JP (2014) IL-33: an alarmin cytokine with crucial roles in innate immunity, inflammation and allergy. Curr Opin Immunol 31C:31–37
32. Kondo Y, Yoshimoto T, Yasuda K, Futatsugi-Yumikura S, Morimoto M, Hayashi N, Hoshino T, Fujimoto J, Nakanishi K (2008) Administration of IL-33 induces airway hyperresponsiveness and goblet cell hyperplasia in the lungs in the absence of adaptive immune system. Int Immunol 20:791–800
33. Bartemes KR, Iijima K, Kobayashi T, Kephart GM, McKenzie AN, Kita H (2012) IL-33-responsive lineage-CD25+ CD44(hi) lymphoid cells mediate innate type 2 immunity and allergic inflammation in the lungs. J Immunol 188:1503–1513
34. Klein Wolterink RG, Kleinjan A, van Nimwegen M, Bergen I, de Bruijn M, Levani Y, Hendriks RW (2012) Pulmonary innate lymphoid cells are major producers of IL-5 and IL-13 in murine models of allergic asthma. Eur J Immunol 42:1106–1116
35. Maazi H, Patel N, Sankaranarayanan I, Suzuki Y, Rigas D, Soroosh P, Freeman GJ, Sharpe AH, Akbari O (2015) ICOS:ICOS-ligand interaction is required for type 2 innate lymphoid cell function, homeostasis, and induction of airway hyperreactivity. Immunity 42:538–551
36. Huang Y, Guo L, Qiu J, Chen X, Hu-Li J, Siebenlist U, Williamson PR, Urban JF Jr, Paul WE (2015) IL-25-responsive, lineage-negative KLRG1(hi) cells are multipotential 'inflammatory' type 2 innate lymphoid cells. Nat Immunol 16:161–169

Chapter 13

Induction and Analysis of Bronchus-Associated Lymphoid Tissue

Henrike Fleige and Reinhold Förster

Abstract

Bronchus-associated lymphoid tissue (BALT) forms spontaneously in the lung after pulmonary infection and has been identified as a highly organized lymphoid structure supporting the efficient priming of T cells in the lung. To explore the mechanisms and instructive signals controlling BALT neogenesis we used both, a single dose of vaccinia virus MVA and repeated inhalations of heat-inactivated *Pseudomonas aeruginosa* (*P. aeruginosa*). Intranasal administration of both pathogens induces highly organized BALT but distinct pathways and molecules are used to promote the development of BALT. Here, we describe the induction and phenotype of the distinct types of BALT as well as the immunofluorescence microscopy-based analysis of the induced lymphoid tissue in the lung.

Key words BALT, Bronchus-associated lymphoid tissue, FDCs, MVA, *P. aeruginosa*

1 Introduction

Tertiary lymphoid organs, also known as ectopic lymphoid tissues, form spontaneously at sites of chronic inflammation during microbial infection, graft rejection, or autoimmune disease (reviewed in [1]). Typically, these structures are named according to the anatomical site of their occurrence, such as the bronchus-associated lymphoid tissue (BALT). BALT represents one of the major constituents of the enormous network of mucosa-associated lymphoid tissues, which plays an important role as a first line of defense against many common pathogens. BALT is characterized as lymphoid tissue consisting of organized B cell compartments, i.e., B cell follicles, in which germinal centers can develop, and T cell areas harboring T cells, antigen-presenting cells as well as high endothelial venules (HEV) specialized in allowing extravasation of lymphocytes from the blood [2–4]. Importantly, perivascular infiltrations of lymphocytes within the lungs are not necessarily equivalent to BALT. In order to meet the definition of BALT, lymphoid aggregates have to be situated adjacent to a bronchus and next to

Björn E. Clausen and Jon D. Laman (eds.), *Inflammation: Methods and Protocols*, Methods in Molecular Biology, vol. 1559, DOI 10.1007/978-1-4939-6786-5_13, © Springer Science+Business Media LLC 2017

a vein and an artery [4]. At sites of infection, BALT can help to eliminate pathogens by providing a microenvironment that supports the local generation of a protective immune response. We and others have demonstrated that BALT does represent an organized and functional lymphoid structure that also serves as a general priming site for T cells in the lung [3, 5].

The lungs of naïve mice and healthy adult humans are typically devoid of (spontaneously developing) BALT. However, viruses like modified vaccinia virus Ankara (MVA), murine Herpes Virus-68 (MHV-68), and Influenza are known to induce BALT formation, and animal infection models utilizing some of these viruses have been established also in our lab [3, 5, 6]. Our group could recently demonstrate that a single intranasal (i.n.) application of the replication-deficient vaccinia virus MVA is sufficient to induce highly organized BALT containing visibly segregated B and T cell zones [5]. Along the same line, repetitive inhalations of heat-killed bacteria such as *Pseudomonas aeruginosa* (*P. aeruginosa*; [7]) or the repeated i.n. administration of lipopolysaccharide (LPS; [8]) have been described to induce BALT in mice. We could recently show that the type of BALT-inducing pathogen determines which key factors are required for the development and maturation of BALT. We identified an IL-17-dependent pathway that induces CXCL12 production by gp38$^+$ stromal cells after i.n. administration of *P. aeruginosa*, and an IL-17-independent pathway that promotes the differentiation of CXCL13-expressing follicular dendritic cells (FDCs) in MVA-induced BALT. The expression of any of these two cytokines allows B cells to aggregate in follicular structures.

In this chapter, we provide a detailed description of the induction and phenotype of both MVA- and *P. aeruginosa*-induced BALT and the quantitative and qualitative immunofluorescence analysis of BALT.

2 Materials

2.1 Induction of BALT

1. 6–12-week-old C57BL/6 mice (*see* **Notes 1–3**).
2. Eye ointment.
3. Paper towels.
4. Pipette + tips.
5. MVA: Modified vaccinia virus Ankara is a highly attenuated orthopoxvirus that lost its capacity to replicate in mammalian cells [9]. Recombinant MVA constructs have been described previously and virus stocks were generated by standard methods [10]. In brief, infect chicken embryo fibroblasts (CEFs) with virus suspension (0.01–1 IU/cell). Remove inoculum 1 h after virus adsorption at 37 °C, wash the cells once and incubate with

fresh medium. Harvest the cells and medium 48 h after infection, freeze-thaw virus material three times, and homogenize it in a cup sonicator. Purify MVA from cell debris by ultracentrifugation for 60 min through sucrose. To determine the infective titer of MVA stock preparation, titrate the resulting lysate on CEFs.

- To induce MVA-BALT, prepare 10^7 IU MVA diluted in 40 μl PBS per mouse.

6. *P. aeruginosa*: *P. aeruginosa* strain PA14 [11] routinely cultured at 37 °C in LB medium. Adjust bacteria to 5×10^9 CFU/ml in PBS and autoclave them at 121 °C for 90 min to heat-inactivate bacteria.
   - To induce *P. aeruginosa*-BALT, dilute 10 μl of a 5×10^9 CFU/ml *P. aeruginosa* stock in 40 μl PBS (final concentration 5×10^7 CFU per mouse).
7. Anaesthesia (such as 0.2 mg of ketamine and 0.02 mg xylazine/g body weight).
8. Warming blanket.

2.2 Isolation of the Lung and Preparation of Cryosections

1. Tissue-Tek OCT.
2. PBS.
3. Kimwipes.
4. Prepare a 1:1 mixture of Tissue-Tek OCT and PBS.
5. Cryomolds.
6. Dry ice.
7. Cryostat.
8. Adhesive microscope slides, such as HistoBond® adhesive slides (Marienfeld-Superior).
9. Ice-cold acetone.

2.3 Immuno histological Staining of Cell Surface Markers on Acetone-Fixed Slides

1. Standard immunofluorescence staining equipment including a slide rack, such as Sequenza™ Slide Rack, Coverplates™ (both Thermo Scientific), coverslips, and Eppendorf tubes.
2. Tris-buffered saline (TBS; 10×): 1.5 M NaCl, 0.1 M Tris–HCl, pH 7.4.
3. 1× TBS containing 0.05 % Tween 20 (TBST).
4. Blocking solution: 5 % mouse or rat serum + 10 % anti-FcR mAb (2.4.G2) in TBST.
5. The specifics of monoclonal antibodies used for immunohistology are provided in Table 1.
6. DAPI staining solution: use 100 μl of 1 μg/ml DAPI per cryosection.
7. Mowiol (Merck Millipore, Darmstadt, Germany): Add 2.4 g of MOWIOL® 4-88 to 6 g of glycerol and stir to mix. Add

Table 1
Monoclonal antibodies used for immunohistological staining of cell surface markers

Specificity	Clone	Species	Isotype	Supplier
B220	RA3-3A1	Rat	IgM	Homemade
CD3	17A2	Rat	IgG2bκ	Homemade
CD21/35	7G6	Rat	IgG2bκ	BD Pharmingen

6 ml of water and stir for several hours at room temperature. Add 12 ml of 0.2 M Tris–HCl (pH 8.5) and heat to 50 °C for 10 min with occasional mixing. After the MOWIOL® 4-88 dissolves, clarify the solution by centrifugation at 5000×g for 15 min.

2.4 Immuno histological Staining of Chemokines on Acetone-Fixed Slides

1. Standard immunofluorescence staining equipment including a slide rack, such as Sequenza™ Slide Rack, Coverplates™ (both Thermo Scientific), coverslips, and Eppendorf tubes.
2. Tris-buffered saline (TBS; 10×): 1.5 M NaCl; 0.1 M Tris–HCl, pH 7.4.
3. 1× TBS containing 0.05% Tween 20 (TBST).
4. Tyramide Signal Amplification (TSA) Kit (PerkinElmer).
5. 0.3–3% H_2O_2 in PBS.
6. TNB blocking buffer: 0.1 M Tris–HCl, pH 7.5; 0.15 M NaCl; 0.5% Blocking Reagent (PerkinElmer).
7. Blocking solution: 5% mouse serum in TNB Blocking Buffer.
8. The specifics and source of antibodies used for chemokine staining are provided in Table 2.

2.5 Immuno fluorescence Imaging

Immunofluorescence imaging can be performed with any fluorescence microscope equipped with 10× and 20× objectives, a sensitive fluorescence camera, a motorized stage, and a software package that allows acquisition of stitched images. For our experiments, we use a BX61 fluorescence microscope (Olympus) equipped with UPlanSApo objectives (10×/0.4 and 20×/0.75) and a motorized XY-stage. Images are taken at room temperature using an F-View II camera and processed with cellSens 1.12 software (all from Olympus).

2.6 Analysis of BALT

For counting and measuring of individual lymphoid structures any software equipped with a counting and polygon tool can be used. For our analysis we used cellSens 1.12 from Olympus. For statistical analysis any statistic software can be used. For our analysis we used Prism 4 (Graph-Pad Software, Inc). All significant values were determined using one-way ANOVA.

Table 2
Polyclonal antibodies used for immunohistological staining of chemokines

Specificity	Clone	Species	Isotype	Supplier
CXCL13	Polyclonal	Goat	Whole IgG	R&D Systems
CXCL12	Polyclonal	Goat	Whole IgG	Peprotech
Anti-goat HRP	Polyclonal	Donkey	Whole IgG	Jackson ImmunoResearch Laboratories, Inc.

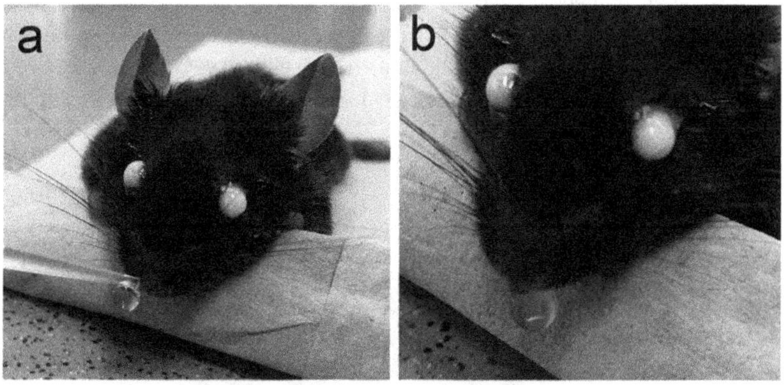

Fig. 1 Intranasal application of MVA or *P. aeruginosa*. (**a**) Transfer of a droplet (containing a volume of 40 μl) from a pipette's tip to the nostrils of a deeply anesthetized mouse. (**b**) Passive inhalation of the droplet by the mouse. Please note eyes of the mice are covered with protective eye ointment to prevent corneal drying or damage

3 Methods

3.1 Intranasal Instillation of MVA or P. aeruginosa to Induce BALT

1. Either dilute 10^7 IU intact MVA or 5×10^7 CFU heat-inactivated *P. aeruginosa* in 40 μl PBS per mouse (*see* **Notes 4** and **5**).
2. Anesthetize mice intraperitoneally with 0.2 mg of ketamine and 0.02 mg xylazine/g body weight.
3. Apply eye ointment to the eyes to prevent corneal drying and damage.
4. Either apply 40 μl of MVA-PBS solution at day 0 or 40 μl of *P. aeruginosa*-PBS solution at day 0 and day 6 to the nostrils of the anesthetized mice (Fig. 1 and *see* **Note 6**).
5. To minimize heat loss during intranasal instillation and recovery place the mice on a 37 °C pre-warmed warming blanket.

3.2 Isolation of the Lung and Preparation of Cryosections

1. Sacrifice mice 12 days after the first instillation of either MVA or *P. aeruginosa*.
2. Open the thorax and perfuse the lung with 10 ml cold PBS via the right heart ventricle (*see* **Note 7**).

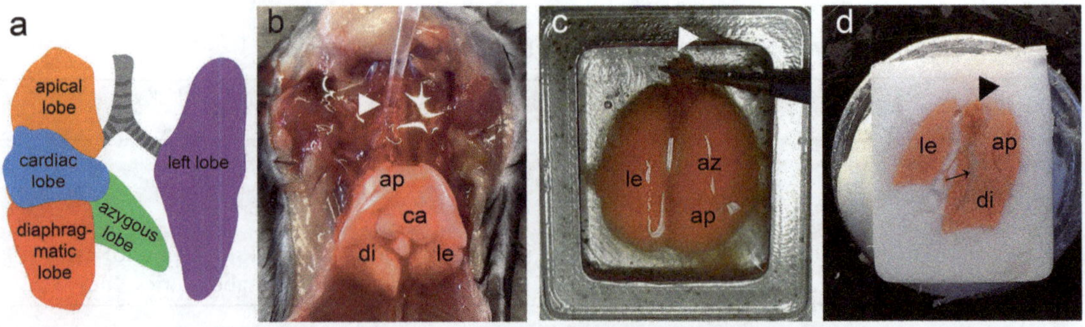

Fig. 2 Isolation, embedding and sectioning of the lung. (**a**) Schematic overview of a murine lung. (**b**) Filling of a perfused lung with a 1:1 mixture of Tissue-Tek OCT and PBS via the trachea. (**c**) Transfer and dorsoventral embedding of an OCT/PBS-filled lung into an OCT-filled cryomold. (**d**) Cross section of a cryopreserved lung at one area of interest. *ap* apical lobe, *az* azygous lobe, *ca* cardiac lobe, *di* diaphragmatic lobe, *le* left lobe, *arrow* bronchus, *arrowheads* trachea

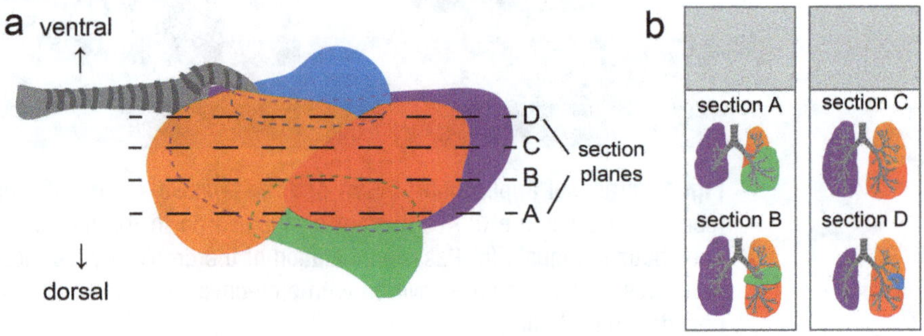

Fig. 3 Schematic overview of the murine lung and section planes. (**a** and **b**) Overview of the four different section planes used for histological analysis

3. Fill the lung with a 1:1 mixture of Tissue-Tek OCT and PBS (Fig. 2b and *see* **Note 8**).
4. Transfer the OCT-filled lung into a cryomold, embed it in OCT (Fig. 2c and *see* **Note 9**) and place it on dry ice to freeze it.
5. Perform 8-μm sections with a cryostat (such as CM3050; Leica).
6. After slicing in a dorsoventral direction, the criterion for the first section to be used for analysis is approval of macroscopically visible bronchi (Fig. 2d and *see* **Note 10**).
7. At distances of 400–1000 μm, three further sections are subjected to analysis (Fig. 3 and *see* **Note 11**).
8. Air-dry the sections and incubate unfixed sections for 10 min in ice-cold (−20 °C) acetone (*see* **Note 12**). Allow the acetone to evaporate from the sections for 20 min at RT.

3.3 Immuno fluorescent Staining of Cell Surface Markers

1. Choose two cryosections per lung/mouse (Fig. 3b) and rehydrate in Tris-buffered saline with 0.05 % Tween 20 (TBST) for 10 min at RT.
2. Transfer the slides assembled with a Coverplate™ into a slide rack and fill the reservoir with TBST 2–3 times (*see* **Note 13**).
3. Block with 5 % rat serum and 10% anti-FcR mAb (2.4.G2) in 200 μl TBST for 20 min at RT.
4. Stain with antibodies by adding 100 μl of TBST containing the mAbs cocktail (Table 1) followed by incubation at RT for 60 min.
5. Wash the slides 2× with TBST.
6. Add 2× 100 μl of TBST containing 1 μg/ml DAPI and incubate for 2 min.
7. Wash the slides 2× with TBST.
8. Remove the slides from staining rack and mount slides by gently adding five drops of MOWIOL to the surface. Gently angle the coverslip over the sample with one edge touching the slide.
9. Dry slides at RT for 12 h.

3.4 Immuno fluorescence Staining of Chemokines

Chemokine staining was performed by using a Tyramide Signal Amplification (TSA) system according to the manufacturer's instructions (PerkinElmer).

Optimized protocol for staining of CXCL13 and CXCL12 on acetone-fixed cryosections:

1. Rehydrate cryosections in TBST for 10 min at RT.
2. Quench endogenous peroxidase activity by incubating slides in 0.3 % H_2O_2 to 3 % H_2O_2 in PBS (*see* **Note 14**).
3. Transfer the slides assembled with a Coverplate™ into a slide rack and fill the reservoir with TBST 2–3 times (*see* **Note 13**).
4. Block with 5 % mouse serum in 200 μl TNB Buffer for 30 min at RT.
5. Label with primary chemokine antibody by adding 100 μl of TNB Buffer containing the primary antibody (Table 2), followed by incubation at 4 °C overnight (*see* **Note 15**).
6. Wash the slides 2× with TBST.
7. Incubate slides with 100 μl horseradish peroxidase (HRP)-labeled secondary antibody diluted in TBST for 60 min at RT.
8. Wash the slides 2× with TBST.
9. Add 100 μl of the Fluorophore Amplification Working Solution (Tyramide-Cy3 or Tyramide-Cy5 1:50 in provided Diluent Reagent) to each slide and incubate for 10 min at RT.
10. Wash the slides 2× with TBST.

11. Counterstain with cell surface markers as required (*see* Subheading 3.4).
12. Remove the slides from staining rack and mount slides by gently adding five drops of MOWIOL to the surface. Gently angle the coverslip over the sample with one edge touching the slide.
13. Dry slides at RT for 12 h.

3.5 Quantification and Categorization of BALT

1. Immunohistological analysis can be done by using any motorized epifluorescence microscope equipped with an image analysis software (such as cellSens from Olympus or AxioVision from Carl Zeiss, Inc.).
2. BALT is typically located along major bronchial airways within the perivascular space identified by densely packed lymphoid aggregates [4]. In addition to BALT, pulmonary infection in mice often results in unorganized interstitial lymphocytic infiltrations not adjacent to a bronchus. Therefore, we define true BALT by the following criteria:
    - Direct proximity to a bronchus and to a vein and an artery (*see* **Note 16**).
    - Organized accumulations of T and B lymphocytes, separated in a densely packed B cell follicle surrounded by a T cell zone.
    - Containing DCs, a network of chemokine-expressing stromal cells and depending on its state of maturation FDCs (*see* **Note 17**).
3. Immunofluorescence analysis of lungs from pathogen-treated wildtype (wt) mice reveals the formation of highly organized BALT 12 days after the induction [5, 12]. One major difference between MVA- and *P. aeruginosa*-induced BALT is the lack of CXCL13-expressing FDCs in the latter situation (Fig. 4a, b, d, e). Here, most likely CXCL12 substitutes for CXCL13 as the central B cell recruiting factor (*see* ref. 5 and Fig. 4c, f).
4. Further qualitative analysis of the induced lymphoid aggregates includes the categorization of all aggregates into three types based on their B cell status (Fig. 5). This can be very helpful to distinguish between typical BALT and unorganized perivascular lymphoid infiltrates:
    - Type I: lymphoid aggregates displaying the characteristic morphology of typical MVA- or *P. aeruginosa*-induced BALT described above (Fig. 5a, d: type I).
    - Type II: lymphoid aggregates situated adjacent to a bronchus, a vein, and an artery but failed to develop densely packed B cell follicles but still containing numerous B cells (Fig. 5b, e: type II).

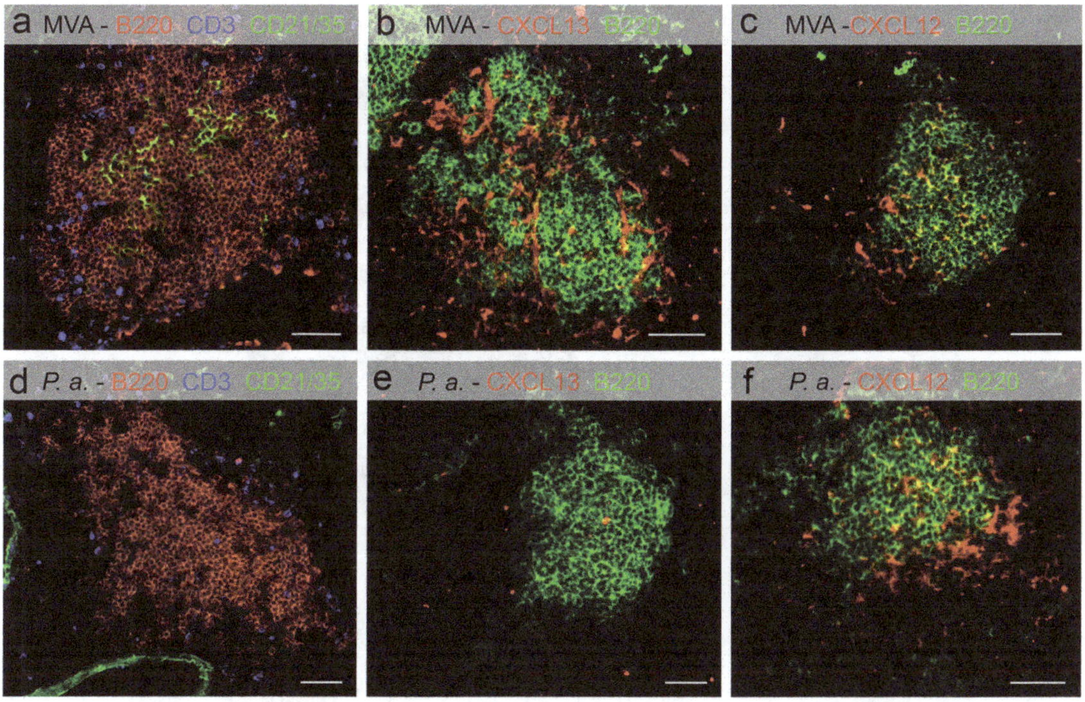

Fig. 4 *P. aeruginosa*-induced BALT lacks CXCL13-expressing FDCs. (**a**–**f**) Immunofluorescence micrograph of BALT 12 days after i.n. administration of intact MVA (**a**–**c**) or heat-inactivated *P. aeruginosa* (*P. a.*; **d**–**f**). Cryosections of adult lungs from 8- to 12-week-old mice stained with the antibodies as indicated. Bars, 100 μm. For further information please *see* ref. 12

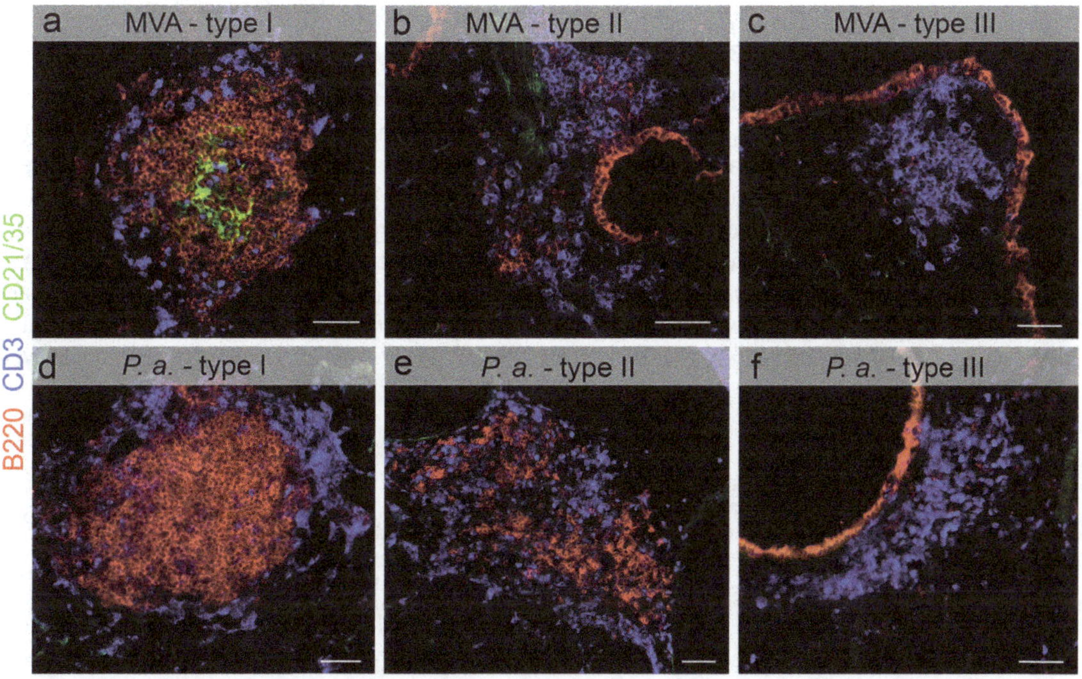

Fig. 5 Categorization of lymphoid aggregates. (**a**–**f**) Immunofluorescence micrograph of three different types of lymphoid aggregates, categorized according to their status of B cells. Cryosections of adult lungs from 8- to 12-week-old mice 12 days after i.n. administration of either intact MVA (**a**–**c**) or heat-inactivated *P. aeruginosa* (*P. a.*; **d**–**f**) stained with the antibodies as indicated. Bars, 100 μm

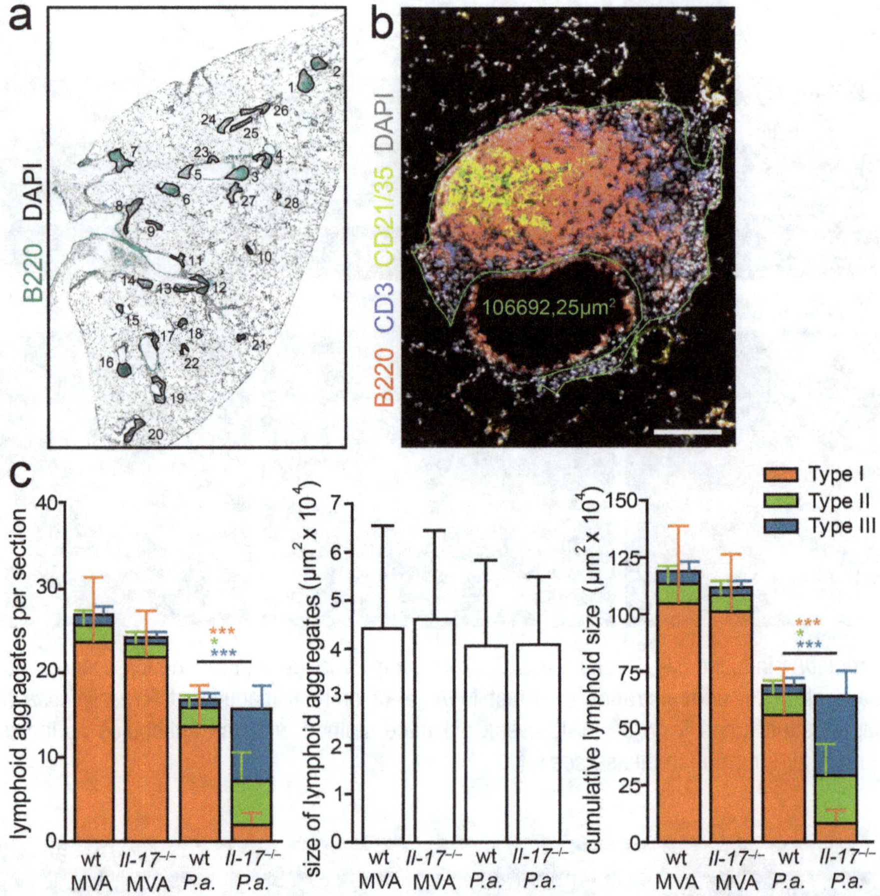

Fig. 6 Quantitative analysis of induced lymphoid aggregates in the lung. Immunofluorescence panoramic overview of a lung containing MVA-induced BALT (**a**) and a detailed micrograph of BALT (**b**) stained with the antibodies as indicated. Shown are representative sections indicating counting (**a**, *numbers*) and area measurement (**b**, *green line* and *value*) of lymphoid aggregates including BALT using cellSens software (Olympus). Bar, 100 μm. (**c**) Quantification and categorization of lymphoid aggregates in the lungs of WT and *Il-17–/–* mice 12 days after i.n. administration of intact MVA or heat-inactivated *Pseudomonas* (*P. a.*). All aggregates of four different panoramic images were counted and categorized (*left*). Individual sizes of all aggregates were measured (*middle*). Cumulative lymphoid size was calculated as the sum of all individual lymphoid aggregates in each category (*right*). Mean and SD; **P*< 0.05; ****P*< 0.001, WT vs. *Il-17–/–*; *color of stars* refers to the type of BALT as indicated

- Type III: lymphoid aggregates situated adjacent to a bronchus, a vein and an artery containing none or only very few B cells, but considerable amounts of T cells (Fig. 5c, f: type III).

5. For quantitative analysis, whole central sections of four different planes of the lung (close to main bronchi and vessels) are analyzed (Fig. 3). Create a single panoramic image of each section (Fig. 6a) and use the counting tool to count all lymphoid

aggregates and the closed polygon tool to measure the individual size of the aggregates (Fig. 6b). Calculate the cumulative lymphoid size of each section as the sum of all individual lymphoid structures. To quantify lymphoid aggregates according to the above mentioned categorization, count and measure all aggregates of the individual types and calculate the cumulative lymphoid size respectively (Fig. 6c).

4 Notes

1. In principle, BALT can be induced in every (inbred) mouse strain, but the degree of induction might vary. Due to the prevalent C57BL/6 background of knockout mice, we preferentially induce and analyze BALT in these mice.
2. In studies designed to investigate the effect of age on BALT formation, it had been observed that neonatal mice (7-days-old) develop more BALT than weanling mice (28-days-old) after intranasal exposure of LPS [8, 13]. However, we did not observe such an effect in MVA-induced BALT formation. Therefore we recommend to preferentially use mice between weeks 6 and 12 after birth to induced BALT by MVA. However, we cannot exclude that younger mice might be more susceptible to develop *Pseudomonas*-induced BALT.
3. The degree of BALT induction might also vary depending on the environment such as housing conditions, food or bedding. In fact, differences in commensal colonization may alter the number or repertoire of regulatory T cells, which are known to interfere with the formation of BALT [14]. Therefore, we recommend to house experimental mice always under the same conditions.
4. For BALT induction by MVA, we use intact virus particles. MVA lost its capacity to replicate in mammalian cells which results in a rapid decrease of infected cells shortly after intranasal infection. Nevertheless, a single intranasal application of MVA induces organized and long-lasting BALT [5].
5. In case of BALT induction by *P. aeruginosa*, we apply inactivated/dead bacteria to circumvent unforced severe lung inflammation including sepsis and death of for example immunodeficient mice. Repetitive application of autoclaved heat-inactivated *P. aeruginosa* leads to equally organized BALT.
6. For intranasal administration, gently form a droplet (containing 40 μl of the solution) at the pipette's tip and apply it to the nostrils of the mice. Do not try to instill it actively but rather let the mice inhale the droplet. To avoid sneezing of the mice leading to loss of BALT-inducing pathogenic material make sure the mice are deeply anesthetized. For convenient applica-

tion to the nostrils, place the mouse flat on the ventral side and position its head on top of a rolled paper towel (Fig. 1).

7. Remove the ribcage and all connective tissue of the mouse. Perfuse 10 ml of cold PBS through the right heart ventricle until the lungs are cleared of blood. Remove the heart and soak up remaining blood with Kimwipes.
8. Expose the trachea, cut away all connective tissue, make a little incision between the cartilage rings and inject ~1 ml of the prepared mix of OCT and PBS until the lung inflates. Keep the trachea closed with a forceps to avoid any leakage of the lung. Dissect out the lung by gently pulling on the trachea and simultaneously separating it from the esophagus (Fig. 2b).
9. For proper analysis of the lung a consistent way of embedding the lung is indispensable. We therefore recommend embedding the lung always in the same dorsoventral orientation (Fig. 2c).
10. 8-μm-thick OCT-embedded cryosections were cut in the dorsoventral plane. Four different section planes covering four (apical, azygous, diaphragmatic, and left lobe) of the five lung lobes were used for analysis (Fig. 3). The first section plane starts at the point of macroscopic visibility of the first bronchus in the azygous lobe [14].
11. The distances of section planes are dependent on the thickness of the individual lung lobes. For further immunohistological analysis, sections of all four planes are included (Fig. 3b).
12. Fixation immobilizes antigens while stabilizing cell morphology and tissue architecture. Immunohistological staining with the antibodies provided in Tables 1 and 2 are optimized for acetone-fixed tissue. Other fixatives may destroy the immunoreactivity of those epitopes.
13. Using the Coverplate™ technology allows liquids to fill the gap between the coverplate and the slide which prevents dehydration of the tissue and waste of staining reagents.
14. HRP catalyzes the activation of the Fluorophore Amplification Reagent. To minimize background signals, quenching of the endogenous peroxidase activity is essential. A quenching protocol according to the tissue being stained needs to be established. For chemokine staining on acetone-fixed lungs, we incubate rehydrated slides for 5 min in 0.5 % H_2O_2 followed by 5 min in 1 % H_2O_2 followed by 10 min in 3 % H_2O_2.
15. Due to potentially high background signals, always run control slides with each experiment. Include at least a negative control without primary antibody but including all other reagents.

16. Perivascular infiltrations of lymphocytes within the lungs are not necessarily equivalent to BALT. A part of the interstitial lymphocytic infiltrations observed in the setting of pulmonary infection are obviously not situated adjacent to a bronchus as well as next to a vein and an artery and have to be excluded from any further analysis consequently.
17. BALT induced by MVA contains a dense network of CXCL13-expressing CD21/35⁺ FDCs 12 days p.i. Regardless of its state of maturation, *P. aeruginosa*-induced BALT fails to develop FDCs or other CXCL13-expressing cells. In the absence of those, other chemokine-expressing stromal cells allow B cell recruitment and follicle formation [12]. Thus, in order to be termed BALT, the presence of FDCs is not necessarily required.

Acknowledgment

We would like to thank Stephan Halle and Tim Worbs for valuable advices in establishing the infection model, Susanne Häußler and Gerd Sutter for providing *P. aeruginosa* and MVA respectively. This work was supported by Deutsche Forschungsgemeinschaft (DFG) grants SFB587-B3 and SFB900-B1 and by ERC grant 322645 LYMPHATICS HOMING to R. Förster.

References

1. Neyt K, Perros F, GeurtsvanKessel CH et al (2012) Tertiary lymphoid organs in infection and autoimmunity. Trends Immunol 33:297–305
2. Xu B, Wagner N, Pham LN et al (2003) Lymphocyte homing to bronchus-associated lymphoid tissue (BALT) is mediated by L-selectin/PNAd, alpha4beta1 integrin/VCAM-1, and LFA-1 adhesion pathways. J Exp Med 197:1255–1267
3. Moyron-Quiroz JE, Rangel-Moreno J, Kusser K et al (2004) Role of inducible bronchus associated lymphoid tissue (iBALT) in respiratory immunity. Nat Med 10:927–934
4. Sminia T, van der Brugge-Gamelkoorn GJ, Jeurissen SH (1989) Structure and function of bronchus-associated lymphoid tissue (BALT). Crit Rev Immunol 9:119–150
5. Halle S, Dujardin HC, Bakocevic N et al (2009) Induced bronchus-associated lymphoid tissue serves as a general priming site for T cells and is maintained by dendritic cells. J Exp Med 206:2593–2601
6. Kocks JR, Adler H, Danzer H et al (2009) Chemokine receptor CCR7 contributes to a rapid and efficient clearance of lytic murine gamma-herpes virus 68 from the lung, whereas bronchus-associated lymphoid tissue harbors virus during latency. J Immunol 182:6861–6869
7. Toyoshima M, Chida K, Sato A (2000) Antigen uptake and subsequent cell kinetics in bronchus-associated lymphoid tissue. Respirology 5:141–145
8. Rangel-Moreno J, Carragher DM, de la Luz Garcia-Hernandez M et al (2011) The development of inducible bronchus-associated lymphoid tissue depends on IL-17. Nat Immunol 12:639–646
9. Meyer H, Sutter G, Mayr A (1991) Mapping of deletions in the genome of the highly attenuated vaccinia virus MVA and their influence on virulence. J Gen Virol 72(Pt 5):1031–1038
10. Kremer M, Volz A, Kreijtz JHCM et al (2012) Easy and efficient protocols for working with recombinant vaccinia virus MVA. Methods Mol Biol 890:59–92
11. Liberati NT, Urbach JM, Miyata S et al (2006) An ordered, nonredundant library of

Pseudomonas aeruginosa strain PA14 transposon insertion mutants. Proc Natl Acad Sci 103:2833–2838

12. Fleige H, Ravens S, Moschovakis GL et al (2014) IL-17-induced CXCL12 recruits B cells and induces follicle formation in BALT in the absence of differentiated FDCs. J Exp Med 211:643–651
13. Foo SY, Zhang V, Lalwani A et al (2015) Regulatory T cells prevent inducible BALT formation by dampening neutrophilic inflammation. J Immunol 194:4567–4576
14. Kocks JR, Davalos-Misslitz ACM, Hintzen G et al (2007) Regulatory T cells interfere with the development of bronchus-associated lymphoid tissue. J Exp Med 204:723–734

Chapter 14

Messenger RNA Sequencing of Rare Cell Populations in the Lung and Lung-Draining Lymph Nodes

Alexander Ulges, Edgar Schmitt, Tobias Bopp, and Matthias Klein

Abstract

Next-generation sequencing (NGS) techniques provide unique prospects for in-depth transcriptome analyses. Nevertheless, the emerging and still growing knowledge about the large diversity and heterogeneity of cells that participate in immunological responses in a tissue- and micromilieu-specific manner calls for advanced isolation and sequencing methods for the accurate quantification of gene expression in small cell populations and even individual cells from any organ or tissue. One of the major limitations in performing transcriptome analyses of rare cell populations was and still is quality and quantity of RNA that often limits analyses of complex mixtures of immune cell populations. Here, we describe a protocol to isolate rare T cell populations from the lung and in particular the subsequent methods to isolate high-grade RNA in order to perform NGS-based transcriptome analyses.

Key words Lung, Rare T cell population, Transcriptome analysis

1 Introduction

Besides of the skin, the lung is probably one of the rare tissues that are constantly exposed to a large variety of extrinsic substances ("antigens") and microorganisms and hence, has to master the difficult task to mount appropriate immune responses against inhaled pathogens, while at the same time preserving tolerance to self and/or harmless antigens. It is becoming apparent that specialized cell populations undertake this task during an immune response. In this respect, especially T cells have the ability to respond in an antigen-specific manner. In this manner, certain T cell subpopulations are capable to tailor immune responses based on their cytokine expression profile. Initially, Mosmann and Coffman recognized that production of different cytokine panels by distinct T cell clones was not stochastic but rather T cells could be subdivided into two distinct subsets according to the production of IFN-γ (T helper (Th)1) and interleukin-4 (Th2) [1]. Inappropriate activation of these Th subsets was shown to lead to allergic (Th2) or

Björn E. Clausen and Jon D. Laman (eds.), *Inflammation: Methods and Protocols*, Methods in Molecular Biology, vol. 1559, DOI 10.1007/978-1-4939-6786-5_14,

autoimmune (Th1) diseases and it was thought that this can be prevented by a balanced cross-regulation of Th1- and Th2-responses [2, 3]. Meanwhile, this Th cell dichotomy was considerably extended and additional $CD4^+$ T cells subsets have been described, among these IL-17-producing T cells (Th17 cells) [4, 5], Th22 cells [6], and Th9 cells [7, 8]. In contrast, regulatory T (T_{Reg}) cells constitute an essential counterbalance to the various Th subsets by their ability to suppress and regulate T cell-dependent adaptive immune responses [9–11]. Adding even more complexity to the system, recent studies have demonstrated that the environmental and tissue-specific context conditions T cells to become specialized effector populations in a micromilieu-dependent manner [12–15]. As a result, seemingly homogeneous T cell populations like distinct Th cells or T_{Reg} cells may indeed comprise a great variety of different specialized Th and T_{Reg} cell subpopulations in a given organ that differ in their function and with that in their transcriptome. Understanding how T cell subpopulations achieve cellular and functional diversity at the transcriptional level especially during inflammation and tolerance preservation is a core challenge in immunological research.

Isolation of total RNA from low cell numbers results in low amounts of total RNA and commonly used protocols and kits (NEBnext ultra RNA and Illumina TruSeq RNA library preparation kits) for library preparation require at least 10 ng of total RNA as starting material. Picelli et al. introduced Smart-seq2 [16, 17] which allows the generation of full-length cDNA and sequencing libraries using standard reagents, thereby providing a highly cost-effective method in generating cDNA libraries even from a single cell.

Here we present a detailed protocol for the isolation of rare T cell subpopulations from the lung and the subsequent procedure to obtain RNA of high quality and final cDNA libraries from small cell numbers (corresponding to <1 ng of RNA) and to perform transcriptome analysis by next-generation sequencing.

2 Materials

2.1 Isolation of Rare Cell Populations from Lung Draining Lymph Nodes

1. Isopropanol (98%).
2. FORENE® 100% (V/V) (active agent: isoflurane).
3. Preparation cutlery.
4. 6-well plate.
5. Minimal Essential Medium (MEM) (Pan Biotech). Medium was supplemented with 50 μM β-mercaptoethanol, 1% penicillin/streptomycin, and 2% FCS.
6. Object slides with rough edges.

7. 50 and 15 ml Falcon tubes.
8. 40 μm cell strainer.
9. FACS buffer: 1× PBS + 0.5 % BSA + 5 mM EDTA + 0.01 % NaN_3.
10. Antibodies for flow cytometry:
    Anti-CD4-Pacific Blue (clone RM4.5; eBioscience).
    Anti-CD25-PE (clone 3C7; eBioscience).
11. Centrifuge.
12. BD FACS ARIA™ II Cell Sorter.

2.2 Isolation of Rare Cell Populations from Lungs

1. Isopropanol (98 %).
2. FORENE® 100 % (V/V) (active agent: isoflurane).
3. Preparation cutlery.
4. Small petri dishes.
5. Scalpel.
6. Incubation shaker.
7. 10 ml syringes and cannulas (18 G; 1.2 × 40 mm).
8. Phosphate buffered saline (PBS).
9. Gey's lysis buffer (0.83% ammonium chloride solution): 8.28 g/l NH_4Cl + 1.0 g/l $KHCO_3$ + 0.037 g/l EDTA.
10. 50 and 15 ml Falcon tubes.
11. 40 μm cell strainer.
12. FACS buffer: 1× PBS + 0.5% BSA + 5 mM EDTA + 0.01 % NaN_3.
13. Antibodies for flow cytometry: anti-CD4-Pacific Blue (clone RM4.5), anti-CD25-PE (clone 3C7).
14. Centrifuge.
15. BD FACS ARIA™ II Cell Sorter.

2.3 Isolation of Total RNA from Lung Draining Lymph Node Cells and Lung Cells

1. RNeasy® Micro Kit (Qiagen).
   RNeasy MinElute® Spin Columns.
   Collection tubes (1.5 and 2 ml).
   RLT buffer.
   RW1 buffer.
   RPE buffer.
   RNase-free water.
2. Ethanol p.a. (70 and 80 %).
3. RNase-free tubes and pipet tips.
4. Microcentrifuge allowing centrifugation of 2 ml tubes.
5. Vinyl or latex gloves.

6. 14.3 M beta-mercaptoethanol.
7. RNase away.
8. Sterile, disposable, RNase-free polypropylene tubes.
9. RNase-free DNase Set (Qiagen): Prepare DNase stock solution by dissolving the lyophilized DNase I (1500 Kunitz units) in 550 μl of RNase-free water. RDD buffer.

2.4 Assessment of Concentration and Quality of Isolated Total RNA

1. Qubit® 2.0 (Invitrogen).
2. Qubit® RNA High-sensitivity (HS) Assay Kit: Qubit RNA HS Reagent, RNA HS buffer, RNA HS Standard#1 (0 ng/μl) and RNA HS Standard#2 (10 ng/μl) in TE buffer.
3. Qubit® Assay tubes.
4. Bioanalyzer 2100 (Agilent).
5. RNA 6000 Pico Kit (Agilent).
6. RNase-free pipet tips.
7. Vinyl or latex gloves.
8. Total RNA.
9. RNase-free 1.5 ml polypropylene tubes. Microcentrifuge allowing centrifugation of 0.5 ml tubes.

2.5 Generation of Full-Length cDNA Using Smart-seq2

2.5.1 Reverse Transcription

1. Total RNA.
2. RNase away.
3. RNase-free pipet tips.
4. Vinyl or latex gloves.
5. RNase-free water.
6. Oligo dT [10 μM].

   5′-AAGCAGTGGTATCAACGCAGAGTACT$^{\times 30}$AC-3′

   The two terminal nucleotide facilitate anchoring the oligonucleotide to the beginning of the polyA tail thereby avoiding unnecessary amplification of a long part of the polyA tail.
7. dNTP [10 mM each].
8. Triton X-100 [0.2%]+4 U RNase inhibitor.
9. Superscript II [200 U/μl].
10. Superscript II buffer.
11. RNase inhibitor [40 U/μl].
12. DTT [100 mM].
13. Betaine [5 M].
14. $MgCl_2$ [100 mM].
15. LNA-modified TSO [5 μM] (Exiqon):

    5′-AAGCAGTGGTATCAACGCAGAGTACATG^{r}G^{r}G*-3′

(G^r) = riboguanosine, (G^*) = LNA-modified guanosine

16. Thermal cycler.
17. Magnetic stand for 96-well plates.
18. Vortexer.
19. Nuclease-free 0.2 ml polypropylene tubes and with caps.
20. Ice.

2.5.2 Amplification

1. KAPA HiFi HotStart ReadyMix (2×) (KAPA biosystems).
2. IS PCR Primer [10 μM]:
   5′-AAGCAGTGGTATCAACGCAGAGT-3′
3. RNase-free water and pipet tips.
4. Thermal cycler.

2.5.3 Purification

1. AMpure XP beads (Beckman Coulter).
2. 96-well plates, nuclease free, 0.2 ml.
3. Magnetic stand for 96-well plates.
4. Ethanol [80 %], freshly prepared.
5. EB solution (10 mM Tris-Cl, pH 8.5, Qiagen).
6. RNase-free water and pipet tips.

2.5.4 Determining the Concentration and Quality of Full-Length cDNA

1. Bioanalyzer 2100 (Agilent).
2. High-sensitivity DNA chip (Agilent).
3. Nuclease-free pipet tips and water.
4. Qubit® 2.0 (Invitrogen).
5. Qubit® dsDNA High-sensitivity Assay Kit: The kit includes concentrated assay reagent, dilution buffer, Qubit dsDNA HS Standard#1 (0 ng/μl) and Qubit dsDNA HS Standard#2 (10 ng/μl) in TE-buffer.
6. Qubit® Assay tubes.

2.6 Preparation of Sequencing Library Employing Nextera XT DNA Sample Preparation Kit

2.6.1 Tagmentation of Input DNA

1. Nuclease-free water.
2. Input DNA (1 ng of ds cDNA).
3. ATM (Amplicon Tagment Mix).
4. TD (Tagment DNA buffer).
5. NT (Neutralize Tagment buffer).
6. 96-well plate, nuclease free, 0.2 ml with cap strips.
7. Nuclease-free pipet tips and water.
8. Thermal cycler.

2.6.2 PCR Amplification

1. NPM (Nextera PCR Master Mix).
2. Index Primers 1 and 2 (N7XX and S5XX).

3. 96-well plate, nuclease free, 0.2 ml with cap strips.
4. Nuclease-free water and pipet tips.
5. Thermal cycler.

2.6.3 PCR Purification

1. RSB (Resuspension buffer).
2. AmpureXP Beads (Beckmann Coulter).
3. Ethanol [80 %], freshly prepared.
4. 96-well plate, nuclease free, 0.2 ml with cap strips.
5. Nuclease-free pipet tips and water.

2.6.4 Checking the Quality and Quantity of the Final cDNA Libraries

1. Bioanalyzer 2100 (Agilent).
2. High-sensitivity DNA chip (Agilent).
3. Nuclease-free pipet tips.
4. Qubit® 2.0 (Invitrogen).
5. Qubit® 2.0 dsDNA High-sensitivity Assay.
6. Qubit® 2.0 Assay tubes.

2.6.5 Pooling of Final cDNA Libraries and Denaturation

1. Barcoded final cDNA libraries.
2. EB solution (10 mM Tris-Cl, pH 8.5, Qiagen).
3. NaOH [0.2 N], freshly prepared from 10 N stock.
4. HT1 buffer (Illumina MiSeq Reagent Kit v3).
5. Nuclease-free water and pipet tips and 1.5 ml tubes.

2.6.6 DNA Sequencing (Illumina MiSeq) and Analysis

1. Denatured cDNA libraries.
2. Flow cell (Illumina MiSeq Reagent v3 kit).
3. Reagent cartridge (Illumina MiSeq Reagent v3 kit).
4. CLC Genomics Workbench (v7) software (Qiagen).
5. Nuclease-free pipet tips.

3 Methods

3.1 Isolation of Rare Cell Populations from Lung Draining Lymph Nodes

Carry out all procedures at room temperature, unless otherwise indicated.

3.1.1 Preparation of Lung-Draining Lymph Node

1. Sacrifice animals using narcotization with isoflurane (*see* **Note 1**).
2. Pin the animal with belly up. Wash the mouse with isopropanol to avoid any contamination with hair. Carefully remove the skin from the belly and chest using a scissor. Avoid harming the underlying muscles.

3. Make an incision at the peritoneum straight below the diaphragm and open the peritoneum without cutting the diaphragm.
4. Make an incision into the diaphragm. The lung should now collapse. Then cut the diaphragm lose from the rib cage. Afterwards cut the rib cage and remove the upper part of the chest with the sternum. Avoid harming any underlying blood vessels.
5. Draw the lung to the right site (from your direction). You should now be able to see the backbone with the vena cava.
6. The tracheal (lung-draining) lymph node is usually located below the connection of vena cava and the axillary blood vessel. Carefully dissect the lymph node using two sharp forceps and store it in a 6-well plate containing 3 ml of ice cold MEM-Medium + 2 % FCS (*see* **Note 2**).

3.1.2 Generation of Single Cell Suspension of Lymph Node Cells

1. Disinfect the rough side of two glass slides by immersing in isopropanol and burning. Let the slides cool down for a few seconds, then moist them with MEM + 2 % FCS medium.
2. Put the lymph node between the rough sides of the glass slides and carefully disrupt the lymph nodes.
3. Wash the glass slides with 3 ml MEM + 2 % FCS and collect the cell suspension in the same 6-well plate, previously used to store the lymph node.
4. Transfer the cell solution into a new 15 ml Falcon tube and thereby filter the cells from any debris using a 40 μm cell strainer.
5. Wash the well of the 6-well plate with another 3 ml MEM + 2 % FCS and transfer them through the cell strainer into the Falcon tube.

3.1.3 Flow Cytometry-Based Isolation of Regulatory T (T_{Reg}) Cells

1. Centrifuge the cells for 5 min at 600 × *g* and 4 °C. Then carefully remove supernatant and wash the cells with 10 ml of ice cold FACS buffer.
2. Prepare staining solution for T_{Reg} cells by diluting the antibodies in FACS buffer to a final concentration of (*see* **Note 3**):

   Anti-CD4-Pacific Blue (clone RM4.5) 1.25 μg/ml.

   Anti-CD25-PE (clone 3C7) 2.5 μg/ml.
3. Centrifuge the washed cells for 5 min at 600 × *g* at 4 °C. Then remove the supernatant and resuspend the cells in the staining solution. We recommend to suspend up to 5×10^7 cells/ml. Incubate the cells for 20 min, 4 °C in the dark.
4. Wash the cells by filling up to 10 ml of FACS buffer. Filter the solution through a 40 μm cell strainer into a new Falcon tube.

Add another 3 ml of FACS buffer to the empty tube. Transfer solution to the tube containing already filtered solution using the same 40 μm cell strainer.

5. Centrifuge the cells for 5 min at 600 × *g* and 4 °C. Remove supernatant and resuspend the cells in FACS buffer (2×10^7 cells/ml).
6. Separate the population of $CD4^+CD25^{hi}$ cells with a FACS sorter (*see* **Note 4**).

3.2 Isolation of Rare Cell Populations from Lungs

Carry out all procedures at room temperature unless otherwise indicated.

3.2.1 Preparation of Lung [18]

1. Please follow **steps 1–4** as described in Subheading 3.1.1.
2. Using a 10 ml syringe with cannula perfuse the lung by injecting 5–10 ml PBS into the dark, right heart chamber (*see* **Note 5**).
3. Remove the lung from the chest and transfer to a small Petri dish. Subsequently move on to Subheading 3.2.2 (*see* **Note 2**).

3.2.2 Generation of Single Cell Suspension of Lung Cells

1. Prepare a digestion solution by solving Collagenase type IA in PBS (1 mg/ml). Prepare 2.6 ml solution per lung.
2. Mince the lung thoroughly in a Petri dish with a scalpel, then transfer the material to a new 50 ml Falcon (*see* **Note 6**).
3. Wash the Petri dish with 2.5 ml PBS and transfer to the 50 ml Falcon tube. Add 2.5 ml of digestion solution to the falcon.
4. Incubate the solution on an incubation-shaker (125 rpm) for 1 h at 37 °C (*see* **Note** 7).
5. Further mince residual tissue by pulling the solution up and down through a 10 ml syringe with cannula.
6. Filter the cell suspension through a 40 μm cell strainer and transfer to a new 50 ml Falcon.
7. Flush the digestion Falcon with 5 ml PBS and transfer through the filter to the cell suspension.
8. Centrifuge the cells for 5 min at 600 × *g* and 4 °C. Then carefully remove supernatant.
9. Remove residual erythrocytes by incubating the cell suspension in Gey's lysis buffer for 1 min on ice. Stop the cell lysis by adding 9 ml PBS. Immediately move on to Subheading 3.2.3.

3.2.3 Flow Cytometry-Based Isolation of Regulatory T (T_{Reg}) Cells

1. Please perform the experiment as described in Subheading 3.1.3.

3.3 Isolation of Total RNA from Lung Draining Lymph Node Cells and Lung Cells

The following section describes the isolation of total RNA from $\leq 1 \times 10^4$ cells using Qiagens RNeasy Micro Kit (*see* **Note 8**).

1. After sorting, immediately centrifuge ($500 \times g$, 5 min) the cells, carefully remove complete supernatant by aspiration and lyse the cell-pellet in 75 μl RLT buffer supplemented with β-mercaptoethanol (10 μl β-ME per 1 ml RLT buffer) (*see* **Note 9**).
2. Carefully pipette up and down until pellet is completely lysed.
3. Add 1 volume (75 μl) of 70% ethanol to the lysate and mix well by pipetting up and down.
4. Place an RNeasy MinElute column in a 2 ml collection tube (supplied with the kit) and transfer sample to the column. Centrifuge for 15 s at $\geq 8000 \times g$.
5. Discard flow-through and add 350 μl buffer RW1 to the column. Centrifuge for 15 s at $\geq 8000 \times g$ to wash the spin column membrane.
6. Discard the flow-through. Prepare DNase I incubation mix by adding 10 μl DNase stock solution to 70 μl RDD buffer per sample. Carefully mix by inverting the tube, do not vortex.
7. Add 80 μl of the prepared DNase I incubation mix to the column membrane and incubate for 15 min at room temperature (20–25 °C).
8. Add 350 μl RW1 buffer to the spin column. Centrifuge for 15 s at $\geq 8000 \times g$ to wash the spin column.
9. Discard collection tube with flow-through.
10. Place column in a new 2 ml collection tube and add 500 μl RPE buffer to the spin column (*see* **Note 10**). Centrifuge for 15 s at $\geq 8000 \times g$ to wash the spin column membrane.
11. Discard the flow-through. Add 500 μl of 80% ethanol to the spin column. Centrifuge for 2 min at $\geq 8000 \times g$ the spin column membrane.
12. Discard collection tube with flow-through and place spin-column in a new 2 ml collection tube. Centrifuge at maximum speed for 5 min.
13. Discard collection tube with flow-through and place spin column in a new 1.5 ml tube. Add 14 μl RNase-free water to the center of the spin column membrane. Centrifuge for 1 min at maximum speed to elute the RNA.

3.4 Assessment of Concentration and Quality of Isolated Total RNA

3.4.1 Concentration

The Qubit HS RNA assay kit (Invitrogen) allows an accurate quantitation of RNA and the RNA assay is highly selective over dsDNA, allowing determining the purity of the sample together with the DNA HS assay kit. It is an easy and very fast method and tolerates common contaminants like salts and detergents. Initial RNA concentrations ranging from 250 pg/μl to 100 ng/μl can be determined.

Calibrating the instrument:

Users have to calibrate the instrument first. For calibration, mix 190 μl of RNA HS buffer with 10 μl Standard#1in one Qubit assay tube and 190 μl RNA HS buffer with 10 μl Standard#2 in another Qubit assay tube. Vortex for 5 s and shortly spin down the tubes in a microcentrifuge. Incubate the tubes for 2 min at room temperature (RT). On the Home Screen of the Qubit 2.0 fluorometer press "RNA" and then choose "RNA high sensitivity". Press "Read Standards" to proceed. Insert the tube for Standard#1, press "read standard#1", remove tube and insert tube with Standard#2. Press "read standard#2"to finalize calibration.

Per sample:

1. Prepare Qubit Working solution in a 1.5 ml polypropylene tube by diluting 1 μl of Qubit RNA HS Reagent in 199 μl RNA HS buffer (1:200).
2. Transfer 198 μl of prepared Working solution into a Qubit assay tube and add 2 μl of the eluted RNA.
3. Vortex for 5 s and shortly spin down the assay tube.
4. Incubate tube for 2 min at RT.
5. On the Home Screen of the Qubit 2.0 fluorometer press "RNA" and then "RNA high sensitivity". Select "No" when asked to "Read new standards".
6. Insert RNA containing assay tube. Press "Read next sample". Press "Calculate stock conc." and choose "2 μl" for volume of sample and choose "ng/μl" as unit.

3.4.2 Quality

Check the quality of isolated RNA on the Bioanalyzer 2100 using a RNA 6000 Pico Kit. The Bioanalyzer 2100 is an electrophoresis device which separates nucleic acid fragments on a chip based on their size. It estimates the integrity of total RNA (RNA integrity number (RIN)) by combining the ratio of the 18S and 28S ribosomal RNA and the entire electrophoretic trace of the RNA sample [19]. A RIN value of ≥8 is strongly recommended for proceeding with generation of full-length cDNA.

Wear latex or vinyl gloves throughout the whole workflow. Adjust the syringe clip to the highest position (for lowest possible pressure).

Preparation of RNA ladder

1. Spin down and heat denature the ladder for 2 min at 70 °C.
2. Immediately cool down the ladder on ice.
3. Add 90 μl of RNase-free water and mix gently.
4. Prepare and store aliquots in RNase-free tubes at −80 °C.
5. Thaw ladder aliquots on ice before use.

Preparing the gel

1. Pipette 550 μl of RNA gel matrix into a spin filter.
2. Centrifuge at 1500 × *g* for 10 min at RT.
3. Aliquot 65 μl filtered gel into RNase-free tubes and store them at 4 °C.

Determining the RIN value

1. Allow RNA dye concentrate to equilibrate to room temperature, vortex it for 10 s, spin down and add 1 μl of dye to 65 μl of the filtered gel aliquot. Vortex, spin down at >8000 × *g* for 2 min and use prepared gel dye mix within 1 day.
2. Pipette 9 μl of gel-dye mix in the appropriate well (white G on black ground) of the RNA pico chip.
3. Close the priming station and press plunger (positioned at 1 ml position) until held by clip.
4. Release clip after 30 s, wait 5 s and open the chip priming station.
5. Pipette 9 μl of gel and 9 μl of RNA conditioning solution in the appropriate (gel: Black G on grey ground; RNA conditioning solution in well CS) wells.
6. Pipette 5 μl of marker into all 11 sample wells and in the ladder well.
7. Pipette 1 μl of heat denatured ladder into the ladder well.
8. Pipette 1 μl of RNA sample in each of the 11 sample wells.
9. Put the chip on the Chip-vortexer (provided with the Bioanalyzer) and vortex for 1 min at 2400 rpm.
10. Run the pico chip on the Bioanalyzer 2100 (*see* Figs. 1 and 2 for examples of high and bad quality total RNA isolated by RNeasy Micro Kit).

3.5 Generation of Full-Length cDNA Using Smart-seq2

Smart-seq2 [16, 17] allows the generation of full-length cDNA and sequencing libraries using standard reagents. It provides a very cheap solution compared to commercially available kits for generation of full-length cDNA starting with ultra low amounts of RNA (even with RNA from a single cell). Although Smart-seq2

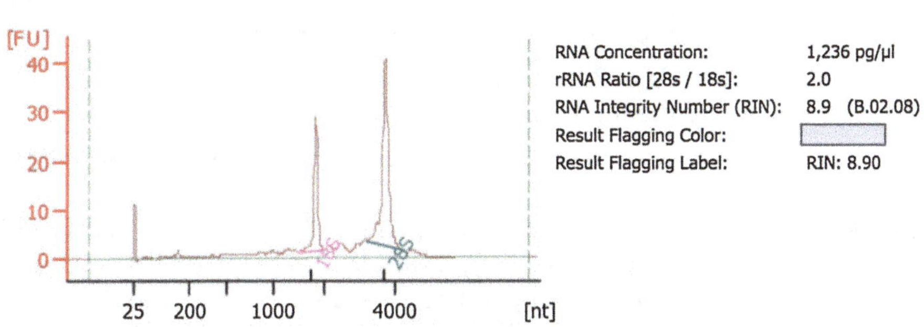

Fig. 1 Example of good quality total RNA eluted by RNeasy Micro-Kit (RIN = 8.9)

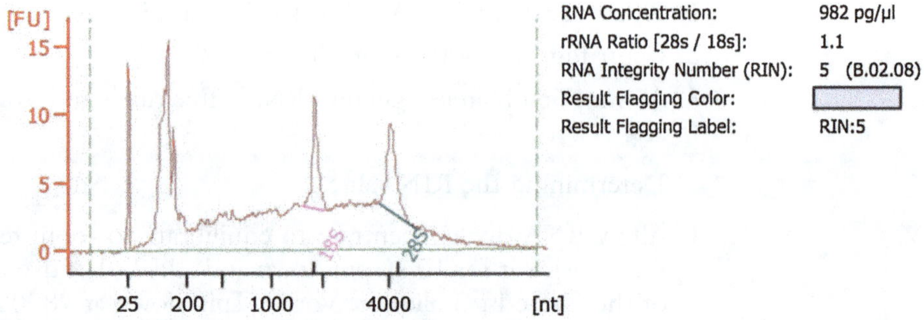

Fig. 2 Example of bad quality total RNA eluted by RNeasy Micro-Kit (RIN = 5)

allows generation of full-length cDNA from single- or oligo-cell samples by directly lysing the cell(s) in 0.5 µl of 0.2 % Triton X-100, it is also possible to pipet an appropriate amount of RNA isolated by RNeasy Micro kit to the reverse transcription reaction. Wear latex or vinyl gloves throughout the whole workflow and destroy RNases on the workbench and on pipettes using RNase away.

3.5.1 Reverse Transcription (1 Sample)

1. Pipette 1 µl Oligo dT [10 µM], 1 µl dNTP mix [10 mM each], and 2 µl of Triton X-100 [0.2 %] into an RNase-free 0.2 ml polypropylene tube.
2. Quickly vortex the tube, spin down the solution and place it on ice immediately.
3. Add 0.5 µl of total RNA sample, pipette solution three times up and down and incubate at 72 °C in a thermocycler for 3 min. Spin down and immediately place tube back on ice.
4. Prepare RT-mix: Pipette 0.5 µl Superscript II Reverse transcriptase [200 U/ml], 0.25 µl RNase inhibitor [40 U/ml], 2 µl Superscript II buffer, 0.25 µl DTT [100 mM], 2 µl Betaine [5 M], 0.9 µl $MgCl_2$ [100 mM], 1 µl TSO [10 µM], and 0.1 µl RNase-free water into an RNase-free 0.2 ml polypropylene tube. Pipette up and down five times to mix.
5. Add 3 µl of the sample incubated at 72 °C (**step 3**) to 7 µl prepared RT mix (**step 4**) and pipette up and down to mix thoroughly. Place sample in thermocycler.
6. Run Reverse transcription on thermal cycler. *See* Table 1 for cycling conditions.
7. Immediately place reversely transcribed sample (RTS) on ice.

3.5.2 Amplification

1. Prepare amplification mix: Pipette 25 µl KAPA HiFi HotStart ReadyMix (2×), 1 µl IS-PCR Primer [10 µM], and 14 µl nuclease-free water into an RNase-free 0.2 ml polypropylene tube. Mix thoroughly by pipetting up and down several times.

Table 1
Cycling conditions for reverse transcription

Cycle	Temperature (°C)	Duration (min:s)
1	42	90:00
2–11	50 42	02:00 02:00
12	70	15:00
13	4	Hold

Table 2
Cycling conditions for amplification of cDNA

Cycle	Temperature (°C)	Duration (min:s)
1	98	03:00
2–13	98 67 72	00:20 00:15 06:00
14	72	5:00
15	4	Hold

2. Transfer amplification mix (40 μl) to 10 μl RTS from **step 7** (Subheading 3.5.1). Pipette up and down five times to mix. Place tube in the thermocycler.
3. Run amplification on thermal cycler. *See* Table 2 for cycling conditions (*see* **Note 11**).

3.5.3 Purification

1. Equilibrate Ampure XP beads at room temperature for 30 min. Before use, vortex Ampure XP beads well for several seconds.
2. Pipette 50 μl of Ampure XP beads (ratio 1:1) to the amplified cDNA (from Subheading 3.4.2) and mix thoroughly by pipetting up and down several times until solution is homogeneous. Transfer solution into a well of a 96-well plate and incubate plate for 8 min at RT.
3. Place plate on magnetic stand. Wait for 5 min until the solution is clear and beads are located at the side adjacent to the magnet.
4. Carefully remove the liquid while plate is still on the magnet (*see* **Note 12**).
5. Leave plate on magnet and wash the beads with 200 μl 80% freshly prepared ethanol. Incubate for 30 s.

6. Repeat **steps 4** and **5** for a total of two washes.
7. Carefully remove the liquid while plate is still on the magnet and let beads dry completely leaving the plate at RT for a minimum of 5 min until a crack can be seen on the surface of the beads (*see* **Note 12**).
8. Take plate off the magnet and add 17.5 μl EB solution and carefully mix until beads are completely resuspended.
9. Incubate at RT for 2 min.
10. Place on magnetic rack for 5 min until solution becomes clear and beads have accumulated at side of magnet.
11. Transfer 15 μl of the supernatant to a new nuclease-free 1.5 ml tube (*see* **Note 13**).

3.5.4 Determining the Concentration and Quality of Full-Length cDNA

Concentration:

The Qubit HS DNA assay kit (Invitrogen) allows an accurate quantitation of dsDNA and the DNA assay is highly selective over RNA. Initial cDNA concentrations ranging from 10 pg/μl to 100 ng/μl can be determined.

Calibrating the instrument:

Users have to calibrate the instrument first. For calibration, mix 190 μl of DNA HS buffer with 10 μl Standard#1 in one Qubit assay tube and 190 μl DNA HS buffer with 10 μl Standard#2 in another Qubit assay tube. Vortex for 5 s and shortly spin down the tubes in a microcentrifuge. Incubate the tubes for 2 min at room temperature (RT). On the Home Screen of the Qubit 2.0 fluorometer press "DNA" and then "DNA high sensitivity". Press "Read Standard" to proceed. Insert the tube for Standard#1, press "read standard#1". Remove standard#1 tube and insert tube with standard#2. Press "read standard#2". The device is now calibrated.

Per sample:

1. Prepare Qubit Working solution in a 1.5 ml polypropylene tube by diluting 1 μl of Qubit DNA HS Reagent in 199 μl DNA HS buffer (1:200).
2. Transfer 198 μl of prepared Working solution into a Qubit assay tube and add 2 μl of the eluted DNA.
3. Vortex for 5 s and shortly spin down the assay tube.
4. Incubate tube for 2 min at RT.
5. On the Home Screen of the Qubit 2.0 fluorometer press "DNA" and then "DNA high sensitivity". Select "No" when asked "Read new standards".
6. Insert DNA containing assay tube. Press "Read next sample". Press "Calculate stock conc." and choose "2 μl" for volume of sample used and choose "ng/μl" as unit.

Quality:

Check the quality of eluted DNA on the Bioanalyzer 2100 using a DNA high sensitivity chip. Wear latex or vinyl gloves throughout the whole workflow. Adjust the syringe clip to the lowest position (for maximum pressure).

Preparing the gel-dye mix

Equilibrate HS DNA dye concentrate and HS DNA gel to room temperature.

1. Pipette 15 μl of HS DNA dye concentrate to HS DNA gel matrix vial.
2. Vortex, spin down and transfer to spin filter.
3. Centrifuge at 2400 × *g* for 10 min and store HS gel-dye mix light-protected at 4 °C (*see* **Note 14**).

Determining quality of eluted DNA

1. Allow prepared gel-dye mix to equilibrate to room temperature.
2. Pipette 9 μl of gel-dye mix in the appropriate well (white G on black ground) of the DNA HS chip placed on the chip priming station.
3. Close the priming station and press plunger (positioned at 1 ml position) until held by clip.
4. Release clip after 60 s, wait 5 s and open the chip priming station.
5. Pipette 9 μl of gel in the remaining gel wells (black G on grey ground).
6. Pipette 5 μl of marker into all sample wells and in the ladder well.
7. Pipette 1 μl of HS DNA ladder into the ladder well.
8. Pipette 1 μl of DNA sample in each of the 11 sample wells.
9. Put the chip on the Chip-vortexer (provided with the Bioanalyzer) and vortex for 1 min at maximum speed (2400 rpm).
10. Run the chip on the Bioanalyzer 2100 (*see* **Note 15**). For an example of an electropherogram of pre-amplified cDNA library (*see* Fig. 3).

3.6 Preparation of Sequencing Library Employing Nextera XT DNA Sample Preparation Kit

3.6.1 Tagmentation of Input DNA

"Tagmentation" is performed by using the Nextera XT sample preparation kit (Illumina). It combines transposon-based fragmentation of input DNA with adding tags, unique adapter sequences, to the DNA. Those tags are used for a PCR-based amplification of the input DNA, which additionally adds indices at both ends of the DNA thereby allowing indexed sequencing of pooled libraries.

Per sample:

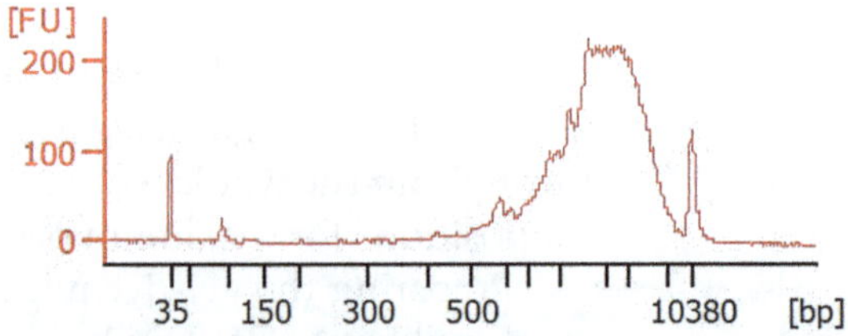

Fig. 3 Electropherogram (bioanalyzer) of pre-amplified cDNA library (14 cycles)

Table 3
Cycling conditions for amplification of library

Cycle	Temperature (°C)	Duration (min:s)
1	72	03:00
2	95	00:30
3–14	95 55 72	00:10 00:30 00:30
15	72	5:00
16	4	Hold

1. Thaw ATM, TD and input DNA on ice and mix gently by inverting the tubes.
2. Based on the concentration measured by Qubit 2.0 in Subheading 3.5.4 dilute eluted DNA (from **step 11**, Subheading 3.5.3) to 0.2 ng/μl with nuclease-free water.
3. Pipette 10 μl TD buffer into a well of a nuclease free 96-well plate.
4. Add 5 μl of diluted DNA (from **step 2**; 1 ng in total).
5. Pipette 5 μl of ATM to the DNA and TD buffer containing well.
6. Gently mix by pipetting up and down several times. Close cap with cap strip.
7. Place plate in the thermal cycler and run at 55 °C for 5 min, hold at 10 °C.
8. Remove cap strip, add 5 μl of NT buffer and mix several times by pipetting up and down, and incubate for 5 min at RT.

3.6.2 PCR Amplification

1. Thaw NPM and index primers 1 and 2 (N7XX and S5XX).
2. Prepare enrichment PCR in 0.2 ml tube of 96-well plate by adding 15 μl NPM, 5 μl Index primers 1 (N7XX), and 5 μl Index primers 2 (N5XX) to 25 μl DNA from Subheading 3.6.1 (**step 8**) (*see* **Note 16**).
3. Perform following program on the thermal cycler: *See* Table 3 (*see* **Note 17**).

3.6.3 PCR Purification

1. Equilibrate Ampure XP beads at room temperature for 30 min. Before use, vortex Ampure XP beads well for several seconds.
2. Add 90 μl of Ampure XP beads to 50 μl PCR reaction (from Subheading 3.6.2, **step 3**) and mix by pipettting up and down ten times.
3. Incubate at RT for 5 min.
4. Place plate on magnetic stand for 3 min until supernatant becomes clear and beads are located at the side of the magnet.
5. Remove and discard supernatant while plate is still on magnet.
6. Leave plate on magnet and wash the beads with 200 μl of freshly prepared 80% ethanol. Incubate for 30 s.
7. Repeat **steps 5** and **6** for a total of two washes.
8. Carefully remove the liquid while plate is still on the magnet and let beads dry completely leaving the plate at RT for a minimum of 5 min until a crack can be seen on the surface of the beads (*see* **Note 12**).
9. Take plate off the magnet and add 35 μl EB solution and carefully mix until beads are completely resuspended.
10. Incubate at RT for 2 min.
11. Place on magnetic rack for 5 min until solution becomes clear and beads have accumulated at side of magnet.
12. Transfer 30 μl of the supernatant to a new nuclease-free 1.5 ml tube (*see* **Notes 13** and **18**).

3.6.4 Checking the Quality and Concentration of the Final cDNA Libraries

See Subheading 3.5.4 for measuring the concentration of each library by Qubit 2.0 DNA HS assay kit and determining the average size distribution on the bioanalyzer 2100 using a high-sensitivity DNA chip. If concentration of final library determined by Qubit exceeds 10 ng/μl dilute final library to a maximum concentration of 10 ng/μl before loading 1 μl of sample on the bioanalyzer high-sensitivity chip. A bioanalyzer-electropherogram of a final sequencing library after tagmentation is depicted in Fig. 4.

3.6.5 Pooling of Final cDNA Libraries and Denaturation

Calculate molarity of the final libraries by using the determined concentration (Qubit) and obtained average library size (bioanalyzer) as follows:

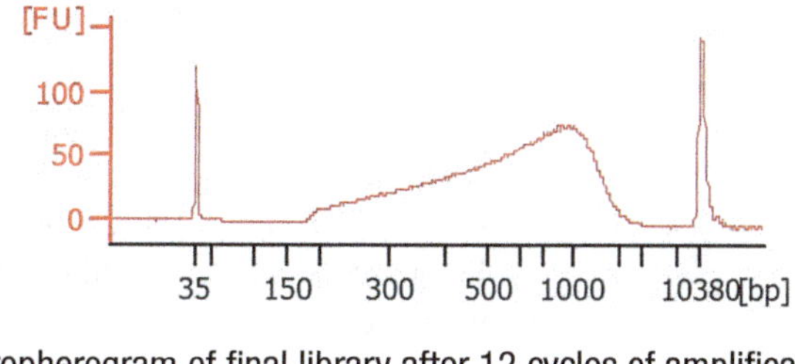

Fig. 4 Electropherogram of final library after 12 cycles of amplification (average size distribution: 700 bp)

(concentration × 1000/1 × (1/649) × (1/average size)) × 1000 = Molarity [nM]

1. Thaw HT1 buffer included in the MiSeq reagent v3 kit.
2. Dilute each library to 4 nM using EB solution and pool 10 μl of each sample in a nuclease-free 1.5 ml tube.
3. Mix by pipetting up and down several times.
4. Transfer 5 μl of pooled libraries to a new, nuclease-free 1.5 ml tube.
5. Add 5 μl of 0.2 N NaOH for denaturing the DNA library and mix gently by pipetting up and down several times. Incubate for 5 min at RT (*see* **Note 19**).
6. Add 990 μl of thawed HT1 buffer (*see* **Note 20**).
7. Dilute 480 μl of 20 pM library-pool with 120 μl HT1 buffer (*see* **Note 21**).

3.6.6 DNA Sequencing (Illumina MiSeq) and Analysis

1. Place MiSeq reagent cartridge in a water bath until all liquid in the wells is completely thawed. Invert the cartridge several times to mix reagents. Load "sample" well of cartridge with 600 μl of 16 pM library pool, put the cartridge in the appropriate place in the MiSeq and start the sequencing run (*see* **Note 22**).
2. Export raw sequencing data (fastq-files) to CLC Genomics Workbench analysis software and align reads to the appropriate reference genome choosing the RNA-Seq analysis from the transcriptomics analysis workflow. Upon mapping of the reads to the reference genome (*see* **Note 23**) choose "Set up experiment" and determine samples to being compared in gene expression levels for each gene.

4 Notes

1. Do not use cervical dislocation or CO_2 as sacrifice method. This will result in bleeding, contaminate your sample and make the tissue preparation more complicated.
2. During the whole preparation procedure avoid injuring any blood vessels. The blood will contaminate your samples and will exacerbate further tissue preparation.
3. T_{Reg} cells are usually defined by the expression of the transcription factor Foxp3. To further increase the purity of T_{Reg} cells consider isolating the cells from appropriate Foxp3 reporter mouse strains which are genetically modified to coexpress fluorescent proteins (like Green Fluorescent Protein) together with Foxp3 [20].

4. Ensure purity of $CD4^+CD25^+Foxp3^+$ T_{Reg} cells of a small fraction of sorted cells by intracellular staining for Foxp3. Do not use cells with a purity of <98 % of $CD4^+CD25^+Foxp3^+$ cells.
5. Perfusion of the lung is necessary to remove blood cells that could contaminate your cell sample. During perfusion the color of the lung should turn to a bright white.
6. Thoroughly mincing the lung is necessary to increase the yield of cells that you obtain from the collagenase digestion step.
7. A water bath including a shaker is most suitable for digestion because of the better thermal replacement.
8. Since ribonucleases (RNases) are very stable enzymes and even minimal amounts are sufficent to destroy RNA it is absolutely essential to clean up the workbench with RNase away and to wear vinyl or latex gloves to prevent contamination of samples with RNase.
9. Work under a fume hood when handling β-ME.
10. Before using RPE buffer for the first time make sure that 96–100 % ethanol has been added as indicated on the bottle.
11. PCR product can be stored at −20 °C for 6 months or longer.
12. Remove liquid very slowly being careful not to aspirate any beads.
13. It is important to remove the supernatant very slowly being careful not to aspirate any beads. If some beads are accidentally removed, pipette sample back into the tube and wait until beads are separated again.
14. Use prepared gel–dye mix within 6 weeks.
15. Run the chip within 5 min.
16. Some experiments require the sequencing of low plexity samples, i.e., comparing only two libraries. Since Illumina's MiSeq uses two different lasers, one to "sequence" G/T and another one to "sequence" C/A, it is highly important to select indices carefully (different bases at each cycle of the index read) to allow proper base calling and demultiplexing. Illumina recommends for a pool of two samples N701 (TAAGGCGA for first sample) and N702 (CGTACTAG for second sample) as index primers#1 together with any index primers#2.
17. If you do not want to immediately proceed with PCR purification, PCR product can be stored at 4 °C over night.
18. Sample can be stored at −20 °C for several months.
19. Adding 5 μl of 0.2 N NaOH to 5 μl of pooled 4 nM libraries results in 2 nM pooled libraries with 100 mM NaOH.
20. Dilution with 990 μl HT1 buffer results in 20 pM pooled libraries with 1 mM NaOH.

21. This dilution results in a final pooled-library concentration of 16 pM with 0.8 mM NaOH. It is of importance that the concentration of NaOH in the final library after dilution with HT1 buffer does not exceed 1 mM (0.001 N) since higher concentrations of NaOH lead to the inhibition of library hybridization and to the decrease of cluster density.
22. Concerning mRNA-Seq we normally perform a 50 bp single-end sequencing run on a MiSeq. It takes less than 8 h and results in 20–30 million reads passing the filter. Demultiplexing is automatically done by the MiSeq (when defined by the user before starting the run).
23. Depending on the number of reads passing the filter and the hardware of the computer on which the analysis software is installed, alignment of reads to the reference genome takes 3–5 h using CLC Genomics workbench (version 7).

References

1. Mosmann TR, Cherwinski H, Bond MW, Giedlin MA, Coffman RL (1986) Two types of murine helper T cell clone. I. Definition according to profiles of lymphokine activities and secreted proteins. J Immunol 136:2348–2357
2. Abbas AK, Murphy KM, Sher A (1996) Functional diversity of helper T lymphocytes. Nature 383:787–793
3. Dong C, Flavell RA (2000) Control of T helper cell differentiation—in search of master genes. Sci STKE 2000:pe1
4. Stockinger B, Veldhoen M, Martin B (2007) Th17 T cells: linking innate and adaptive immunity. Semin Immunol 19:353–361
5. Miossec P, Korn T, Kuchroo VK (2009) Interleukin-17 and type 17 helper T cells. N Engl J Med 361:888–898
6. Eyerich K, Pennino D, Scarponi C, Foerster S, Nasorri F, Behrendt H, Ring J, Traidl-Hoffmann C, Albanesi C, Cavani A (2009) IL-17 in atopic eczema: linking allergen-specific adaptive and microbial-triggered innate immune response. J Allergy Clin Immunol 123:59–66.e4
7. Veldhoen M, Uyttenhove C, Van Snick J, Helmby H, Westendorf A, Buer J, Martin B, Wilhelm C, Stockinger B (2008) Transforming growth factor-beta "reprograms" the differentiation of T helper 2 cells and promotes an interleukin 9-producing subset. Nat Immunol 9:1341–1346
8. Dardalhon V, Awasthi A, Kwon H, Galileos G, Gao W, Sobel RA, Mitsdoerffer M, Strom TB, Elyaman W, Ho I-C, Khoury S, Oukka M, Kuchroo VK (2008) IL-4 inhibits TGF-beta-induced Foxp3+ T cells, and together with TGF-beta, generates IL-9+ IL-10+ Foxp3(−) effector T cells. Nat Immunol 9:1347–1355
9. Shevach EM (2002) CD4+ CD25+ suppressor T cells: more questions than answers. Nat Rev Immunol 2:389–400
10. Sakaguchi S, Yamaguchi T, Nomura T, Ono M (2008) Regulatory T cells and immune tolerance. Cell 133:775–787
11. Josefowicz SZ, Rudensky A (2009) Control of regulatory T cell lineage commitment and maintenance. Immunity 30:616–625
12. Burzyn D, Kuswanto W, Kolodin D, Shadrach JL, Cerletti M, Jang Y, Sefik E, Tan TG, Wagers AJ, Benoist C, Mathis D (2013) A special population of regulatory T cells potentiates muscle repair. Cell 155:1282–1295
13. Ulges A, Klein M, Reuter S, Gerlitzki B, Hoffmann M, Grebe N, Staudt V, Stergiou N, Bohn T, Brühl T-J, Muth S, Yurugi H, Rajalingam K, Bellinghausen I, Tuettenberg A, Hahn S, Reißig S, Haben I, Zipp F, Waisman A, Probst H-C, Beilhack A, Buchou T, Filhol-Cochet O, Boldyreff B, Breloer M, Jonuleit H, Schild H, Schmitt E, Bopp T (2015) Protein kinase CK2 enables regulatory T cells to suppress excessive TH2 responses in vivo. Nat Immunol 16:267–275
14. Gray DHD, Liston A (2014) Uhrf to Treg cells: reinforcing the mucosal peacekeepers. Nat Immunol 15:533–534

15. Thome JJC, Farber DL (2015) Emerging concepts in tissue-resident T cells: lessons from humans. Trends Immunol 36:428–435
16. Picelli S, Faridani OR, Björklund ÅK, Winberg G, Sagasser S, Sandberg R (2014) Full-length RNA-seq from single cells using Smart-seq2. Nat Protoc 9:171–181
17. Picelli S, Björklund ÅK, Faridani OR, Sagasser S, Winberg G, Sandberg R (2013) Smart-seq2 for sensitive full-length transcriptome profiling in single cells. Nat Methods 10:1096–1098
18. Bopp T, Dehzad N, Reuter S, Klein M, Ullrich N, Stassen M, Schild H, Buhl R, Schmitt E, Taube C (2009) Inhibition of cAMP degradation improves regulatory T cell-mediated suppression. J Immunol 182:4017–4024
19. Schroeder A, Mueller O, Stocker S, Salowsky R, Leiber M, Gassmann M, Lightfoot S, Menzel W, Granzow M, Ragg T (2006) The RIN: an RNA integrity number for assigning integrity values to RNA measurements. BMC Mol Biol 7:3
20. Lahl K, Loddenkemper C, Drouin C, Freyer J, Arnason J, Eberl G, Hamann A, Wagner H, Huehn J, Sparwasser T (2007) Selective depletion of Foxp3+ regulatory T cells induces a scurfy-like disease. J Exp Med 204:57–63

Part III

Inflammatory Diseases of the Intestinal and Oral Mucosa

Chapter 15

Isolation and Identification of Intestinal Myeloid Cells

Charlotte L. Scott, Calum C. Bain, and Allan McI Mowat

Abstract

The identification of conventional dendritic cells (cDCs) and macrophages (mϕ) in the intestinal mucosa has been hampered by the difficulties associated with isolating cells from the intestine and by the fact that overlapping markers have made it complicated to discriminate them accurately from each other and from other intestinal myeloid cells. Here we detail the protocols we have developed to isolate live leukocytes from steady state mouse small and large intestines and describe reliable strategies which can be used to identify bona fide cDCs, monocytes and macrophages in such preparations.

Key words Dendritic cells, Identification, Intestine, Isolation, Macrophages, Subsets

1 Introduction

1.1 Dendritic Cells, Macrophages, and the Intestinal Immune Response

Given the large surface area of the gut and its continual exposure to a wide variety of agents including dietary constituents, commensal bacteria, and pathogens, the intestine has evolved to be the largest compartment of the immune system [1]. The intestinal immune system must be able to discriminate between harmless and harmful antigens. Whereas tolerance must be induced to harmless materials such as commensal, self or dietary antigens, active immunity must be generated for the eradication of pathogens. When this decision making process breaks down, aberrant responses to innocuous antigens may lead to a number of pathologies including food allergies, celiac disease, and inflammatory bowel diseases such as Crohn's disease and ulcerative colitis [2].

Conventional dendritic cells (cDCs) and macrophages (mϕ) are crucial to these immunological processes, playing distinct, but complementary roles. As the primary sentinels of the immune system, cDCs in the intestine continually sample antigens in their environment and migrate constitutively to the draining mesenteric lymph nodes (MLNs). Here they present the antigen to naïve T cells and initiate tolerance or active immunity as appropriate by specifying the differentiation of effector or regulatory T cells. cDCs

Björn E. Clausen and Jon D. Laman (eds.), *Inflammation: Methods and Protocols*, Methods in Molecular Biology, vol. 1559,
DOI 10.1007/978-1-4939-6786-5_15, © Springer Science+Business Media LLC 2017

are also responsible for inducing the expression of gut homing markers on responding T cells, ensuring they migrate back to the intestinal mucosa once they have differentiated [3–6]. In contrast, although mϕ may sample antigen locally, they do not migrate to the draining lymph nodes or prime naïve T cells. Instead they are sessile phagocytes that scavenge bacteria and damaged cells, and maintain an anti-inflammatory environment in the mucosa via constitutive production of IL10 [7]. If intestinal mϕ do interact with T cells, this is likely to be a local interaction in the gut wall and involve T cells that have migrated there after initial activation by cDCs in the draining LNs [8]. However, mϕ may also contribute to the initial priming of T cells through the transfer of antigen to neighboring cDCs for subsequent presentation to T cells [9, 10].

1.2 Anatomical Aspects of the Intestinal Immune System

The gastrointestinal tract consists of the stomach, small intestine (SI), caecum, large intestine (colon), and rectum, and it is associated with a number of organized lymphoid tissues including the Peyer's patches (PPs), microscopic isolated lymphoid follicles (ILFs) and the draining mesenteric lymph nodes (MLNs). PP and ILFs are important for the generation of immune responses against bacteria and viruses, while the MLNs are essential for all aspects of tolerance and immunity in the gut [11]. cDCs are found in all these organized lymphoid tissues, from which they can usually be isolated and characterized using the same methods that are used for other secondary lymphoid organs. Conversely, mϕ are rare in the organized lymphoid tissues associated with the intestine under steady state conditions and for these reasons, we concentrate on the large populations of myeloid cells found in the wall of the intestine itself (the mucosa). Most of these are found in the lamina propria (LP), the layer of connective tissue immediately below the epithelium.

1.3 Mononuclear Phagocyte Heterogeneity in the Intestine

Together, cDCs and mϕ are referred to as mononuclear phagocytes and those in the intestinal mucosa have many unusual properties. Despite being first identified many years ago [12], their isolation and subsequent characterization presents several challenges to the researcher. As well as being difficult to obtain in substantial numbers, it is now clear that intestinal cDCs and mϕ share many phenotypic markers such as CD11b, CD11c, and MHCII, meaning these cannot be used to discriminate between them as has been done in the past (reviewed in [7]). Furthermore, the advent of multiparameter flow cytometric techniques has revealed considerable heterogeneity among both populations.

As we discuss below, a number of subsets of cDCs are present in the LP of both small and large intestine and can be separated on the basis of their expression of CD103 and CD11b. All share the abilities to acquire antigen in LP and migrate to the draining MLNs, where they encounter and present antigen to naïve T cells. As a result, the "migratory" subset of cDCs in MLNs contains analogous populations to those seen in LP and similar phenotypic groups can also be found in PPs ([13–17] and our own unpublished observations). Plasmacytoid DCs (pDCs) are also found in the LP of the small intestine of both mice and humans, but they do not migrate to the draining lymph nodes and are absent from the normal colon [11].

Intestinal mϕ are also more heterogeneous than once thought. While at birth these derive from embryonic progenitors, recent studies have shown that these do not maintain themselves through self-renewal and are instead replaced by monocyte-derived mϕ within the first few weeks of life [18]. Mature resident mϕ in the adult intestine are then continuously replenished by circulating $Ly6C^{hi}$ monocytes that differentiate locally after arrival in the mucosa. As a result, small numbers of monocytes and intermediary stages in the development continuum are present even in the steady state intestine [18–20]. Different stages within this so-called "monocyte waterfall" can be identified based on their expression levels of Ly6C, MHCII, F4/80 and CX3CR1, with newly arrived monocytes being $Ly6C^{hi}$ $MHCII^{-}$, $CX3CR1^{int}$ before acquiring MHCII, then losing Ly6C and finally becoming $CX3CR1^{hi}$ $MHCII^{hi}$ $F4/80^{hi}$. This generates mature mϕ with characteristic anti-inflammatory and homeostatic properties including IL10 production, hyporesponsiveness to stimulation, expression of scavenger receptors, avid phagocytic activity, and production of tissue remodeling enzymes ([19–22] and our own unpublished data). Together, these adaptations allow intestinal mϕ to remodel the mucosa and clear away effete tissue cells and bacteria without causing inflammation. This is prevented by IL10R signaling on mϕ, with the main source of IL10 being local T cells, although there is also the clear potential for autocrine effects from the constitutive production of IL10 by the mϕ themselves [21]. Mϕ IL10 is also important for maintaining the survival of regulatory T cells in the mucosa [8]. During active immunity or inflammation, the normal differentiation process is disrupted, leading to the accumulation of $Ly6C^{hi}$ monocytes and production of pro-inflammatory cytokines [23]. Thus, phenotypic characterization of the monocyte–macrophage waterfall is a powerful tool in defining the role of this lineage in the intestine under both physiological and pathological conditions.

Here we describe how to isolate and characterize cDCs and mϕ from the small and large intestinal mucosa of steady state mice using precise phenotypic gating strategies.

2 Materials

2.1 Reagent Preparation (See Note 1)

1. Calcium and magnesium free (CMF) Hank's buffered salt solution (HBSS) containing 2% fetal calf serum (FCS): stored at 4 °C.

2. CMF HBSS containing 2 mM ethylenediamine tetra-acetic acid (EDTA) solution: pre-warmed and stored at 37 °C.
3. CMF HBSS; pre-warmed and stored at 37 °C.
4. Complete RPMI (cRPMI): RPMI supplemented with 10% FCS, 2 mM L-glutamine, 100 U/ml penicillin, 100 μg/ml streptomycin, and 50 μM 2-mercaptoethanol, pre-warmed and maintained at 37 °C.
5. FACS buffer: phosphate buffered saline (PBS) containing 2% FCS and 1 mM EDTA; stored at 4 °C.
6. Enzymatic cocktails specific for tissue to be digested (Table 1) in complete RPMI should be made up fresh immediately prior to use.
7. Antibodies for flow cytometry (Tables 2 and 3).

3 Methods

3.1 Isolation of Leukocytes from Small Intestinal Lamina Propria

1. Kill mouse according to appropriate ethical guidelines and immediately remove SI from pyloric outlet of stomach to end of ileum and place in a 9 ml petri dish filled with CMF HBSS containing 2% FCS (*see* **Note 2**).
2. Place SI on tissue, soak with PBS and remove fat with tweezers.
3. Carefully remove all Peyer's patches from SI with scissors (*see* **Note 3**).
4. Open SI longitudinally using scissors.
5. Wash thoroughly in CMF HBSS 2% FCS in a 9 ml petri dish.
6. Cut SI into 0.5 cm segments.
7. Transfer SI segments to 50 ml Falcon tube containing 10 ml CMF HBSS 2% FCS and keep on ice (*see* **Note 4**).
8. Manually shake tubes vigorously and then discard supernatant (*see* **Note 5** and Fig. 1).

Table 1
Enzyme cocktails for intestinal digestions

Tissue	Vol. (ml)	Enzymes	Supplier	Cat. No	Conc.
Small intestine	10	Collagenase VIII DNase	Sigma Roche	C2139 101104159001	0.6 mg/ml 30 μg/ml
Colon	10	Collagenase V Collagenase D Dispase DNase	Sigma Roche Invitrogen Roche	C9623 11088882001 17105-041 101104159001	0.425 mg/ml 0.625 mg/ml 1 mg/ml 30 μg/ml

Table 2
Typical staining panel used for flow cytometric analysis of intestinal conventional dendritic cells

Antibody	Clone	Supplier	Cat. No	Isotype	Fluorochrome
Fc Block (anti-CD16/CD32)	2.4G2	Biolegend	101320	N/A	N/A
CD45	30-F11	Biolegend	103128	Rat IgG2b	AF700
CD11c	N418	Biolegend	117318	Ham IgG1	PE-Cy7
CD11b	M1/70	eBioscience	47-0112-82	Rat IgG2b	APC-eFluor780
CD103	M290	BD	557493	Rat IgG2a	Biotin
MHCII	M5/114.15.2	eBioscience	48-5321-82	Rat IgG2b	eFluor450
CD64	X54-5/7.1	BD	558539	Mouse IgG1	AF647 (*see* **Note 14**)
F4/80	BM8	Biolegend	123120	Rat IgG2a	AF488 (*see* **Note 14**)
Fixable Live/Dead	N/A	eBioscience	65-0866-18	N/A	eFluor506 (*see* **Note 17**)
Streptavidin	N/A	Invitrogen	Q10101MP	N/A	QDot605
Lineage (CD3, CD19, B220, NK1.1)	145-2C11, 1D3, RA3-6B2, PK136	Tonbo Biosciences, eBioscience, BD, Biolegend	TONB55-0031-U100, 15-0193-83, 553091, 108716	Ham IgG1, Rat IgG2a, Rat IgG2a, Mouse IgG2a	PECy5 (*see* **Note 18**)
CD45R (B220)	RA3-6B2	BD	553087	Rat IgG2a	FITC (*see* **Note 18**)

Table 3
Typical staining panel used for flow cytometric analysis of intestinal monocytes and macrophages

Antibody	Clone	Supplier	Cat. No	Isotype	Fluorochrome
Fc Block (anti-CD16/ CD32)	2.4G2	Biolegend	101320	N/A	N/A
CD45	30-F11	Biolegend	103138	Rat IgG2b	BV510
CD11c	N418	Biolegend	117318	Ham IgG1	PE-Cy7
CD11b	M1/70	Biolegend	101226	Rat IgG2b	APC-eFluor780
MHCII	M5/114.15.2	Biolegend	107622	Rat IgG2b	AF700
CD64	X54-5/7.1	BD	558539	Mouse IgG1	AF647 (*see* **Notes 14** and **20**)
F4/80	BM8	eBioscience	13-4801-85	Rat IgG2a	Biotin (*see* **Notes 14** and **20**)
Ly6C	HK1.4	eBioscience	48-5932-82	RatIgG2c	eFluor450
Ly6G	1A8	BD	551461	Rat IgG2a	PE (*see* **Note 22**)
Siglec F	E50-2440	BD	552126	Rat IgG2a	PE (*see* **Note 19**)
Streptavidin	N/A	Invitrogen	Q10101MP	N/A	QDot605
7-AAD	N/A	Biolegend	420404	N/A	PE-Cy5 or PerCP/ PerP-Cy5.5 (*see* **Note 17**)

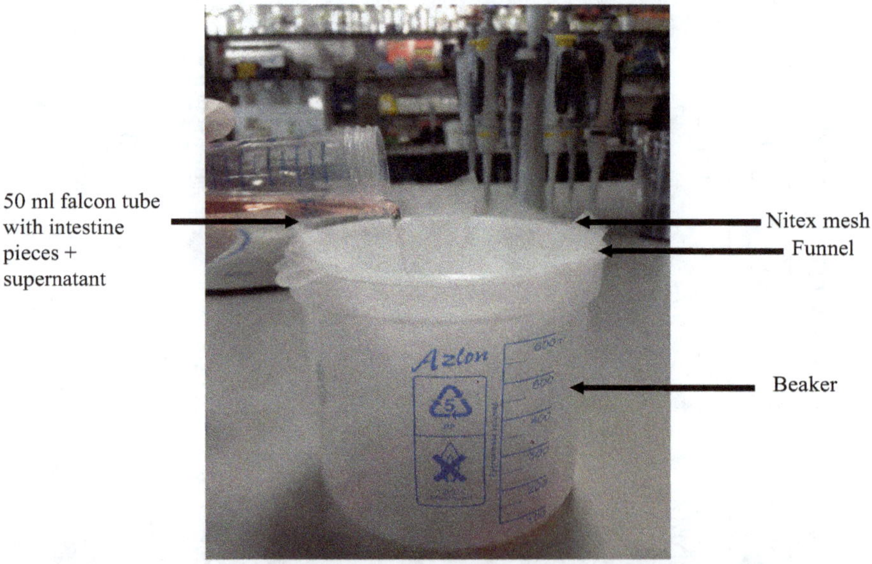

Fig. 1 Removal of supernatants during digestion of murine intestine and resected human material. Supernatants are removed by pouring tube contents through Nitex nylon mesh inserted in a funnel, allowing supernatant waste to drain into a connecting beaker, while tissue is retained on the Nitex nylon mesh

9. Add 10 ml CMF HBSS 2 mM EDTA to remaining pieces of SI and transfer to a shaking water bath/incubator at 37 °C for 20 min (*see* **Notes 6** and **7**).
10. Manually shake tubes vigorously and then discard supernatant.
11. Wash pieces of SI by adding 10 ml warmed CMF HBSS, manually shake tubes vigorously and discard supernatant.
12. Add 10 ml CMF HBSS 2 mM EDTA and transfer to a shaking water bath/incubator at 37 °C for 20 min.
13. Prepare appropriate enzyme cocktail (Table 1) in 10 ml complete RPMI.
14. Manually shake tubes vigorously and discard supernatant.
15. Wash by adding 10 ml warmed CMF HBSS, then manually shake tubes vigorously and remove supernatant.
16. Add 10 ml of the prepared enzyme cocktail to each tube.
17. Transfer to a shaking water bath/incubator at 37 °C, for approximately 20 min, or until all tissue pieces are almost completely digested, with manual vigorous shaking performed every 5 min (*see* **Notes 8** and **9**).
18. Add 10 ml cold FACS buffer and store on ice.
19. Pass single cell suspension through 100 μm cell strainer.
20. Pass single cell suspension through a 40 μm cell strainer.
21. Centrifuge at 400×*g* for 5 min and resuspend in 5 ml FACS buffer.
22. Count cells (*see* **Note 10**) and keep on ice until use.

3.2 Isolation of Leukocytes from Colonic Lamina Propria

1. Kill mouse according to appropriate ethical guidelines and immediately remove colon from top of caecum to rectum, place on tissue, soak in PBS and remove caecum and as much fat and feces as possible using tweezers (*see* **Notes 2** and **11**).
2. Open colon longitudinally with scissors (*see* **Note 3**).
3. Wash thoroughly in CMF HBSS 2% FCS in a 9 ml petri dish.
4. Cut colon into 0.5 cm segments.
5. Transfer colon to a 50 ml Falcon tube with 10 ml CMF HBSS 2% FCS on ice (*see* **Note 4**).
6. Manually shake tubes vigorously and discard supernatant (*see* **Note 5** and Fig. 1).
7. Add 10 ml CMF HBSS 2 mM EDTA and transfer to a shaking water bath/incubator at 37 °C for 15 min (*see* **Notes 6** and 7).
8. Manually shake tubes vigorously and discard supernatant.
9. Wash by adding 10 ml warmed HBSS then manually shake tubes vigorously and discard supernatant.

10. Add 10 ml CMF HBSS 2 mM EDTA and transfer to a shaking water bath/incubator at 37 °C for 30 min.
11. Prepare appropriate enzyme cocktail as per Table 1 in 10 ml cRPMI.
12. Manually shake tubes vigorously and discard supernatant.
13. Wash by adding 10 ml warmed CMF HBSS then manually shake tubes vigorously and discard supernatant.
14. Add 10 ml of the enzyme cocktail.
15. Transfer to a shaking water bath/incubator at 37 °C, for approximately 45 min, or until all tissue pieces are almost completely digested, with manual vigorous shaking performed every 5 min (*see* **Notes 8** and **9**).
16. Add 10 ml cold FACS buffer and store on ice.
17. Pass single cell suspension through 40 μm cell strainer.
18. Centrifuge at 400 × *g* for 5 min and resuspend in 5 ml FACS buffer.
19. Count cells (*see* **Note 12**) and keep on ice until use.

3.3 Preparation of Cells for FACS Analysis

1. Add 3–5 × 10^6 cells in FACS buffer to individual 6 ml FACS tubes; alternatively, 2–3 × 10^6 cells can be added to each well of a 96-well plate.
2. Centrifuge at 400 × *g* for 5 min at 4 °C and discard supernatant.
3. Block Fc receptors by incubating with purified anti-CD16/32 'Fc block' (1:200 dilution) for 20 min at 4 °C in FACS buffer (*see* Tables 2 and 3).
4. Wash cells by adding FACS buffer (1 ml if using tubes for staining, 100 μl if using plates), centrifuge at 400 × *g* for 5 min at 4 °C and discard supernatant.
5. Incubate cells with primary antibodies at 4 °C for 20–30 min in the dark (*see* Tables 2 and 3; **Notes 13–16**).
6. Wash cells by adding FACS buffer (1 ml if using tubes for staining, 100 μl if using plates), centrifuge at 400 × *g* for 5 min at 4 °C and discard supernatant.
7. Where necessary, incubate with fluorochrome conjugated streptavidin for 15 min at 4 °C in the dark.
8. Wash cells by adding FACS buffer (tubes 1 ml, plate 100 μl), centrifuge at 400 × *g* for 5 min, and remove supernatant.
9. Add 12 μl per tube 7-AAD (7-aminoactinomycin D) to discriminate live and dead cells (*see* **Note 17**).
10. Analyze on flow cytometer (*see* **Notes 18–22**).

3.4 Phenotypic Identification of Dendritic Cells and Macrophages in the Intestine

3.4.1 General Comments

As we have discussed, investigating the biology of intestinal mononuclear phagocytes has been stifled by a number of factors, many relating to the use of inappropriate and overlapping phenotypic markers [7]. The main aims of our work have been to establish reliable protocols for obtaining suitable numbers of cells of high viability, and then to apply rigorous flow cytometric techniques that can be used to characterize and distinguish mucosal cDCs and mϕ precisely. Here we describe the gating strategies and staining panels that we have found most useful for doing this in murine intestine.

3.4.2 Identifying cDCs in the Intestinal Mucosa

Having obtained suspensions of LP cells by enzymatic digestion as described above, the first step is to identify live CD45^{+} single cells in a broad FSC/SSC gate, using a live/dead marker (*see* **Note 17**) and CD45 expression. Next, lineage^{-} MHCII^{+} cells are gated before mϕ are excluded as F4/80^{+}CD64^{+} cells and cDCs are identified among the remaining cells as CD11c^{hi} cells (Fig. 2a). In the past, CD11c and MHCII co-expression alone was often used to identify cDCs, but as CD64^{+}F4/80^{+} mϕ also express MHCII and varying levels of CD11c, it is clear that exclusion of these cells is first necessary before a pure population of cDCs can be obtained (Fig. 2b) [15, 17, 24, 25]. In addition to CD64 and F4/80, the pan mϕ marker CD14 can also be used to exclude mϕ (Fig. 2b). A further marker to discriminate between cDCs and mϕ is CD26 (Fig. 2b) [26]. Our work confirms that the CD64^{-} F4/80^{-} CD11c^{+} CD26^{+} MHCII^{+} cells are *bona fide* cDCs as they express CD135 (flt3) and the cDC-specific gene *Zbtb46*; their development in vivo is dependent on the flt3L growth factor and they are derived from committed cDC precursors, (pre-cDCs) [17]. Unlike LP mϕ, the

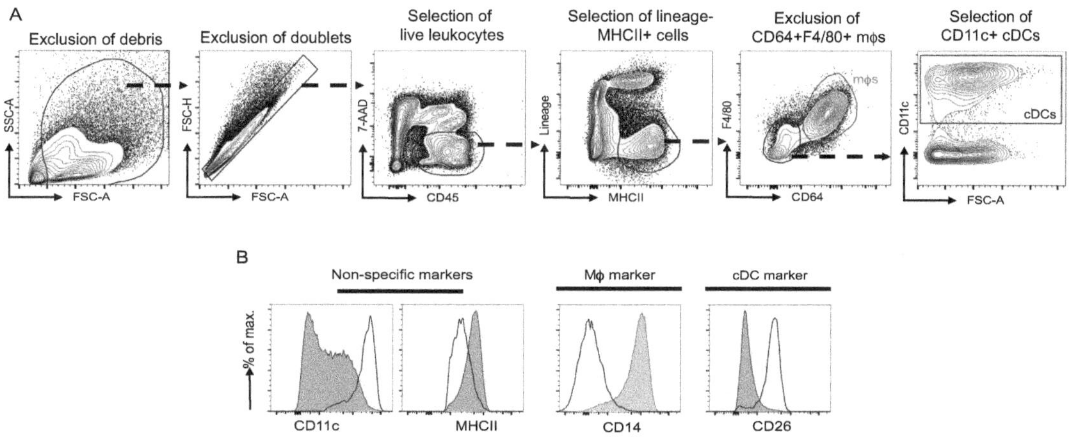

Fig. 2 Identification of cDCs in the murine intestine. (**a**) Single live leukocytes are identified among total cells on the basis of FSC and SSC, followed by exclusion of dead cells and of non-hematopoietic CD45^{-} cells. Lineage^{-}MHCII^{+} cells are then identified and cDCs identified as CD64^{-}F4/80^{-}CD11c^{+}. (**b**) Expression of CD11c, MHCII, CD14, and CD26 by CD64^{+}F4/80^{+} mϕ and CD64^{-}F4/80^{-}CD11c^{+} cDCs. cDCs are shown in *black* and mϕ are depicted in *grey*

CD64⁻/F4/80⁻ CD11c⁺MHCII⁺ cells also express CCR7, migrate via lymphatics to draining lymph nodes and are capable of retinoic acid production [7, 16, 17, 27]. Notably, although often considered to define cells of the monocyte/macrophage lineage, CCR2 expression is not sufficient to discriminate between these cells and cDCs in the gut, as at least some mature LP cDCs express this receptor [17]. It should be noted that cDCs are relatively more numerous in the small intestine, whereas mϕ are more frequent in the large intestine [11]. The pDCs found in the small intestine can be identified among live CD45⁺ cells as CD317⁺ (PDCA1) Siglec H⁺ Ly6C⁺ B220⁺ CD11b⁻ CD11c^{lo} MHCII^{lo} (*see* **Note 18**).

3.4.3 cDC Subsets in the Intestinal Mucosa

The cDC population can be separated into four distinct groups defined on the basis of CD103 and CD11b expression, revealing CD103⁺CD11b⁺, CD103⁺CD11b⁻, CD103⁻CD11b⁺, and CD103⁻CD11b⁻ subsets (Fig. 3a). Their proportions vary depending on the segment of the gut, with the CD103⁺CD11b⁺ cDC subset predominating in the upper small intestine and CD103⁺CD11b⁻ cDCs being most abundant in the colon (Fig. 3b) [11].

The cDC subsets can also be characterized further using additional markers [16, 17]. CD103⁺CD11b⁺ and CD103⁻CD11b⁺ DCs all express CD172a (SIRPα) and the transcription factor IRF4, as do some of the CD103⁻CD11b⁻ cDCs. The development of the CD103⁺CD11b⁺ subset requires IRF4 and Notch 2

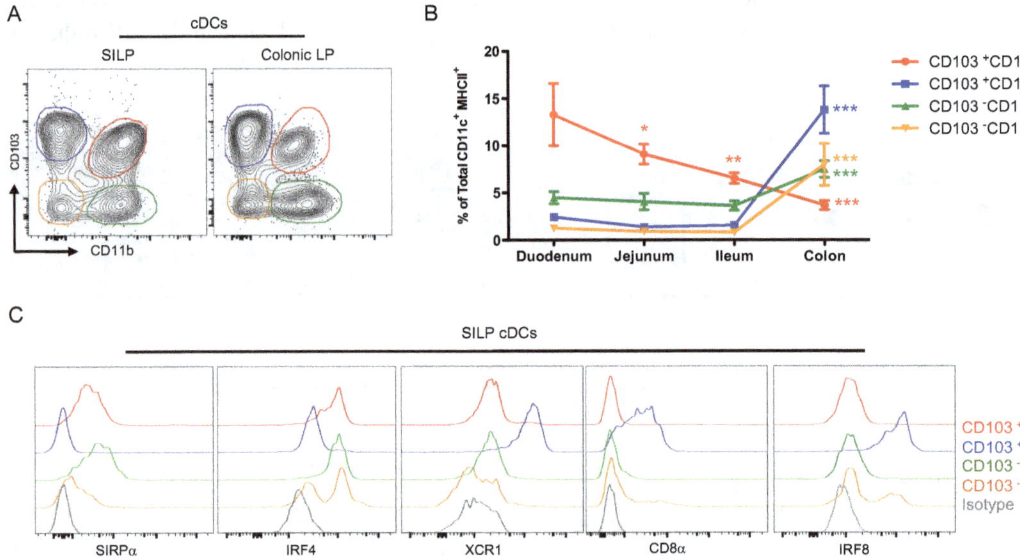

Fig. 3 Subsets of murine intestinal cDCs. (**a**) Expression of CD103 and CD11b on cDCs from mouse small and large intestines, identified as shown in Fig. 2. (**b**) The relative frequencies of cDC subsets in mouse LP varies along the length of the intestine. (**c**) Expression of CD172a (SIRPα), IRF4, XCR1, IRF8, and CD8α by the subsets of cDCs in mouse small intestinal LP

signaling in vivo [14, 28]. In contrast, the CD103$^+$CD11b$^-$ cDCs lack CD172a and IRF4, but express XCR1, CD8α and the transcription factor IRF8 (Fig. 3c). Their development is dependent on IRF8 and Batf3 [29, 30]. The CD103$^-$CD11b$^-$ cDCs are heterogeneous for CD172a, IRF4, CD8α, and IRF8 but lack XCR1 expression (Fig. 2c). The exact nature of this population is unknown. Some may represent precursor cells, while others may be contaminants of LP preparations derived from isolated lymphoid follicles (ILFs) [16]. The CD103$^-$CD11b$^-$ and CD103$^-$CD11b$^+$ cDCs are also heterogeneous for expression of CCR2 ([17] and our unpublished observations).

Much remains to be understood regarding the in vivo functions of the individual populations. While the CD103$^+$CD11b$^-$ cDCs appear to be equivalent to the lineage of Batf3-dependent IRF8$^+$XCR1$^+$CD103$^+$ cDCs that cross-present exogenous antigen to CD8$^+$ T cells in other murine tissues [31–33], the functions of the other subsets are less well defined. The CD103$^+$CD11b$^+$ cDCs have only been reported in the intestine and they have been shown to drive the differentiation of FoxP3$^+$ regulatory T cells in vitro. However depletion of CD103$^+$CD11b$^+$ cDCs in vivo leads to a defect in T_h17 cells in the intestine [13–15, 28, 34], and the numbers of regulatory T cells are only reduced under conditions when both CD103$^+$ cDC populations are absent [35]. The CD103$^-$CD11b$^+$ subset of intestinal cDCs may have a relatively enhanced ability to prime T_h17 cells in vitro and this is especially true of the CCR2$^+$ subset of these cDCs [16, 17]. The relationship of these CD103$^-$CD11b$^+$ cDCs to the CD103$^+$CD11b$^+$ subset and to CD11b$^+$ cDCs in other mouse tissues is unclear.

3.4.4 Macrophages in the Intestinal Mucosa

Once single, live CD45$^+$ cells have been gated in lamina propria isolates as described above, identification of the mϕ lineage is best achieved by first taking all cells expressing CD11b (*see* **Note 20**) and then excluding neutrophils and eosinophils on the basis of their expression of Ly6G and Siglec F respectively (Fig. 4a and **Notes 19–22**). Alternatively, eosinophils can be gated out based on their distinctive SSC^{hi} property (Fig. 4a).

The expression of CD64 can then be used to identify cells of the monocyte–macrophage lineage and exclude the smaller number of *bona fide* CD11b$^+$ DCs (Fig. 4a) (*see* **Note 20**). Ly6C and MHCII expression can then be used to delineate the different maturation stages of the monocyte–macrophage "waterfall" within the total CD64$^+$ compartment (Fig. 4b). Ly6C^{hi} MHCII$^-$ cells are phenotypically and morphologically identical to circulating blood monocytes, whereas transcriptional and functional studies indicate Ly6C^{hi} MHCII$^+$ cells are a more mature stage of differentiation; both of these populations are present only in small numbers in healthy intestine and express low/intermediate levels of the pan-mϕ markers CD64 and F4/80 (Fig. 4b–e). They produce only low

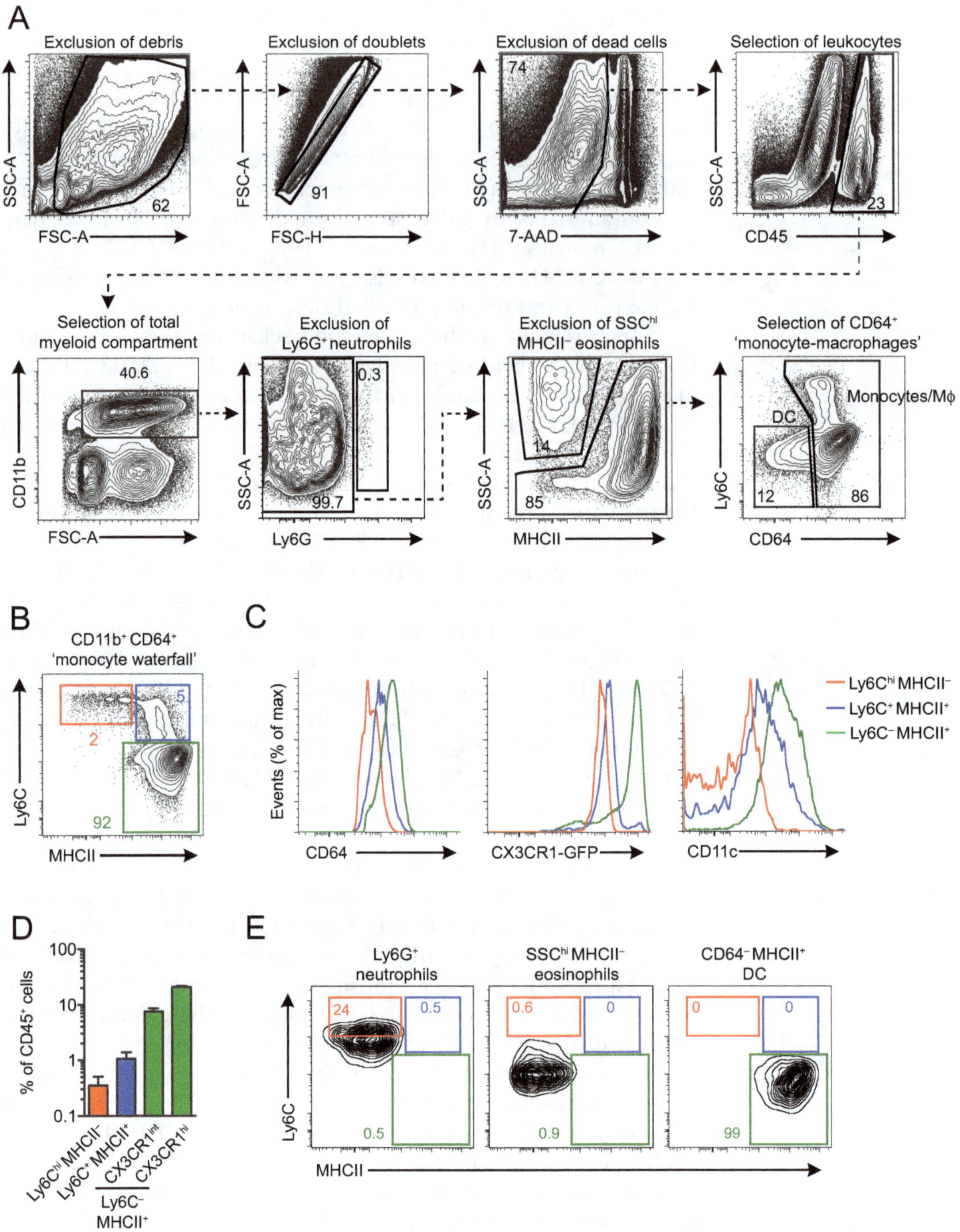

Fig. 4 Identification of monocytes and macrophages in the murine intestine. (**a**) Gating strategy used to identify the monocytes and mϕ in steady state mucosa of *Cx3cr1*$^{+/GFP}$ reporter mice. (**b**) Expression of Ly6C and MHCII by live CD45$^+$ CD11b$^+$ Ly6G$^-$ SSC^{lo} CD64$^+$ cells reveals the 'monocyte waterfall'. (**c**) Expression of CD64, CX3CR1-GFP, and CD11c by Ly6C^{hi} MHCII$^-$, Ly6C$^+$ MHCII$^+$, and Ly6C$^-$ MHCII$^+$ cells. (**d**) The frequency of Ly6C^{hi} MHCII$^-$, Ly6C$^+$ MHCII$^+$, CX3CR1^{int} Ly6C$^-$ MHCII$^+$, and CX3CR1^{hi} Ly6C$^-$ MHCII$^+$ cells among total CD45$^+$ leukocytes. (**e**) The expression of Ly6C and MHCII by CD11b$^+$ Ly6G$^+$ neutrophils, SSC^{hi} MHCII$^-$ eosinophils and CD64$^-$ DC, illustrating the potential of other myeloid cells to affect the analysis of the monocyte waterfall if not excluded

levels of IL10, have poor phagocytic activity and low expression of scavenger molecules [18]. Their numbers expand markedly during inflammation, where their ability to respond to for example TLR stimulation and produce cytokines such as TNFα and IL1 allows them to contribute to immunopathology [19, 20, 23].

The majority population in steady state mucosa consists of Ly6C$^-$ MHCII^{hi} cells, many of which co-express CD11c at relatively high levels (*see* **Note 23**). The use of *Cx3cr1*$^{+/GFP}$ reporter mice [36] (*see* **Note 24**) allows the separation of the Ly6C$^-$ MHCII^{hi} compartment into CX3CR1^{int} and CX3CR1^{hi} subsets, with the latter being the dominant and most mature population in the steady state mucosa. CX3CR1^{hi} Ly6C$^-$ MHCII^{hi} cells have the morphological appearance of mature macrophages with large 'foamy' cytoplasm and an abundance of cytoplasmic vacuoles, and are characterized by the anti-inflammatory and scavenger properties described above. The CX3CR1^{int} Ly6C$^-$ MHCII^{hi} cells are short-lived intermediaries between recently arrived monocytes and CX3CR1^{hi} macrophages.

F4/80^{hi} CD64^{hi} cells that lack both Ly6C and MHCII expression may also be present in the mucosa depending on microbiological status, although in fully colonized, SPF mice these are rare.

4 Notes

1. Reagents for each experiment can be prepared the night before they are required and stored at 4 °C, except for enzymes which must be freshly prepared on the day of the experiment. On the day of the experiment, all digestion reagents should be placed at 37 °C prior to use.
2. One SI/colon provides sufficient cells for multi-parameter FACS analysis of adult mice cDCs and mϕ. If cDC subset purification is required, six SIs or ten colons are needed to obtain approx. 30,000 cells per subset. If monocyte–macrophage population purification is required, three SIs or five colons are needed to obtain approx. 30,000 cells per population. If necessary, SIs or colons can be pooled into one 50 ml Falcon tube, but reagents must be scaled up appropriately and no more than three intestines should be pooled per tube. Each volume mentioned in the above protocols is for one intestine per tube.
3. PPs must be removed carefully, as they contain cDCs that are distinct from those in LP. This can be done easily, as PPs are macroscopically visible structures. However many 1000s of isolated lymphoid follicles (ILFs) are also found in the intestine, particularly the colon. As ILFs cannot be visualized with the naked eye, it is impossible to remove them and cDCs from these tissues are likely to be present in small numbers in preparations of LP.

4. In our experience, once excised and cleaned, intestinal segments can be kept on ice for up to 6 h before digestion with minimal effect on cell yield and viability.
5. Supernatants are removed by pouring cell suspensions into a beaker through 50 μm nylon mesh inserted in a funnel (Fig. 1).
6. EDTA is used to remove the surface epithelial layer, allowing access of enzymes to the LP in the next steps.
7. All shaking steps should be performed at 250 rpm to aid digestion.
8. Some tissue should remain in the 50 ml Falcon tube to prevent over-digestion, which can compromise the viability of the cells isolated.
9. Try to leave the intestines in the enzyme cocktail for as short a time as possible. Move on to the next step as soon as the tissue has been digested.
10. Typical cell yield from a murine small intestine digestion is $1–5 \times 10^6$ total cells.
11. The caecum is usually not included for the purposes of isolating large intestinal leukocytes, but may be useful to include under certain conditions such as specific infections that involve the caecum.
12. Typical cell yield from a murine colon digestion is $5–8 \times 10^6$ total cells.
13. We typically acquire $1–2 \times 10^6$ total cells to be able to visualize sufficient numbers of all subsets.
14. For identification of cDCs, CD64 and F4/80 are used to exclude mϕ in mouse tissues. Either marker will suffice for mϕ exclusion. However, the combination of both is preferable.
15. We use a broad FSC-A/SSC-A gate to identify cells and a stringent FSC-A/FSC-H gate to identify single cells prior to identifying live $CD45^+$ cells.
16. We do not use Percoll or any other pre-enrichment strategy prior to FACS analysis or sorting, as we find this can result in a significant loss of multiple cells types including DCs and mϕ. Enrichment procedures of this kind should be assessed carefully before being used routinely.
17. Alternative live/dead dyes can be used depending on the panel in use. If 7-AAD or DAPI are used, they should be added a few minutes prior to FACS analysis and not left on the cells for a prolonged period of time. Fixable Live/Dead dyes can also be used and should be added to the first staining step. However this should be performed in PBS without FCS, as per manufacturer's guidelines.

18. Plasmacytoid DCs (pDCs) are present in the small intestine and can be identified as $B220^{+}CD11c^{int}MHCII^{int}$. If pDCs are to be analyzed, B220 should be included in a separate channel from other lineage markers (CD3, CD19, and NK1.1). PDCA-1 can be used as an additional marker for pDCs.
19. Eosinophils are relatively abundant in normal intestinal mucosa and are a further population of myeloid cells that needs to be excluded carefully, as they are $CD11b^{+}$ and can also express intermediate levels of CD11c and F4/80. However they are universally Siglec F^{hi}, distinguishing them from other cells of the myeloid lineage.
20. For identification of cells of the monocyte–macrophage lineage in the mucosa, CD64 and F4/80 expression alone are not sufficient, as the early stages of monocyte differentiation do not express high levels of these markers. Thus total $CD11b^{+}$ cells are taken as the starting population.
21. Newly arrived $Ly6C^{hi}$ monocytes express CD64 at lower levels than mature mϕ. Allow for this when gating the $CD64^{+}$ compartment (*see* Fig. 4a, b).
22. Neutrophils are rare in healthy intestine and are characteristically $Ly6C^{int}$ $Ly6G^{hi}$, distinguishing them from monocytes which are $Ly6C^{hi}$ $Ly6G^{-}$.
23. Circulating $Ly6C^{hi}$ monocytes express little or no CD11c, which appears as the cells begin to acquire MHCII in the mucosa and its expression continues to increase as the mϕ mature in the mucosa. The proportion of mature mϕ that expresses CD11c and the levels of expression can vary substantially depending on the antibody clone used (e.g., HL3 vs. N418) and the microbiological status of the mice.
24. *Cx3cr1*$^{+/GFP}$ reporter mice are extremely useful in the analysis of cells of the monocyte/macrophage lineages in the intestine, as they allow the mature $Ly6C^{-}$ $MHCII^{hi}$ mϕ to be separated into different stages of maturation. While anti-CX3CR1 antibodies exist, the expression levels obtained with these often do not parallel GFP expression and they should be used with caution.

References

1. Mowat AM (2003) Anatomical basis of tolerance and immunity to intestinal antigens. Nat Rev Immunol 3:331–341
2. Pabst O, Mowat AM (2012) Oral tolerance to food protein. Mucosal Immunol 5:232–239
3. Johansson-Lindbom B, Agace WW (2007) Generation of gut-homing T cells and their localization to the small intestinal mucosa. Immunol Rev 215:226–242
4. Iwata M, Hirakiyama A, Eshima Y et al (2004) Retinoic acid imprints gut-homing specificity on T cells. Immunity 21:527–538
5. Johansson-Lindbom B, Svensson M, Pabst O et al (2005) Functional specialization of gut CD103+ dendritic cells in the regulation of tissue-selective T cell homing. J Exp Med 202:1063–1073
6. Zeng R, Oderup C, Yuan R et al (2013) Retinoic acid regulates the development of a

gut-homing precursor for intestinal dendritic cells. Mucosal Immunol 6(4):847–856

7. Cerovic V, Bain CC, Mowat AM et al (2014) Intestinal macrophages and dendritic cells: what's the difference? Trends Immunol 35:270–277
8. Hadis U, Wahl B, Schulz O et al (2011) Intestinal tolerance requires gut homing and expansion of FoxP3+ regulatory T cells in the lamina propria. Immunity 34:237–246
9. Mazzini E, Massimiliano L, Penna G et al (2014) Oral tolerance can be established via gap junction transfer of fed antigens from CX3CR1$^+$ macrophages to CD103$^+$ dendritic cells. Immunity 40:248–261
10. Schulz O, Jaensson E, Persson EK et al (2009) Intestinal CD103+, but not CX3CR1+, antigen sampling cells migrate in lymph and serve classical dendritic cell functions. J Exp Med 206:3101–3114
11. Mowat AM, Agace WW (2014) Regional specialization within the intestinal immune system. Nat Rev Immunol 14:667–685
12. Mayrhofer G, Pugh CW, Barclay AN (1983) The distribution, ontogeny and origin in the rat of Ia-positive cells with dendritic morphology and of Ia antigen in epithelia, with special reference to the intestine. Eur J Immunol 13:112–122
13. Scott CL, Murray TFPZ, Beckham KSH et al (2014) Signal Regulatory Protein alpha (SIRPα) regulates the homeostasis of CD103(+) CD11b(+) DCs in the intestinal lamina propria. Eur J Immunol 44(12):3658–3668
14. Persson EK, Uronen-Hansson H, Semmrich M et al (2013) IRF4 transcription-factor-dependent CD103(+)CD11b(+) dendritic cells drive mucosal T helper 17 cell differentiation. Immunity 38:958–969
15. Schlitzer A, McGovern N, Teo P et al (2013) IRF4 transcription factor-dependent CD11b(+) dendritic cells in human and mouse control mucosal IL-17 cytokine responses. Immunity 38:970–983
16. Cerovic V, Houston SA, Scott CL et al (2013) Intestinal CD103(−) dendritic cells migrate in lymph and prime effector T cells. Mucosal Immunol 6:104–113
17. Scott CL, Bain CC, Wright PB et al (2015) CCR2(+)CD103(−) intestinal dendritic cells develop from DC-committed precursors and induce interleukin-17 production by T cells. Mucosal Immunol 8(2):327–339
18. Bain CC, Bravo-Blas A, Scott CL et al (2014) Constant replenishment from circulating monocytes maintains the macrophage pool in the intestine of adult mice. Nat Immunol 15(10):929–937
19. Bain CC, Scott CL, Uronen-Hansson H et al (2013) Resident and pro-inflammatory macrophages in the colon represent alternative context-dependent fates of the same Ly6Chi monocyte precursors. Mucosal Immunol 6:498–510
20. Tamoutounour S, Henri S, Lelouard H et al (2012) CD64 distinguishes macrophages from dendritic cells in the gut and reveals the Th1-inducing role of mesenteric lymph node macrophages during colitis. Eur J Immunol 42(12):3150–3166
21. Zigmond E, Bernshtein B, Friedlander G et al (2014) Macrophage-restricted interleukin-10 receptor deficiency, but not IL-10 deficiency, causes severe spontaneous colitis. Immunity 40:720–733
22. Platt AM, Bain CC, Bordon Y et al (2010) An independent subset of TLR expressing CCR2-dependent macrophages promotes colonic inflammation. J Immunol 184:6843–6854
23. Zigmond E, Varol C, Farache J et al (2012) Ly6C(hi) monocytes in the inflamed colon give rise to proinflammatory effector cells and migratory antigen-presenting cells. Immunity 37:1076–1090
24. Guilliams M, Ginhoux F, Jakubzick C et al (2014) Dendritic cells, monocytes and macrophages: a unified nomenclature based on ontogeny. Nat Rev Immunol 14:571–578
25. Schraml BU, van Blijswijk J, Zelenay S et al (2013) Genetic tracing via DNGR-1 expression history defines dendritic cells as a hematopoietic lineage. Cell 154:843–858
26. Miller JC, Brown BD, Shay T et al (2012) Deciphering the transcriptional network of the dendritic cell lineage. Nat Immunol 13:888–899
27. Persson EK, Scott CL, Mowat AM et al (2013) Dendritic cell subsets in the intestinal lamina propria: ontogeny and function. Eur J Immunol 43(12):3098–3107
28. Lewis KL, Caton ML, Bogunovic M et al (2011) Notch2 receptor signaling controls functional differentiation of dendritic cells in the spleen and intestine. Immunity 35:780–791
29. Edelson BT, KC W, Juang R et al (2010) Peripheral CD103+ dendritic cells form a unified subset developmentally related to CD8alpha+conventional dendritic cells. J Exp Med 207:823–836
30. Ginhoux F, Liu K, Helft J et al (2009) The origin and development of nonlymphoid tissue CD103+ DCs. J Exp Med 206:3115–3130

31. Bachem A, Hartung E, Güttler S et al (2012) Expression of XCR1 characterizes the Batf3-dependent lineage of dendritic cells capable of antigen cross-presentation. Front Immunol 3:214
32. Hildner K, Edelson BT, Purtha WE et al (2008) Batf3 deficiency reveals a critical role for CD8alpha + dendritic cells in cytotoxic T cell immunity. Science (New York, NY) 322:1097–1100
33. Cerovic V, Houston SA, Westlund J et al (2015) Lymph borne CD8a + DCs are uniquely able to cross-prime CD8+ T cells with antigen acquired from intestinal epithelial cells. Mucosal Immunol 8(1):38–48
34. Satpathy AT, Briseño CG, Lee JS et al (2013) Notch2-dependent classical dendritic cells orchestrate intestinal immunity to attaching-and-effacing bacterial pathogens. Nat Immunol 14(9):937–948
35. Welty NE, Staley C, Ghilardi N et al (2013) Intestinal lamina propria dendritic cells maintain T cell homeostasis but do not affect commensalism. J Exp Med 210:2011–2024
36. Jung S, Aliberti J, Graemmel P et al (2000) Analysis of fractalkine receptor CX3CR1 function by targeted deletion and green fluorescent protein reporter gene insertion. Mol Cell Biol 20(11):4106–4114

Chapter 16

Monitoring and Modulation of Inducible Foxp3$^+$ Regulatory T-Cell Differentiation in the Lymph Nodes Draining the Small Intestine and Colon

S. Veenbergen, L.A. van Berkel, M.F. du Pré, A.E. Kozijn, and Janneke N. Samsom

Abstract

The mucosa-draining lymphoid tissue favors differentiation of inducible Foxp3$^+$ regulatory T cells. Adoptive transfer of T-cell receptor (TCR) transgenic (Tg) T cells is a powerful tool to study antigen-specific regulatory T-cell differentiation in lymphoid tissues in vivo. The kinetics and nature of the T-cell response largely depend on the route of antigen administration and degree of clonal competition. Here, we describe that adoptive transfer of CD4$^+$ DO11.10 TCR Tg T cells can be used for monitoring Foxp3$^+$ regulatory T-cell differentiation in the gut-draining lymph nodes. We describe two routes of mucosal antigen administration, e.g., the oral and intracolonic route known to induce T-cell responses in the small intestine-draining mesenteric lymph nodes (MLN) and distal colon-draining caudal and iliac lymph nodes (ILN), respectively. In particular, we discuss differences in frequency of inducible Foxp3$^+$ regulatory T cells after adoptive transfer of variable numbers of Tg T cells and various amounts of orally gavaged ovalbumin (OVA), and explain how Foxp3$^+$ regulatory T-cell differentiation can be modulated by coadministration of the adjuvant cholera toxin (CT) with OVA using this adoptive transfer system.

Key words Adoptive transfer, Clonal competition, Tregs, iTregs, Foxp3, Small intestine and colon, Mucosal immune regulation, OT-II TCR transgenic

1 Introduction

Adoptive transfer of T cells with the same T-cell receptor (TCR) specificity, originally developed by Kearney et al. [1] is widely used to study T-cell differentiation in vivo. In this system, high numbers of T cells from TCR transgenic mice are transferred into wild type syngeneic recipient mice that are subsequently exposed to antigen in vivo. By fluorescently labeling the TCR transgenic cells with a proliferation marker, the antigen-specific response can easily be visualized and subsequent analysis of lineage-specific transcription factors and cytokine expression reveals the type of immune response generated. The obvious advantage of the adoptive transfer system is

Björn E. Clausen and Jon D. Laman (eds.), *Inflammation: Methods and Protocols*, Methods in Molecular Biology, vol. 1559, DOI 10.1007/978-1-4939-6786-5_16,

the presence of increased numbers of antigen-specific responders within the pool of naive T cells, which allows for the quantitation of the T-cell response. In wild type mice, the frequency of antigen-specific T cells lies below 1/1000, making analysis of a tailored response for a specific antigen very difficult [1]. However, an important disadvantage of the adoptive transfer system is that introduction of an artificial number of TCR transgenic cells in vivo can cause clonal competition due to clonal abundance [2]. Activation of antigen-reactive T cells becomes less efficient with increasing numbers of transferred cells. In addition, T cells activated in a state of clonal abundance go through fewer divisions and show an accelerated decline in survival [2–5]. Therefore, the adoptive transfer system does not always reflect physiological activation.

Despite these disadvantages, the adoptive transfer system is often the only method available to determine the effect of an immunological intervention on T-cell differentiation. The behavior of the antigen-specific T cells and whether antigen-specific immunity or tolerance is induced depends on the type of antigen and route of antigen administration. Differentiation of regulatory T cells (Treg) is often studied in the context of oral tolerance. Oral ovalbumin (OVA) feed preferentially induces differentiation of inducible Forkhead box protein 3 (Foxp3)$^+$ Treg cells in the mesenteric lymph nodes (MLNs) and liver-draining lymph nodes [6–9], while after intramuscular injection of OVA, Foxp3$^+$ Treg differentiation in the thigh-draining popliteal and inguinal lymph nodes (PLN) is far less efficient. Using the adoptive transfer system, we have recently identified the caudal and iliac lymph nodes (ILNs) as inductive sites for antigen-specific T-cell responses to harmless protein antigen that is encountered in the distal part of the colon [10]. In this chapter, we provide a detailed description of the induction of Foxp3$^+$ Treg cells in MLNs and ILNs after adoptive transfer of CD4$^+$ DO11.10 TCR Tg T cells. We describe the effect of varying the total number of adoptively transferred T cells, the antigen dose and the administration route on Treg differentiation, and will explain how Foxp3$^+$ Treg differentiation can be modulated by coadministration of the adjuvant cholera toxin (CT).

2 Materials

2.1 Adoptive Transfer of Ovalbumin-Specific T Cells

2.1.1 Isolation and Fluorescent Labeling of CD4$^+$KJ1.26$^+$Rag$^{-/-}$ T Cells

1. 8–12-week-old DO11.10 transgenic (Tg) × *Rag*$^{-/-}$ donor mice having a T-cell receptor specific for the ovalbumin (OVA) 323–339 peptide (*see* **Note 1**).
2. Phosphate-buffered saline (PBS).
3. PBS supplemented with 2 or 10% heat-inactivated (30 min, 56 °C) newborn calf serum (NBCS) (*see* **Note 2**).
4. Scissors and forceps.

5. 70-μm nylon cell strainers.
6. Sterile 1 ml syringe plunger.
7. Erythrocyte lysis buffer consisting of 0.16 M NH_4Cl, 0.17 M Tris–HCl; pH 7.2.
8. Normal mouse serum or unlabeled anti-CD16/32 antibody.
9. Anti-CD4 and anti-DO11.10 Tg TCR (KJ1.26) antibodies.
10. 5,6-carboxyfluorescein succinimidyl ester (CFSE).
11. Sterile solution of 0.9 % sodium chloride.
12. Trypan blue 0.4 % solution.

2.1.2 Intravenous Injection of CD4+KJ1.26+Rag−/− T Cells

1. 8–12-week-old BALB/c recipient mice (*see* **Note 1**).
2. Sterile 27 gauge needles and 1 ml syringes.
3. Infrared heat lamp.
4. Restrainer for mice specifically designed for tail vein injection (Fig. 1a).
5. Ethanol 70 %.

2.2 Analysis of Foxp3+ Treg Induction by Flow Cytometry

1. Scissors and forceps.
2. PBS supplemented with 2 % heat-inactivated NBCS.
3. 70-μm nylon cell strainers.
4. Sterile 1 ml syringe plunger.
5. Normal mouse serum or unlabeled anti-CD16/32 antibody.
6. Fixation/permeabilization concentrate, fixation/permeabilization diluent, and permeabilization buffer.

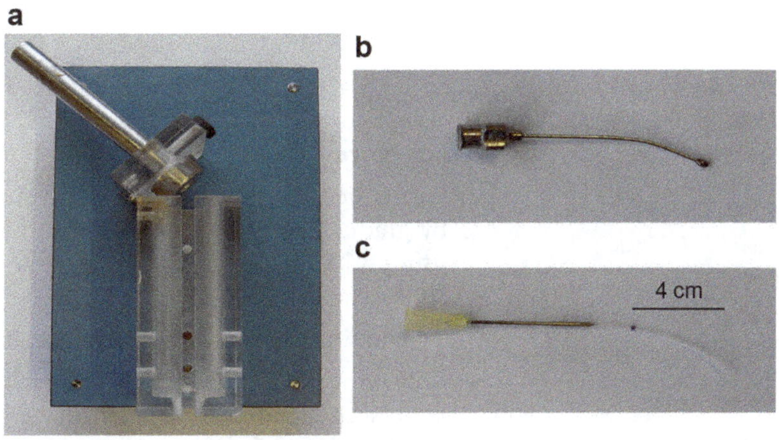

Fig. 1 Instruments needed for intravenous injection, oral gavage, and intracolonic administration. (**a**) Mouse restrainer specifically designed for tail vein injections. (**b**) Reusable needles for oral gavage. (**c**) Cannula for intracolonic administration

Table 1
Antibodies used for flow cytometry[a]

Specificity	Clone	Species	Isotype
CD4	GK1.5	Rat	IgG2b, κ
CD25	PC61	Rat	IgG1, λ
CD62L	MEL-14	Rat	IgG2a, κ
Foxp3	FJK-16s	Rat	IgG2a, κ
DO11.10 TCR	KJ1-26	Mouse	IgG2a

[a]Dilution depends on vendor and lot number, and needs to be optimized for each antibody

7. Anti-Foxp3, anti-CD62L, anti-CD25, anti-CD4 monoclonal antibodies (*see* Table 1).
8. BD FACSCanto II and FlowJo software.

2.3 Intramuscular, Oral, and Intracolonic Administration of Protein Antigen and Adjuvant

1. Ovalbumin (*see* **Note 3**).
2. Cholera toxin (CT, azide-free).
3. Anesthesia isoflurane vaporizer with nose cone circuit.
4. Sterile solution of 0.9 % sodium chloride.
5. Commercially available gavage needles (Fig. 1b).
6. Polyethylene tubing (inside diameter 0.86 mm, outside diameter 1.27 mm) and sterile 19 gauge needle (Fig. 1c).
7. Insulin 30 gauge, 8 mm syringe.
8. 1 ml syringes.

3 Methods

3.1 Adoptive Transfer of Ovalbumin-Specific T Cells

3.1.1 Isolation of CD4⁺KJ1.26⁺Rag$^{-/-}$ T Cells

1. Spleens are isolated from DO11.10 Tg × *Rag*$^{-/-}$ mice and kept on ice in PBS supplemented with 2 % heat-inactivated NBCS (*see* **Note 2**).
2. Subsequently, spleens are cut into small pieces and dissociated by gradually pressing them through 70-μm nylon cell strainers using a sterile 1 ml syringe plunger to obtain single-cell suspensions (*see* **Note 4**).
3. The strainer is rinsed thoroughly using PBS/2 % NBCS.
4. Following preparation of single-cell suspensions, cell pellets are resuspended in 1 ml erythrocyte lysis buffer per spleen and incubated for 5 min on ice. Lysing of the erythrocytes is stopped by adding PBS/2 % NBCS in excess (*see* **Note 5**).

5. After washing, cells are resuspended in PBS/2% NBCS, and the number of viable cells are counted using trypan blue exclusion.
6. A small cell aliquot is transferred into FACS tubes to determine CD4+KJ1.26+*Rag*$^{-/-}$ T-cell purity. In order to block Fcγ receptors, cell suspensions are preincubated on ice for 10 min with saturating amounts of anti-mouse CD16/32 or normal mouse serum. Next, cells are washed with PBS/2% NBCS, and stained in 50 μl of PBS/2% NBCS containing anti-CD4 and anti-DO11.10 Tg TCR antibodies, followed by incubation on ice for 20 min in the dark (Table 1).
7. Following incubation, cells are washed with 200 μl PBS/2% NBCS.
8. Subsequently, cells are resuspended in 200 μl PBS/2% NBCS and acquired on a BD FACSCanto II flow cytometer. Lymphocytes are gated according to their FSC-A/SSC-A profile (gate G1, Fig. 2a). A dot plot of KJ1.26/CD4 is used to quantify the lymphocytes that are double positive for the DO11.10 Tg TCR and co-receptor CD4 (gate G2, Fig. 2a).

3.1.2 Fluorescent Labeling with 5,6-Carboxyfluorescein Succinimidyl Ester

1. The remaining cells are washed twice in PBS to remove contaminating extracellular protein.
2. Subsequently, cells are resuspended in PBS at a concentration of 1×10^7 cells/ml before CFSE is added to the cells in a final concentration of 2 μM. To ensure homogeneous labeling, CFSE has to be added just above fluid level and the cell suspension must be thoroughly mixed by gently swirling for 10 s, but not vortexing.
3. Cells are incubated at 37 °C (water bath or incubator) for 10 min in the dark. After 3 and 7 min, cell suspension should be swirled to ensure optimal labeling (*see* **Note 6**).
4. Staining reaction is stopped by washing the cell suspension sequentially with ice-cold PBS/10% NBCS, PBS/2% NBCS and 0.9% sodium chloride, respectively.
5. The cells are resuspended in sterile endotoxin-free 0.9% sodium chloride for intravenous injection.

3.1.3 Intravenous Injection of CD4+KJ1.26+Rag$^{-/-}$ T Cells

1. Prior to the intravenous injection, BALB/c recipient mice are warmed to dilate the veins by placing a heat lamp above the cage (*see* **Note 7**).
2. After 5–10 min, the mice are placed in a restrainer specifically designed for tail vein injection (Fig. 1a).
3. The tail may be wetted with 70% ethanol to increase contrast between tail vein and skin, after which the needle is inserted

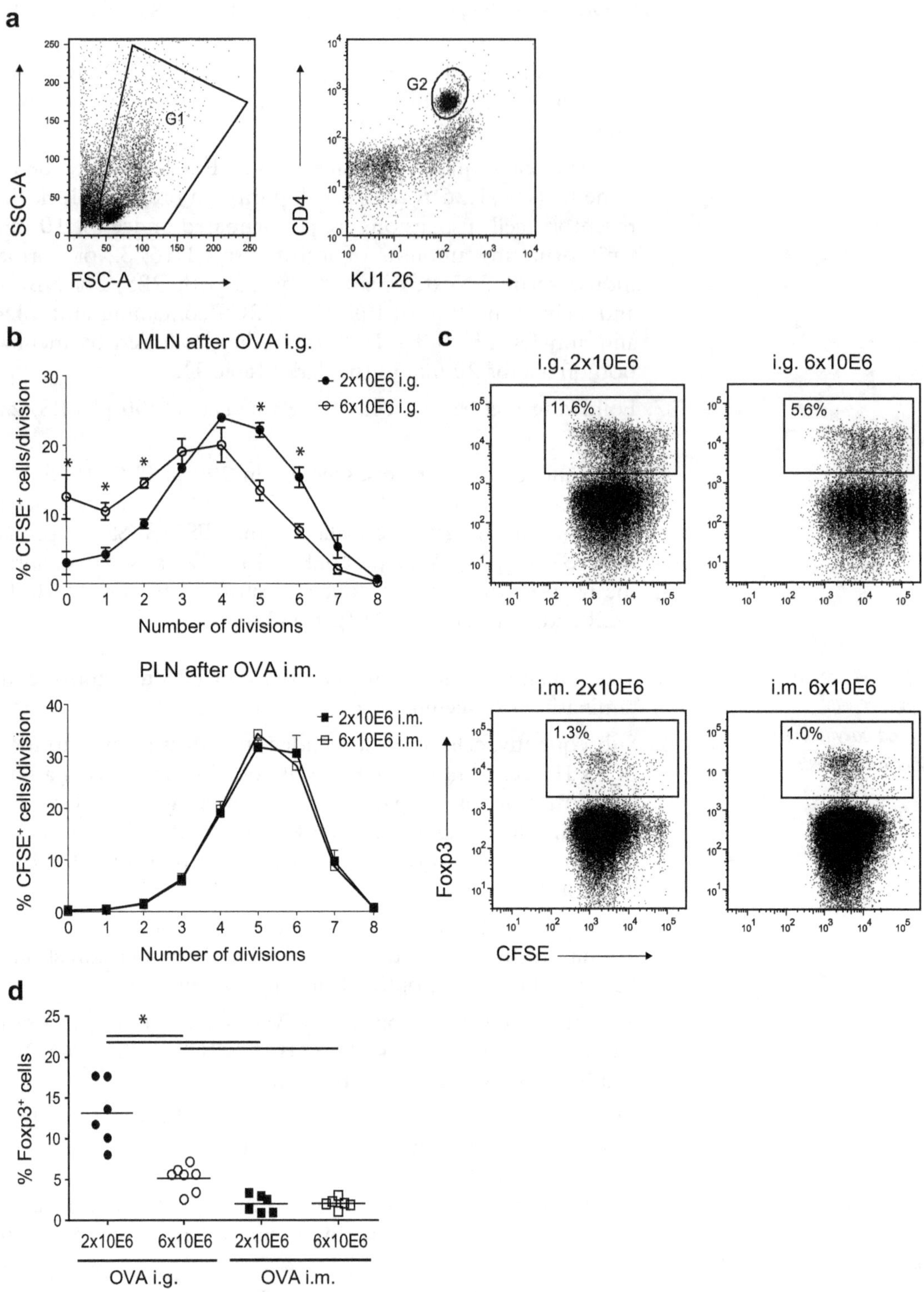

Fig. 2 Adoptive transfer of lower numbers of OVA-specific T cells induces an increased percentage of Foxp3⁺ cells and changes T-cell proliferation kinetics. (**a**–**c**) BALB/c recipient mice were injected intravenously with 2×10^6 or 6×10^6 CFSE-labeled CD4⁺KJ1.26⁺*Rag*$^{-/-}$ T cells and either received 70 mg OVA i.g. or 400 μg OVA i.m. the next day. Draining lymph nodes (MLN for i.g., PLN for i.m.) were isolated at 72 h after antigen administration and analyzed by flow cytometry for proliferation kinetics and phenotype (gated on KJ1.26⁺CFSE⁺ cells). (**a**) Flow cytometry gating strategy to define the purity of the isolated CD4⁺KJ1.26⁺*Rag*$^{-/-}$ T cells. (**b**) Proliferation kinetics

into the vein while holding the tail under tension. Keep the needle and syringe parallel to the tail to avoid perforation.

4. Either 2×10^6 or 6×10^6 CD4+KJ1.26+ cells in 100 μl 0.9% sodium chloride are injected slowly in the lateral tail vein (*see* **Note 8**).

3.2 Analysis of Foxp3+ Treg Induction by Flow Cytometry

Peripheral induction of Foxp3+ Treg cells upon adoptive transfer can be detected in the gut-draining lymph nodes within 48–72 h after administration of soluble antigen via the mucosa [7]. The lymphoid inductive site for Foxp3+ Treg induction largely depends on the route of antigen administration (*see* Subheading 3.3). At times later than 72 h, detection of Foxp3+ Treg in the draining lymph nodes is hindered by egress of fully differentiated lymphocytes into the circulation. As a result, antigen-specific T cells in third or fourth division will be detected in lymphoid tissues other than their inductive site such as spleen and peripheral lymph nodes.

3.2.1 Preparation of Lymph Node Single-Cell Suspension

1. Draining lymph nodes are isolated and kept on ice in PBS/2% NBCS.
2. Subsequently, lymph nodes are cut into small pieces and dissociated by gradually pressing them through 70-μm nylon cell strainers using a sterile 1 ml syringe plunger to obtain single-cell suspensions.
3. The strainer is rinsed thoroughly using PBS/2% NBCS.
4. Following preparation of single-cell suspensions, cell pellets are resuspended in PBS/2% NBCS, transferred into FACS tubes, and the number of viable cells are counted using trypan blue exclusion.

3.2.2 Flow Cytometry

1. Cell pellets are preincubated on ice for 10 min with saturating amounts of anti-mouse CD16/32 or normal mouse serum in order to block Fcγ receptors.
2. Following incubation, cells are washed with PBS/2% NBCS, and stained on ice for 20 min in the dark with 50 μl of PBS/2% NBCS containing anti-CD4, anti-CD25, and anti-CD62L antibodies (Table 1).
3. Cells are washed with 200 μl PBS 2%/NBCS before they are resuspended in 100 μl Fixation/Permeabilization Buffer from eBioscience. Prepare fresh Foxp3 Fixation/Permeabilization

Fig. 2 (continued) after intragastric (i.g.) and intramuscular (i.m.) administration of OVA, based on CFSE dilution. Data are representative for two independent experiments ($n=3$ per group). (**c**) Representative dot plot showing Foxp3 expression in the KJ1.26+CFSE+ T cell population. (**d**) Percentages of Foxp3+ cells in the KJ1.26+CFSE+ T cell population. Each *symbol* represents one animal and the *bars* represent the mean per group. Data are pooled from two independent experiments. *$P<0.05$ using one-way analysis of variance (ANOVA). *i.g.* intragastric, *i.m.* intramuscular, *OVA* ovalbumin, *MLN* mesenteric lymph nodes, *PLN* popliteal and inguinal lymph nodes working solution by diluting Fixation/Permeabilization Concentrate (1 part) with Fixation/Permeabilization Diluent (3 parts).

4. Cell suspensions are incubated on ice for 30 min in the dark.
5. Following this incubation, cells are washed with 200 μl 1× permeabilization buffer and stained with anti-Foxp3 antibody (Table 1) in 50 μl 1× permeabilization buffer for 30 min at 4 °C. Prepare a 1× solution of permeabilization buffer by diluting the 10× concentrate with distilled water prior to use.
6. After the staining, cells are washed sequentially with 200 μl 1× permeabilization buffer and 200 μl PBS 2%/NBCS before acquiring them on a BD FACSCanto II flow cytometer.

3.3 Intramuscular, Oral, and Intracolonic Administration of Protein Antigen and Adjuvant

One day after the transfer of CD4[+]KJ1.26[+] *Rag*$^{-/-}$ cells, BALB/c recipient mice receive protein antigen with or without adjuvant via intramuscular, oral, or intracolonic route (*see* **Notes 9–11**).

3.3.1 Intramuscular Administration of OVA

1. The mice are restrained by one person who steadies the leg to be injected.
2. The second person swabs the area with 70 % ethanol and inserts the needle of the insulin syringe into the caudal thigh at a 45° angle.
3. The mice receive 400 μg OVA resuspended in 15 μl 0.9 % sodium chloride in both hind legs (*see* **Note 12**).

3.3.2 Oral Administration of OVA

1. Animals are restrained and held in a vertical position.
2. The gavage needle is inserted into the right side of the animal's mouth (Fig. 1b).
3. The needle can be used to raise the head so the esophagus is in a straight line.
4. The needle should slide down the esophagus easily after which the fluid can be administered slowly.
5. After administration, remove the gavage needle from the esophagus slowly (*see* **Note 13**).

Three days after antigen administration, draining lymph nodes (mesenteric lymph nodes (MLN) for i.g., popliteal and inguinal lymph nodes (PLN) for i.m.) can be isolated and analyzed for Foxp3[+] Treg induction by flow cytometry. In contrast to the PLN, note that the proliferation kinetics of T cells in the MLN of mice receiving an adoptive transfer of either 2×10^6 or 6×10^6 CD4[+]KJ1.26[+]*Rag*$^{-/-}$ T cells is significantly different (Fig. 2b). In particular, adoptive transfer of 2×10^6 T cells induces more cells to proceed into division, and more cells reach a higher number of divisions when compared to adoptive transfer of 6×10^6 T cells. These findings are in agreement with previous reports that show an increase in proliferation and survival upon adoptive transfer of a lower frequency of naive CD4+ T cells [2–5]. Besides proliferation, the number of transferred T cells also affects the differentiation of Foxp3+ T cells in the MLN, as adoptive transfer of 2×10^6 T cells induces a higher percentage of Foxp3+ T cells compared to adoptive transfer of 6×10^6 T cells (Fig. 2c, d). These differences are not seen in the PLN after i.m. injection. It should be noted that choosing adoptive transfer of lower numbers of CD4+KJ1.26+*Rag*−/− T cells to enhance the frequency of inducible Foxp3+ Treg will entail a lower cellular yield and therefore limits the extensiveness of the FACS panel for further analysis.

With regard to varying antigen dose, the proliferation kinetics in mice that received either 35 or 70 mg of OVA follows the same pattern, with the majority of the Tg T cells dividing up to 4–5 times (Fig. 3a). Foxp3 expression, as determined by flow cytometry, can be detected in all rounds of T-cell division and the percentage of Foxp3+ T cells does not significantly differ after gavage of 35 or 70 mg OVA (Fig. 3b). Moreover, no significant differences in the percentage of Foxp3+CD25+ or Foxp3+CD62L+ T cells are observed when comparing mice that received 35 or 70 mg of OVA. Thus, expression of Foxp3, CD25 and CD62L as well as the T-cell proliferation kinetics upon oral OVA administration are not dose-dependent within the range of 35–70 mg of OVA.

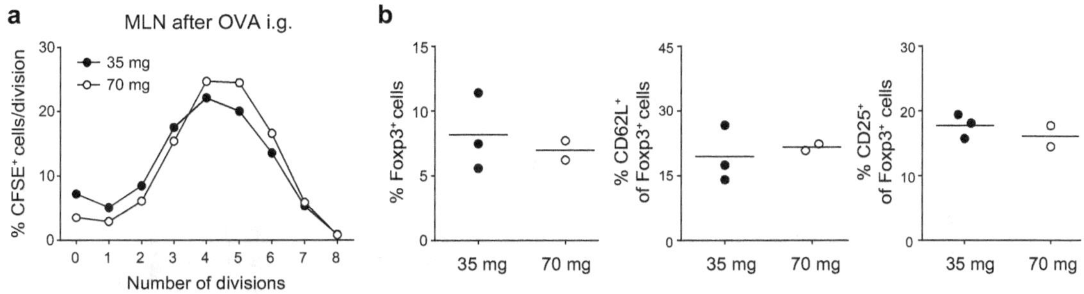

Fig. 3 Proliferation kinetics and expression of Foxp3 by CD4+KJ1.26+*Rag*−/− T cells in the MLN upon OVA administration are not dose-dependent. (**a** and **b**) BALB/c recipient mice were injected intravenously with 2×10^6 CFSE-labeled CD4+KJ1.26+*Rag*−/− T cells and either received 35 or 70 mg OVA i.g. the next day. MLN were isolated at 72 h after antigen administration and analyzed by flow cytometry for proliferation kinetics and phenotype (gated on KJ1.26+CFSE+ cells). (**a**) Cell proliferation kinetics of CD4+KJ1.26+*Rag*−/− T cells in the MLN 72 h after oral administration of 35 or 70 mg of OVA, based on CFSE dilution. The results shown are from one of two experiments with $n = 2$–3 mice per group. (**b**) Percentages of Foxp3+ cells, Foxp3+CD25+ cells and Foxp3+CD62Lhi cells of the KJ1.26+CFSE+ cell population in the MLN. Each *symbol* represents one animal and the *bars* represent the mean per group. The results shown are from one of two experiments with $n = 2$–3 mice per group. *i.g.* intragastric, *OVA* ovalbumin, *MLN* mesenteric lymph nodes

3.3.3 Intracolonic Administration of OVA

1. The mice are anesthetized with 2–5 % isoflurane in oxygen. Induction is performed in an induction chamber after which the mice are positioned in a nose cone (*see* **Note 14**). Two persons are required to perform this procedure. To prevent droplets from coming out of the anus during intracolonic administration, mice should be handled or restrained before anesthesia in order to stimulate the mice to defecate. Overnight starvation can be an alternative option.
2. The cannula (Fig. 1c) is wetted with 0.9 % sodium chloride and gently inserted into the anus to maximally 4 cm (*see* **Notes 15** and **16**).
3. The fluid should be administered very slowly to prevent droplets from coming out of the anus (*see* **Notes 17** and **18**).

While oral OVA administration results in antigen-specific proliferation and de novo Foxp3⁺ Treg induction in the MLN, such Foxp3⁺ Treg differentiation after colonic OVA administration occurs in the iliac and caudal lymph nodes (ILN) ([10], Fig. 4a, b). However, irrespective of whether OVA is applied orally or colonically, Foxp3⁻ inflammatory cytokine-secreting T cells differentiate simultaneously to the Foxp3⁺ Treg response in the draining lymph nodes. Using the adoptive transfer system, frequencies of differentiating inflammatory cytokine-secreting T cells and Foxp3⁺ Treg can be quantified, since their ratio is often altered in disease. In this context, we define two ways of restimulation to detect intracellular cytokines. Cells can be stimulated polyclonally meaning that

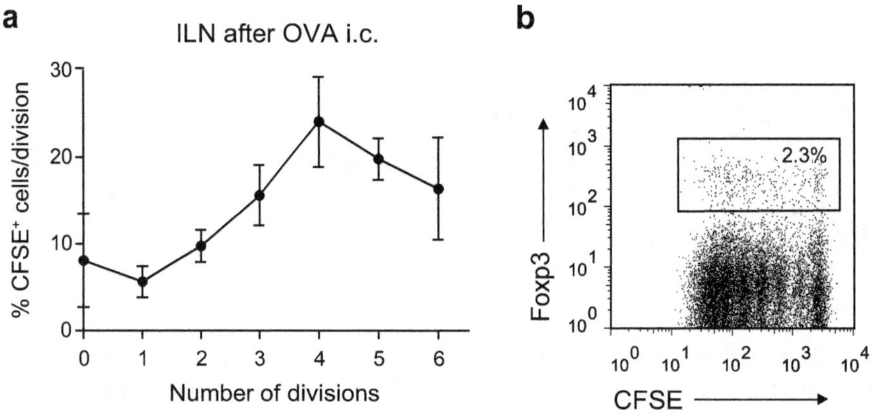

Fig. 4 Intracolonic OVA administration induces Foxp3⁺ Treg differentiation in the ILN. (**a** and **b**) CD4⁺KJ1.26⁺*Rag*$^{-/-}$ T cells were purified from DO11.10 transgenic × *Rag*$^{-/-}$ mice and labeled with CFSE. Subsequently, BALB/c mice were given 6 × 10^{6} CFSE-labeled T cells intravenously and 1 day later, received 70 mg OVA i.c. Seventy-two hour after OVA administration, draining lymph nodes were isolated and analyzed for CD4⁺KJ1.26⁺CFSE⁺Foxp3+ T cells by flow cytometry. (**a**) Percentage proliferating cells in each division peak. Values are depicted as mean plus SEM of three mice. (**b**) Representative dot plot showing staining for Foxp3 in the KJ1.26⁺CFSE⁺ T cell population. *i.c.* intracolonic, *OVA* ovalbumin, *ILN* caudal and iliac lymph nodes

approximately every cell in the population (donor CD4⁺KJ1.26⁺*Rag*$^{-/-}$ T cells and host BALB/c cells) is activated. Examples are αCD3/αCD28, PHA, PMA/ionomycin. Alternatively, restimulation with OVA can be considered as a way to reactivate only antigen-specific CD4⁺KJ1.26⁺*Rag*$^{-/-}$ T cells in the population. The range of OVA concentration can be 0.5–2 mg/ml, but depends on the TCR transgenic model and should be titrated.

3.3.4 Adjuvant Administration

1. Mice are given a single oral gavage of 70 mg OVA in combination with 20 μg cholera toxin (CT). Control animals are given a single gavage of OVA alone (*see* Subheading 3.3.2).
2. A single intramuscular injection can be used as a non-tolerogenic control (*see* Subheading 3.3.1).
3. Draining lymph nodes (MLN for i.g., PLN for i.m.) are isolated at 72 h after antigen administration and analyzed for proliferation kinetics and Foxp3⁺ Treg induction by flow cytometry (*see* Subheading 3.2).

Coadministration of CT with OVA induces more cells to proceed into division when compared to OVA alone (Fig. 5a) and affects T-cell differentiation, as the percentage of Foxp3⁺ T cells in the MLN is significantly reduced (Fig. 5b). The differentiation of Foxp3⁺ T cells is not fully blocked by CT as the percentage of Foxp3⁺ T cells remains higher than the non-tolerogenic i.m.

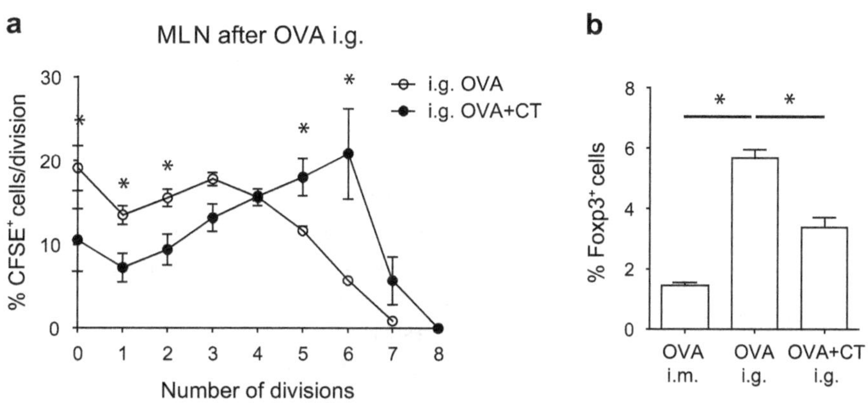

Fig. 5 Coadministration of CT with OVA enhances OVA-specifc T-cell proliferation in the MLN and reduces differentiation of Foxp3⁺ T cells. (**a** and **b**) BALB/c recipient mice were injected intravenously with 6×10^6 CFSE-labeled CD4⁺KJ1.26⁺*Rag*$^{-/-}$ T cells and received a single gavage of 70 mg OVA with or without 20 μg of CT or a single i.m. injection of 400 μg of OVA the next day. MLN were isolated at 72 h after antigen administration and analyzed by flow cytometry for proliferation kinetics and phenotype (gated on KJ1.26⁺CFSE⁺ cells). (**a**) Proliferation kinetics of transferred cells based on CFSE dilution. The results shown are from one of three experiments with $n=3$ mice per group. (**b**) Percentage of Foxp3⁺ cells of the KJ1.26⁺CFSE⁺ cell population in the MLN. The results shown are from one of three experiments with $n=3$ mice per group. *$P<0.05$ using one-way analysis of variance (ANOVA). *i.m.* intramuscular, *OVA* ovalbumin, *CT* cholera toxin, *MLN* mesenteric lymph nodes

control. The same results on T-cell kinetics and Foxp3$^+$ T-cell differentiation are obtained when 2×10^6 CFSE-labeled CD4$^+$KJ1.26$^+$*Rag*$^{-/-}$ T cells are transferred (our unpublished observations).

4 Notes

1. All mice are kept under specific pathogen-free housing conditions and fed a standard diet and water ad libitum.
2. New Born Calf Serum is a high quality, cost-effective replacement for Fetal Calf Serum.
3. The endotoxin level in OVA should be low and preferably endotoxin-free OVA should be used. Be aware of the OVA content in the diet, as it can interfere in the procedure.
4. The yield of cells is determined during the procedure of single cell-suspension preparation. Manual dissociation of the tissue can cause cell damage and sometimes results in clotting. These clots can be removed without affecting the procedure.
5. All washing steps are performed at $423 \times g$ for 10 min at 4 °C. Unless stated otherwise, cells should be kept on ice at all times.
6. Optimal labeling with CFSE is reflected by clearly defined peaks following division.
7. Extra care must be taken to prevent overheating of the animals while using the heat lamp during intravenous injection.
8. It is pivotal to be aware that clonal competition perturbs T-cell differentiation when using adoptive transfer of TCR Tg T cells. T-cell division can be affected due to clonal competition between T cells of the same specificity. Reducing the number of adoptively transferred TCR Tg T cells increases the proliferation and the percentage of differentiating cells. In our system, transfer of 2×10^6 TCR Tg cells is sufficient to yield a reliable proliferation profile and results in consistent detection of Foxp3$^+$ conversion, but one should realize that a lower number of transferred cells limits comprehensive FACS analysis.
9. It is recommended to pre-warm the OVA solution (room temperature or body temperature) before application, because injection of cold fluid will be painful.
10. Ovalbumin should preferably be dissolved in sodium chloride rather than phosphate-buffered saline (PBS), because phosphates can have adverse effects in vivo.
11. The protocol is applicable to the OT-II TCR transgenic mouse system. However, it should be noted that differences exist

between the DO11.10 and OT-II TCR transgenic system and OVA dosage, number of adoptively transferred T cells and timing should be optimized when using OT-II T cells.

12. Injection volumes should not exceed 50 μl in the thigh muscle.
13. The gavage needle is reusable and should be cleaned immediately after use with 0.9 % sodium chloride and can be stored in 70 % ethanol. Inspect the gavage needle to ensure that there are no burrs or points that could damage the esophagus.
14. The use of ketamine as anesthetic during intracolonic OVA administration should be avoided as it impairs intestinal OVA absorption.
15. Inspect the cannula to ensure that there are no burrs or points that could damage the intestine.
16. To detect antigen-specific T-cell responses in the ILN after intracolonic OVA administration, the cannula needs to be inserted 2.5 cm (C57BL/6) to maximally 4 cm (BALB/c) proximal to the anus.
17. To reach the maximum absorbance during intracolonic administration, the OVA solution should be administered very slowly to prevent droplets from coming out of the anus. The amount of 70 mg OVA should be injected intracolonically in a maximum volume of 150 μl. Be aware that the whole procedure of intracolonic administration will take approximately 10 min per mouse.
18. Droplets coming out of the anus can be carefully collected and reintroduced without causing any damage to the intestine.

Acknowledgments

This work was supported by the Dutch Digestive Foundation grant (WO 10-37) and Sophia Foundation grant 470.

The authors have no conflicting financial interests.

References

1. Kearney ER, Pape KA, Loh DY, Jenkins MK (1994) Visualization of peptide-specific T cell immunity and peripheral tolerance induction in vivo. Immunity 1:327–339
2. Hataye J, Moon JJ, Khoruts A, Reilly C, Jenkins MK (2006) Naive and memory CD4+ T cell survival controlled by clonal abundance. Science 312:114–116
3. Ford ML, Koehn BH, Wagener ME, Jiang W, Gangappa S, Pearson TC, Larsen CP (2007) Antigen-specific precursor frequency impacts T cell proliferation, differentiation, and requirement for costimulation. J Exp Med 204:299–309
4. Foulds KE, Shen H (2006) Clonal competition inhibits the proliferation and differentiation of adoptively transferred TCR transgenic CD4 T cells in response to infection. J Immunol 176:3037–3043
5. Garcia Z, Pradelli E, Celli S, Beuneu H, Simon A, Bousso P (2007) Competition for antigen determines the stability of T cell-dendritic cell

interactions during clonal expansion. Proc Natl Acad Sci U S A 104:4553–4558

6. Coombes JL, Siddiqui KR, Arancibia-Carcamo CV, Hall J, Sun CM, Belkaid Y, Powrie F (2007) A functionally specialized population of mucosal CD103+ DCs induces Foxp3+ regulatory T cells via a TGF-beta and retinoic acid-dependent mechanism. J Exp Med 204:1757–1764
7. Hauet-Broere F, Unger WW, Garssen J, Hoijer MA, Kraal G, Samsom JN (2003) Functional CD25− and CD25+ mucosal regulatory T cells are induced in gut-draining lymphoid tissue within 48 h after oral antigen application. Eur J Immunol 33:2801–2810
8. Siewert C, Lauer U, Cording S, Bopp T, Schmitt E, Hamann A, Huehn J (2008) Experience-driven development: effector/memory-like alphaE+Foxp3+ regulatory T cells originate from both naive T cells and naturally occurring naive-like regulatory T cells. J Immunol 180:146–155
9. Sun CM, Hall JA, Blank RB, Bouladoux N, Oukka M, Mora JR, Belkaid Y (2007) Small intestine lamina propria dendritic cells promote de novo generation of Foxp3 T reg cells via retinoic acid. J Exp Med 204:1775–1785
10. Veenbergen S, van Berkel LA, du Pré MF, He J, Karrich JJ, Costes LMM, Luk F, Simons-Oosterhuis Y, Raatgeep HC, Cerovic V, Cupedo T, Mowat AM, Kelsall BL, Samsom JN (2016) Colonic tolerance develops in the iliac lymph nodes and can be established independent of CD103 dendritic cells. Mucosal Immunol 9(4):894–906. doi:10.1038/mi.2015.118

Chapter 17

Isolation and Flow Cytometry Analysis of Innate Lymphoid Cells from the Intestinal Lamina Propria

Konrad Gronke*, Michael Kofoed-Nielsen*, and Andreas Diefenbach

Abstract

The intestinal mucosa constitutes the biggest surface area of the body. It is constantly challenged by bacteria, commensal and pathogenic, protozoa, and food-derived irritants. In order to maintain homeostasis, a complex network of signaling circuits has evolved that includes contributions of immune cells. In recent years a subset of lymphocytes, which belong to the innate immune system, has caught particular attention. These so-called innate lymphoid cells (ILC) reside within the lamina propria of the small and large intestines and rapidly respond to environmental challenges. They provide immunity to various types of infections but may also contribute to organ homeostasis as they produce factors acting on epithelial cells thereby enhancing barrier integrity. Here, we describe how these cells can be isolated from their environment and provide an in-depth protocol how to visualize the various ILC subsets by flow cytometry.

Key words Innate lymphoid cells, ILC, Mucosa, Lamina propria, Mucosal inflammation

1 Introduction

Mucosal surfaces are the main entry route for pathogens but also a large surface often peacefully inhabited by a complex microbiota and exposed to myriads of nutrient compounds. In particular the intestinal mucosa is challenged every day, needing to differentiate between commensal and harmful bacteria [1, 2]. Uncontrolled activation of the immune system to commensal bacteria may lead to severe pathological inflammation, while an insufficient response to pathogens puts the entire organism at risk. An important decision maker at barrier surfaces is the innate immune system, which is particularly multifaceted in the gut. During the recent years, a new player in mucosal immune responses has emerged, innate lymphoid cells (ILC) [3]. ILC belong to the lymphoid lineage but do not express any recombined antigen receptors. They are generated in the fetal liver during embryogenesis [4] and the bone marrow

* Author contributed equally with all other contributors.

Björn E. Clausen and Jon D. Laman (eds.), *Inflammation: Methods and Protocols*, Methods in Molecular Biology, vol. 1559, DOI 10.1007/978-1-4939-6786-5_17, © Springer Science+Business Media LLC 2017

during adult life [5], from where they home to different mucosal tissues and organs. Based on their expression of key transcription factors, four different groups of ILC can be differentiated, which all can be found within the lamina propria of the intestine [6]. Group 1 ILC express T-bet, produce IFN-γ and contribute to the defense against intracellular pathogens [5]. Group 2 ILC are dependent on GATA-3 and RORα [7, 8] and fend off helminths by the production of IL-5 and IL-13 [9, 10]. The third subset of ILC expresses RORγt and is particularly important for the mucosal defense against extracellular bacteria. Their main effector cytokines are IL-17 and IL-22 [11, 12]. IL-22 belongs to the IL-10 family and acts on epithelial cells because of the restriction of IL-22 receptor expression to non-hematopoietic cells such as epithelial cells and stroma cells [13]. IL-22 is expressed even during steady-state and induces the production of anti-bacterial proteins, which are constantly secreted into the gut lumen. It also promotes the fucosylation of proteins [14], which are shed from the surface of epithelial cells and support commensal microbiota, thus making it a bona fide homeostatic cytokine. The last subset of ILC is probably the best known but least abundant at mucosal surfaces. These are the cytotoxic ILC expressing T-bet and Eomes, which likely represent the mucosal counterpart of conventional NK cells and contribute to the killing of virus-infected and tumor cells [15, 16].

As these cells are tightly entangled with extracellular matrix components, their extraction is challenging and requires a multistep procedure involving enzymatic digestion releasing lamina propria cells from their environment. Here we provide a step-by-step protocol to isolate lymphocytes as well as myeloid cells from the lamina propria of the murine intestine. The isolation procedure is based on an EDTA-mediated dissociation of the epithelium and subsequent enzymatic digestion of the extracellular matrix. The separation of leukocytes from epithelial cells and extracellular matrix components is achieved by Percoll density gradient centrifugation. We also suggest a staining protocol to identify the various ILC subsets within the lamina propria. While there are certainly various ways to identify the known ILC subsets, we propose a strategy that can easily identify most relevant ILC subsets within a limited number of stains without the use of any specific genetic mouse models (e.g., reporter mice for lineage-defining transcription factors).

2 Materials

For 3.1 Tissue Harvest

Pre-made solutions Phosphate buffered saline (PBS).

General supplies 50 mL conical test tubes.

Scissors (straight 23 mm edge) and scalpels (blade size #21).

Petri Dishes.

For 3.2 Cell Isolation

General supplies 50 mL conical test tubes.
Scissors (straight 23 mm edge) and scalpels (blade size #21).
70 μm cell strainer.
Cell Dissociation Medium Hank's balanced salt solution (HBSS) with phenol red without calcium or magnesium. Supplement HBSS with 10 mM HEPES buffer and 5 mM EDTA. We recommend to prepare a sterile 0.5 M EDTA stock and dilute it 1:100.
Digestion Solution HBSS without phenol red (with calcium and magnesium) supplemented with 500 μg/mL collagenase D, 500 μg/mL DNase1, dispase (0.5 U/mL), and 2% FCS (*see* **Note 5**).
DMEM-10 Dulbecco's modified Eagle medium (DMEM) with 10% fetal calf serum (FCS) and 80 mM 2-mercaptoethanol, 8 mg/mL glutamine, 100 U/mL penicillin, 0.4 mg/mL gentamicin, and 100 mg/mL streptomycin.

For 3.3 Cell Purification
Pre-made solutions Percoll.
10× PBS.

General supplies 50 and 15 mL conical test tubes.

Pasteur pipettes.
DMEM-10 Dulbecco's modified Eagle medium (DMEM) with 10% fetal calf serum (FCS) and 80 mM 2-mercaptoethanol, 8 mg/mL glutamine, 100 U/mL penicillin, 0.4 mg/mL gentamicin, and 100 mg/mL streptomycin.

For 3.4 Flow Cytometry
General supplies V-bottom 96-well plates.
Staining buffer for flow cytometry PBS supplemented with 2% FCS.
Formaldehyde based fixation and permeabilization solution (we recommend "Foxp3/Transcription Factor Staining Buffer Set" from eBioscience; *see* also **Note 15**).
Fluorochrome-coupled antibodies.

3 Methods

As lamina propria lymphocytes are extremely sensitive, all steps are carried out on ice, unless specified otherwise.

3.1 Tissue Harvest

1. Prepare 10 cm petri dishes with ice-cold PBS before the beginning of the experiment and place on ice. Keep the lids for **step 12**.
2. After opening the peritoneal cavity, dislodge the small intestine and colon gently with forceps out of the peritoneal cavity. Try to already remove the mesenteric fat during this process. Cut off the caecum and place the small intestine and colon into separate petri dishes with PBS (Fig. 1). If preparation of cecal leukocytes is planned, the caecum can be processed in a similar

fashion. If the intestines have been separated, treat every piece as a distinct entity during the following protocol.

3. Since we are interested in the ILC of the lamina propria, remove the Peyer's patches (of the small intestine) with your scissors (*see* **Note 1**). All leftover fat tissue should be removed meticulously (*see* **Note 2**).
4. Cut open the intestine longitudinally with straight 23 mm-edge scissors and swirl it quickly in the petri dish to remove large parts of the feces.
5. Fill up a 50 mL conical tube with approximately 25 mL ice-cold PBS and transfer the gut into it. Repeat **steps 2–5** for every mouse that will be analyzed (*see* **Note 3**).
6. Close the tube and shake it intensely. Replace the PBS with fresh one and repeat this step until no macroscopic feces can be detected on the tissue anymore.

3.2 Cell Isolation

7. Prepare a 50 mL conical tube with 5 mL cell dissociation medium. Transfer the clean gut into this tube.
8. Incubate the samples at 37 °C agitating (120 rpm) in a shaker for 20 min (*see* **Note 6**).
9. Remove from shaker and vortex the tube containing the gut and the cell dissociation medium for 15 s at maximal intensity. Discard the supernatant (contains epithelial cells) and refill it with fresh 5 mL cell dissociation medium (*see* **Note 4**). Repeat the incubation from **step 8** and vortex again as in **step 9**.

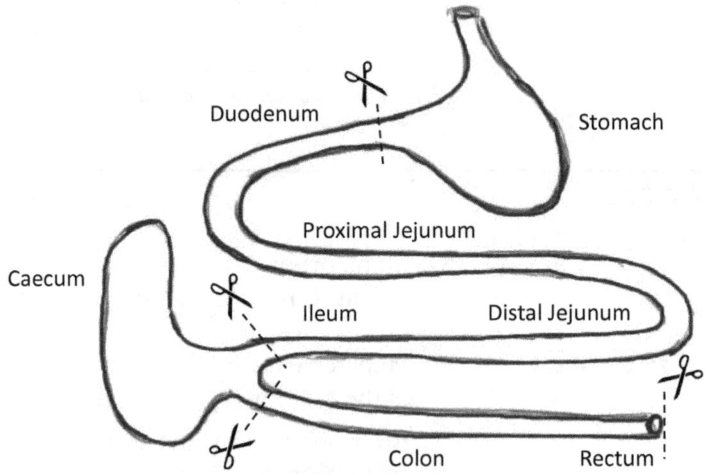

Fig. 1 Sketch of the murine gastrointestinal system (not proportional). Within the peritoneal cavity the following intestinal sections can be found from cranial to caudal: stomach, small intestine (consisting of duodenum, proximal and distal jejunum, ileum), caecum and colon. *Scissors mark* possible incision points for the separate preparation of different compartments (e.g., small intestine and colon)

10. After vortexing the gut for a second time, immediately transfer the gut into ice-cold PBS.
11. Prepare digestion solution during the last incubation step. You will need 15 mL digestion solution per sample (small intestine and colon count as two samples!) (*see* **Note 5**).
12. Take the tissue out of the PBS and shortly dab it on a paper towel. Then transfer it to a petri dish lid. Use the scissors to cut the gut into small pieces and mince it further with a scalpel. Transfer the gut-mash into a 50 mL conical tube with 5 mL digestion solution.
13. Incubate the samples at 37 °C agitating in a shaker for 20 min (*see* **Note 6**).
14. Prepare collection tubes by placing 70 μm cell strainers on 50 mL conical tubes. Add 15 mL of DMEM-10 to each tube.
15. Remove sample from shaker and vortex for 20 s at maximal force. Pour the supernatant through the cell strainer into the collection tube. Collect the gut mash from the strainer surface and retransfer it into the digestion tube. Add 5 mL fresh digestion solution and repeat **steps 13–15** two more times (*see* **Note 7**). To increase the cell yield, flush the strainer with 2 mL DMEM-10.

3.3 Cell Purification

16. Pellet the cells for 10 min at 800 × *g* at 20 °C (*see* **Note 8**).
17. Prepare a Percoll density gradient by adding first 1 vol. of 10× PBS to 9 vol. Percoll solution. We regard this 90% Percoll solution as stock solution. Per sample prepare 3 mL "80%" Solution by adding 600 μL DMEM-10 to 2.4 mL Percoll stock solution and 5 mL "40%" solution by adding 3 mL DMEM-10 to 2 mL Percoll stock (*see* **Note 9**). Fill 3 mL of "80%" solution into a 15 mL conical tube.
18. Resuspend the pellet in 1 mL "40%" Percoll solution and afterwards add the remaining 4 mL and resuspend it shortly again. Now slowly overlay the 3 mL "80%" with the 5 mL "40%" solution containing your harvested cells (*see* **Note 10**).
19. Now centrifuge the gradient for 20 min at 1300 × *g* without break. This step has to be carried out at room temperature, since temperature differences will affect the gradient. Be sure to disable the break function of your centrifuge, as it would disrupt the gradient.
20. Remove the upper phase containing fat and cell debris with a suction pump or a Pasteur pipette. Use a fresh Pasteur pipette to collect the ring interphase between the "80%" and "40%" phases and transfer it into a fresh 15 mL conical tube.
21. Fill up the tube with flow cytometry buffer, invert it shortly and centrifuge it for 10 min at 800 × *g*. From now on, all centrifugation steps can be done at 4 °C (*see* **Note 11**).

3.4 Flow Cytometry

22. Resuspend cells in ~500 μL flow cytometry buffer containing Fc-Block (CD16/CD32 IgG2b). At this step you can count the cells.
23. Aliquot 2.5 million cells into each well of a V-bottom 96-well plate. Spin down at 450 × *g* for 5 min at 4 °C. The cells should be kept on ice or at 4 °C throughout the staining procedure and all centrifugation steps are done as described in this step (*see* **Note 12**).
24. Wash the cells by resuspending them in 200 μL flow cytometry staining buffer. Spin down.
25. Resuspend the cells in 50 μL staining buffer containing the lineage staining cocktail antibodies and incubate for 25 min on ice or at 4 °C (*see* **Note 13**).
26. Wash the cells twice by adding staining buffer up to 200 μL each time.
27. Resuspend the cells in 50 μL staining buffer containing the surface staining cocktail antibodies and incubate for 25 min on ice or at 4 °C in the dark (*see* **Note 14**).
28. Wash the cells twice by adding up to 200 μL staining buffer each time.
29. Fix the cells in 100 μL formaldehyde-based fixation and permeabilization solution overnight at 4 °C in the dark (*see* **Note 15**).
30. Wash the cells twice by adding staining buffer (or permeabilization buffer if the "FoxP3 Kit" is used) up to 200 μL each time.
31. Resuspend the cells in 50 μL staining buffer (or permeabilization buffer if "FoxP3 Kit" is used) containing the transcription factor staining cocktail antibodies and incubate for 2 h on ice at 4 °C in the dark (*see* **Note 16**).
32. Wash the cells twice by adding 200 μL staining buffer (or permeabilization buffer if "FoxP3 Kit" is used).
33. Resuspend the cells in 200 μL staining buffer and acquire at the flow cytometer.
34. The gating strategy to identify all currently known ILC populations using the stainings listed within this protocol can be seen in Fig. 2.

4 Notes

1. The Peyer's patches can be found at the contra-mesenteric side of the gut. These patches can also be collected and processed like normal lymph nodes.
2. Be careful not to dry out or warm up the gut during this step. Leftover fat will affect the efficiency of the Percoll gradient later on.

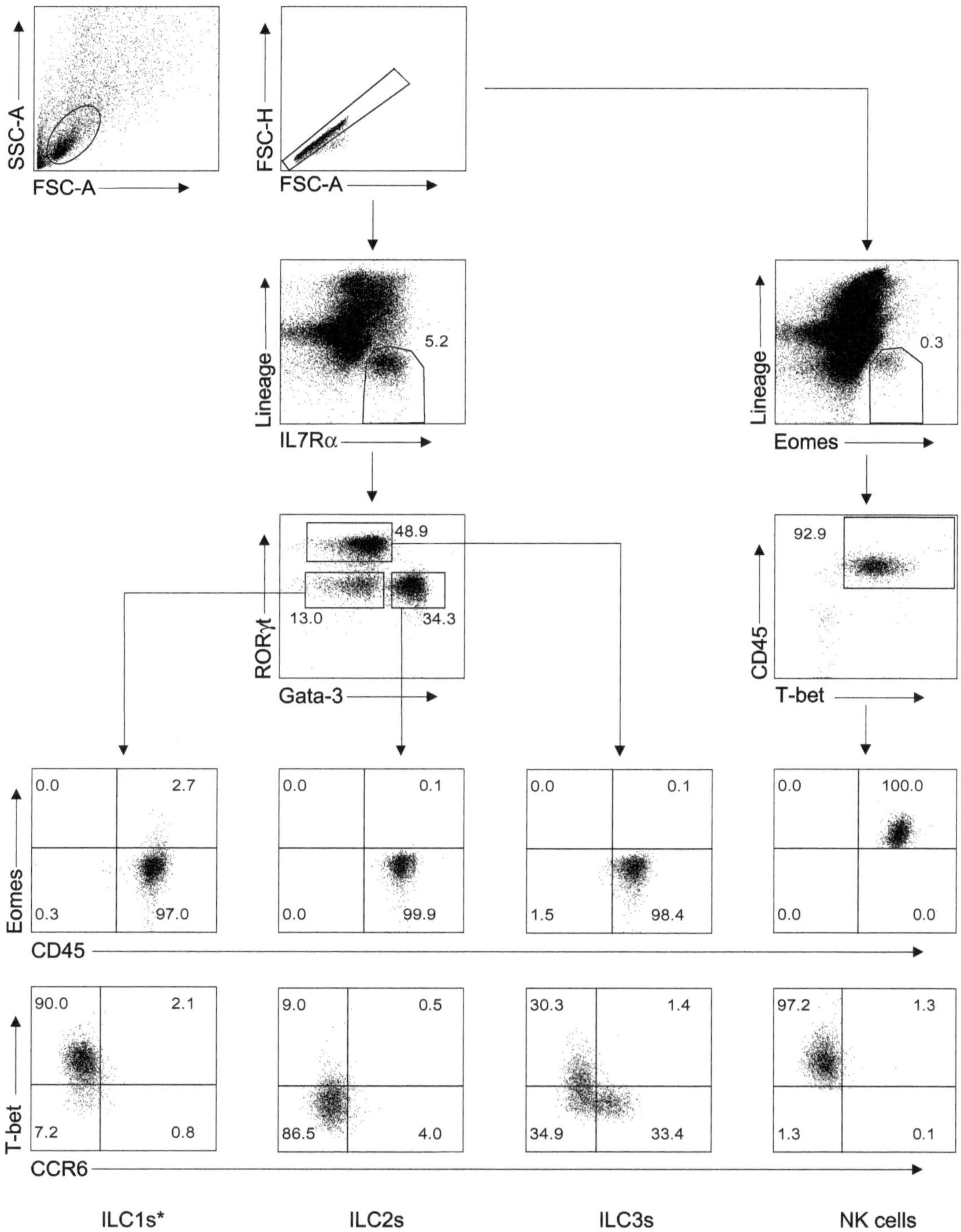

Fig. 2 Analysis of ILC subsets based on lineage defining transcription factors and IL-7 receptor expression. Lymphocytes from the small intestinal lamina propria were isolated, stained, and analyzed by flow cytometry. Percentages of cells in the respective gates may vary according to genetic background and health status of the mouse. As CD45.2 is not expressed in all mouse strains, anti-CD45 or anti-CD90 can be used instead (*see* **Note 14**). *ILC1: this population includes ex-RORγt+ ILC3 [17], which can be distinguished using genetic models or by co-staining with CD27 in the small intestine [5]

3. As the removal of the gut, the clearance of mesenteric fat, Peyer's Patches and the longitudinal opening are time intensive and represent a very vulnerable phase at the same time, we recommend to process one mouse at a time until the pre-cleaned gut is put into cold PBS. Due to the high sensitivity to timing, we recommend to start with no more than four gut equivalents (i.e., two small intestines and two colons) during the first runs of this protocol. More experienced users will be able to increase this number to up to eight guts.
4. The EDTA from the cell dissociation medium will sequester the divalent ions (mostly Calcium) from epithelial cell-junctions, making it possible to remove the epithelial layer by mechanical force. Depending on the mouse model you can shorten the incubation time from 20 to 15 (or even less) minutes. Have an eye on the color of the cell dissociation medium, if it turns bright-orange or yellow immediately replace it with fresh cell dissociation medium. A low pH will result in massive apoptosis of lamina propria lymphocytes. If you are interested in epithelial cells of the gut as well, you can also collect the supernatant after **step 9** and proceed with it as needed (e.g., put it into Trizol for RNA extraction).
5. You will need three times 5 mL digestion solution for the preparation of one sample. Since the enzymes are heat sensitive, this solution should be kept on ice until use. In order to increase viability of your cells, you can raise FCS levels up to 5%. But be aware that higher FCS concentrations will reduce digestion efficiency. Some antigens (such as CD27) will be cleaved off by dispase. If your molecule of interest cannot be found on the surface, try leaving out the dispase from the digestion solution. Although extracted cell numbers will drop dramatically, some antigens can be identified this way.
6. Place the tubes into the shaker in a way that the solutions are constantly mixed thoroughly. We recommend a speed of 120 rpm and an angle of approximately 30° (0° being horizontal). Optimal conditions will differ from one model to another.
7. In order to increase your yield, you can flush the strainer after the first digestion with 2–3 mL DMEM-10. During the first digestion you will collect approximately 60–70% of your total lymphocytes. More and longer digestion periods will increase the number of cells you dissociate from the lamina propria, but will negatively affect your cell viability.
8. A good indication of a successful gut preparation is a slight pink to red color of the tissue. The color originates from erythrocytes, which are very sensitive to cell death. At the end of **step 16** you should be able to see a small red ring

within your pellet. If you do not see it, most likely your cells died during the previous steps.

9. The "80%" and "40%" refer to percentage of Percoll stock solution. The actual Percoll dilutions are 72% and 36%, respectively.
10. Resuspension in 1 mL using a 1000 μL pipette will result in a more homogenous cell suspension. Single cells are more likely to traffic through the gradient undisturbed and end up in the right density layer. In order to overlay the "80%" solution with your "40%" Percoll containing the lamina propria lymphocytes, tilt the tube to an almost horizontal angle, decrease your pipette boy strength and slowly pipette the solution into the tube. The speed should be determined by gravity and not by the pump of your pipette boy as it will disrupt the layers. Be particularly careful when releasing the last drop of the solution as most pipette boy models will push it out with a certain force.
11. Inverting the tube is important as just filling it up might not disturb the Percoll layer. This would inhibit pellet formation. When removing the supernatant after centrifugation, it is advisable to remove it with a pipette boy until there is less than 1 mL left. Remove that last bit completely with a 1000 μL pipette.
12. 2.5×10^6 cells per staining is enough to accurately analyze populations and subpopulations of ILC in the small intestine and colon. More cells can be used but we advice not to use more than 5×10^6 cells per well. If five million cells are used, the volumes used for the staining steps should also be doubled.
13. The antibody cocktail to exclude T cells, B cells, and neutrophils/monocytes includes the following antibodies:

Antigen	Clone	Dilution
CD3	145-2C11	1:600
CD5	53-7.3	1:1000
CD19	MB19-1	1:100
Ly6C/G (Grl)	RB6-8C5	1:600

We recommend using biotinylated antibodies for the lineage cocktail, which can then be visualized by fluorophore-coupled streptavidin. In general, regular resuspension of cells in the staining solution will positively affect your staining efficiency (also for the surface and transcription factor stainings).

14. The following surface staining cocktail, in combination with subsequent staining for transcription factors, enables the visualization of most populations of ILC in the gut. It includes the following antibodies:

Antigen	Clone	Dilution
IL7Rα	A7R34	1:100
CD45.2[a]	104	1:200
CCR6	29-2L17	1:100
Streptavidin[b]	–	1:800

[a]This will work for C57BL/6, all 129 strains, BALB/c and CBA mice. For all other mouse strains, anti-CD45 (clone 30-F11) or anti-CD90 (clone G7) can be used.

[b]Streptavidin coupled to a fluorochrome of your choice.

15. We recommend fixing the cells in the "Foxp3/Transcription Factor Staining Buffer Set" from eBioscience overnight as it gives the brightest transcription factor staining, but any other formaldehyde based fixation should work as well. A minimum of 30 min fixation at 4 °C is needed, but better results can be obtained by fixing overnight.
16. Transcription factor staining cocktail:

Antigen	Clone	Dilution
RORγt	B2D	1:200
T-bet	4B10	1:200
GATA-3	TWAJ	1:200
Eomes	DAN11mag	1:200

References

1. Belkaid Y, Hand TW (2014) Role of the microbiota in immunity and inflammation. Cell 157:121–141. doi:10.1016/j.cell.2014.03.011
2. Mowat AM, Agace WW (2014) Regional specialization within the intestinal immune system. Nat Rev Immunol 14:667–685. doi:10.1038/nri3738
3. Walker JA, Barlow JL, McKenzie ANJ (2013) Innate lymphoid cells—how did we miss them? Nat Rev Immunol 13:75–87. doi:10.1038/nri3349
4. Mebius RE et al (2001) The fetal liver counterpart of adult common lymphoid progenitors gives rise to all lymphoid lineages, CD45+CD4+CD3− cells, as well as macrophages. J Immunol 166:6593–6601
5. Klose CSN et al (2014) Differentiation of type 1 ILCs from a common progenitor to all helper-like innate lymphoid cell lineages. Cell 157:340–356. doi:10.1016/j.cell.2014.03.030
6. Diefenbach A, Colonna M, Koyasu S (2014) Development, differentiation, and diversity of innate lymphoid cells. Immunity 41:354–365. doi:10.1016/j.immuni.2014.09.005
7. Wong SH et al (2012) Transcription factor RORα is critical for nuocyte development. Nat Immunol 13:229–236. doi:10.1038/ni.2208
8. Hoyler T et al (2012) The transcription factor GATA-3 controls cell fate and maintenance of type 2 innate lymphoid cells. Immunity 37:634–648. doi:10.1016/j.immuni.2012.06.020
9. Moro K et al (2009) Innate production of TH2 cytokines by adipose tissue-associated c-Kit+Sca-1+ lymphoid cells. Nature 463:540–544. doi:10.1038/nature08636
10. Neill DR et al (2010) Nuocytes represent a new innate effector leukocyte that mediates type-2 immunity. Nature 464:1367–1370. doi:10.1038/nature08900

11. Cella M et al (2009) A human natural killer cell subset provides an innate source of IL-22 for mucosal immunity. Nature 457:722–725. doi:10.1038/nature07537
12. Sonnenberg GF, Monticelli LA, Elloso MM, Fouser LA, Artis D (2011) CD4(+) lymphoid tissue-inducer cells promote innate immunity in the gut. Immunity 34:122–134. doi:10.1016/j.immuni.2010.12.009
13. Sonnenberg GF, Fouser LA, Artis D (2011) Border patrol: regulation of immunity, inflammation and tissue homeostasis at barrier surfaces by IL-22. Nat Immunol 12:383–390. doi:10.1038/ni.2025
14. Goto Y et al (2014) Innate lymphoid cells regulate intestinal epithelial cell glycosylation. Science (New York, NY) 345:1254009. doi:10.1126/science.1254009
15. Gordon SM et al (2012) The transcription factors T-bet and Eomes control key checkpoints of natural killer cell maturation. Immunity 36:55–67. doi:10.1016/j.immuni.2011.11.016
16. Sun JC, Lanier LL (2011) NK cell development, homeostasis and function: parallels with $CD8^+$ T cells. Nat Rev Immunol 11:645–657. doi:10.1038/nri3044
17. Vonarbourg C et al (2010) Regulated expression of nuclear receptor RORγt confers distinct functional fates to NK cell receptor-expressing RORγt(+) innate lymphocytes. Immunity 33:736–751. doi:10.1016/j.immuni.2010.10.017

Chapter 18

Analysis of Leukocytes in Oral Mucosal Tissues

Asaf Wilensky, Gabriel Mizraji, Yaara Tabib, Hafez Sharawi, and Avi-Hai Hovav

Abstract

The oral mucosa is constantly exposed to an immense amount of microorganisms, while some colonize the various anatomical niches existing in the oral cavity. To deal with such a complex challenge, the oral mucosal immune system must tolerate commensal microorganisms but prevent invasion of pathogens. Such activity is likely to be achieved by a wide range of mechanisms that could be similar or different to those employed by other mucosal tissues. The dental biofilm represents a unique challenge to the mucosal immune system, and inadequate immune responses might lead to periodontal diseases and the associated adverse systemic complications. It is thus crucial to study the mechanisms by which the oral mucosal immune system maintains homeostasis, and also induces protective immune responses against pathogens. To facilitate probing oral mucosal immunity, we describe here methods allowing immunological analysis of murine oral tissues using flow cytometry and immunofluorescence techniques.

Key words Oral, Mucosa, Immunity, Flow cytometry, Periodontitis

1 Introduction

The oral cavity is a unique anatomical structure, containing both soft and hard tissues that are continuously challenged by foreign antigens from air, food, and microorganisms. The major function of the local immune system is to protect the various tissues of the oral cavity such as teeth, gingiva, and jaws. This is achieved by maintaining immunological and microbial homeostasis, enabling the survival of commensals in the oral cavity while controlling their load and ability to invade the mucosa [1]. Upon infection with a pathogen, the oral mucosal immune system should induce an effective immune response that will prevent invasion with a minimal damage to the mucosa [2]. However, the presence of teeth, the only hard tissue in the body exposed to the hostile external environment, makes these immunological tasks highly complicated. Bacteria colonizing the tooth surface develop a complex and chronic biofilm, which puts a difficult challenge to the adjacent

Björn E. Clausen and Jon D. Laman (eds.), *Inflammation: Methods and Protocols*, Methods in Molecular Biology, vol. 1559, DOI 10.1007/978-1-4939-6786-5_18,

gingiva responsible to maintain local homeostasis [3, 4]. Nevertheless, this equilibrium is often disrupted, resulting in an excessive inflammatory response destructing soft and hard tissues [5]. Moreover, this can also facilitate intravascular dissemination of microorganisms throughout the body associated with adverse systemic conditions [6].

During the past decades much progress has been made in our understanding of the oral mucosal immune system. This is mainly attributed to work involving mouse studies, and the development of various models of experimental periodontitis. These studies revealed the important role of innate immunity components such as complement, neutrophils, and dendritic cells, as well as elements of adaptive immunity, particularly $CD4^+$ T cells, in inducing and regulating mucosal immunity against various oral immunological challenges [7–10]. Still, our knowledge regarding the mechanisms utilized by the oral mucosal immune system to fight pathogens is quite limited. Furthermore, the mechanism by which oral immunological and microbial homeostasis is maintained remains largely unexplored.

In this chapter, we provide a detailed description of methods enabling examination of oral mucosal immunity at steady state and inflammatory conditions. To induce inflammation we choose to describe the clinically relevant experimental periodontitis model, a technique by which an oral pathogen such as *Porphyromonas gingivalis* is inoculated by oral gavage to induce inflammation-driven bone loss. The chapter also describes how to excise and process various oral tissues, thus facilitating immunological analysis in other experimental settings.

2 Materials

2.1 Murine Model of Periodontitis

1. 8–10-week-old, sex- and weight-matched mice.
2. Anaerobic Wilkins media (Wilkins-Chalgren Anaerobe Broth—Oxoid).
3. *Porphyromonas gingivalis* (*P. gingivalis*).
4. Carboxymethyl cellulose (CMC).
5. Anaerobic sterile saline solution.
6. Gavage needle No. 22.

2.2 Isolation of Murine Oral Tissues

1. Sharp tissue scissors.
2. Scalpel holder and No. 10, 15C blades.
3. Tissue pliers.
4. Working solution: 2% FCS in PBS (Ca^+ and Mg^+ free).

2.3 Epithelial Sheet Separation

1. Dispase II.
2. PBS (Ca^+ and Mg^+ free).

2.4 Flow Cytometry

1. Working solution: 2 % FCS in PBS (Ca^+ and Mg^+ free), pH 7.2.
2. Propidium Iodide solution or 7-AAD for live/dead cell discrimination.
3. 70-μm nylon cell strainers.
4. The specifics and source of monoclonal antibodies used for flow cytometry are provided in Table 1.

2.5 Immuno fluorescence Microscopy

1. Hoechst stain.
2. 4 % paraformaldehyde or 95 % ethanol.
3. Optimal Cutting Temperature (O.C.T.) compound (Sakura).
4. Liquid nitrogen.
5. Working solution: 2 % FCS in PBS (Ca^+ and Mg^+ free), pH 7.2.
6. Dispase II solution—2 mg/ml in Working solution.
7. Blocking solution: 8 % FCS and 5 % Triton in PBS.
8. The specifics and source of monoclonal antibodies used for immunofluorescence staining are provided in Table 2.

Table 1
Antibodies used for FACS analysis of leukocytes present in murine oral mucosa

Specificity	Clone	Species	Isotype	Supplier
CD45	104	Mouse (SJL)	IgG2a, κ	Biolegend
MHC II	M5/114.15.2	Rat	IgG2b, κ	Biolegend
CD11c	N418	Armenian Hamster	IgG	Biolegend
CD3	17A2	Rat	IgG2b, κ	Biolegend
CD19	6D5	Rat	IgG2a, κ	Biolegend
NK1.1	PK136	Mouse	IgG2a, κ	Biolegend
CD11b	M1/70	Rat	IgG2b, κ	Biolegend
Ly6C	HK1.4	Rat	IgG2c, κ	Biolegend
Ly6G	1A8	Rat	IgG2a, κ	Biolegend
CD4	GK1.5	Rat	IgG2b, κ	Biolegend
CD8α	53-6.7	Rat	IgG2a, κ	Biolegend
EpCAM	G8.8	Rat	IgG2a, κ	Biolegend

Table 2
Antibodies used for immunofluorescence analysis in this study

Specificity	Clone	Species	Isotype	Supplier
Langerin	eBioL31	Rat	IgG2a	eBioscience
MHC II	M5/114.15.2	Rat	IgG2b, κ	Biolegend
Hoechst				Sigma

3 Methods

3.1 Murine Model of Periodontitis

There are various models to induce experimental periodontitis. In this section we describe a widely used method involving an oral gavage to administer the oral pathogen *P. gingivalis* (other oral pathogens can be also inoculated this way). In this model the mice are inoculated several times with the pathogen, however, the number of gavages and the intervals between them varies among the different groups employing this method. Here, we describe an approach successfully used in our laboratory in which the mice receive three consecutive gavages with 2-day intervals (*see* **Note 10**).

3.1.1 Growing of P. gingivalis

Prior to growing *P. gingivalis* prepare Wilkins media as indicated by the manufacturer, and place in an anaerobic jar at 37 °C for at least 6 h.

1. Grow frozen *P. gingivalis* in 9 ml of anaerobic Wilkins medium. Incubate in anaerobic conditions, 37 °C for 24 h.
2. Check the bacteria in the microscope. If there are no signs of contamination (for instance, shape and motility), transfer 1 ml of *P. gingivalis* to new 9 ml of anaerobic Wilkins medium. Incubate for 24 h at 37 °C.
3. Check the bacteria in the microscope. If there are no signs of contamination add 90 ml of anaerobic Wilkins medium. Incubate at 37 °C for 1 day.

3.1.2 Preparation of P. gingivalis for Oral Gavage

Prepare anaerobic sterile saline solution (250 ml approximately).

1. Spin down bacteria in a pre-cold centrifuge at 4500 × *g* at 4 °C for 20 min.
2. Discard supernatant, add 40 ml of cold anaerobic saline solution and mix the bacteria.
3. Centrifuge at 4500 × *g* at 4 °C for 20 min.
4. Repeat **steps 2** and **3**.
5. Add 2 ml of cold anaerobic saline solution, mix well and place the bacteria on ice.

6. Quantify bacterial number using spectrophotometer.
7. Prepare 4% CMC with saline solution (2 g of CMC in 50 ml of saline solution), on a hot plate at 56 °C with magnetic stirrer. Once the powder has dissolved place the CMC on ice.
8. Mix equal volume of 4% CMC with *P. gingivalis* to obtain bacteria in 2% CMC.
9. Aspirate the prepared bacteria with a 2 ml syringe and cap it with the gavage needle.
10. Hold the mouse, insert the needle into the oral cavity and drop 200 μl of the bacteria in 2% CMC (Fig. 1a) (*see* **Note 11**).
11. Repeat Subheadings 3.1.1 and 3.1.2 two more times with 48 h intervals.

3.2 Isolation of Oral Tissues

The oral cavity has distinct anatomical niches, each with its unique leukocyte content, thus suggesting an immunological functional specification. To isolate each niche properly, one should have a deep understanding of the anatomy of the murine oral cavity (Fig. 1b) (*see* **Note 1**).

3.2.1 Isolation of the Buccal Mucosa

The buccal mucosa is located at the sides of the oral cavity posterior to the commissure, anterior to the anterior pillar and between the upper and lower vestibule (Fig. 2a).

1. Using scissors, cut the buccal mucosa in the lower vestibule until the mandibular ramus.
2. Cut the ramus of the mandible, in a deep and strong cut (externally of the anterior pillar).
3. Repeat this step on the other side of the mouth and then pull down the mandible.

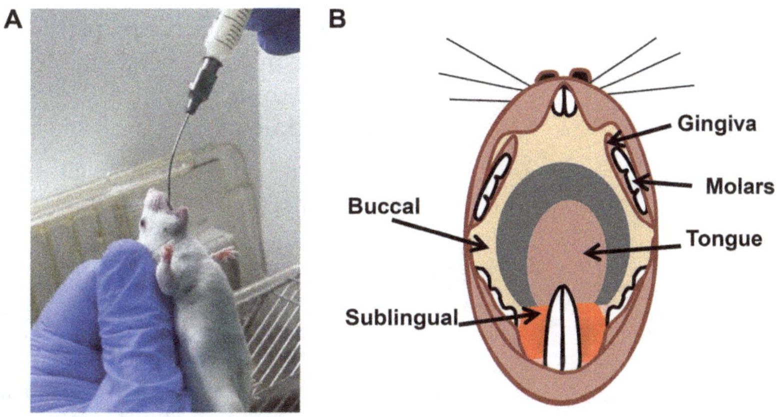

Fig. 1 (**a**) Representative photograph demonstrating the inoculation of a mouse with *P. gingivalis* in 2% CMC solution by oral gavage using a syringe No. 22. (**b**) Schematic representation of the oral mucosal surfaces described in this study

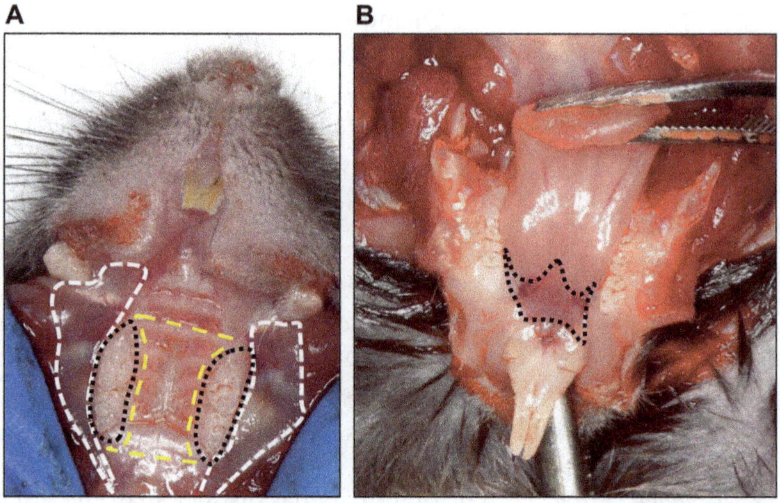

Fig. 2 Representative photographs demonstrating the anatomical location of the (**a**) buccal mucosa (*white lines*), gingiva (*black lines*), palate mucosa (*yellow lines*) and (**b**) sublingual mucosa

4. Using scissors, incise upper vestibule.
5. Using a No. 15C blade delineate the anterior and the posterior limits of the oral mucosa (*see* **Note 4**).
6. Peel off and place the tissue in 1 ml of Working solution in a plate.

3.2.2 Upper Gingiva and Palatal Mucosa

The gingiva covers the alveolar bone. We describe the isolation of the gingiva surrounding the upper molars (Fig. 2a) (*see* **Note 2**).

1. Perform **steps 1–3** of buccal mucosa isolation (Subheading 3.2.1).
2. Using sharp bladed scissors, placed perpendicular to the plane of the palate, make a lateral cut (from right to left) 1 mm posterior to the third molar (it is important to cut through both soft and hard tissues).
3. With the same scissors, make another lateral cut 2 mm posterior to the incisors.
4. Expose the nasal cavity by pulling down the nose (anterior to the last cut).
5. Detach the palatal and the maxillary bone from the skull using scissors placed parallel to the plane of the palate, one blade inside the nasal cavity and the other laterally (on the mucogingival line) and then make the incision (*see* **Note 3**).
6. Repeat the last step in the other side of the mouth.
7. Detach the palatal and maxillary bone.

8. Peel off the soft tissue from the bone using tissue pliers. It is easier to begin from the anterior aspect.
9. Place the soft tissue on paper (the epithelial side toward it). With a No. 15C blade separate the gingival tissue from the palatal mucosa.
10. Place the tissue in 1 ml of Working solution in a plate.

3.2.3 Sublingual Mucosa

The sublingual mucosa covers the floor of the mouth and it is situated beneath the tongue, limited by the gingiva laterally and anteriorly and with the ventral aspect of the tongue base posteriorly (Fig. 2b).

1. Perform **steps 1–3** of buccal mucosa isolation (Subheading 3.2.1).
2. Separate the mandible from the mouse and secure it with needles. One needle in the tongue stretching it backward. Place two additional needles on the sides.
3. With a No. 15C blade incise next to the mandibular bone separating the gingiva from the sublingual tissue at both sides.
4. With Dumont #5c forceps penetrate from the lateral cut and separate the mucosa from the subjacent muscular tissue.
5. Make anterior and posterior incisions with small scissors.
6. Peel off the sublingual mucosa and place it in working media.

3.2.4 Tongue

1. Grasp the tongue with Adson forceps and cut the tongue at its base.
2. To separate the dorsal and ventral aspect cut the tongue transversally with a No. 10 blade.
3. Place the tissue in 1 ml of Working solution in a plate.

3.3 Epithelial Sheet Separation

Soft tissues of the oral cavity are frequently exposed to bacteria and other microorganisms. Host-microbe homeostasis is considered to involve interaction between the outermost layers (i.e., the epithelium) and oral microbiota. The oral mucosal epithelium is stratified, allowing simple separation from the underneath lamina propria layer while leaving both layers intact.

3.3.1 Separation of the Epithelial Layer (see Note 5)

1. Incubate the oral tissues in 2 ml of Dispase II solution per sample for 35 min at 37 °C. For sublingual and buccal tissues, incubate for 1 h. To separate the tongue epithelium, dissect it to dorsal and ventral halves and then incubate in 1 mg/ml of Dispase II solution at 4 °C for 4 h.
2. Under a stereoscope, place the samples with the epithelium side facing up. Use delicate forceps in order to remove the epithelium from the underlining submucosa (*see* **Note 6**).

3.4 Processing Murine Oral Tissues for Preparation of a Single Cell Suspension

1. Mince the tissue to tiny pieces using a blade, and transfer it to a 15 ml test tube (*see* **Note 8**).
2. Rinse the plate with 1 ml of digestion solution and transfer it to the same 15 ml test tube.
3. Incubate for 20 min at 37 °C in a shaker.
4. Add 20 μl of 0.5 M EDTA per 2 ml sample to the digested tissue and incubate for an additional 10 min in order to stop the enzymatic activity.
5. Wash the cells with 10 ml of Working solution and spin down for 8 min at 400 × *g*.
6. Remove the supernatant and add 2 ml of Working solution.
7. Filter the samples through a 70-μm cell strainer and then spin down the sample for 6 min at 300 × *g*.
8. Remove the supernatant leaving 300 μl for further staining.
9. Count the cells.

3.5 Flow Cytometry Staining (see Note 7)

1. Prepare the antibodies for staining: add the total volume of the antibodies required to stain all samples to washing medium (100 μl of washing medium per sample).
2. Add 100 μl of the antibody solution to each sample, vortex and keep on ice for 15 min in the dark (*see* **Note 9**).
3. Wash the cells with 2 ml of Working solution and spin down for 6 min at 300 × *g*.
4. Remove the supernatant and add 300 μl of Working solution.
5. Filtrate each sample through a 70-μm nylon cell strainer into a FACS tube.
6. Add 2 μl of the propidium iodide solution 10 min before acquiring the sample in a flow cytometer.
7. Please *see* Figs. 3 and 4 for gating strategies and representative results obtained from mice infected with *P. gingivalis*.

3.6 Whole Mount Immunofluorescence Staining

1. Separate the epithelial and lamina propria layers as described in Subheading 3.3.
2. Transfer the separated tissues into 4% paraformaldehyde at 4 °C for 1 h or into ice-cold 95% ethanol at −20 °C for 45 min.
3. Soak the samples in PBS for 15 min at room temperature on a shaker, and repeat this step three times.
4. Incubate the samples in blocking solution for 1 h at room temperature on a shaker.
5. Transfer the samples into primary antibody solution (diluted 1:100 in blocking solution) at 4 °C overnight.
6. Wash the samples with PBS for 15 min at room temperature on a shaker, and repeat it three times.

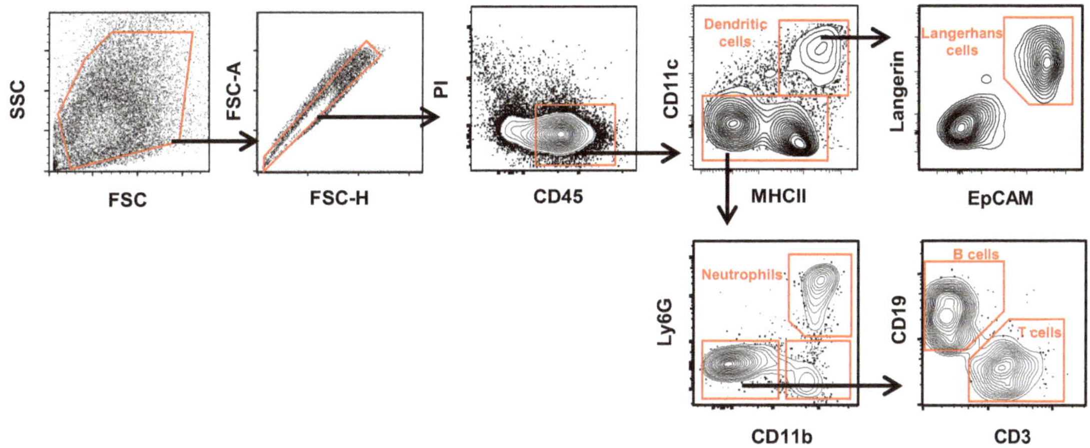

Fig. 3 Gating strategy for the analysis of leukocyte subsets in the oral mucosa. A general gate is performed on SSC/FSC plot to discard cell debris. Doublets are then excluded by gating on the events positioned on a diagonal of FSC-A (area) and FSC-H (height). Live leukocytes are selected by gating on cells that are CD45$^+$ but negative for propidium iodide. The various leukocyte subsets can then be identified using common surface markers

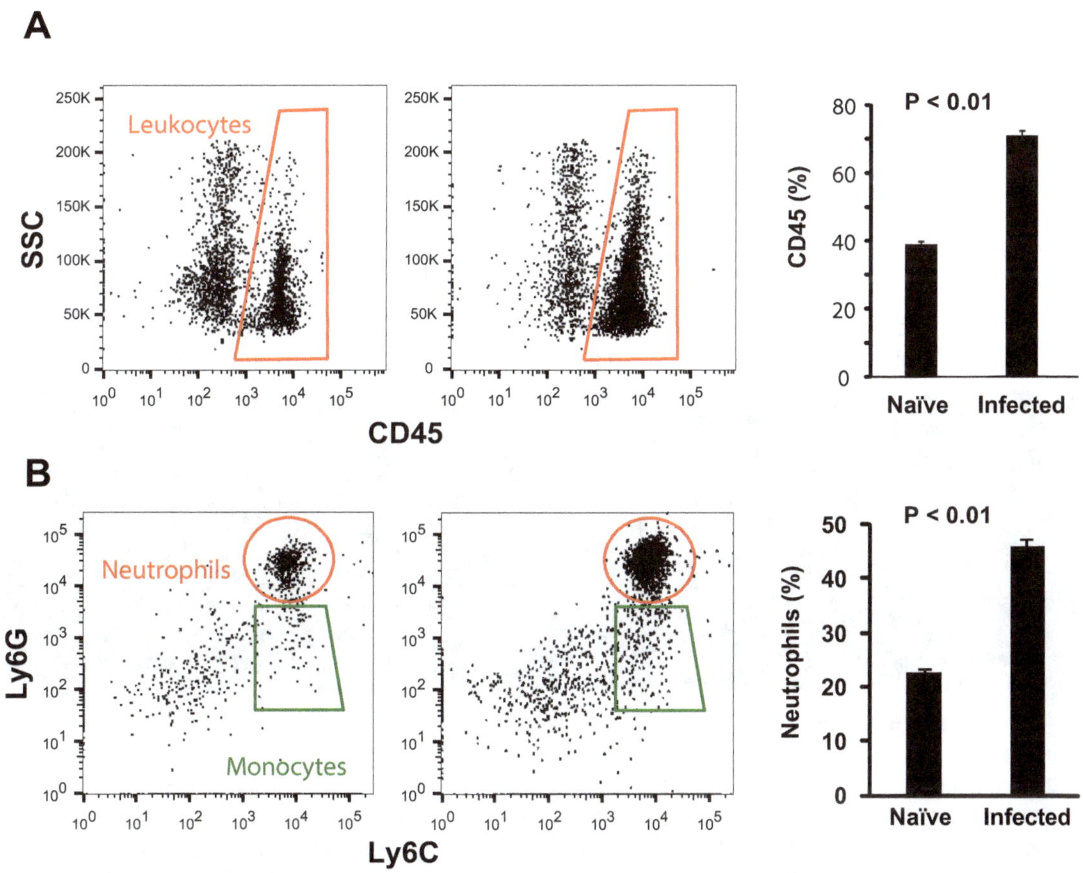

Fig. 4 Inoculation of *P. gingivalis* by oral gavage induces a local inflammatory response in the gingiva. Mice were inculcated with *P. gingivalis* and 3 days later the frequency of (**a**) total leukocytes and (**b**) neutrophils was determined in the gingiva by flow cytometry

7. Transfer the samples into secondary antibody solution (1:200 in blocking solution) at room temperature for 1.5 h on a shaker.
8. Wash the samples with PBS for 15 min at room temperature on a shaker, and repeat it three times.
9. Incubate in Hoechst solution (1 μl in 10 ml PBS) at room temperature for 10 min on a shaker.
10. Wash the samples with PBS for 15 min at room temperature on a shaker, and repeat it three times.
11. Under a stereoscope, using thin brushes flatten the samples on slides in the desired orientation, dry the slides carefully without touching the tissues, add fluorescence mounting medium and close the slides with a cover glass.
12. Refer to Fig. 5 for representative results.

3.6.1 Immuno fluorescence Staining: Cross Sections

1. Extract one side of the lower jaw from each mouse so all three molars will be included as one part, and insert the tissue into 4% paraformaldehyde at 4 °C overnight.
2. To discard the bone and the enamel tissues transfer the samples into 0.5 M EDTA pH 8.5 and incubate at 4 °C for 7 days. Refresh with new solution every 2 days.
3. Immerse the samples into OCT, snap-freeze in liquid nitrogen, and store at −80 °C until use.

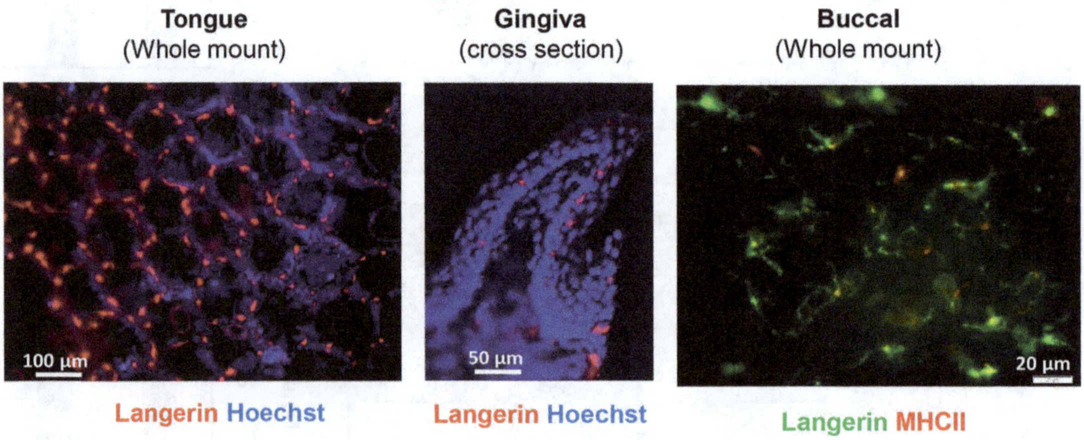

Fig. 5 Immunofluorescence analysis of oral mucosal tissues. (**a**) An epithelial layer from the dorsal aspect of the tongue from a naive B6 mouse was stained for langerin (*red*), and Hoechst (nuclei, *blue*) and analyzed by confocal microscopy. (**b**) Gingival cross section of a naive B6 mouse was stained with antibodies against langerin (*red*) and Hoechst (*blue*) for immunofluorescence analysis. (**c**) An epithelial layer from the buccal of a naive B6 mouse was stained for langerin (*green*), MHCII (*red*), and Hoechst (nuclei, *blue*) and analyzed by confocal microscopy

4. Using a cryostat cut 8 μm cryosections of the jaw and incubate in a closed chamber at room temperature overnight. The next day store at −80 °C until use or begin the staining.
5. Section can be stained with H&E using standard procedures, or by immunofluorescence using the protocol indicated in Subheading 3.6.1 (**steps 3–10**).
6. Dry the slides carefully without touching the tissues, add fluorescence mounting medium and close the slides with a cover glass.
7. Please *see* Fig. 5 for representative results.

4 Notes

1. In this study, we did not specify the strain of *P. gingivalis* used to induce inflammation. Several strains of *P. gingivalis* are described in the literature, and each one of them can be used to induce local inflammation by oral gavage. Nevertheless, the various strains might differ in their capacity to cause periodontal bone loss.
2. When performing an oral gavage, most of the bacterial solution should be placed in the oral cavity of the mouse. Hence, pull out the needle slowly while injecting the solution.
3. Excision of the oral mucosal tissues described above requires a profound understanding of the anatomy of the oral cavity. We highly recommend including a dentist or an expert of the oral cavity when executing for the first time the protocols described in this study.
4. Regarding Subheading 3.2.1 (Isolation of the buccal mucosa) after the anterior and posterior incision the tissue retracts itself. Take into consideration that the oral mucosa has a pallid pink color and the muscle underneath is red.
5. It is highly recommended to use magnifying lenses (Loupes) when isolating oral mucosal tissues.
6. Regarding Subheading 3.3.1, after the separation of the epithelial sheet, you can use the cells for the distinct oral mucosal tissues are located close to each other, and each tissue might contain different types and frequencies of leukocyte subsets. It is very important to precisely isolate the oral tissues, as failing to do so will probably lead to inconsistent results.
7. When separating epithelial layers, it is important to use the recommended incubation times in a Dispase solution for each tissue. Separation of the mucosal epithelium is relatively easy but requires some practice.
8. Regarding step 3.3.1, after the separation of the epithelial sheet, you can use the cells for further RNA or protein isolation.

9. When processing large numbers of mice, keep the tissues on ice until processing.
10. Due to the small size of the oral mucosal tissues, it is necessary to pool tissues from at least 2–3 mice in order to obtain sufficient cell numbers for flow cytometry analysis.
11. Regarding step 3.5, it is recommended to stain cells inside a hood, without light. Keeping the cells and the solutions on ice throughout the procedure will increase cell viability.

References

1. Hovav AH (2014) Dendritic cells of the oral mucosa. Mucosal Immunol 7:27–37. doi:10.1038/mi.2013.42
2. Ebersole JL et al (2013) Periodontal disease immunology: 'double indemnity' in protecting the host. Periodontology 2000(62):163–202. doi:10.1111/prd.12005
3. Kolenbrander PE, Palmer RJ Jr, Periasamy S, Jakubovics NS (2010) Oral multispecies biofilm development and the key role of cell-cell distance. Nat Rev Microbiol 8:471–480. doi:10.1038/nrmicro2381
4. Socransky SS, Haffajee AD, Cugini MA, Smith C, Kent RL Jr (1998) Microbial complexes in subgingival plaque. J Clin Periodontol 25:134–144
5. Garlet GP (2010) Destructive and protective roles of cytokines in periodontitis: a re-appraisal from host defense and tissue destruction viewpoints. J Dent Res 89:1349–1363. doi:10.1177/0022034510376402
6. Hajishengallis G (2015) Periodontitis: from microbial immune subversion to systemic inflammation. Nat Rev Immunol 15:30–44. doi:10.1038/nri3785
7. Arizon M et al (2012) Langerhans cells down-regulate inflammation-driven alveolar bone loss. Proc Natl Acad Sci U S A 109:7043–7048. doi:10.1073/pnas.1116770109
8. Hajishengallis G, Abe T, Maekawa T, Hajishengallis E, Lambris JD (2013) Role of complement in host-microbe homeostasis of the periodontium. Semin Immunol 25:65–72. doi:10.1016/j.smim.2013.04.004
9. Hajishengallis G, Chavakis T, Hajishengallis E, Lambris JD (2014) Neutrophil homeostasis and inflammation: novel paradigms from studying periodontitis. J Leukoc Biol. doi:10.1189/jlb.3VMR1014-468R
10. Wilensky A et al (2014) Dendritic cells and their role in periodontal disease. Oral Dis 20:119–126. doi:10.1111/odi.12122

Chapter 19

Optimized Mouse Models for Liver Fibrosis

Yong Ook Kim, Yury Popov, and Detlef Schuppan

Abstract

Fibrosis is the excessive accumulation of extracellular matrix components due to chronic injury, with collagens as predominant structural components. Liver fibrosis can progress to cirrhosis, which is characterized by a severe distortion of the delicate hepatic vascular architecture, the shunting of the blood supply away from hepatocytes and the resultant functional liver failure. Cirrhosis is associated with a highly increased morbidity and mortality and represents the major hard endpoint in clinical studies of chronic liver diseases. Moreover, cirrhosis is a strong cofactor of primary liver cancer. In vivo models are indispensable tools to study the cellular and molecular mechanisms of liver fibrosis and to develop specific antifibrotic therapies towards clinical translation. Here, we provide a detailed description of select optimized mouse models of liver fibrosis and state-of-the-art fibrosis readouts.

Key words Biliary fibrosis, Carbon tetrachloride (CCL_4), Cirrhosis, Collagen, Extracellular matrix (ECM), Fibrosis, Hydroxyproline (HYP), Liver fibrosis, Mdr2-knockout, Metavir staging, Panlobular fibrosis, Picrosirius Red, Thioacetamide (TAA)

1 Introduction

Fibrosis is defined as excessive deposition of extracellular matrix (ECM) components resulting from a protracted wound-healing response. Fibrosis is the default response to continuing tissue injury and associated with most chronic inflammatory diseases. Advanced fibrosis leads to replacement of functional by scar tissue, a distortion of the normal vascular architecture and organ dysfunction or even demise. Moreover, advanced fibrosis is a predisposition for the development of cancers, especially in epithelial organs. Therefore fibrotic diseases are responsible for up to 45 % of overall mortality worldwide [1, 2]. Liver fibrosis and its advanced stage cirrhosis are characterized by vascular architectural distortion and liver dysfunction resulting from chronic liver injury [3]. Major etiologies of liver fibrosis and cirrhosis are chronic viral hepatitis B or C, toxic (e.g., alcoholic) liver disease, autoimmune and biliary diseases, e.g., primary biliary cirrhosis (PBC) and primary sclerosing

Björn E. Clausen and Jon D. Laman (eds.), *Inflammation: Methods and Protocols*, Methods in Molecular Biology, vol. 1559, DOI 10.1007/978-1-4939-6786-5_19, © Springer Science+Business Media LLC 2017

cholangitis (PSC), and increasingly nonalcoholic steatohepatitis (NASH), which is linked to obesity, type 2 diabetes, and metabolic syndrome [2–5].

Notably, even advanced fibrosis is not considered any longer static and irreversible, but rather a dynamic process due to a dysbalance of fibrolysis (removal of excessive ECM) tilted in favor of enhanced ECM synthesis and deposition (fibrogenesis). Thus long-term suppression of the hepatitis B virus or elimination of the hepatitis C virus by effective antiviral therapies have shown that even (clinically still compensated) cirrhosis can reverse to a noncirrhotic liver over several years [6, 7]. Combined with the increasing understanding of the cellular and intercellular signaling underlying fibrogenesis or fibrolysis, a relevant focus of translational research is now aimed at (organ specific) antifibrotic therapies that do not only inhibit progression but also induce reversal of advanced fibrosis. Here not only the fibrogenic effector cells that produce the excess ECM (mainly activated myofibroblasts), but also injured epithelia, activated immune cells, and vascular cells, and their molecular specifics have become important pharmacological targets [1–5, 8]. In basic and translational research the use of rodent models of liver fibrosis has become indispensable. There exist more fibrosis models for liver than for other organs, and several of these mirror important facets of human pathology. Importantly, it appears that the fibrotic responses in humans can be replicated fairly well by a good selection of rodent (mainly mouse) models, and that differences of involved downstream effector cells (mainly myofibroblasts) and ECM molecules between species are less obvious than for example for immune cells and cyto/chemokines [2, 4, 5, 9, 10].

Here we present a selection of rodent liver fibrosis models that we optimized for mechanistic studies and especially for testing and validation of antifibrotic therapies, as an important step before clinical translation [8, 9]. Among a variety of rodent models [11] we prefer to use mouse models that incur much lower costs for maintenance and reagents, and that permit broad mechanistic studies due to the broad availability of transgenic animals. Here we describe Mdr2 (Abcb4, bile canalicular phospholipid flippase) knockout mice as a model of spontaneously progressive secondary biliary fibrosis [12, 13], and the refined models of toxin-induced parenchymal liver damage and fibrosis, induced by carbon tetrachloride (CCL_4) and thioacetamide (TAA) [14]. When performed properly, the latter two models can be used to study both fibrosis progression and its regression (after discontinuation of the toxin). A combination of three of these models ($Mdr2^{-/-}$ and toxin-induced progression as well as regression) is a fairly good predictor of fibrosis scenarios that occur in human livers, despite the usually more aggressive and faster evolution of fibrosis in the experimental models [1, 9]. Moreover, in our experience their combination is a good predictor of antifibrotic drug effects in patients (own unpublished data). These (optimized) models have been characterized extensively by us and key readouts related to fibrosis, fibrogenesis, and fibrolysis are well established [2, 9, 12–21]. While mechanism and phenotype underlying fibrosis in the $Mdr2^{-/-}$ knockout (accumulation of toxic bile acids in hepatocytes and initiation of a profibrogenic cholangiocyte response) are well defined and have a human correlate (progressive familial intrahepatic cholestatasis type 3, PFIC-3; resembling also secondary sclerosing cholangitis, PSC) [13, 22, 23], the mechanisms of fibrosis induced by CCL_4 and TAA have not been fully elucidated. CCL_4, like other haloalkanes, is activated by oxidases to yield the trichloromethyl (CCl3) radical, which initiates lipid peroxidation and can react with the sulfhydryl groups of proteins leading to hepatocyte necrosis, apoptosis, and necroapoptosis [24, 25], with defective repair and liver fibrosis that increases with the intensity and duration of toxin exposure. Notably, fibrosis starts from the hepatic centrilobular zone 3 and progresses towards the portal tracts of zone 1, opposite to the biliary fibrosis in $Mdr2^{-/-}$ mice. Likewise, the thiono-sulfur-compound TAA is oxidatively bioactivated in hepatocytes leading to reactive S and S-S oxides that react with amine-lipids and amino groups of proteins. They are likely to be responsible for TAA hepatoxicity [26], yielding a liver damage and fibrosis pattern similar to the CCL_4, model, but with a more prominent zone 1 injury. Importantly, the advanced toxin models as performed by us do not show a significant fibrosis regression (despite a favorable architectural remodeling) after toxin discontinuation over up to 36 weeks, which makes them excellent predictors of "true antifibrotic drug effects" for translation towards human studies. In this chapter, we provide an indepth description of these models including detailed experimental protocols for state-of-the-art fibrosis related readouts including liver collagen quantification, general histomorphometry, and qRT-PCR.

2 Materials

2.1 Mouse Models

2.1.1 Model of Hepatotoxin (CCL_4 or TAA)-Induced Panlobular Fibrosis Progression and Fibrosis Regression

1. 7–8-week-old sex- and weight-matched C57BL/6 or BALB/c mice (*see* **Note 1**).
2. Hepatotoxic reagent: Carbon tetrachloride (CCL_4) or thioacetamide (TAA), mineral oil and distilled water as vehicle for CCL_4 or TAA, respectively.
3. 1 ml syringe and gavage needle.

2.1.2 Model of Portal/Periductular Fibrosis ($Mdr2^{-/-}$ Mice)

1. 6 week old female (male) $Mdr2^{-/-}$ mice (C57BL/6) and their wild type controls (*see* **Note 2**).

2.2 Mouse Anesthesia and Organ Collection

1. Anesthetics (e.g., isoflurane, ketamine–xylazine mixture), injection needle, and devices for mouse autopsy.
2. Balance.
3. Liquid nitrogen.

2.3 Hydroxyproline (HYP) Assay

All solutions are made with ultrapure water (using deionized water with a resistance of 18 MΩ cm at 25 °C) and analytical grade reagents. Preparation and storage of all reagents at room temperature (RT) (unless indicated otherwise).

2.3.1 Large Volume Assay

1. Hand homogenizer or tissuelyser.
2. Dry oven.
3. Spectrophotometer.
4. 6 N HCl.
5. 50% isopropanol.
6. 0.84% chloramine-T: 42 mM sodium acetate, 2.6 mM citric acid, 39.5% (v/v) isopropanol, pH 6.0. Store at 4 °C.
7. 12% Ehrlich's reagent: 0.248 g of *p*-dimethylamino-benzaldehyde in 0.27 ml of 60% perchloric acid and 0.73 ml isopropanol. Should be prepared immediately before use.
8. High purity hydroxyproline (HYP) for standards: 0, 0.1, 0.2, 0.4, 0.6, 0.8, 1.0, and 1.6 μg HYP/ml water.

2.3.2 Microplate Assay

1. Hand homogenizer or tissuelyser.
2. Dry oven.
3. Spectrophotometer.
4. 96-well microplate.
5. 6 N HCl.
6. Citrate-acetate acid buffer: 5% citric acid, 7.24% sodium acetate, 3.4% NaOH, 1.2% glacial acetic acid, pH 6.0. Can be stored for several months at 4 °C, but should be used at RT before assay.
7. 1.3% Chloramine-T: 32 ml citrate-acetate buffer pH 6.0, 4 ml distilled water, 4 ml isoropanol, 564 mg Chloramine-T hydrate (*see* **Note 3**). Store at 4 °C.
8. 14% Ehrlich's reagent: 4.5 g of *p*-dimethylamino-benzaldehyde, 7.8 ml of 70% perchloric acid, and 18.6 ml isopropanol. Should be prepared immediately before use.
9. High purity HYP for standards: 10, 20, 40, 60, 80, 100, and 200 μg HYP/ml water.

2.4 Histology

2.4.1 Preparation of Paraffin Sections

1. Tissue processor.
2. Tissue embedder.
3. Microtome.

4. Water bath.
5. Glass slides and cover glass.
6. Mounting medium.
7. 4% formaldehyde, a series of graded isopropanol/water, xylene, paraffin wax.
8. Histology cassette and metal mold.

2.4.2 Picrosirius Red Staining

1. Mayer's hematoxylin solution.
2. Picrosirius Red solution: 0.5 g Sirius red, e.g., Direct Red 80, 500 ml of 1.3% saturated aqueous solution of picric acid. The reagent can be stored at RT for at least 3 years.
3. Acidified water: 5 ml glacial acetic acid, 1 l distilled water.
4. Isopropanol and xylene.
5. Xylene-based mounting medium.
6. Light microscope, Image analyzer (ImageJ; NIH, Bethesda, MD).

2.4.3 Hematoxylin and Eosin Staining

1. Mayer's hematoxylin solution.
2. 0.25% eosin Y solution: 250 ml eosin Y stock solution, 750 ml 80% ethanol, 5 ml glacial acetic acid. 1% stock solution: 10 g eosin Y, 200 ml distilled water, 800 ml 95% ethanol.
3. Ethanol and xylene.
4. Xylene-based mounting medium.

3 Methods

3.1 Model of Hepatotoxin (CCL_4 or TAA)-Induced Panlobular Fibrosis Progression and Regression

1. Mice are maintained in specific pathogen-free conditions on a 12-h light–12-h dark cycle in an air conditioned room at 25 °C and provided water and standard mouse pellet chow ad libitum.
2. Mice receive escalating doses of CCL_4 (50/50 vol. mixed with mineral oil) three times per week via oral gavage, starting with 0.875 ml/kg (1st dose, week 1), 1.75 ml/kg (2nd to 9th dose, week 1–4), 2.5 ml/kg (10th to 23rd dose, week 4–8), and 3.25 ml/kg (after week 8). The working solution can be stored at RT (*see* Fig. 1).
3. Alternatively, fibrosis is induced by escalating doses of TAA dissolved in 200 μl PBS, intraperitoneally three times a week, starting with 50 mg/kg (1st and 2nd dose, week 1) (*see* **Note 4**), 100 mg/kg (2nd to 5th dose, week 1–2), 200 mg/kg (6th to 10th dose, week 2–4), 300 mg/kg (11th to 15th dose, week 4–5), and 400 mg/kg (16th dose onwards, after week 6). The working solution is stored at 4 °C. Prepare fresh solution every week (*see* Fig. 2).

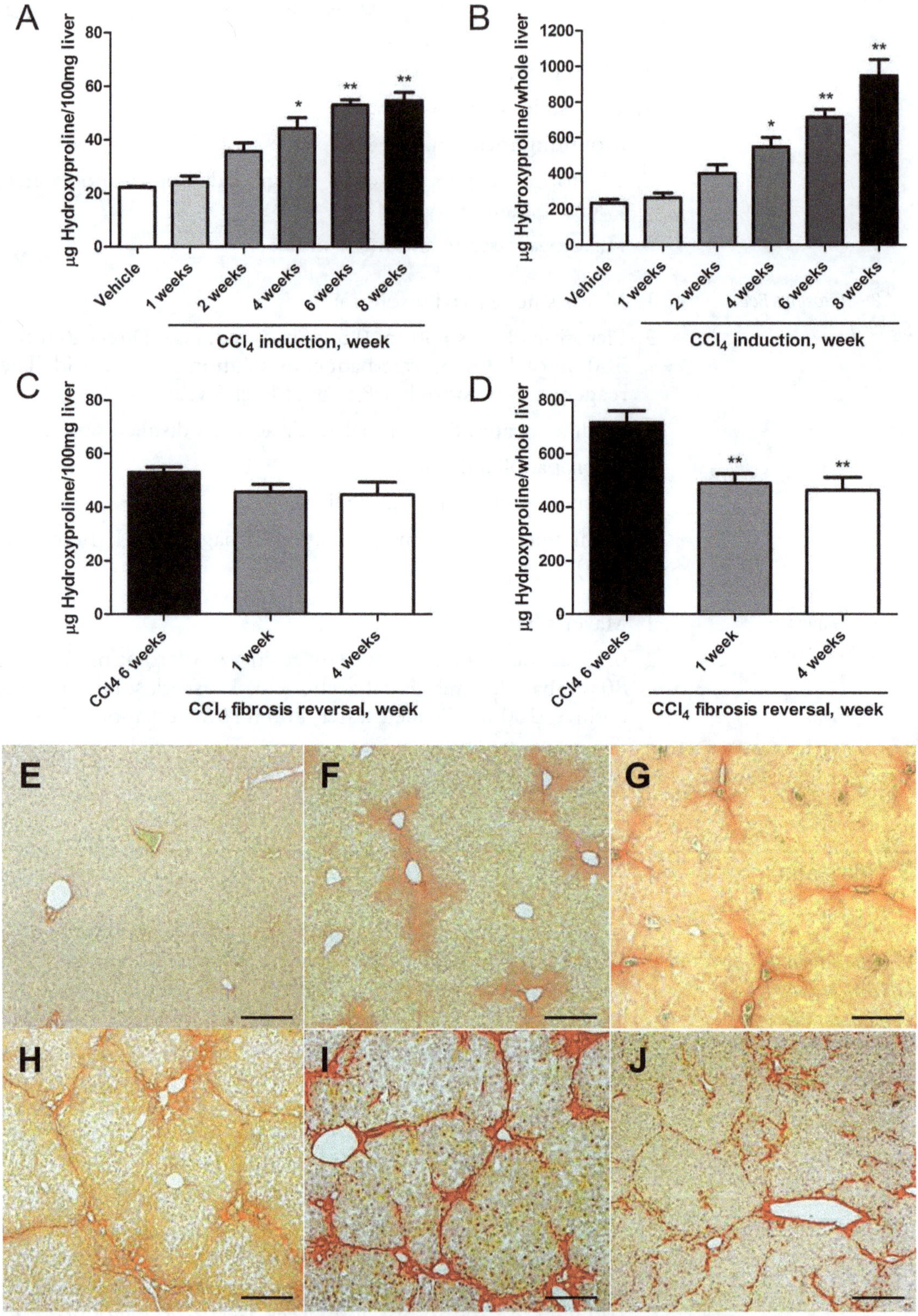

Fig. 1 Changes of liver HYP content and Picrosirius Red stained area in the CCL_4-induced fibrosis progression and regression models in C57BL/6 mice. (**a**–**d**) HYP content per 100 mg liver and per whole liver. HYP content expressed as (**a**) relative (μg per 100 mg liver, derived from the left and median lobes) at week 1, 2, 4, 6, and 8 of fibrosis induction, and (**b**) total hepatic HYP expressed as μg per liver, at week 1, 2, 4, 6, and 8 of fibrosis

4. For the generation of an advanced fibrosis progression model, mice are treated for at least 6 weeks, for induction of bridging fibrosis/cirrhosis treatment is given for 10–12 weeks (*see* **Note 5**). To study (advanced or cirrhotic) fibrosis regression, toxins are applied for 6 or 10–12 weeks, respectively, and the mice are followed for 2–4 or up to 36 weeks off the toxin, with little or no spontaneous regression, respectively [14] (*see* Figs. 1 and 2).
5. Mice are sacrificed 1–2 days after the last CCL_4 or TAA application by cervical dislocation under general anesthesia, livers and spleens (plus other organs of interest) are excised and weighed. Liver specimens from two lobes (e.g., left and right/median) are either fixed in 4% buffered formalin or snap-frozen in liquid nitrogen for further analysis.

3.2 Model of Portal/Periductular Fibrosis (Mdr2$^{-/-}$ Mice)

1. Mdr2$^{-/-}$ mice are maintained under specific pathogen-free conditions on a 12-h light–12-h dark cycle in an air conditioned room at 25 °C and provided water and standard mouse pellet chow ad libitum.
2. These mice develop spontaneously progressive biliary fibrosis until 15–18 week of age, with a maximal progression rate from week 4–12 (*see* Fig. 3 and **Note 6**).
3. Mice sacrifice and organ sampling are performed as described in Subheading 3.1.

3.3 Hepatic Collagen Quantification (HYP Assay) (See Note 7)

3.3.1 Protocol for Large Volume Assay (See Note 8)

1. Homogenize the liver tissue (150–300 mg liver samples from two different lobes; these amounts of tissue are necessary for optimal reproducibility due to the inhomogeneity of the fibrosis) in 5 ml of 6 N HCl and hydrolyze at 110 °C for 16 h (*see* **Note 9**).
2. After hydrolysis, let samples cool and filter the hydrolysate, then evaporate 50 μl aliquots under vacuum and remove residual HCl via evaporation after addition of methanol (*see* **Note 10**).
3. Dissolve the sediment in 1.2 ml of 50% isopropanol.
4. Incubate with 0.2 ml of 0.84% chloramine-T for 10 min at RT.
5. Add 1.0 ml of 12% Ehrlich's reagent and incubate the mixture at 50 °C for 90 min.

Fig. 1 (continued) induction. (**c**) Relative HYP content (μg per 100 mg liver) at week 1 and 4 after cessation of a 6-week treatment with CCL_4 (fibrosis regression), (**d**) total hepatic HYP (μg per whole liver) at week 1 and 4 of regression. Results are expressed as means ± SEM ($n = 6$–10 per group). $^{*}p < 0.01$, $^{**}p < 0.001$ as compared to vehicle (**a** and **b**) and to 6 weeks fibrosis control (**c** and **d**) (ANOVA). (**e**–**j**) represent the respective Picrosirius Red stained livers during the course of fibrosis progression and regression. (**e**) Week 0 control (Ishak 0), (**f**) week 1 (Ishak 1), (**g**) week 2 (Ishak 2), (**h**) week 4 (Ishak 3), (**i**) week 8 (Ishak 4, with full developed septal fibrosis), (**j**) incipient degradation of septal fibrosis at 4 weeks of regression following 6 weeks of CCL_4 induction. Magnification ×100, scale bar 100 μm

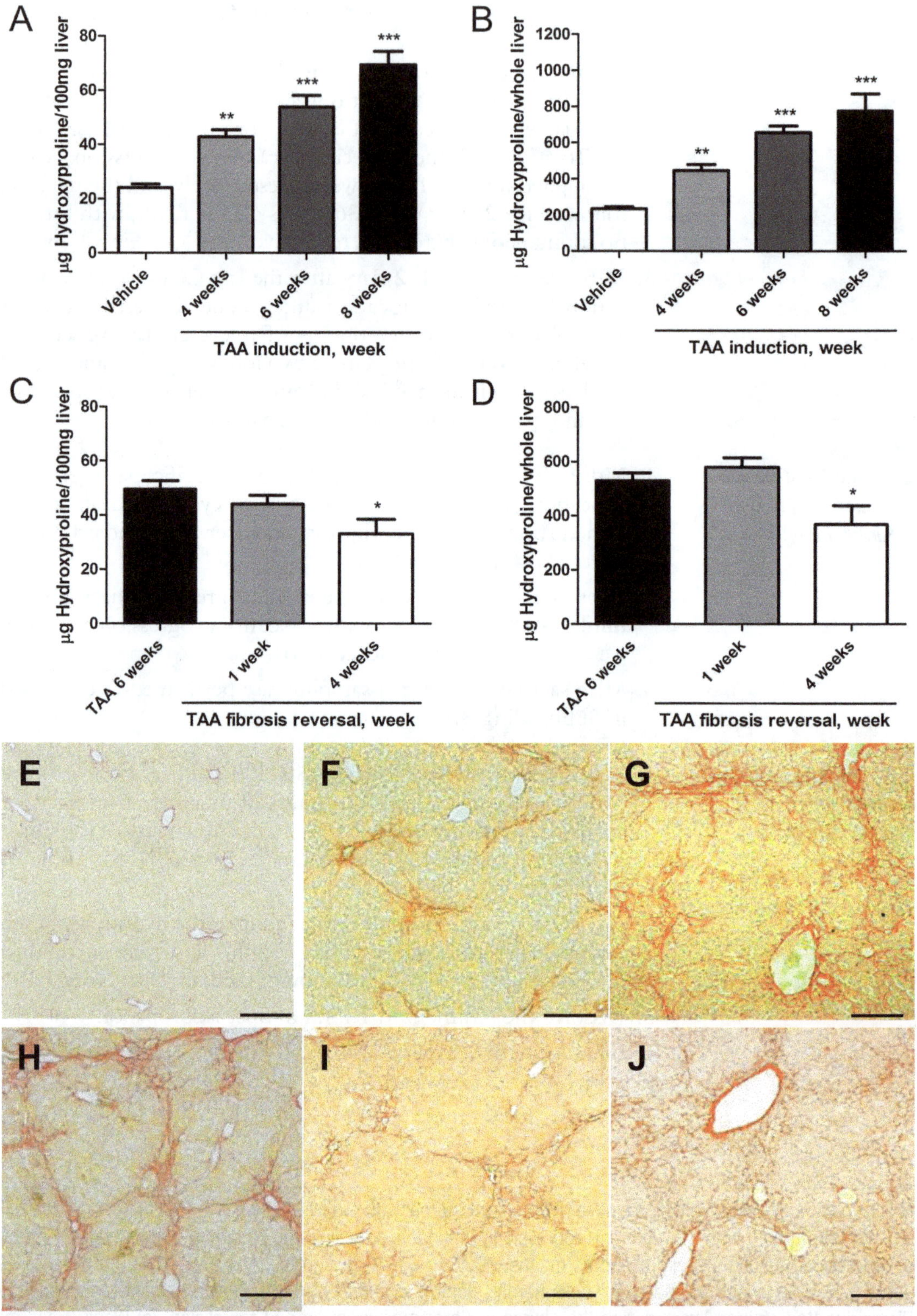

Fig. 2 Changes of liver HYP content and Picrosirius Red stained area in the TAA-induced fibrosis progression and regression models in C57BL/6 mice. (**a–d**) HYP content per 100 mg liver and per whole liver. HYP content expressed as (**a**) relative (μg per 100 mg liver, derived from the left and median lobes) at week 4, 6 and 8 of fibrosis induction, and (**b**) total hepatic HYP expressed as μg per liver, at week 4, 6 and 8 of fibrosis induction.

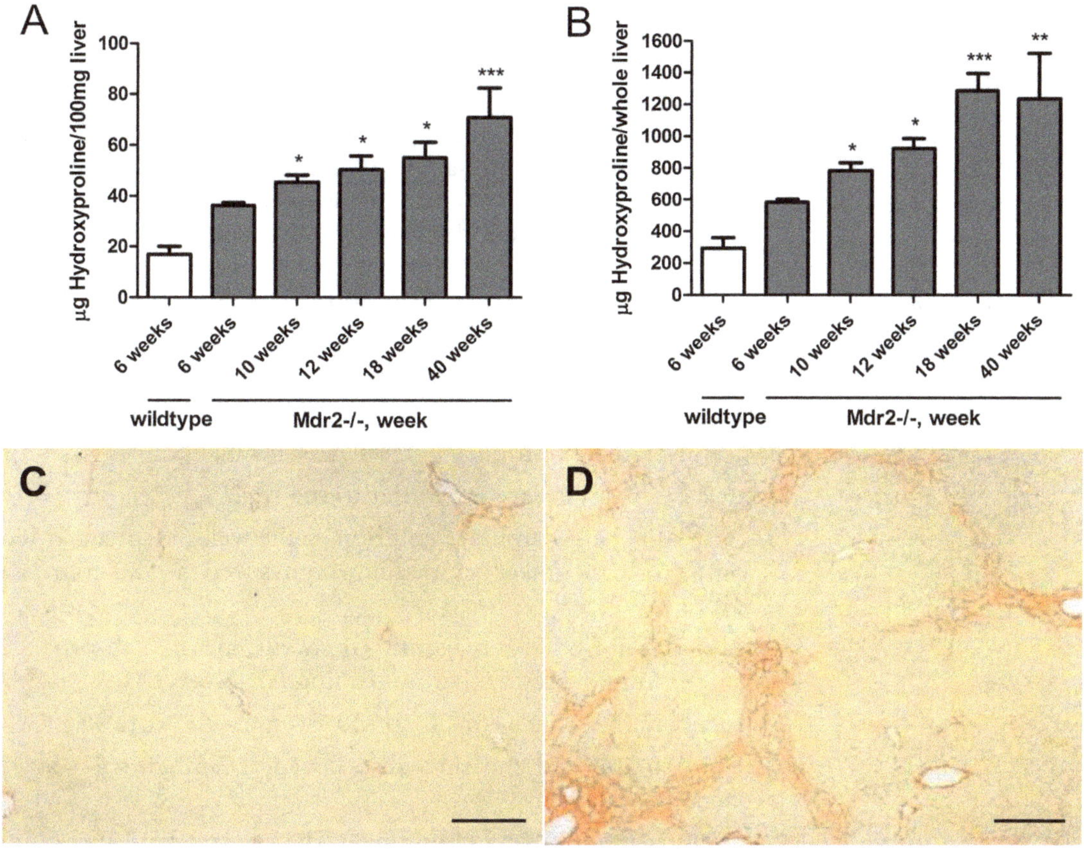

Fig. 3 $Mdr2^{-/-}$ mice develop spontaneous progressive hepatic collagen accumulation. (**a**) HYP content expressed as relative (μg per 100 mg liver, derived from the left and median lobes) at week 6, 10, 18, 24 and 40 of age, (**b**) total hepatic HYP expressed as μg per liver, as calculated by multiplication of individual liver weights with the relative HYP content. Results are expressed as means ± SEM ($n = 6$–10 per group). $^{*}p < 0.05$, $^{**}p < 0.01$ and $^{***}p < 0.001$ as compared to 6 weeks $Mdr2^{-/-}$ mice (ANOVA). (**c**) and (**d**) Represent the Picrosirius Red stained livers of FVB wildtype and FVB $Mdr2^{-/-}$ mice at age 6 (FVB wt, Ishak 0) and 10 weeks (FVB $Mdr2^{-/-}$, Ishak 3, with proliferating bile ductular cells in the portal area). Magnification ×100, scale bar 100 μm

Fig. 2 (**c**) Relative HYP content (μg per 100 mg liver) at week 1 and 4 after cessation of a 6 week treatment with TAA (fibrosis regression), (**d**) total hepatic HYP (μg per whole liver) at week 1 and 4 of regression. Results are expressed as means ± SEM ($n = 6$–10 per group). $^{*}p < 0.05$, $^{**}p < 0.01$ and $^{***}p < 0.001$ as compared to vehicle (**a** and **b**) and to 6 weeks fibrosis control (**c** and **d**) (ANOVA). (**e**–**j**) Represent the respective Picrosirius Red stained livers during the course of fibrosis progression and regression. (**e**) Week 0 control (Ishak 0), (**f**) week 4 (Ishak 2), (**g**) week 6 (Ishak 3), (**h**) week 8 (Ishak 4, with full developed septal fibrosis), (**i** and **j**) incipient degradation of septal fibrosis at 1 week (**i**), and 4 weeks (**j**) of regression following 6 weeks of TAA induction. Magnification ×100, scale bar 100 μm

6. Place briefly on crushed ice to chill.
7. HYP is then quantitated photometrically at 550 nm compared to a standard curve (*see* **Note 11**).
8. Calculate the HYP content of the liver sample using the formula: [Absorption of sample/0.26] × 400 = μg HYP/g liver. Multiplication of this value by the whole liver weight in g yields the total HYP content per liver.

3.3.2 Protocol for 96-Well Plate Assay (See Note 12)

1. Homogenize liver tissue (150–300 mg) in 5 ml 6 N HCl, and hydrolyse samples at 110 °C for 16 h.
2. After hydrolysis, let samples cool.
3. Aliquot 5 μl of standards, samples and blanks into the wells of a 96 well plate in triplicate. Use water for blank.
4. Add 50 μl citrate-acetate buffer to the wells.
5. Add 100 μl chloramine-T solution to the wells, incubate at RT on an orbital shaker at medium-high speed for 20 min (*see* **Note 13**).
6. Add 100 μl Ehrlich's reagent to the wells, measure absorbance at 550 nm for pre-incubation reading (*see* **Note 14**).
7. Incubate the plate at 65 °C for 20–30 min (*see* **Note 15**).
8. Cool to RT and measure absorbance at 550 nm for post-incubation reading.
9. Subtract the post-incubation from the pre-incubation reading for each well, including standards, and obtain mean value of the three wells.
10. Plot the means into the equation for the standard curve. This yields the μg/ml of HYP in the hydrolysates.
11. Multiply this value by the total volume of hydrolysate, then divide it by the tissue weight used. This is the relative HYP content of each sample (μg HYP per g liver). Multiply this by the whole liver weight. This is the total HYP content (μg HYP per liver).

3.4 Histology

3.4.1 Preparation of Slides

1. The left and median (or right) liver lobes are fixed in 4% formaldehyde at 4 °C for 48 h, after which tissues are moved into 70% ethanol for long term storage or dehydrated through a series of graded alcohol, and finally infiltrated with paraffin wax. This is usually carried out by an automated tissue processor, e.g., with a programmed gradient of 40, 60, 80, 90% isopropanol for 1 h each, 100% two times for 1 h and once for 2 h, 100% xylene three times for 1 h, and 100% paraffin two times for 3 h each. The thus paraffinized tissues are pressed into a metal mold generally using a paraffin embedding machine. These blocks can be stored at RT for years.

2. For histology the paraffinized tissue is sectioned using a microtome. Blocks to be sectioned are placed face down on ice for 10 min (or overnight). Trimming is done with 10 μm thick cuts, once cutting is smooth, proceed with 5–6 μm sections. Sections are floated on the surface of the 37 °C water bath and taken up on clean glass slides. Place the slide with paraffin section in a 65 °C oven for 20 min to bond the tissue to the glass.
3. Paraffinized tissues must be rehydrated before the staining by deparaffination, i.e., after melting the paraffin in 65 °C in a dry oven for 30 min, the paraffinization procedure is reversed, using 100 % xylene two times for 3 min, 100 % isopropanol two times for 5 min, 90 % and 75 % for 5 min each, dipping in distilled water two times.

3.4.2 Sirius Red Staining (See Note 16)

1. Deparaffinize the tissue and stain in Picrosirius Red solution for 1 h and rinse in distilled water, and wash in acidified water two times for 5 min.
2. Dehydrate the slides again, e.g., in 90 % isopropanol for 5 min, 100 % isopropanol two times for 5 min, 100 % xylene two times for 5 min. Drop the xylene-based mounting reagent on the tissue and cover with a cover glass.
3. Collect the images using a light microscope (×100 magnification) (*see* **Note 17**). The red stained collagen area is calculated as the % stained area using an image analyzer, e.g., ImageJ (NIH, Bethesda, MD) (*see* **Note 18**).

3.4.3 Hematoxylin and Eosin (H&E) Staining (See Note 19)

1. Deparaffinize the tissue.
2. Stain the tissue with Mayer's hematoxylin for 3–5 min, and wash in running tap water until the water is no longer colored (5–10 min).
3. Counterstain with Eosin Y working solution for 10–30 s (*see* **Note 20**).
4. Place in 95 % ethanol for 30 s and rinse in four changes of distilled water.
5. Dehydrate the slides, e.g., using 90 % isopropanol for 5 min, 100 % isopropanol two times for 5 min; 100 % xylene two times for 5 min. Drop the xylene-based mounting reagent on the tissue and cover with a cover glass.
6. Capture images using light microscope observation (×200 magnification) (*see* Fig. 4 and **Note 21**).

3.4.4 Staging of Liver Fibrosis Using the Metavir Scoring System (See Note 22)

The Ishak staging is simple but broadly validated in clinical samples, especially for viral hepatitis B and C, but is also used increasingly in rodent fibrosis studies. A major reason is that histological staging, although being semiquantitative, provides important additional information on the architectural derangement of the

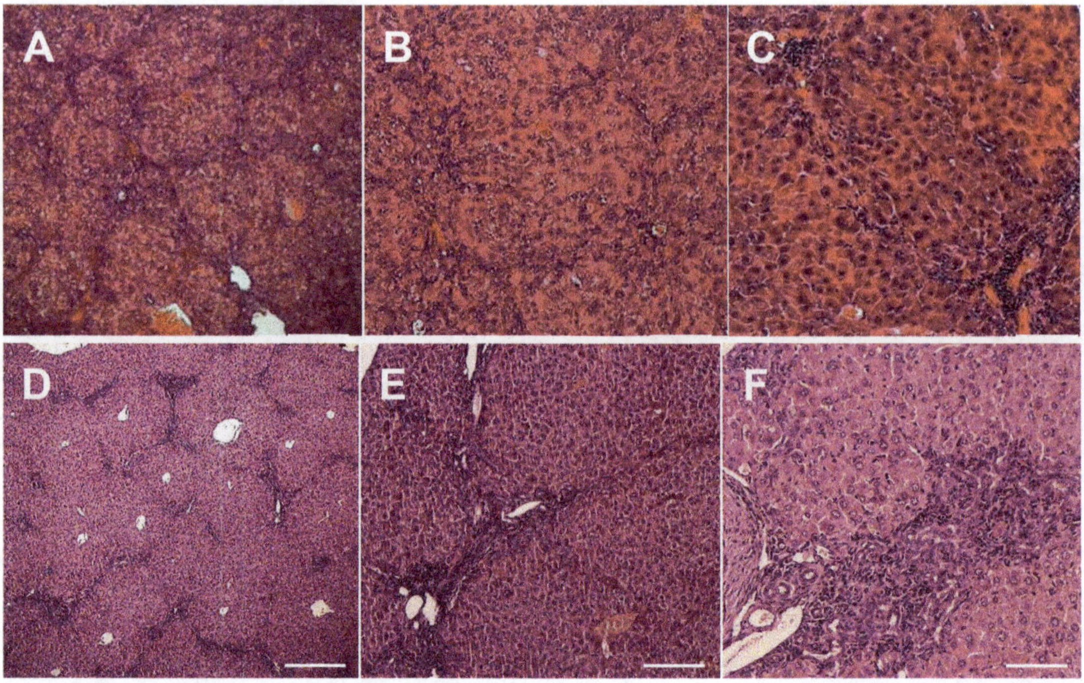

Fig. 4 Hematoxylin and eosin stain of necroinflammation in fibrotic livers. (**a–c**) Panlobular liver fibrosis after 6 weeks of intraperitoneal TAA induction. (**d–f**) biliary fibrosis in 10 week old Mdr2$^{-/-}$ mice. (**a**) Infiltrating leukocytes (monocytes) as stained with hematoxylin appear in a septal pattern. Magnification: (**a** and **d**) ×50, (**b** and **e**) ×100, (**c** and **f**) ×200, scale bar 100 μm

liver, which often does not correlate well with the mere accumulation of ECM. Ishak staging uses seven categories ranging from normal to cirrhosis based on collagen staining, such as the preferred Picrosirius Red staining. It correlates with another frequently used scoring system according to Metavir (five categories from normal to cirrhosis). Both staging systems also include frequently used grading scores for inflammation, which are not discussed here [27, 28]. In the following the Ishak system is matched to the corresponding morphometrical collagen proportional area and the Metavir score;

Stage 0, No fibrosis (normal) (1.9 % stained; Metavir F0).

Stage 1, Fibrous expansion of some portal area, with or without short fibrous septa (3.0 % stained; Metavir F1).

Stage 2, Fibrous expansion of most portal areas, with or without short fibrous septa (3.6 % stained; Metavir F2).

Stage 3, Fibrous expansion of most portal areas with occasional portal to portal (P-P) bridging (6.5 % stained; Metavir F2).

Stage 4, Fibrous expansion of portal areas with marked bridging (portal to portal (P-P) as well as portal to central (P-C)) (13.7 % stained; Metavir F3).

Stage 5, Marked bridging (P-P and/or P-C), with occasional nodules (incomplete cirrhosis) (24.3% stained; Metavir F3).

Stage 6, Cirrhosis, probable of definite (27.8% stained; Metavir F4).

All images of each tissue should be staged, like Picrosirius Red stain analysis, including more than 10 (–15) images per slide is recommended to minimize the errors (*see* **Note 23**).

3.5 Further Readouts

A rigorous fibrosis assessment requires further, refined readouts, such as (1) quantitative reverse transcription PCR for transcript levels related to fibrogenesis, fibrolysis, and inflammation, (2) immunohistochemistry on frozen or paraformaldehyde fixed sections, (3) fluorescence associated cell sorting, (4) bioactivity determinations, e.g., for proteolytic enzymes such as matrix metalloproteinases (MMPs) or for kinase activities. Moreover, any in vivo fibrosis study should be accompanied by determination of a set of routine (alanine aminotransferase, bilirubin, creatinine and others) specific (fibrosis or immune related markers) serum parameters and surrogates relevant to the study. These will not be detailed here but can be found in publications of our and of other groups [13–16, 21, 29–32].

4 Notes

1. The susceptibility to CCL_4 and TAA-induced fibrosis relies considerably on the genetic background of mouse strain. While FVB/N mice are less susceptible, BALB/c inbred mice are more responsive to CCL_4 [26], displaying occasional mortality, and C57BL/6 mice develop intermediate levels of fibrosis. We mostly use C57BL/6 mice, due to the availability of knockout strains.
2. $Mdr2^{-/-}$ mice begin to develop biliary fibrosis 4 weeks after birth [7]. Male FVB background $Mdr2^{-/-}$ mice develop less fibrosis compared to females (30% less at 10 weeks). Therefore, also for easier cohousing we recommend to preferentially use females and to avoid using both males and females in a single experiment.
3. This volume of reagent will suffice for two microplates. Chloramine-T is hardly dissolved by vortex mixing. If needed, the suspension can be heated to below 50 °C using a heat block or water bath to dissolve. This reagent needs to be prepared freshly before each experiment.
4. The intraperitoneal application of TAA frequently results in higher mortality (<5%) than oral CCL_4. This animal loss can be utmost avoided by applying lower dose(s) for adaptation (e.g., two doses of 50 or 25 mg/kg as a starting doses) especially in cases of excessive weight loss (greater than 10%).

5. With escalating doses of these hepatotoxins, incipient fibrosis (two to threefold increased liver collagen) is evident at 3 weeks, advanced fibrosis (three to fourfold increased liver collagen) at 6 weeks, and bridging fibrosis/cirrhosis (five to sixfold increased liver collagen) at 12 weeks [14]. For testing the effect of antifibrotics on fibrosis progression, the drugs are administered during either the whole period of fibrosis induction or (preferably) during the last 4 weeks before sacrifice. Hepatotoxin and drug treatment should be spaced apart at least 8 h if administered on the same day. In proof-of-concept studies for antifibrotics the test drug can also be given for shorter periods (1–2 weeks), with mainly qRT-PCR based fibrosis readouts [15, 18].
6. For testing antifibrotics in $Mdr2^{-/-}$ mice, the test drug is administered preferably either from age of 4–8, or 6–10 weeks of age before sacrifice (*see* Fig. 3).
7. Hydroxyproline (HYP) is an amino acid that is almost exclusively expressed in collagens, representing between 10 and 14% in the predominant, fibril forming collagens (types I > III > V in liver) [33–35]. The biochemical determination of hepatic HYP content is the 'gold standard' to quantify collagen accumulation in fibrotic tissues, and an essential prerequisite to detect antifibrotic drug effects in animal models. Since the assay is based on the measurement of the HYP oxidized by Chloramine-T to permit a reaction with the chromophore of Ehrlich's reagent [36], this method must be used with caution for tissues in which excessive free radicals have been produced. i.e., at least 1 day after the last dose of CCL_4 or TAA.
8. Reliable measurements can only be obtained with larger amounts of sample, especially in cases of biliary fibrosis. Exceptionally 30–50 mg of liver tissue can be used but results must be interpreted with care and higher numbers per group will be needed to achieve statistical significance. The large volume assay is a more reliable HYP quantification than the micro-well plate based assay [37–39].
9. Hydrolysis can either be performed with wet (frozen) or dry (fixed and deparaffinized) tissue with similar results. The homogenization step can be omitted for small-sized samples, and replacement of room air in the reaction flask with nitrogen yields more reproducible results. Screw cap flasks are recommended and the cap should be tightly sealed before hydrolysis to prevent evaporation. Take caution right after the hydrolysis when handling the 'boiling' acid hydrolysate.
10. Some charred residue is often produced during acid settling to the bottom once the sample is stored in the cold room for a few hours. After the assay, the rest of the acid hydrolysate can be stored at −20 °C or at RT after drying. However, in solu-

tion the HYP is slowly (within a few days to weeks) degraded at RT or at 4 °C.

11. Liver hydrolysates with high absorptions that reach the nonlinear range of the standard curve need to be further diluted.
12. This microplate assay is suitable for high throughput analysis for large numbers of samples [31, 40]. However, because this assay is quite sensitive to for example pipetting errors, the assay may need to be repeated to ensure the reading is stable and the back calculated values of standards match the expected values. Especially, generation of an accurate linear regression standard curve is essential. The result should be consistent with the result of the large volume assay, and also correlate with the results of the Picrosirius Red morphometry and for example procollagen mRNA expression.
13. Only a few minutes before the incubation period ends Ehrlich's reagent should be prepared. Mixing the reagents produces an exothermic reaction. Place briefly on ice to chill to RT as soon as the reagents are completely mixed. Wear a mask/gloves handling this toxic reagent and work in a fume hood.
14. Take the reading right after the mixture stops looking opaque, which takes approximately 2–3 min.
15. If incubated for >30 min, the standard curve becomes nonlinear and should not be used for the calculation.
16. The Picrosirius Red stain is for the histological visualization of collagen. The strongly cationic dye binds to the [Gly-X-Y]*n* triple helical structure found in all types of collagens [41]. The advantage of this stain is the higher specificity for collagen binding than the Masson's trichrome stain and the clearer delineation from other tissue structures. Moreover, it can be observed both in bright field and polarized light [42], with the color of the fibers under polarized light reflecting the density of the collagen fibrils.
17. When collecting the images for morphometrical analysis, taking more than 10 (–15) images per slide is recommended. This will encompass almost the whole tissue area on the slide, which is critical to prevent biased selection of stained areas. Thus, the collagen-dense large portal tracts in fibrosis should be omitted or quantified separately from the parenchymal collagen deposits that are functionally more relevant and often represent the bulk of liver collagen. Unfortunately, in most publications, this is not analyzed separately.
18. The results should be correlated and compared with the results of fibrosis scoring [28] and the gold standard of HYP quantification.

19. Hematoxylin and eosin staining is commonly used as a principal stain in histology. It is commonly used for grading inflammatory infiltration, fatty changes (micro- and macro-vesicular), hepatocyte degeneration (necrosis and apoptosis), and for an assessment of fibrosis. The staining method involves application of hematoxylin which binds to basophilic substances (e.g., DNA/RNA) staining them blue. The nuclear staining is followed by counterstaining with eosin Y which binds to acidophilic substances (e.g., proteins) and stains them pink.
20. The required staining time is determined by the thickness of the tissue, the age of the solution and the depth of the counterstain desired.
21. In fibrotic livers the immune cell infiltration can be specified and semi-quantified (graded); at high magnification orange colored phagocytosized pigments are often observed in Kupffer cells; apoptotic hepatocytes are hypereosinophilic and angular with fragmented and condensed nuclear material within the cytoplasm; the apoptotic bodies in dark pink may be free or contained within Kupffer cells; collagen is colored in pale pink (*see* Fig. 4). However, for the precise identification of cell populations, immunohistochemistry or flow cytometry are needed.
22. There are several histologic scoring systems developed for human livers, i.e., the Ishak, the Knodell and the related Metavir score, originally developed to assess the severity of chronic viral hepatitis, which includes descriptions of both necroinflammatory activity (grade) and the stage of fibrosis. The Knodell score assigns stages from one of four [43], the Metavir score from zero to four [28], and the Ishak score from one to six [27]. There are specific scoring systems for biliary liver diseases (e.g., the Scheuer score) and for nonalcoholic steatohepatitis (e.g., the Brunt and the NAS score). Scoring systems that include more stages for describing fibrosis are better able to document small changes in fibrosis over time. In this chapter, we describe the Ishak and Metavir stages with a focus on fibrosis.
23. In principle at least two experienced pathologists should be involved in the scoring after a pre-trial consensus meeting to clarify the boundaries between the categories. Independent blinded assessment (without knowledge of sample information) of the complete samples should be performed by each of the pathologists. Assessments should be carried out in as short a time as possible. Stage scoring is not a measurement, but a categorical assignment; thus any statistical analysis should take this into account [28]. The results complement HYP and morphometrical (Picrosirius Red stained samples) measurements.

Acknowledgments

This work was supported by NIH U19 AI066313-04 Hepatitis C Cooperative Research Centers, EU ERC Advanced Grant titled "Quantitative Imaging of Liver Fibrosis and Fibrogenesis," and a grant within the EU Project "European Study of Steatohepatitis" to DS.

References

1. Mehal WZ, Schuppan D (2015) Antifibrotic therapies in the liver. Semin Liver Dis 35:184–198
2. Schuppan D, Kim YO (2013) Evolving therapies for liver fibrosis. J Clin Invest 123:1887–1901
3. Schuppan D, Afdhal NH (2008) Liver cirrhosis. Lancet 371:838–851
4. Friedman SL (2010) Evolving challenges in hepatic fibrosis. Nat Rev Gastroenterol Hepatol 7:425–436
5. Friedman SL, Sheppard D, Duffield JS et al (2013) Therapy for fibrotic diseases: nearing the starting line. Sci Transl Med 5:167sr161
6. D'ambrosio R, Aghemo A, Rumi MG et al (2012) A morphometric and immunohistochemical study to assess the benefit of a sustained virological response in hepatitis C virus patients with cirrhosis. Hepatology 56:532–543
7. Marcellin P, Gane E, Buti M et al (2013) Regression of cirrhosis during treatment with tenofovir disoproxil fumarate for chronic hepatitis B: a 5-year open-label follow-up study. Lancet 381:468–475
8. Schuppan D, Pinzani M (2012) Anti-fibrotic therapy: lost in translation? J Hepatol 56(Suppl 1):S66–S74
9. Popov Y, Schuppan D (2009) Targeting liver fibrosis: strategies for development and validation of antifibrotic therapies. Hepatology 50:1294–1306
10. Schuppan D (2015) Liver fibrosis: common mechanisms and antifibrotic therapies. Clin Res Hepatol Gastroenterol 39(Suppl 1):S51–S59
11. Liedtke C, Luedde T, Sauerbruch T et al (2013) Experimental liver fibrosis research: update on animal models, legal issues and translational aspects. Fibrogenesis Tissue Repair 6:19
12. Ikenaga N, Liu SB, Sverdlov DY et al (2015) A new Mdr2(−/−) mouse model of sclerosing cholangitis with rapid fibrosis progression, early-onset portal hypertension, and liver cancer. Am J Pathol 185:325–334
13. Popov Y, Patsenker E, Fickert P et al (2005) Mdr2 (Abcb4)−/− mice spontaneously develop severe biliary fibrosis via massive dysregulation of pro- and antifibrogenic genes. J Hepatol 43:1045–1054
14. Popov Y, Sverdlov DY, Sharma AK et al (2011) Tissue transglutaminase does not affect fibrotic matrix stability or regression of liver fibrosis in mice. Gastroenterology 140:1642–1652
15. Jimenez Calvente C, Sehgal A, Popov Y et al (2015) Specific hepatic delivery of procollagen alpha1(I) small interfering RNA in lipid-like nanoparticles resolves liver fibrosis. Hepatology 62:1285–1297
16. Patsenker E, Popov Y, Stickel F et al (2008) Inhibition of integrin alphavbeta6 on cholangiocytes blocks transforming growth factor-beta activation and retards biliary fibrosis progression. Gastroenterology 135:660–670
17. Patsenker E, Popov Y, Stickel F et al (2009) Pharmacological inhibition of integrin alphavbeta3 aggravates experimental liver fibrosis and suppresses hepatic angiogenesis. Hepatology 50:1501–1511
18. Popov Y, Patsenker E, Stickel F et al (2008) Integrin alphavbeta6 is a marker of the progression of biliary and portal liver fibrosis and a novel target for antifibrotic therapies. J Hepatol 48:453–464
19. Schattenberg JM, Nagel M, Kim YO et al (2012) Increased hepatic fibrosis and JNK2-dependent liver injury in mice exhibiting hepatocyte-specific deletion of cFLIP. Am J Physiol Gastrointest Liver Physiol 303:G498–G506
20. Sedlaczek N, Jia JD, Bauer M et al (2001) Proliferating bile duct epithelial cells are a major source of connective tissue growth factor in rat biliary fibrosis. Am J Pathol 158:1239–1244
21. Yoshida S, Ikenaga N, Liu SB et al (2014) Extrahepatic platelet-derived growth factor-beta, delivered by platelets, promotes activation of hepatic stellate cells and biliary fibrosis in mice. Gastroenterology 147:1378–1392

22. Fickert P, Zollner G, Fuchsbichler A et al (2002) Ursodeoxycholic acid aggravates bile infarcts in bile duct-ligated and Mdr2 knockout mice via disruption of cholangioles. Gastroenterology 123:1238–1251
23. Smit JJ, Schinkel AH, Oude Elferink RP et al (1993) Homozygous disruption of the murine mdr2 P-glycoprotein gene leads to a complete absence of phospholipid from bile and to liver disease. Cell 75:451–462
24. Shi J, Aisaki K, Ikawa Y et al (1998) Evidence of hepatocyte apoptosis in rat liver after the administration of carbon tetrachloride. Am J Pathol 153:515–525
25. Slater TF, Cheeseman KH, Ingold KU (1985) Carbon tetrachloride toxicity as a model for studying free-radical mediated liver injury. Philos Trans R Soc Lond B Biol Sci 311:633–645
26. Hajovsky H, Hu G, Koen Y et al (2012) Metabolism and toxicity of thioacetamide and thioacetamide S-oxide in rat hepatocytes. Chem Res Toxicol 25:1955–1963
27. Ishak K, Baptista A, Bianchi L et al (1995) Histological grading and staging of chronic hepatitis. J Hepatol 22:696–699
28. Standish RA, Cholongitas E, Dhillon A et al (2006) An appraisal of the histopathological assessment of liver fibrosis. Gut 55:569–578
29. De Meijer VE, Sverdlov DY, Popov Y et al (2010) Broad-spectrum matrix metalloproteinase inhibition curbs inflammation and liver injury but aggravates experimental liver fibrosis in mice. PLoS One 5:e11256
30. Kornek M, Lynch M, Mehta SH et al (2012) Circulating microparticles as disease-specific biomarkers of severity of inflammation in patients with hepatitis C or nonalcoholic steatohepatitis. Gastroenterology 143:448–458
31. Popov Y, Patsenker E, Bauer M et al (2006) Halofuginone induces matrix metalloproteinases in rat hepatic stellate cells via activation of p38 and NFkappaB. J Biol Chem 281:15090–15098
32. Popov Y, Sverdlov DY, Bhaskar KR et al (2010) Macrophage-mediated phagocytosis of apoptotic cholangiocytes contributes to reversal of experimental biliary fibrosis. Am J Physiol Gastrointest Liver Physiol 298:G323–G334
33. Neuman RE, Logan MA (1950) The determination of hydroxyproline. J Biol Chem 184:299–306
34. Schuppan D (1990) Structure of the extracellular matrix in normal and fibrotic liver: collagens and glycoproteins. Semin Liver Dis 10:1–10
35. Schuppan D, Ruehl M, Somasundaram R et al (2001) Matrix as a modulator of hepatic fibrogenesis. Semin Liver Dis 21:351–372
36. Prockop DJ, Udenfriend S (1960) A specific method for the analysis of hydroxyproline in tissues and urine. Anal Biochem 1:228–239
37. Boigk G, Stroedter L, Herbst H et al (1997) Silymarin retards collagen accumulation in early and advanced biliary fibrosis secondary to complete bile duct obliteration in rats. Hepatology 26:643–649
38. Cho JJ, Hocher B, Herbst H et al (2000) An oral endothelin-A receptor antagonist blocks collagen synthesis and deposition in advanced rat liver fibrosis. Gastroenterology 118:1169–1178
39. Gerling B, Becker M, Staab D et al (1997) Prediction of liver fibrosis according to serum collagen VI level in children with cystic fibrosis. N Engl J Med 336:1611–1612
40. Fujita M, Shannon JM, Irvin CG et al (2001) Overexpression of tumor necrosis factor-alpha produces an increase in lung volumes and pulmonary hypertension. Am J Physiol Lung Cell Mol Physiol 280:L39–L49
41. Junqueira LC, Bignolas G, Brentani RR (1979) Picrosirius staining plus polarization microscopy, a specific method for collagen detection in tissue sections. Histochem J 11:447–455
42. Whittaker P, Kloner RA, Boughner DR et al (1994) Quantitative assessment of myocardial collagen with picrosirius red staining and circularly polarized light. Basic Res Cardiol 89:397–410
43. Knodell RG, Ishak KG, Black WC et al (1981) Formulation and application of a numerical scoring system for assessing histological activity in asymptomatic chronic active hepatitis. Hepatology 1:431–435

Chapter 20

Monitoring of Chemically Induced Colitis

Sonja Reißig and Benno Weigmann

Abstract

Inflammation is a common symptom of inflammatory bowel disease (IBD). Actually, many experimental models of colitis exist and try to mimic the human situation in order to understand the pathogenesis of Crohn's disease and ulcerative colitis. These experimental models of inflammation can be characterized by specific parameters, which illustrate the proceeding inflammatory process. By use of these models potentially new reagents for improved therapeutic approaches can be analyzed. Here, we describe the TNBS-mediated colitis model and specify different parameters for the detailed characterization of the inflammatory process in experimental colitis models.

Key words Colitis, Inflammatory bowel disease, Lamina propria, Mucosal immunology

1 Introduction

Inflammatory bowel diseases like Crohn's disease and ulcerative colitis are chronic inflammatory disorders of the intestinal tract [1]. The cause of the inflammation is unclear but in the last years progress to reveal the mechanism has been made by using experimental colitis models. To this aim, different models of IBD are used, like for instance the T-cell transfer, the hapten-induced colitis, the dextran-induced inflammation and even the spontaneous developing colitis in specific gene-deficient mice [2, 3]. All of these models try to mimic inflammation or specific inflammatory aspects in patients but cannot fully substitute the situation in humans. One of the most widely used chemically induced models of intestinal inflammation is the TNBS-mediated colitis model, which is useful to study T helper cell dependent mucosal immune responses. The TNBS-mediated colitis model resembles a human acute Th1-related inflammation as CD4+ T cells have been shown to play a central role in this model [4]. Nevertheless, it is important to recognize and understand the inflammatory process during the course of disease. Therefore different parameters of inflammation should be analyzed during the progression of disease by the researcher

Björn E. Clausen and Jon D. Laman (eds.), *Inflammation: Methods and Protocols*, Methods in Molecular Biology, vol. 1559, DOI 10.1007/978-1-4939-6786-5_20, © Springer Science+Business Media LLC 2017

[5]. One common and first sign of inflammation is the loss of body weight during the course of the experimental models. If animals lose weight, the induction of inflammation should be examined firstly by mini-endoscopy. The major advantage of this method is, that mice can be examined quickly and without interfering with the inflammatory process. The detailed mini-endoscopic investigations exactly define the status of disease and allow morphological grading of inflammation. Because inflammation is a multistep process, another possibility to analyze inflammatory signs is the luminol-based in vivo imaging bioluminescence. The substrate luminol in accordance with the myeloperxoidase (MPO) enzymatic activity` of effector cells like neutrophils and monocytes in the inflamed area, allows visualization in a noninvasive manner, which can be easily performed. In addition, the extent of the colonic inflammatory response can be assessed by macroscopic measurement of the colon. Inflammation leads to a shortening of the length and thickening of the colon wall compared to healthy mice. By analyzing cryo- or paraffin-sections of the intestine further parameters of inflammation can be investigated. Appropriate immunohistochemical staining of the intestinal biopsies reveals inflammation-driven MPO production by neutrophils and monocytes, clearly underlining the inflammatory status. Moreover, ulcerations, infiltration of neutrophils and the destruction of the villi/crypt structure in the colon are additional signs of inflammation and can be investigated by standard hematoxylin and eosin staining of sections from the intestine. Here, a grading system based on these results can be applied and help to characterize and quantify the inflammatory status. Finally, the expression of specific mRNA molecules from interstinal tissue involved in T_H-driven inflammation can be quantified by quantitative RT-PCR analysis (qPCR) to further define the inflammatory process in these experimental models. Together, all these parameters will define and analyze the complex inflammatory process in experimental colitis models and might help to translate the obtained results to the human situation of IBD.

2 Materials

2.1 Equipment

1. Balance (optimal for the range from 1 to 50 g).
2. Coloview system (Karl Storz, Germany) for Subheading 3.3.2.
3. Cryostat.
4. Cryo-tubes.
5. Electric clipper for animals.
6. Flexible catheter (3.5 F, length 20 cm) with soft tip.
7. Forceps.

8. Scissors.
9. 20 G needle.
10. Syringe 1 ml.
11. Glass slides.
12. In vivo imaging system (IVIS Lumina, PerkinElmer) for Subheading 3.6.
13. Oxygen concentrator (e.g., OxyVet) for Subheading 3.3.1.
14. Vaporizer (e.g., Vapor) for Subheading 3.3.1.

2.1.1 Reagent Setup

1. 70 and 45 % ethanol.
2. Acetone.
3. Fixation solution: paraformaldehyde (PFA) 4% in PBS (pH 6.9).
4. Formalin solution 10 %.
5. Ice-cold phosphate-buffered saline (PBS), pH 7.4.
6. Luminol.
7. Olive oil.
8. TNBS (2,4,6-trinitrobenzenesulfonic acid).
9. TNBS challenge solution: Dissolve 1 mg TNBS in 1 ml of 45 % ethanol to obtain a 1 % (w/v) solution. Mix the solution carefully.
10. TNBS sensitization solution: Mix acetone and olive oil in a 4:1 v/v ratio. Dissolve 2.5 mg TNBS in 1 ml of this solution to obtain a 2.5 % (w/v) TNBS sensitization solution. Mix the solution carefully.
11. Isoflurane.
12. Ketamine (e.g., Ketavest 100 mg/ml).
13. Xylazine (e.g., Rompun 2 %).
14. Anesthetic solution: Use a mixture of ketamine and xylazine. Mix 0.6 ml ketamine (100 mg/ml), 0.4 ml xylazine (20 mg/ml) and 4 ml PBS.

2.2 Animals

Usually 8–16-week-old sex- and age-matched littermate mice, at least five mice per experimental group are recommended. The animals should be kept under same conditions in order to keep identical gut microbiota, which can influence experimental outcome.

3 Methods

3.1 Induction of Inflammation with TNBS

The procedure of inducing TNBS-mediated colitis consists of a sensitization phase, a challenge phase and the analysis of the resulting intestinal inflammation. The described protocol requires approximately 8 days for the induction of colonic inflammation, starting with animal sensitization on day 0 and challenge on day 6 (*see* **Note 1**).

3.1.1 Sensitization

1. On day 0, carefully shave an approximately 3 cm × 2 cm field on the skin of the back of the mouse by using an electric clipper.
2. To apply the solution, hold the mouse with one hand and use the other hand to administer 150 μl of the TNBS sensitization solution on the shaved skin. The solution is quickly absorbed by the skin. As a control group, mice are treated with sensitization solution without TNBS.
3. Wait until the solution is absorbed, then return the animals to their cages. Leave the mice until day 6.

3.1.2 Challenge

1. On day 6, weigh and label the sensitized animals.
2. Anesthetize the mice before TNBS challenge. To achieve this, use an intraperitoneal injection of 80 μl of a ketamine–xylazine solution per 10 g body weight. Alternatively, use an isoflurane inhalation anesthetic system (*see* Subheading 3.3.1).
3. Connect a 3.5 F catheter to a 1 ml syringe and fill the syringe with the TNBS challenge solution.
4. Before TNBS administration, carefully position the catheter into the murine colon (insertion depth about 3–4 cm proximal to the anus). Remove stool pellets by flushing the colon carefully with a pipette filled with PBS (*see* **Note 2**).
5. Administer approximately 100 μl of the TNBS challenge solution into the colonic lumen via the catheter. Administration should be performed slowly and carefully (*see* **Note 3**).
6. Remove the catheter and keep the mouse in a vertical position (head down) for 2–3 min to avoid spilling out the injected solution.
7. Return animals carefully back to their cages.

3.2 Body Weight

1. Take the baseline weight of each mouse obtained before starting the experiment. Depending on the experiment, the mice are weighed either daily or weekly.
2. Make a graph of the body weight measurement by calculating the average of each mouse group. The body weight should be illustrated as percentage, using the baseline body weight as 100% (Fig. 1a).
3. Make a statistical analysis of the values in order to determine significance by ANOVA test.

3.3 Mini-Endoscopy

This procedure is divided into three parts, the anesthesia, the endoscopy and the analysis.

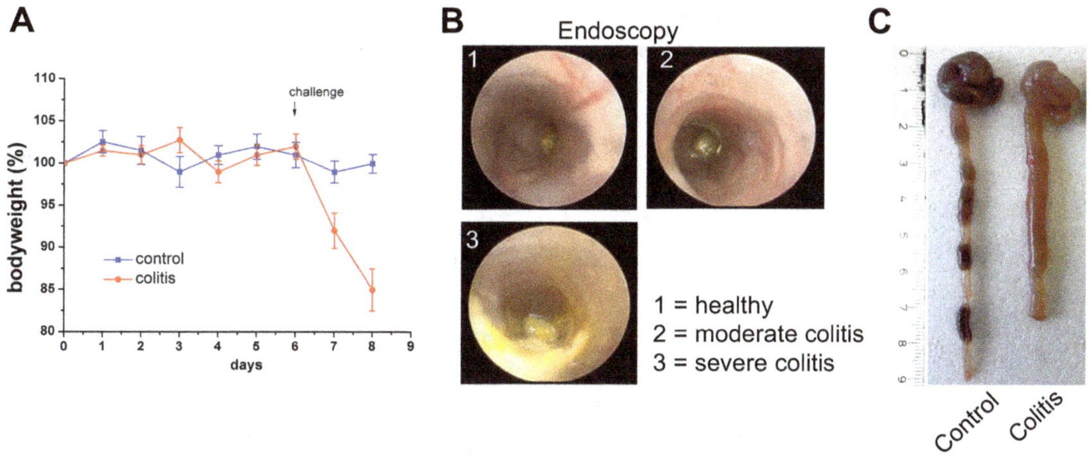

Fig. 1 (**a**) Graph displays the body weight as percentage of healthy control and colitic mice measured at the indicated time points ($n = 3$). (**b**) Photographs of colons isolated from healthy (*1*), moderate (*2*), and severe inflamed colitic (*3*) mice. (**c**) Macroscopic examination of colons from healthy (*left*) and inflamed mice (*right*)

3.3.1 Anesthesia

Before the endoscopy procedure starts, mice are anesthetized either by ketamine–xylazine injection or isoflurane inhalation.

1. Ketamine–xylazine anesthesia: Inject intraperitoneally a volume of approximately 80 μl ketamine–xylazine per 10 g body weight. Use the lowest possible dose necessary for anesthesia for your experiments.
2. Isoflurane inhalation: A vaporizer should be used in order to provide a constant gas concentration. Isoflurane is administered at a final concentration of 4% in a mixture of 36% oxygen/60% nitrogen suspension with a steady flow of 1 l/min. Place the mouse in a container of 20 cm diameter and 10 cm height, which is linked with the vaporizer. The anesthesia is induced in 15–30 s, allowing the mouse to be placed in a supine position. The isoflurane concentration provides a deep anesthesia with no movement of the legs or abdomen, no pain signs, and a stable blood pressure combined with steady respiratory rate (*see* **Note 4**) [6].

3.3.2 Endoscopy

1. Switch the endoscope on and test the airflow of the pump by holding the top of the endoscope into a cup of water. The uprising air bubbles should be steady and slow-going with middle size (one small bubble in water per second).
2. Take the anesthetized mouse and lay it with its ventral side up on an absorbent paper or mat. Take the tail with the left hand and the grip of the endoscope with the right hand or other way round if you are a left-handed researcher.

3. Insert cautiously the top of the endoscope into the rectum of the mouse and control the behavior of the mouse. The breathing of the mouse should be calm and steady during the procedure.
4. Then move the endoscope carefully as far as possible into the colon. During this procedure the researcher controls the process at the monitor. Since the top of the endoscope is often fixed the researcher has to be careful if stool pellets are visible to avoid perforation of the colon.
5. Approximately 5 cm into the colon it makes a curve (flexure), which cannot be passed with a rigid scope. Reaching this endpoint start the recording process while slowly moving the endoscope back to the anus. The movie can be saved in a common file format as MP4 or AVI. Try to avoid image compressing of the movie that reduces the quality of the pictures.
6. Upon reaching the anus, stop the recording process and lay the mouse carefully back into the cage.
7. Clean the endoscope by using 70% ethanol and control the breathing of the mouse. In case of isoflurane anesthesia, the animal should be awake within about 20 s after setting it back to normal air (*see* **Note 5–7**).

3.3.3 Analysis

1. The recorded endoscopy movie should be opened with a movie application, often delivered by the operating system. Then start watching the endoscopic examination again. To grade the inflammation of the colon, use the MEICS score (murine endoscopic index of colitis severity) consisting of five endoscopic parameters: translucency of the colon wall, vascularity of the mucosa, granularity of the mucosal surface, stool consistency, and the presence of fibrin production [6]. Here, you can discriminate between four stages of inflammation, which are numerated as 0–3. The degree of severity is determined as follows: 0 = no inflammation, 1 = mild inflammation, 2 = moderate inflammation, 3 = severe inflammation. Overall you can sum up all five parameters to a highest cumulative score of 15 as maximum score of inflammation (Table 1).
2. By using a picture grabbing movie application you can take an image of the most representative colon. The image can be saved as a TIF or JPG file and easily be integrated into a presentation.
3. Translate the numerical scoring system to a diagram illustration by using adequate statistical analysis software and combine it with the image from the endoscopy movie (Fig. 1b).

3.4 Harvesting Colonic Tissue Samples

1. Sacrifice the mice and open their abdomen longitudinal with scissors.

Table 1
List of five parameters for endoscopic score of inflammation

MEICS	Score
Translucency	0–3
Granularity	0–3
Fibrin production	0–3
Vascularity	0–3
Stool consistency	0–3
Total	0–15

2. Identify the small intestine, caecum, and colon. Dissect the colon from the surrounding mesentery carefully. Cut the pelvis to dissect the distal colon and rectum. Transect the colon at the rectum and colonocecal margin to harvest the colon from rectum till caecum.
3. Measure the length of the colon from the rectum till the caecum, as shortening of the colon is another indicator of inflammation [7].
4. Illustrate the intestinal inflammation and accompanied shortening of the colon by taking a picture of it (Fig. 1c).
5. For histological analysis and qPCR, cut a small fragment of the colon (0.5 cm), from the proximal, mid-colon and distal section. Flush colon pieces with ice-cold PBS by using a 20 G needle and a 1 ml syringe until the eluate is clear of stool and fibrin. Dry the biopsies carefully on an absorbent paper and place them straight into a labeled cryo-tube. Be sure to maintain the correct orientation of the colon sample. Snap freeze the samples by using liquid nitrogen and store them at −80 °C (*see* **Note 8**).

3.5 Evaluation of Colitis by Histology and Quantitative RT-PCR Analysis

The severity of the inflammatory response can be assessed by alterations in the histology of the colon and increased expression of inflammatory cytokines as well as enzymes. Morphology of the intestinal tissue can be investigated by hematoxylin and eosin (H&E) staining of cryo or paraffin sections (*see* **Note 6**). In general, paraffin sections can be cut easier and exhibit a better morphology than cryo-sections. To examine which cells are responsible for the inflammatory response, cryo-section are analyzed by immunohistochemistry. Here, the expression of inflammatory enzymatic activity from activated neutrophils is measured by myeloperoxidase (MPO) staining in combination with or without the macrophage surface marker F4/80, T-cell infiltration by CD4 and invasion of myeloid-derived cells by CD11c staining. Finally, the expression of pro-inflammatory mRNA molecules like IL-6 or TNF-α can be determined by the isolation of mRNA from tissue with subsequent transcription to cDNA and qPCR analysis in relation to a housekeeping gene.

3.5.1 H&E Staining and Immunohistochemistry

1. Cut sections 5–15 μm thick from frozen colonic tissue using a cryostat and fix them with 4 % PFA fixation solution for 10 min.
2. Wash the fixed sections with PBS one time.
3. Proceed directly with the H&E or immunofluorescence staining (Fig. 2a, b; Table 2) (*see* **Note 9**).
4. For evaluation and scoring of inflammation by means of H&E and immunostaining use the described criteria (*see* **Note 10**) [3].
5. Cryo-sections should be stained for the analysis of specific surface cell markers with denoted antibodies (*see* Table 2) (*see* **Note 11**) [8].

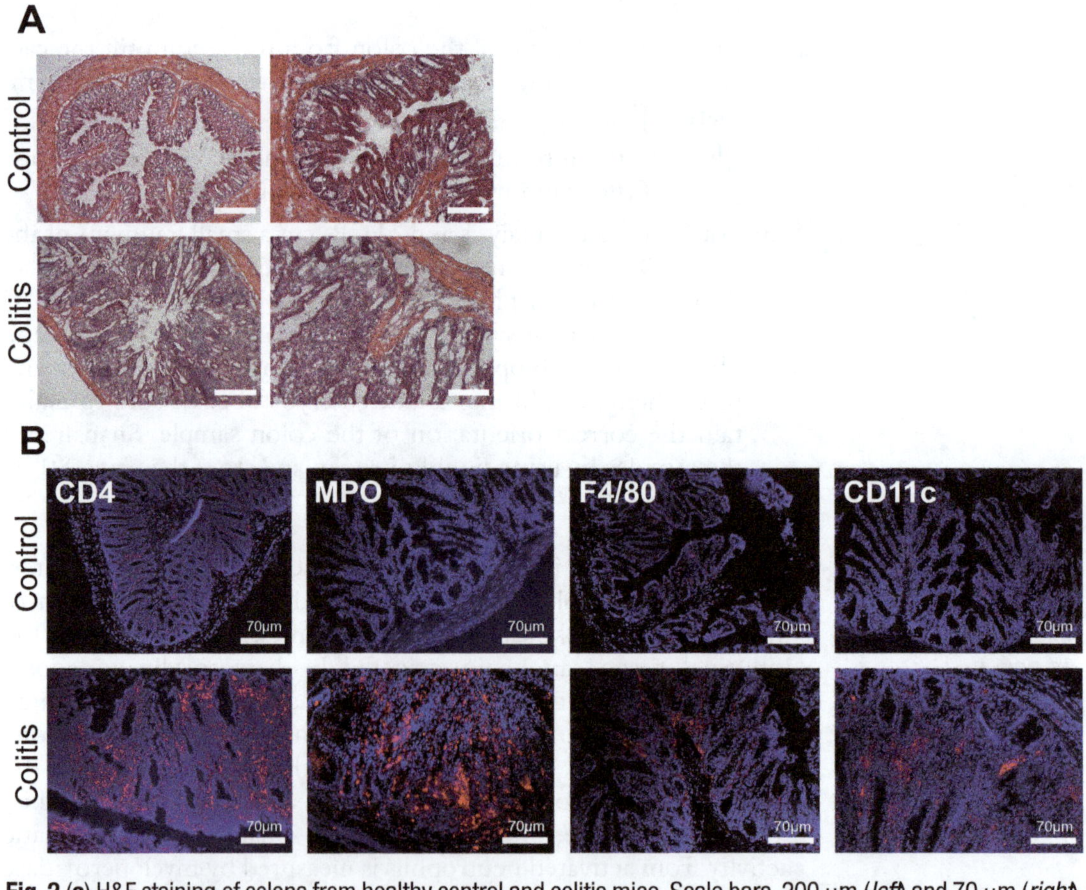

Fig. 2 (**a**) H&E staining of colons from healthy control and colitis mice. Scale bars, 200 μm (*left*) and 70 μm (*right*). (**b**) Immunofluorescence staining of colonic cryo-sections from healthy control and colitis mice, stained for CD4, MPO, F4/80, and CD11c (*red*). Nuclei were counterstained with Hoechst 3342 (*blue*). Scale bars, 70 μm

Table 2
List of antibodies used for immunofluorescence staining

Primary antibody	Dilution	Secondary antibody	Dilution
α-mouse CD4 (Clone RM4-5)	1:1000	α-hamster-biotin labeled	1:1000
α-mouse CD11c (Clone HL3)	1:200	α-hamster-biotin labeled	1:1000
α-mouse myeloperoxidase (Clone 8F4)	1:20	α-rabbit-biotin labeled	1:1000
α-mouse F4/80 (Clone BM8)	1:1000	α-rat-biotin labeled	1:1000

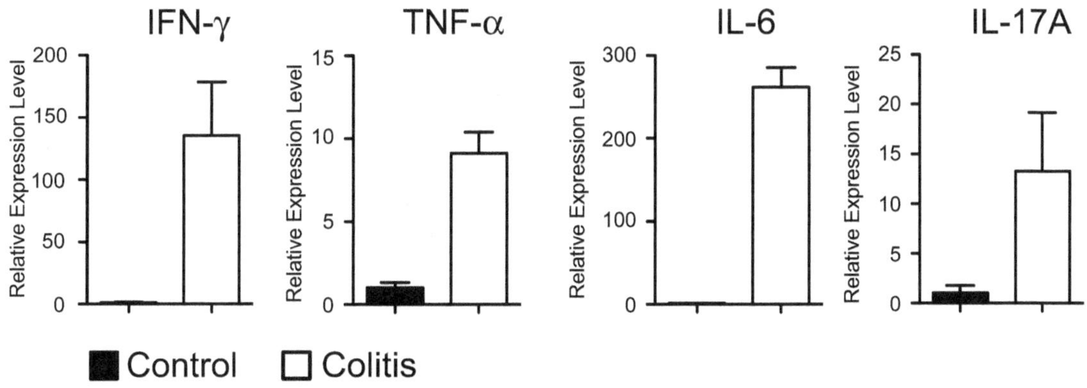

Fig. 3 Colonic tissues from healthy control and colitis mice were analyzed by qPCR for the indicated transcripts of pro-inflammatory cytokines. Gene expression levels were normalized and set in relation to HPRT gene expression

3.5.2 Quantitative RT-PCR Analysis

1. Take 0.3–0.5 cm of the frozen colon and isolate RNA by using a total RNA isolation kit according to manufacturer's instructions.
2. Use mRNA as template and convert it into cDNA by using random primers and reverse transcriptase.
3. Dilute cDNA 1:3 and use quantitative RT-PCR method for the analysis of inflammatory cytokines (Fig. 3). Gene-specific primers can be ordered with the following sequences (Table 3) (*see* **Note 12**) [9].

3.6 In Vivo Imaging of Inflammation

The use of in vivo imaging systems can visualize signs of inflammatory by detecting reactive oxygen and nitrogen species produced by the enzymatic activity of activated neutrophils. The chemiluminescent signal is produced in the colon by an activated luminol agent and can be detected by the imaging system in the green light range. For monitoring colitis the IVIS system consists of a tight chamber with a cooled camera.

Table 3
List of primers used for qPCR

q-PCR gene	Upstream forward primer	Downstream reverse primer
IL-6	CTCTGGGAAATCGTGGAAAT	CCAGTTTGGTAGCATCCATC
IL-17A	ATCCCTCAAAGCTCAGCGTGTC	GGGTCTTCATTGCGGTGGAGAG
IFN-γ	TCAAGTGGCATAGATGTGGAAGAA	TGGCTCTGCAGGATTTTCATG
TNF-α	CATCTTCTCAAAATTCGAGTGACAA	TGGGAGTAGACAAGGTACAACCC

1. Anesthetize the animals as described in Subheading 3.3.1 with an isoflurane/oxygen gas mixture. Only in this way it is ensured that the mice are not moving during the measurement.
2. Shave the mouse on the abdominal area by using a depilatory cream or an electric clipper, because mice have strong background autofluorescent signals originating from the hair. The IVIS system has a heated platform to avoid cooling down of the animals during the anesthesia (*see* **Note 13**).
3. Dissolve the chemiluminescent probe luminol in sterile H_2O to a final concentration of 20 mmol/l.
4. Inject the luminol solution intraperitoneally in a 100 μl volume into the mouse.
5. Lay the mouse quickly into the IVIS chamber and start measuring the light emission beginning 30 s after the injection. The luminol chemiluminescence is visible in the blue light range of 435 nm. The detector filter set should be switched to this wavelength (Fig. 4) [10].
6. Take several images, as sometimes the bloodstream of the mouse needs time to distribute the luminol evenly across the abdomen.
7. After taking the images, place the mouse back into the cage and control awakening of the animal.

4 Notes

1. Typically, signs of the acute inflammation will develop on day 8, 9, and 10 post TNBS sensitization. Each investigator should experimentally determine the working concentration of TNBS, given a different sensitivity of a variety of different mouse strains and a distinct composition of the commensal microflora of the local animal facilities.
2. Move the catheter very carefully to avoid the damage or perforation of the mucosal colon wall by the instillation.

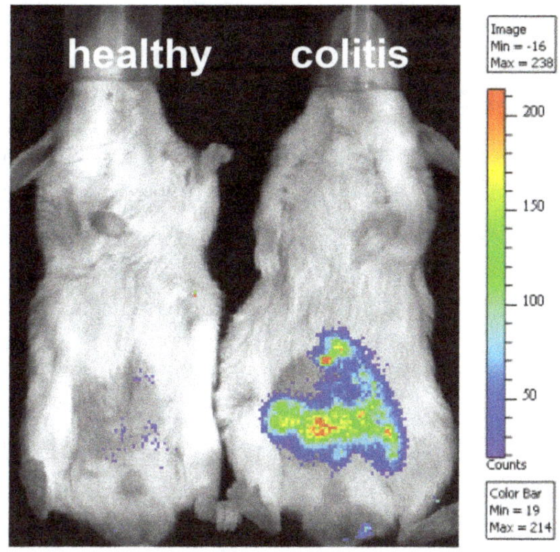

Fig. 4 In vivo imaging of colitis by IVIS instrument. Representative images of a healthy mouse (*left*) and a mouse with colonic inflammation (*right*) are shown. The color scale on the *right* shows the severity of inflammation from *blue* to *red* as highest inflammation

3. To get comparable results, ensure that the TNBS solution remains trapped in the colon lumen by careful handling and avoiding abrupt moving.
4. Supervise the breathing of the animals. It should be steady and calm. When anesthetized animals get low breathing, stop the endoscopy procedure and set animals in a preheated cage for 10 min.
5. Sometimes poor optical visibility during the endoscopy process is resulting from massive fibrin production, stool and contact bleeding. To avoid this, withdraw the mini-endoscope and clean it with 70% ethanol before inserting it again. By using ketamine–xylazine anesthesia, mice should be kept warm after the endoscopic procedure to ensure recovery from the anesthesia. Mice should be awake within 10–30 min after ketamine–xylazine injection, depending on the dose and healthiness of the mice.
6. Mortality of animals can be prevented by avoiding perforation of the colon during the endoscopy procedure. Perforation of the colon wall results in a peritonitis. Be always careful and try to avoid abrupt movements with the endoscope. Do not push the endoscopy with force forward if you feel resistance.
7. Be aware that inflamed animals are very susceptible to perforation due to thin or bleeding mucosa. Try to reduce the air pressure of the endoscope in order to avoid intense tension of the mucosa.

8. Alternatively to cryo-sections, also paraffin sections can be used for H&E staining. Therefore, do not freeze colon samples. Instead, fix the tissue samples in neutral buffered formalin solution for 48 h before embedding in paraffin. When colon samples are fixed with paraffin, thinner sections can be sliced and analyzed as compared to frozen samples, sliced with a cryostat.
9. If cryo-sections will not be used directly for staining, store them at −80 °C for up to 6 months. When using frozen cryo-sections, allow them to thaw briefly at room temperature before the fixation step. After thawing, never freeze sections for a second time.
10. The inflammation scoring system for the histological evaluation of H&E stained colonic sections should be performed in a blinded manner. The tissue injury index should be calculated by the following parameters: mucosal erosion and ulceration, loss of crypt architecture, submucosal spread and transmural involvement, loss of goblet cells and infiltration of neutrophils. These parameters are graded as follows: grade 0 = normal tissue architecture; grade 1 = minimal scattered mucosal inflammatory cell infiltrates, with or without minimal epithelial hyperplasia; grade 2 = mild scattered to diffuse inflammatory cell infiltrates, cell infiltrates sometimes extend into the submucosa associated with erosions, minimal to mild epithelial hyperplasia, minimal to mild mucin depletion from goblet cells; grade 3 = mild to moderate inflammatory cell infiltrate, sometimes transmural and often associated with ulceration, moderate epithelial hyperplasia and mucin depletion; grade 4 = marked inflammatory cell infiltrate which is often transmural and associated with ulceration, marked epithelial hyperplasia and mucin depletion; grade 5 = marked transmural inflammation with severe ulceration, loss of intestinal glands, and massive infiltration of neutrophils. The scoring of inflammation based on the H&E staining of colon tissue cryo-sections needs some training, in order to obtain reproducible results.
11. The antibodies for immunofluorescence staining (Table 2) are recommended for cryo-sections, but not paraffin-sections. For surface immunostaining of paraffin sections a pioneer experiment is required to identify optimal antibodies and their dilutions. Here no specific suggestions can be made.
12. For qPCR analysis relative expression factors are always denoted. For evaluating mRNA expression levels of genes of interest in intestine tissue, normalize them to a housekeeping gene like 18S-rRNA or HPRT mRNA [11].
13. When using fluorescence dyes in green light range, like FITC, it is recommended to place the animals on an alfalfa-free diet (*Medicago sativa* L.) for 2 days in order to reduce autofluorescence signals from the background.

Acknowledgment

B.W. was supported by DFG grants WE4656/2-2 and SFB 1181-B02.

References

1. Strober W, Fuss I, Mannon P (2007) The fundamental basis of inflammatory bowel disease. J Clin Invest 117:514–521
2. Neurath MF (2012) Animal models of inflammatory bowel diseases: illuminating the pathogenesis of colitis, ileitis and cancer. Dig Dis 30(1):91–94
3. Weigmann B (2014) Induction of colitis in mice (T-cell transfer model). Methods Mol Biol 1193:143–151
4. Wirtz S, Neurath MF (2000) Animal models of intestinal inflammation: new insights into the molecular pathogenesis and immunotherapy of inflammatory bowel disease. Int J Colorectal Dis 15:144–160
5. Neurath MF, Fuss I, Kelsall BL, Stüber E et al (1995) Antibodies to interleukin-12 abrogates established experimental colitis in mice. J Exp Med 182(5):1281–1290
6. Becker C, Fantini MC, Wirtz S, Nikolaev A et al (2005) In vivo imaging of colitis and colon cancer development in mice using high resolution chromoendoscopy. Gut 54:950–954
7. Boirivant M, Fuss IJ, Chu A, Strober W (1998) Oxazolone colitis: a murine model of T helper cell type 2 colitis treatable with antibodies to interleukin 4. J Exp Med 188(10):1929–1939
8. Eschborn M, Weigmann B, Reissig S, Waisman A et al (2015) Activated glycoprotein A repetitions predominant (GARP)-expressing regulatory T cells inhibit allergen-induced intestinal inflammation in humanized mice. J Allergy Clin Immunol 136(1):159–168
9. Reissig S, Hövelmeyer N, Weigmann B, Nikolaev A et al (2012) The tumor suppressor CYLD controls the function of murine regulatory T cells. J Immunol 189(10):4770–4776
10. Gerlach K, Hwang Y, Nikolaev A, Atreya R et al (2014) TH9 cells that express the transcription factor PU.1 drive T cell-mediated colitis via IL-9 receptor signaling in intestinal epithelial cells. Nat Immunol 15:676–686
11. Banda M, Bommineni A, Thomas RA, Luckinbill LS et al (2008) Evaluation and validation of housekeeping genes in response to ionizing radiation and chemical exposure for normalizing RNA expression in real-time PCR. Mutat Res 649(1–2):126–134

Chapter 21

Oxazolone-Induced Intestinal Inflammation in Adult Zebrafish

Sylvia Brugman and Edward E.S. Nieuwenhuis

Abstract

Zebrafish are an excellent model for the study of intestinal immunity. The availability of several transgenic reporter fish for different innate and adaptive immune cells and the high homology in terms of gut function and morphology enables in depth analysis of the process of intestinal inflammation. Here, we describe a method to induce intestinal inflammation by intra-rectal injection of the hapten oxazolone in adult zebrafish.

Key words Zebrafish, Intestinal inflammation, Oxazolone, Intra-rectal injection, IBD, Crohn's disease, Gut barrier function, Ulcerative colitis, Granulocytes

1 Introduction

Starting out as a model for developmental biology, in the last decade the zebrafish received more and more attention as a model organism to study immunity. The availability of several immune-gene transgenic reporter zebrafish, the high fecundity and transparency early in life has made the zebrafish a unique model. Interestingly, since zebrafish develop from fertilized eggs and hatch at 2 days post fertilization (2 dpf), development of the immune system can be studied in great detail. Macrophages, neutrophils, eosinophils, mast cells, and dendritic cells have all been identified, with neutrophils and macrophages being present as early as 30 and 48 h post fertilization respectively [1–5]. There is still debate on the timing of adaptive immune development. Previously, it was shown that T cell-dependent and independent immunity was only functional from 4 weeks of age as measured by specific IgM responses [6]. However, new transgenic reporter zebrafish show the presence of T and B cells in the periphery as early as 9 days and expression of the newly discovered IgZ (mucosal Ig) already at 2 weeks post fertilization [7]. This IgZ (also termed IgT) appears to be the fish equivalent of mucosal antibody IgA [8, 9]. We have observed small percentages

Björn E. Clausen and Jon D. Laman (eds.), *Inflammation: Methods and Protocols*, Methods in Molecular Biology, vol. 1559, DOI 10.1007/978-1-4939-6786-5_21,

of T lymphocytes in the intestines from 3 weeks of age onwards [10]. Therefore, it is currently believed that at least until 2 weeks of life, zebrafish do not have mature adaptive immunity and totally rely on innate immunity for their survival.

Although zebrafish do not have five intestinal segments like mammals (i.e., jejunum, duodenum, ileum, cecum (appendix), and colon), there is functional homology. Zebrafish are stomachless and have three different gut segments that are discriminated on the basis of morphology and gene expression: the intestinal bulb (anterior gut segment), the midgut, and the posterior gut segment [11]. Digestive enzymes are strongly expressed in the intestinal bulb segment where the villi (called folds) are longest. The presence of these digestive enzymes and solute transporters in the anterior and mid intestines underlines the function of nutrient absorption in these two segments [12]. The last part of the mid intestine contains vacuolated M-like cells which might indicate that besides nutrient absorption this region plays a role in mucosal immunity [13–15]. The epithelial villi of the posterior region are short and this part does not contain absorptive enterocytes, but is likely involved in water absorption [16].

Several models for intestinal inflammation have been developed for larvae (2,4,6-trinitrobenzenesulfonic acid (TNBS), dextran sulfate sodium (DSS), glafenine) as well as adults (oxazolone, TNBS) [17–20]. Here we describe a method to induce oxazolone enterocolitis in adult zebrafish [21].

2 Materials

2.1 Zebrafish of 14 wpf (Adult)

Different transgenic reporter lines currently exist (mpx:eGFP myeloperoxidase, neutrophils; mpeg1:mCherry macrophage expressed gene 1, macrophages; lck:GFP, lymphocyte cell-specific protein-tyrosine kinase, T lymphocytes; Ighm:GFP, IgM, B lymphocytes; Cd4:GFP, CD4, T helper cells) next to the different wildtype lines such as AB or TL. Depending on your research question you can use either wildtype or transgenic fish. We have used both females and males. We did not observe obvious differences between males and females in this protocol.

2.2 Anesthetizing Fish

1. Preparing stock solution anesthesia

   Tricaine (3-amino benzoic acid ethyl ester also called ethyl 3-aminobenzoate) comes in a powdered form. Make a tricaine solution for anesthetizing fish by combining the following in a glass bottle with a screw cap: 400 mg tricaine powder, 97.9 mL double distilled water and ~2.1 mL 1 M Tris (pH 9). Adjust pH to 7. Store this solution in the freezer (protocol from Zebrafish Handbook [22], 4th edition, available online at http://zfin.org/zf_info/zfbook/). Keep the work solution in the fridge in a dark bottle (light sensitive).

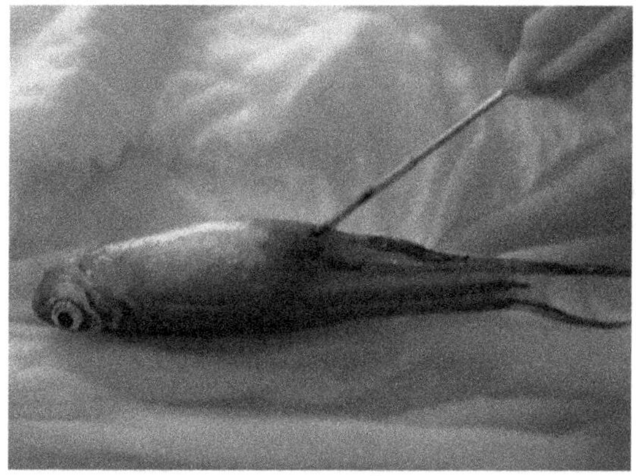

Fig. 1 Intra-rectal injection of adult zebrafish. Gently squeeze the abdomen to locate the anal opening and angle the needle with silicone tubing at the end at 45°

2. Prepare a zebrafish tank for anesthesia

   Use a separate tank to anesthetize the zebrafish (one by one). Add 4.2 mL tricaine stock solution per 100 mL clean tank (system) water.

2.3 Intra-rectal Injection of Zebrafish

1. To perform the injection after the fish is anesthetized, prepare a petri dish-lid mounted with a tissue soaked in clean tank water. Fold the tissue into a small wet mold as to hold the fish belly-up and keep it wet (*see* Fig. 1).
2. Prepare a fresh solution of 20 mg oxazolone (4-ethoxymethylene-2-phenyl 2 oxazolin-5-one) in 5 mL 100% ethanol. Make sure the oxazolone is fully dissolved, and then add 5 mL PBS (0.8% NaCl, 0.02% KCl, 0.02 M PO_4, pH 7.3; protocol from Zebrafish Handbook [22], 4th edition, available online at http://zfin.org/zf_info/zfbook/). As a control solution prepare 50% ethanol solution in PBS.
3. Since we inject per bodyweight, a scale that can measure in the milligram range is needed to be able to inject the right amount of oxazolone or ethanol.
4. For the injection a small syringe is needed, preferably a Hamilton gastight syringe (100 μL; Chrompack; Hamilton Company, Bonaduz, Switzerland) of a low volume with blunt end. As an alternative, a 1 mL syringe can be used connected to a small needle covered with silicon tubing of a diameter of less than 1 mm. The disadvantage of using normal 1 mL syringe is the resistance of the plunger and difficulty to inject similar small volumes consistently.

2.4 Recovery of Zebrafish

1. Prepare a separate tank with clean tank (system) water.

2.5 Euthanasia

1. Use of 4 mg tricaine/mL tank (system) water to euthanize the zebrafish.

2.6 Fixation for Histology

1. Prepare 4% paraformaldehyde in PBS, pH 7.4.

2.7 Cell Suspension for Flow Cytometry

1. Prepare PBS with 2% (heat inactivated) FBS. Use 70 and 40 μm cell strainers per intestine.

3 Methods

1. Anesthetizing zebrafish

   Wear gloves. Transfer the zebrafish from their tank to a separate tank where they can be easily caught with a net. Be careful not to stress them by gently taking them out with the net. Catch a zebrafish and transfer it to the tank containing the anesthetic. Wait for the fish to stop swimming and watch the gill movements. Once the movement of the gills stops, carefully use the net to see whether the fish still reacts to mechanical stimulation (gently tapping the table will also show whether the fish is fully anesthetized or not). Take the fish out of the tank, weigh the fish and transfer it to the wet tissue on the petri dish lid, belly up (Fig. 1).

2. Injection of oxazolone or ethanol control solution

   Gently squeeze the proximal part of the belly to locate the anal opening. Gently inject 0.6–1.0 μL per 0.1 g of zebrafish (Fig. 1). Quickly transfer the fish to the recovery tank and wait for all of the fish to recover before putting them back in the husbandry system. The faster this procedure is performed the better. We take approximately 2–3 s to inject the anesthetized fish and return it to the recovery tank.

3. Dynamics of intestinal inflammation

   In our hands, intestinal damage will be visible on histology within 5 h after injection. The resulting inflammation can be observed until 1 week after the injection. At 2 weeks after injection the zebrafish that are left have normal gut morphology.

4. Scoring system to quantify intestinal inflammation

   At the desired time points, zebrafish are euthanized using an overdose of tricaine (<4 mg/mL). The intestines can be removed and directly placed in 4% paraformaldehyde. Samples are kept overnight in 4% paraformaldehyde at 4 °C. The next day the tissue needs to be transferred to 70% ethanol and kept at 4 °C for further processing. Embed the tissue in paraffin and cut 5 μm sections. Perform an Alcian-Blue Periodic Acid Schiff (PAS) staining that will stain mucus-producing goblet cells and eosinophilic granulocytes (PAS-positive cells). Intestinal bulb, anterior mid-intestine, and posterior mid-intestine are assessed separately. In Table 1 a description of the scores is given and in Fig. 2 examples of the different scores per parameter can be found. Total

Table 1
Enterocolits scoring system

Parameter	Score 1	Score 2	Score 3
Bowel wall thickening	Slightly thickened ~25 µm	Moderately thickened ~45 µm	Severely thickened ~75 µm
Intestinal-fold architecture disruption	Slight disruption – Disruption of the barrier – Slight increase villus width	Moderate disruption – Increased inter-villus distance and/or gaps between cells – Increased villus width – Decreased villus height	Severe disruption – Gaps between epithelial cells – Loss of villi/flattening of the villi – Increase in villus width
Goblet cell appearance	Slightly decreased or increased number of goblet cells	One or two goblet cells per villus or increased numbers (>20) with increased mucus production	Complete disappearance of goblet cells
Infiltration of PAS-positive eosinophils	Some scattered cells	Clusters of infiltrating cells at the base of the folds	Massive infiltrates and clusters at base and along the entire villi

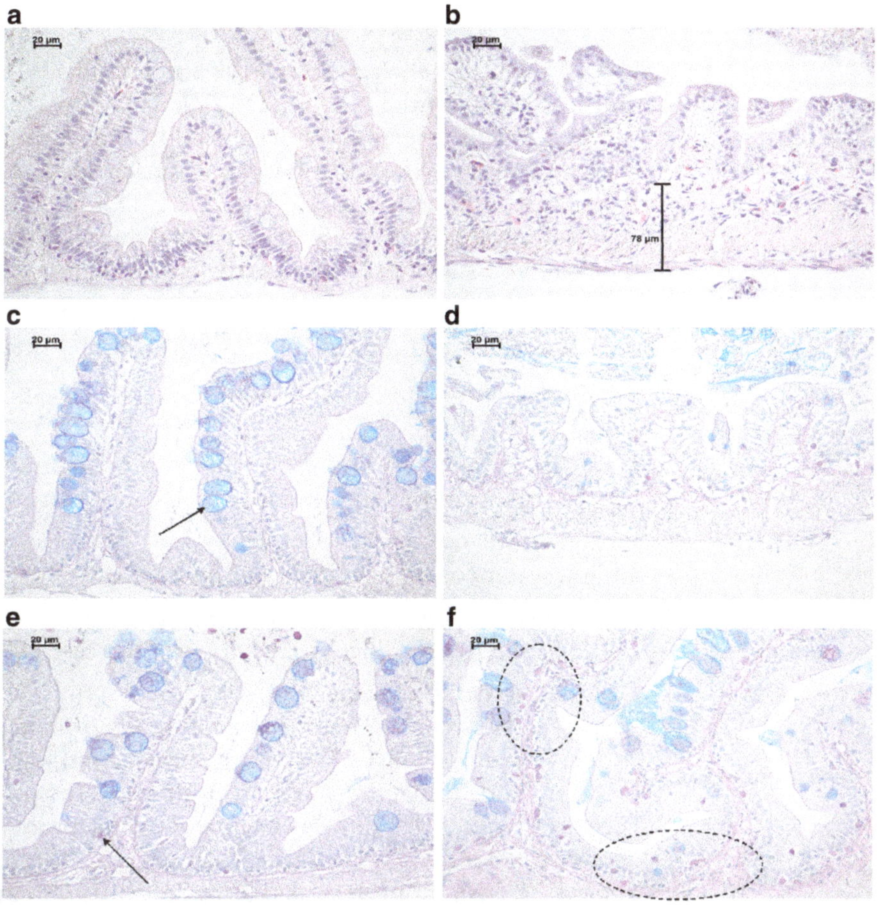

Fig. 2 Representative pictures of oxazolone-induced gut pathology. (**a**) Healthy intestines (anterior mid gut), (**b**) Bowel wall thickening (score 3, maximum score), (**c**) Normal number of Goblet cells (*black arrow*), (**d**) Depleted Goblet cells (score 3, maximum score), (**e**) normal numbers of eosinophils (*black arrow*), (**f**) Increased numbers of eosinophils (score 3, maximum score). For detailed description of the score please refer to Table 1 and [21]

enterocolitis score represents the cumulative values of these separate parameters for all three segments of the intestine.

5. Flow cytometric quantification of immune cells

   When using transgenic zebrafish, quantification of the desired cell type's presence in the intestines can be achieved by homogenizing the intestinal tissue by teasing it through a 70-μm filter (Greiner One). Use the back of a syringe plunger to disrupt the tissue. After rinsing in phosphate-buffered saline (PBS) containing 2% heat-inactivated newborn calf serum (NBCSi), tissue is further separated using 40-μm filter (Greiner One). After centrifugation (1350 rpm (300 × *g*), 4 °C, 10 min, Hereaus Multifuge 3S-R; Thermo Scientific, Waltham, MA), cells are taken up in 200 μL PBS containing 2% heat-inactivated NBCSi and 1 μL 7-amino-actinomycin D (Beckman Coulter, Fullerton, CA) to stain dead cells. The desired cell type can now be measured by flow cytometry using the appropriate channel.

4 Notes

1. Like in mammals the severity of the enterocolitis is dependent on the diversity of the microbiota [21]. Therefore, the absence of enterocolitis after oxazolone injection might indicate that your husbandry system is too clean. Transferring the zebrafish to separate tank with separate filter system without UV irradiated water will help diversify the intestinal microbiota and make the fish more susceptible to intestinal inflammation induction.
2. Be careful to use a blunt needle or silicone tubing around the needle not to harm the fish and assess the entire intestine.
3. Keep fish wet during injection and try to inject as quickly (but gently) as possible.
4. If fish are fed you can find the anal opening much easier when squeezing the abdomen.
5. First dissolve oxazolone completely in 100% ethanol before adding water (oxazolone does not dissolve otherwise).
6. Buy the smallest amount of tricaine as possible, and store the bottle in the freezer since its activity will decrease rapidly.
7. Do not use demi or normal tap water as system water for the zebrafish. It usually contains too high levels of metals such as copper killing the fish. For more information on zebrafish breeding and husbandry please consult Westerfield [22]. The zebrafish book, 5th Edition; A guide for the laboratory use of zebrafish (*Danio rerio*), Eugene, University of Oregon Press. Paperback (4th Edition available online: http://zfin.org/zf_info/zfbook/).

Acknowledgments

The authors would like to thank the Wilhelmina Children's Hospital Utrecht (WKZ research fund) and the Sophia Children's Hospital Research Fund (Vrienden van Sophia) Rotterdam for generously supporting this work.

References

1. Balla KM, Lugo-Villarino G, Spitsbergen JM, Stachura DL, Hu Y, Banuelos K, Romo-Fewell O, Aroian RV, Traver D (2010) Eosinophils in the zebrafish: prospective isolation, characterization, and eosinophilia induction by helminth determinants. Blood 116(19):3944–3954. doi:10.1182/blood-2010-03-267419
2. Renshaw SA, Loynes CA, Trushell DM, Elworthy S, Ingham PW, Whyte MK (2006) A transgenic zebrafish model of neutrophilic inflammation. Blood 108(13):3976–3978. doi:10.1182/blood-2006-05-024075
3. Lugo-Villarino G, Balla KM, Stachura DL, Banuelos K, Werneck MB, Traver D (2010) Identification of dendritic antigen-presenting cells in the zebrafish. Proc Natl Acad Sci U S A 107(36):15850–15855. doi:10.1073/pnas.1000494107
4. Ellett F, Pase L, Hayman JW, Andrianopoulos A, Lieschke GJ (2011) mpegl promoter transgenes direct macrophage-lineage expression in zebrafish. Blood 117(4):e49–e56. doi:10.1182/blood-2010-10-314120
5. Zapata A, Diez B, Cejalvo T, Gutierrez-de Frias C, Cortes A (2006) Ontogeny of the immune system of fish. Fish Shellfish Immunol 20(2):126–136. doi:10.1016/j.fsi.2004.09.005
6. Lam SH, Chua HL, Gong Z, Lam TJ, Sin YM (2004) Development and maturation of the immune system in zebrafish, Danio rerio: a gene expression profiling, in situ hybridization and immunological study. Dev Comp Immunol 28(1):9–28
7. Hu YL, Xiang LX, Shao JZ (2010) Identification and characterization of a novel immunoglobulin Z isotype in zebrafish: implications for a distinct B cell receptor in lower vertebrates. Mol Immunol 47(4):738–746. doi:10.1016/j.molimm.2009.10.010
8. Hansen JD, Landis ED, Phillips RB (2005) Discovery of a unique Ig heavy-chain isotype (IgT) in rainbow trout: implications for a distinctive B cell developmental pathway in teleost fish. Proc Natl Acad Sci U S A 102(19):6919–6924. doi:10.1073/pnas.0500027102
9. Zhang YA, Salinas I, Li J, Parra D, Bjork S, Xu Z, LaPatra SE, Bartholomew J, Sunyer JO (2010) IgT, a primitive immunoglobulin class specialized in mucosal immunity. Nat Immunol 11(9):827–835. doi:10.1038/ni.1913
10. Brugman S, Witte M, Scholman RC, Klein MR, Boes M, Nieuwenhuis EE (2014) T lymphocyte-dependent and -independent regulation of Cxcl8 expression in zebrafish intestines. J Immunol 192(1):484–491. doi:10.4049/jimmunol.1301865
11. Wallace KN, Pack M (2003) Unique and conserved aspects of gut development in zebrafish. Dev Biol 255(1):12–29
12. Mudumana SP, Wan H, Singh M, Korzh V, Gong Z (2004) Expression analyses of zebrafish transferrin, ifabp, and elastaseB mRNAs as differentiation markers for the three major endodermal organs: liver, intestine, and exocrine pancreas. Dev Dyn 230(1):165–173. doi:10.1002/dvdy.20032
13. Oehlers SH, Flores MV, Hall CJ, O'Toole R, Swift S, Crosier KE, Crosier PS (2010) Expression of zebrafish cxcl8 (interleukin-8) and its receptors during development and in response to immune stimulation. Dev Comp Immunol 34(3):352–359. doi:10.1016/j.dci.2009.11.007
14. Oehlers SH, Flores MV, Chen T, Hall CJ, Crosier KE, Crosier PS (2011) Topographical distribution of antimicrobial genes in the zebrafish intestine. Dev Comp Immunol 35(3):385–391. doi:10.1016/j.dci.2010.11.008
15. Gebert A, Jepson MA (1996) Is the epithelial origin of M cells controversial? Gastroenterology 111(4):1163
16. Wallace KN, Akhter S, Smith EM, Lorent K, Pack M (2005) Intestinal growth and differentiation in zebrafish. Mech Dev 122(2):157–173. doi:10.1016/j.mod.2004.10.009
17. Oehlers SH, Flores MV, Hall CJ, Okuda KS, Sison JO, Crosier KE, Crosier PS (2013) Chemically induced intestinal damage models in zebrafish larvae. Zebrafish 10(2):184–193. doi:10.1089/zeb.2012.0824
18. Geiger BM, Gras-Miralles B, Ziogas DC, Karagiannis AK, Zhen A, Fraenkel P, Kokkotou E (2013) Intestinal upregulation

of melanin-concentrating hormone in TNBS-induced enterocolitis in adult zebrafish. PLoS One 8(12):e83194. doi:10.1371/journal.pone.0083194

19. Goldsmith JR, Cocchiaro JL, Rawls JF, Jobin C (2013) Glafenine-induced intestinal injury in zebrafish is ameliorated by mu-opioid signaling via enhancement of Atf6-dependent cellular stress responses. Dis Model Mech 6(1):146–159. doi:10.1242/dmm.009852

20. Brugman S (2016) The zebrafish as a model to study intestinal inflammation. Dev Comp Immunol. doi:10.1016/j.dci.2016.02.020

21. Brugman S, Liu KY, Lindenbergh-Kortleve D, Samsom JN, Furuta GT, Renshaw SA, Willemsen R, Nieuwenhuis EE (2009) Oxazolone-induced enterocolitis in zebrafish depends on the composition of the intestinal microbiota. Gastroenterology 137(5):1757–1767, e1751. doi:10.1053/j.gastro.2009.07.069

22. Westerfield M (2007) The zebrafish book, 5th edn. A guide for the laboratory use of zebrafish (Danio rerio). Eugene: University of Oregon Press. Paperback (4th edition available online: http://zfin.org/zf_info/zfbook)

Part IV

Inflammation of the Brain, Joint and Vasculature

Chapter 22

High Dimensional Cytometry of Central Nervous System Leukocytes During Neuroinflammation

Dunja Mrdjen, Felix J. Hartmann, and Burkhard Becher

Abstract

Autoimmune diseases like multiple sclerosis (MS) develop from the activation and complex interactions of a wide network of immune cells, which penetrate the central nervous system (CNS) and cause tissue damage and neurological deficits. Experimental autoimmune encephalomyelitis (EAE) is a model used to study various aspects of MS, including the infiltration of autoaggressive T cells and pathogenic, inflammatory myeloid cells into the CNS. Various signature landscapes of immune cell infiltrates have proven useful in shedding light on the causes of specific EAE symptoms in transgenic mice. However, single cell analysis of these infiltrates has thus far been limited in conventional fluorescent flow cytometry methods by 14–16 parameter staining panels. With the advent of mass cytometry and metal-tagged antibodies, a staining panel of 35–45 parameters is now possible. With the aid of dimensionality reducing and clustering algorithms to visualize and analyze this high dimensional data, this allows for a more comprehensive picture of the different cell populations in an inflamed CNS, at a single cell resolution level. Here, we describe the induction of active EAE in C56BL/6 mice and, in particular, the staining of microglia and CNS invading immune cells for mass cytometry with subsequent data visualization and analysis.

Key words Central nervous system, Autoimmunity, EAE, Inflammation, Mass cytometry, High dimensional data

1 Introduction

Inflammation of the central nervous system (CNS), or neuroinflammation, can occur in response to a variety of cues. These include infection, traumatic brain injury, and degenerative diseases like multiple sclerosis (MS), Alzheimer's disease [1] and Parkinson's disease [2]. MS is initiated by autoreactive T cells that mount aberrant responses against CNS autoantigens, and is characterized by the infiltration of immune cells from the periphery across the blood brain barrier (BBB). This promotes inflammation and demyelination of neurons, resulting in neuroaxonal degeneration [3, 4].

Understanding the complex cellular interactions in the pathogenesis of MS critically relies on the use of mouse models, one of which is experimental autoimmune encephalomyelitis (EAE) [5].

Björn E. Clausen and Jon D. Laman (eds.), *Inflammation: Methods and Protocols*, Methods in Molecular Biology, vol. 1559, DOI 10.1007/978-1-4939-6786-5_22, © Springer Science+Business Media LLC 2017

EAE manifests as an acute, chronic and relapsing-remitting disease in different mouse strains [6]. In wild type C57BL/6 mice EAE is a chronic disease, which results in ascending paralysis of the animal. It is driven by helper T (TH) cells specific for myelin oligodendrocyte glycoprotein (MOG) which are primed in the periphery after subcutaneous immunization with an emulsion of MOG peptide or recombinant protein in Complete Freund's Adjuvant (CFA). MOG-specific, activated TH cells migrate to the CNS and are reactivated by vessel-proximal antigen presenting cells (APCs) and invade early in lesion formation where they secrete pro-inflammatory cytokines. These cytokines attract an abundant infiltration of myeloid cells [7]. Multiple populations of myeloid cells have been proposed to be involved in the effector phase of the disease, however recent reports indicated monocyte-derived dendritic cells or macrophages as the direct cause of eventual tissue damage and the critical perpetuator of the neuroinflammation during chronic disease [8, 9].

In order to study the role of specific cytokines and cell types in the progression and possible treatment of EAE and MS, numerous transgenic mice have been studied. One important readout during such a study is the landscape of infiltrating cells within the CNS at the peak of EAE symptoms. Conventional fluorescent flow cytometry has shed much light on the nature of these cell population landscapes under various knockout conditions but has been limited to an average of 14–16 parameters (depending on the cytometer) per staining panel. With the advent of mass cytometry and metal-tagged antibodies without the need for extensive compensation, this number has increased to 35–45 parameters (and continues to increase) [10]. Along with the application of dimensionality reduction and clustering algorithms to handle such large data, it is now possible to obtain a more comprehensive picture of the different infiltrating cell populations. In this chapter, we provide a detailed description of the induction and scoring of EAE in C57BL/6 mice, the isolation of the CNS at peak disease and preparation of a single cell suspension of microglia and infiltrating immune cells, the staining of cell markers with metal-tagged antibodies for mass cytometry, and finally the visualization and analysis of the resulting high dimensional data.

2 Materials

2.1 Experimental Autoimmune Encephalomyelitis (EAE) Induction

1. Rubber free Luer lock syringe with female Luer-to-closed part and Luer-to-Luer connector part.
2. MOG_{35-55} peptide (amino acid sequence: MEVGWYRS PFSRVVHLYRNGK).
3. Complete Freund's Adjuvant (CFA).

4. 24-G × 1″ Luer needle and 1 ml Luer lock syringe with rubber plunger head.
5. Pertussis toxin.
6. Insulin syringe.
7. Cage grid.
8. Gel-packet food.

2.2 CNS Isolation and Preparation of Single-Cell Suspension

1. 35-G butterfly needle attached to a 50 ml syringe for perfusion.
2. PBS.
3. Clamp.
4. Standard laboratory equipment including 70 μm nylon cell strainers, 50 ml Falcon tubes, eppendorf tubes, 12-well plate.
5. Digestion medium: RPMI complemented with 2 % FBS, 2 mM HEPES, 0.4 mg/ml Collagenase D and 2 mg/ml DNAse.
6. EDTA.
7. A 5 ml syringe with a 20-G needle for homogenizing.
8. Fixed angle rotor for centrifuge and fitting 16 ml tubes for one CNS sample, or 30 ml tubes when two samples are pooled.

2.3 Mass Cytometry Staining

1. Cell staining medium (CSM): PBS complemented with 0.5 % bovine serum albumin (BSA).
2. Horizontal shaker (optional).
3. Cisplatin (Sigma Aldrich) solution (1 μM in PBS).
4. Heavy-metal tagged antibodies (Fluidigm).
5. Cell-ID Intercalator-Ir (Fluidigm).
6. Maxpar® Fix and Perm Buffer (Fluidigm).
7. Intercalation solution: Maxpar® Fix and Perm Buffer supplemented with 1:4000 Cell-ID Intercalator-Ir.

2.4 Acquisition

1. Milli-Q ultra-pure deionized water.
2. Cell counter or microscope with hemocytometer.
3. Maxpar® EQ™ Four Element Calibration beads, diluted 1:10 in Milli-Q water.
4. Mass cytometer.

2.5 Data Analysis

1. Cytobank: https://www.cytobank.org/cytobank/
2. De-barcoding software (optional): https://github.com/nolan-lab/single-cell-debarcoder
3. FlowJo (optional).

3 Methods

3.1 Experimental Autoimmune Encephalomyelitis (EAE) Induction

3.1.1 Active Induction of EAE

1. An emulsion of MOG_{35-55} peptide in CFA is prepared using a rubber-free Luer-Lok syringe and connector system. A total of 200 μg of MOG_{35-55} peptide per mouse is diluted in PBS as required and mixed with an equal volume of CFA, to a final concentration of 100 μg/100 μl. The mixture is prepared directly in a rubber free Luer lock syringe which is then connected to a second Luer lock syringe and the mixture is mixed until a thick white emulsion forms (*see* **Note 1**).
2. Male or female C57BL/6 mice are anesthetized and injected subcutaneously (s.c.) with 100 μl of emulsion into each flank (200 μl in total) using a 24-G × 1″ Luer needle attached to a 1 ml Luer lock syringe with a rubber plunger head.
3. Following s.c. injection, mice are given 200 ng pertussis toxin intraperitoneally (i.p.) at the time of immunization (Day 0), and again 48 h later (Day 2), to aid in activation of a systemic inflammatory response.

3.2 Soring of EAE Disease Symptoms

EAE mice are assessed for disease symptoms according to our laboratory scoring criteria (*see* Fig. 1 and [11]): No disease: 0; distal limp tail: 0.5; complete limp tail: 1.0; limp tail and hind limb weakness: 1.5; unilateral partial hind limb paralysis: 2; bilateral partial hind limb paralysis: 2.5; complete bilateral hind limb paralysis: 3; complete bilateral hind limb paralysis and partial forelimb paralysis: 3.5; moribund (mouse completely paralyzed): 4; death: 5. Mice scoring 4 or between 4 and 5 are euthanized immediately. Disease symptoms commonly appear between day 7 and day 10 after immunization (*see* Fig. 1) (*see* **Note 2**).

3.3 CNS Isolation and Preparation of Single-Cell Suspension

1. Mice are euthanized with CO_2 and perfused with PBS through the left ventricle of the heart using a 25-G butterfly needle attached to a 50 ml syringe. The spinal cord is removed by flushing the spinal column with PBS after clamping the butterfly needle into the spinal column. The brain and brain stem are removed by dissecting the skull.
2. All the CNS tissues are then pooled and cut into small pieces using scissors in an empty eppendorf tube, transferred to a 12-well plate with 3 ml digestion medium (*see* Subheading 2.2 and **Note 3**) and digested at 37 °C for 30 min. Enzymatic digestion is stopped by adding EDTA to a final concentration of 5 mM.
3. To homogenize the tissue, the suspension is repeatedly sucked up and ejected using a 5 ml syringe with a 20-G needle until a uniform milky homogenate is formed, avoiding excessive foaming. Thereafter the homogenate is filtered through a

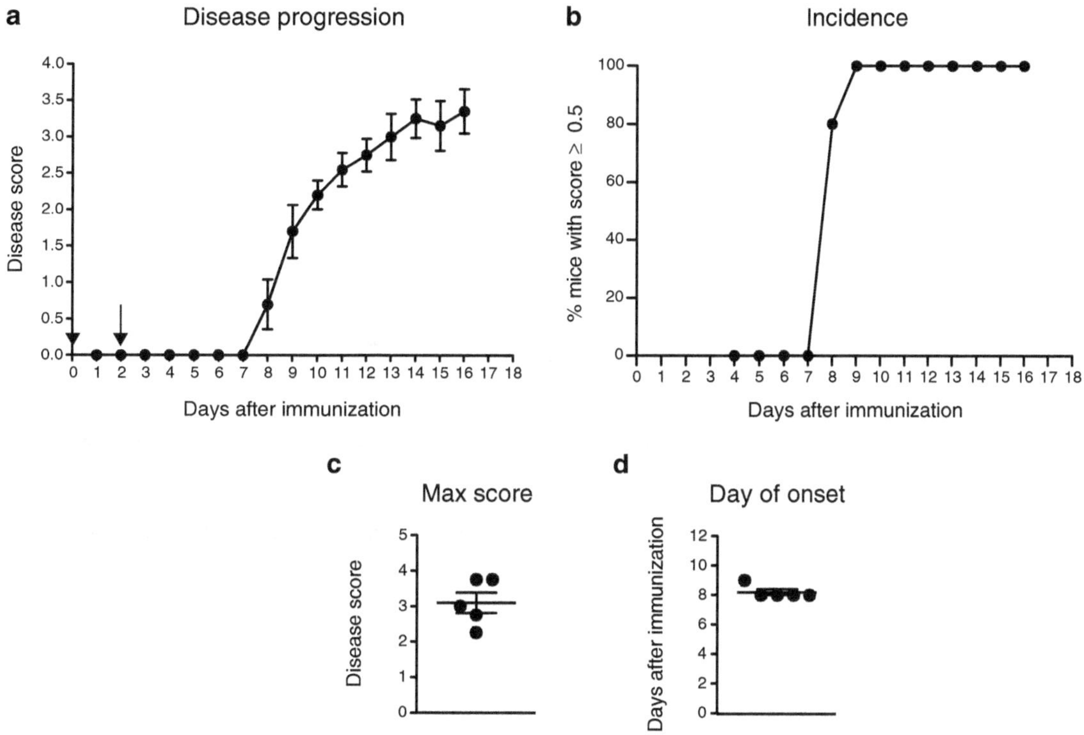

Fig. 1 EAE disease progression in wild type C57BL/6 mice. (***a***) Mice were immunized s.c. with 200 μg MOG peptide emulsified in CFA and 200 ng Pertussis toxin i.p. on Day 0, and with 200 ng Pertussis toxin again on Day 2. Mice were then scored for symptoms of EAE and sacrificed at Day 16 when the disease score was still at its peak. (***b***) Incidence of EAE as determined by the percentage of mice with a disease score of ≥0.5. (***c***) The mean day of onset of disease symptoms. (***d***) The mean maximum score reached after 16 days of EAE progression

70 μm nylon cell strainer into a 50 ml Falcon tube which is then filled up with PBS and centrifuged at 450 ×*g* for 8 min at 4 °C to pellet the cells and myelin.

4. The supernatant is discarded by pouring it off gently, and the pellet is resuspended in a final volume of 10.5 ml PBS to which 4.5 ml of Percoll is added (15 ml total volume, 30% Percoll). This is mixed to create a uniform distribution of Percoll and transferred to a 16 ml tube with a lid for a fixed angle rotor fitting in a centrifuge and centrifuged at 23,500 ×*g* for 30 min at 4 °C, without brakes (*see* **Note 4**). This step separates the cells from the myelin by density gradient centrifugation.
5. After centrifugation, a PBS-Percoll gradient will have formed, each layer containing a specific fraction of the homogenate (*see* Fig. 2). The myelin is carefully sucked off using a suction pump or pipette. The large middle layer containing the leukocytes (microglia and cell infiltrates in an EAE CNS or predominantly microglia in a naïve CNS) is transferred without the bottom

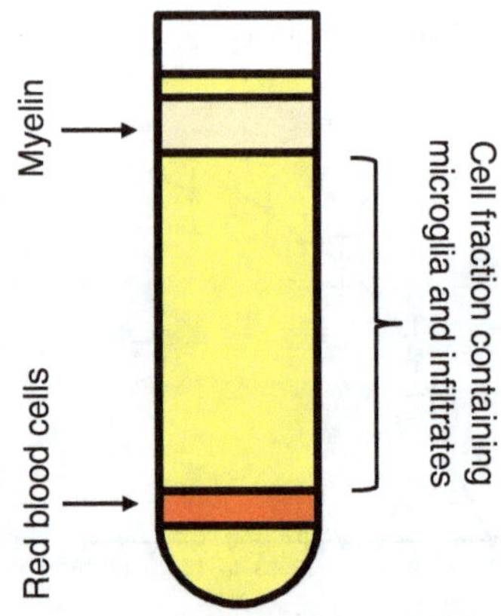

Fig. 2 The PBS-Percoll gradient layer formation after centrifugation. Three clear layers can be seen and contain specific parts of the CNS homogenate: the top layer is white and comprises the myelin just beneath the surface of the PBS-Percoll and can be sucked off with a suction pump; the large middle layer is transparent and comprises microglia and immune cell infiltrates; the bottom layer is red and comprises the red blood cells which can be left behind or taken along with the middle layer of immune cells

layer of red blood cells into a Falcon tube and filtered once more through a 70 μm nylon cell strainer (*see* **Note 5**). This is topped up with more PBS and centrifuged at 450×*g* for 10 min to pellet the cells. The supernatant is discarded and the cells are resuspended in 1 ml cell staining medium (CSM). The cell suspension is transferred to 1.5 ml eppendorf tubes and centrifuged at 300×*g* for 5 min. The supernatant is decanted and the cells are now ready for barcoding (optional) or directly for surface staining.

3.4 Mass Cytometry

3.4.1 Cell Surface Staining and Live/Dead Discrimination

Optionally, in a first step individual samples can be barcoded and combined into a single sample tube (*see* **Note 6**). Then the antibody mix for the cell surface staining is prepared by adding the appropriate concentration of each surface antibody in the panel to 100 μl/sample of CSM. In case more than 20×10^6 cells are present in the sample, this volume is adjusted so that the concentration of cells in the antibody mixture does not exceed 200×10^6/ml. Cells are incubated for 30 min at 4 °C, preferably on a horizontal shaker with 500 rpm (*see* **Note 7**). Subsequently, 400 μl of cisplatin solution (1 μM in PBS) are added to the samples on top of the surface antibody mix and incubated for a further 2 min at room temperature to allow for the exclusion of dead cells [12]. Lastly, 800 μl of CSM is added and the samples are centrifuged at 300×*g* for 5 min. The supernatant is decanted and the samples are now ready for optionalg intracellular staining (*see* **Note 8**) or DNA intercalation.

3.4.2 Cell Fixation and DNA Intercalation

First, the cell pellet is loosened in the remaining volume. Next, 400 µl of intercalation solution is added and the samples are incubated for at least 1 h at room temperature, or overnight at 4°C (*see* **Note 9**). DNA-intercalated iridium allows for the identification of cells during analysis, and separation from leftover myelin and debris.

3.4.3 Acquisition

The samples should be left in intercalation solution until the day of acquisition to prevent leakage of Iridium from the cells. On the day of acquisition, samples are pulse-vortexed and washed twice with 1 ml of CSM at 600×*g*, and lastly once with Milli-Q water. They should be left in pellet form and at 4 °C until the mass cytometer has been started up and tuned for acquisition. Immediately prior to injection of the sample, cells are resuspended in 500 µl of acquisition beads, counted, the cell concentration is adjusted to 1–2 million cells per ml, and injected into the mass cytometer (this is the optimal cell concentration when using the CyTOF Helios and varies between mass cytometer models).

3.5 Data Analysis

3.5.1 Data Quality Check

After acquisition, bead normalization and randomization of the data using the CyTOF software, the data can be stored in the FCS file format. In case barcoding has been performed, the combined file can now be debarcoded into single FCS files (*see* **Note 10**). Next, a manual quality check is performed for each antibody that was used to stain the cells. This can either be done by uploading the FCS files onto the web-based analysis platform cytobank [13] (*see* **Note 11**) or by using standard FCS file analysis software such as FlowJo. Antibodies that failed to give an identifiable positive signal for their particular marker are excluded from further analysis.

3.5.2 Data Visualization and Analysis

As a first step in data analysis, a suitable visualization of the high-dimensional data makes it more accessible to the researcher for further analysis. Such dimensionality reduction and visualization of the data can be achieved using a variety of existing algorithms [14, 15]. One of these is the t-Distributed Stochastic Neighbor Embedding (t-SNE) [16, 17] algorithm which displays the high dimensional data in a two dimensional plot where cells which are very similar in the high-dimensional space are located closely together. We will here describe the computation of the two t-SNE dimensions using the cytobank platform, however there are plenty of alternative implementations of the t-SNE algorithm, e.g., within the R-environment, now also available as a FlowJo add-on, or matlab (included in the cyt analysis platform [17]).

Before the generation of a t-SNE map, a few manual pre-gating steps should be performed. In case a visualization of all the immune cells within the CNS is the aim, then a simple gating on live, single, and optionally CD45$^+$, cells is required (*see* Fig. 3a). Using the viSNE feature within cytobank, the pre-gated population, the

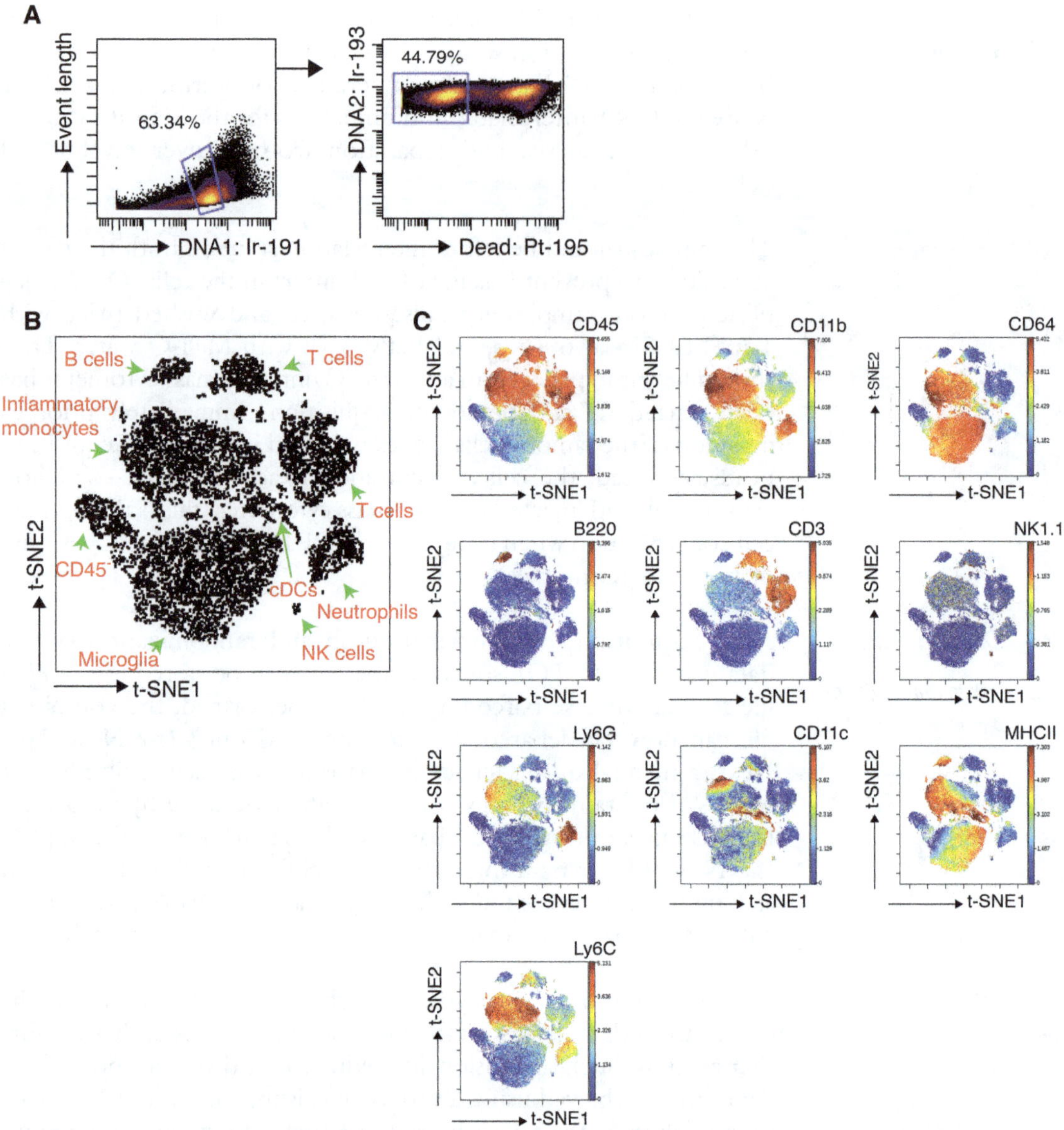

Fig. 3 Gating and data visualization with t-SNE. (***a***) Live cells are identified by the two DNA intercalating isotopes of Iridium, Ir-191 (DNA1) and Ir-193 (DNA2). Some doublet cells can be identified as DNA^{high} in the DNA1 channel and are excluded. Dead cells are identified by the dead cell marker Cisplatin, Pt-195, and are also excluded. The resulting gate comprises live, single cells and can further be gated on CD45^{+} cells. (***b***) The two dimensional t-SNE map depicting a landscape of various cell populations. Cells which are similar in the high dimensional space are positioned closely together on the two dimensional t-SNE map. (***c***) Identification of the cell populations in (***b***) by displaying relative expression levels of markers within the panel in the Working Illustration feature of cytobank. Based on these expression levels, we can identify microglia (CD45^{low} CD11b^{+} CD64^{+}), monocytes (CD45^{high} CD11b^{+} CD64^{+}), B cells (B220^{+}), T cells (CD3^{+}), NK cells (NK1.1^{+}), and neutrophils (Ly6G^{+}) in this sample of CNS from mice at peak EAE

according FCS files and the markers to be included in this visualization are selected (*see* **Note 12**). If a comparison between two groups of samples is desired, we recommend to include both sets of FCS files into one single analysis to allow the direct comparison of the two groups on the resulting t-SNE map.

Once the two t-SNE dimensions have been calculated, cytobank's Gating feature and the Working Illustration feature can display the FCS files separately as well as the expression levels of different markers across the map to get an instant overview and identify all immune populations present within the samples (*see* Fig. 3b, c). Visualization of the high-dimensional data using t-SNE thus helps to make high-dimensional data more accessible to researchers for further exploration, but it is only the first step in a more comprehensive analysis. For further analysis of the data, the FCS files can be exported from cytobank and imported into a clustering algorithm or an algorithm that identifies stratifying populations between two groups (*see* **Note 13**).

4 Notes

1. MOG_{35-55} peptide CFA emulsion: The syringe is connected to a second syringe ensuring that there are no air bubbles in the mixture. The mixture is repeatedly injected from one connected syringe to the other (left and right), for approximately 15 min (depending on the volume) during which time the color turns to white, the mixture feels denser and the emulsion is formed.
2. Unilateral hind limb paralysis is positive when one hind leg falls through the cage grid. While there is no world standard for scoring EAE symptoms, the commonly used scores are 0–5 or 0–6 point scales. Within these scales there is also variation between laboratories in evaluating the severity of EAE (reviewed in [18]), and between individual researchers, due to the subjective nature of the scoring. Variation in the day of onset of disease symptoms is common and can even vary from day 7 to day 14. The reason for this variation is not completely understood and may be a result of the potency of the CFA used. Mice should be monitored after immunization every second day until visible signs of EAE manifest, thereafter mice should be monitored daily. A gel-packet of food should be provided inside the cage when mice reach a score of 1.5 or more.
3. Collagenase IV and D purchased from Sigma or Worthington are used with comparable efficiency in our lab to prepare single cell suspensions. To prevent over-digestion and potential loss of cell surface epitopes, we recommend not exceeding the 30 min digestion time and adding EDTA to a final concentration of 5 mM at the end of the digestion to stop the reaction.

4. The ratio of PBS and Percoll must be maintained to create the correct density gradient during centrifugation. These volumes can be upscaled to accommodate pooled CNS samples. Tubes of 30 ml for fixed angle rotors are also available. Each closed tube should be inverted a couple of times before being placed into the centrifuge to ensure a uniform distribution or PBS, Percoll and homogenate. It is important to centrifuge samples with no brakes (or low brakes, depending on the centrifuge) set on the centrifuge to maintain the PBS-Percoll separation at the end of the run.
5. The bottom layer of red blood cells can also be included in the main leukocyte fraction to avoid loss of cells of interest. However, in this case it is recommended to include an erythrocyte specific antibody in the staining panel (e.g. Ter119).
6. The concept of live cell barcoding comprises labeling of the individual samples with a unique combination of dedicated heavy-metal isotopes by which they can be identified unambiguously later in the analysis [19–21]. Employing barcoding significantly reduces antibody consumption, renders possible sample carry-over during acquisition irrelevant, helps to exclude inter-sample doublet cells from the analysis and most importantly it eliminates non-biological inter-sample staining variability. A possible implementation of this concept is to label each sample with a unique combination of two or three anti-CD45 antibodies, conjugated to different heavy-metal isotopes. This can be achieved by incubating the samples with the respective combination of barcoding antibodies diluted in 100 μl CSM for 15–30 min at 37 °C on a horizontal shaker with 500 rpm. In case CD45 is essential for later discrimination of CD45 low and high expressing cell populations in the CNS such as microglia and infiltrates, a further anti-CD45 antibody conjugated to the same heavy-metal isotope (e.g., CD45-147 Sm from Fluidigm) for all samples can be added to the barcoding mix, however it is important to determine the maximum number of CD45 antibodies that can be used together per sample without loss of signal due to epitope saturation. After incubation, barcoded samples are washed by adding 1 ml of CSM and centrifuging for 5 min at 300 × *g*. The supernatant is discarded, the individual samples are resuspended in 100 μl CSM and then combined into a single 1.5 ml eppendorf tube. The combined sample is washed again by centrifuging the tube for 5 min at 300 × *g*. All subsequent steps, starting with the surface staining can now be performed on the combined sample.
7. Staining for several antigens, especially chemokine receptors, can usually be enhanced by performing the cell surface staining step for 20–30 min at 37 °C. However, it has to be ensured

that background staining for other cell surface antigens does not considerably increase using this approach.

8. In case a staining against intracellular antigens is desired in addition to surface antigens, cells are loosened and fixed by resuspending them in 300 μl of 1.6 % paraformaldehdye (PFA) in PBS for 30 min at 4 °C (or the preferred fixation buffer). Alternatively, fixation can be performed for 10 min at room temperature which we found to give comparable results. Cells are washed by adding 1 ml of perm buffer (PBS supplemented with 0.5 % saponin, 2 % BSA, and 0.05 % sodium azide) and centrifuging at 600 × *g* for 5 min, and decanting the supernatant. The antibody mix for the intracellular staining is prepared by adding the appropriate concentration of each antibody to 100 μl/sample of perm buffer. In case more than 20 million cells are present in the sample, this volume is adjusted so that the concentration of cells in the antibody mixture does not exceed 200×10^6/ml. Cells are incubated for 1 h at 4 °C, preferably on a horizontal shaker with 500 rpm. Afterwards, cells are washed by adding 1 ml of perm buffer and centrifuging at 600 × *g* for 5 min and decanting the supernatant.
9. We found that cells can be stored up to 2 weeks in intercalation solution without any significant impact on the quality of the staining.
10. Debarcoding of combined samples can either be performed using dedicated debarcoding software [19] or Boolean gates on the barcoding channels in FlowJo with subsequent export of the identified samples.
11. In addition, cytobank.org offers further tools for data visualization and analysis, such as t-SNE and SPADE. However, in order to use these functions, a fee-based premium account has to be purchased.
12. The number of cells used to generate the t-SNE map can either be proportional or equal between FCS files and should be optimized. However, the more cells used, the more the time required to generate the map. Another consideration is the selection of markers used which requires careful thought and optimization, since markers that are expressed in a broadly uniform manner across cell populations will not contribute to the resolution of cell populations in the t-SNE map. Conversely, markers that are expressed discretely by specific cell population and not by others will allow the separation of these populations and create clear pseudo-borders in the t-SNE map.
13. While t-SNE generates visually appealing maps of high dimensional data, it does not output clusters of populations with defined borders or an analysis of the differences between any two groups of samples. The clustering algorithm PhenoGraph

[22] is also available via the cyt platform for matlab and can output clusters and metaclusters of cell populations whose frequencies could then be calculated and compared between samples. Citrus [23], on the other hand, is available as a clickable R interfaced algorithm and runs clustering of data and outputs stratifying populations between two or more groups of samples.

References

1. Heppner FL, Ransohoff RM, Becher B (2015) Immune attack: the role of inflammation in Alzheimer disease. Nat Rev Neurosci 16: 358–372
2. Hirsch EC, Vyas S, Hunot S (2012) Neuroinflammation in Parkinson's disease. Parkinsonism Relat Disord 18:S210–S212
3. Compston A, Coles A (2008) Multiple sclerosis. Lancet 372:1502–1517
4. Dendrou CA, Fugger L, Friese MA (2015) Immunopathology of multiple sclerosis. Nat Rev Immunol 63:S3–S7
5. Ransohoff RM (2012) Animal models of multiple sclerosis: the good, the bad and the bottom line. Nat Neurosci 15:1074–1077
6. Terry RL, Ifergan I, Miller SD (2014) Experimental autoimmune encephalomyelitis in mice. In: Weissert R (ed) Multiple sclerosis : methods and protocols, vol 1304, Methods Mol Biol. Springer, New York, pp 145–160
7. Codarri L, Greter M, Becher B (2013) Communication between pathogenic T cells and myeloid cells in neuroinflammatory disease. Trends Immunol 34:114–119
8. Yamasaki R, Lu H, Butovsky O et al (2014) Differential roles of microglia and monocytes in the inflamed central nervous system. J Exp Med 211:1533–1549
9. Croxford AL, Lanzinger M, Hartmann FJ et al (2015) The cytokine GM-CSF drives the inflammatory signature of CCR2+ monocytes and licenses autoimmunity. Immunity 43: 502–514
10. Bendall SC, Nolan GP, Roederer M, Chattopadhyay PK (2012) A deep profiler's guide to cytometry. Trends Immunol 33: 323–332
11. Miller SD, Karpus WJ, Davidson TS (2007) Experimental autoimmune encephalomyelitis in the mouse. Curr Protoc Immunol 15(1): 1–26
12. Fienberg HG, Simonds EF, Fantl WJ et al (2012) A platinum-based covalent viability reagent for single-cell mass cytometry. Cytometry A 81(6):467–475
13. Kotecha N, Krutzik PO, Irish JM (2010) Web-based analysis and publication of flow cytometry experiments. In: Data processing and analysis. Curr Protoc Cytom 53: 10.17.1–10.17.24. John Wiley & Sons, Inc, pp 1–24.
14. Diggins KE, Ferrell PB, Irish JM (2015) Methods for discovery and characterization of cell subsets in high dimensional mass cytometry data. Methods 82:55–63
15. Chester C, Maecker HT (2015) Algorithmic tools for mining high-dimensional cytometry data. J Immunol 195:773–779
16. Van Der Maaten L, Hinton G (2008) Visualizing data using t-SNE. J Mach Learn Res 9:2579–2605
17. Amir ED, Davis KL, Tadmor MD et al (2013) viSNE enables visualization of high dimensional single-cell data and reveals phenotypic heterogeneity of leukemia. Nat Biotechnol 31:545–552
18. Takeuchi C, Yamagata K, Takemiya T (2013) Variation in experimental autoimmune encephalomyelitis scores in a mouse model of multiple sclerosis. World J Neurol 3:56–61
19. Zunder ER, Finck R, Behbehani GK et al (2015) Palladium-based mass tag cell barcoding with a doublet-filtering scheme and single-cell deconvolution algorithm. Nat Protoc 10:316–333
20. Mei HE, Leipold MD, Schulz AR et al (2015) Barcoding of live human peripheral blood mononuclear cells for multiplexed mass cytometry. J Immunol 194:2022–2031
21. Lai L, Ong R, Li J, Albani S (2015) A CD45-based barcoding approach to multiplex mass-cytometry (CyTOF). Cytometry A 87: 369–374
22. Levine JH, Simonds EF, Bendall SC et al (2015) Data-driven phenotypic dissection of AML reveals progenitor-like cells that correlate with prognosis. Cell 162:184–197
23. Bruggner RV, Bodenmiller B, Dill DL et al (2014) Automated identification of stratifying signatures in cellular subpopulations. Proc Natl Acad Sci U S A 111:E2770–E2777

Chapter 23

Isolation of Microglia and Immune Infiltrates from Mouse and Primate Central Nervous System

Thais F. Galatro*, Ilia D. Vainchtein*, Nieske Brouwer, Erik W.G.M. Boddeke, and Bart J.L. Eggen

Abstract

Microglia are the innate immune cells of the central nervous system (CNS) and play an important role in the maintenance of tissue homeostasis, providing neural support and neuroprotection. Microglia constantly survey their environment and quickly respond to homeostatic perturbations. Microglia are increasingly implicated in neuropathological and neurodegenerative conditions, such as Alzheimer's disease, Parkinson's disease, and glioma progression. Here, we describe a detailed isolation protocol for microglia and immune infiltrates, optimized for large amounts of *post mortem* tissue from human and rhesus macaque, as well as smaller tissue amounts from mouse brain and spinal cord, that yield a highly purified microglia population (up to 98% purity). This acute isolation protocol is based on mechanical dissociation and a two-step density gradient purification, followed by fluorescence-activated cell sorting (FACS) to obtain pure microglia and immune infiltrate populations.

Key words Microglia, Ex vivo, Acute isolation, FACS, Neuroinflammation, CNS, Multiple sclerosis, Glioma

1 Introduction

Microglia are the macrophages of the central nervous system (CNS), originating from erythro-myeloid progenitors in the yolk sac [1]. Microglia are highly specialized and adapted to their CNS environment, involved in CNS development and homeostasis [2–4]. Although microglia and other tissue macrophages, like liver Kupffer cells and skin Langerhans cells, arise from erythro-myeloid progenitors, they differ in their developmental programs and their respective tissue environment plays a major role in determining their unique gene expression profiles and functions [1, 5, 6].

Under healthy conditions, microglia are the only immune cells present in the CNS parenchyma. However, under neuropathological

*These authors contributed equally to this work.

Björn E. Clausen and Jon D. Laman (eds.), *Inflammation: Methods and Protocols*, Methods in Molecular Biology, vol. 1559, DOI 10.1007/978-1-4939-6786-5_23, © Springer Science+Business Media LLC 2017

and neurodegenerative conditions, various other immune and antigen-presenting (AP) cells, such as macrophages and dendritic cells, infiltrate the CNS tissue [7–9], where they modulate further immune cell infiltration and phenotypes. To elucidate the role of such immune cells in both normal conditions and disease, it is crucial to obtain sizable cell numbers and purity. Here, we present a fluorescence-activated cell sorting (FACS)-based protocol yielding highly pure immune cell populations from the CNS of mammals. The flexibility of this procedure allows diversity in sample origin (mouse, human and nonhuman primates) and tissue type (brain or spinal cord).

Contrary to enzymatic dissociation protocols, mechanical dissociation does not require a 37 °C incubation, hence maintaining the cell surface markers integrity and allowing for phenotype investigation [10]. The isolation procedure described here consists of three main steps: (1) mechanical dissociation of the tissue to obtain a single-cell suspension; (2) separation of cells from debris and myelin using Percoll gradient centrifugation; and (3) purification of immune cell types based on cell surface marker expression using FACS sorting (Fig. 1).

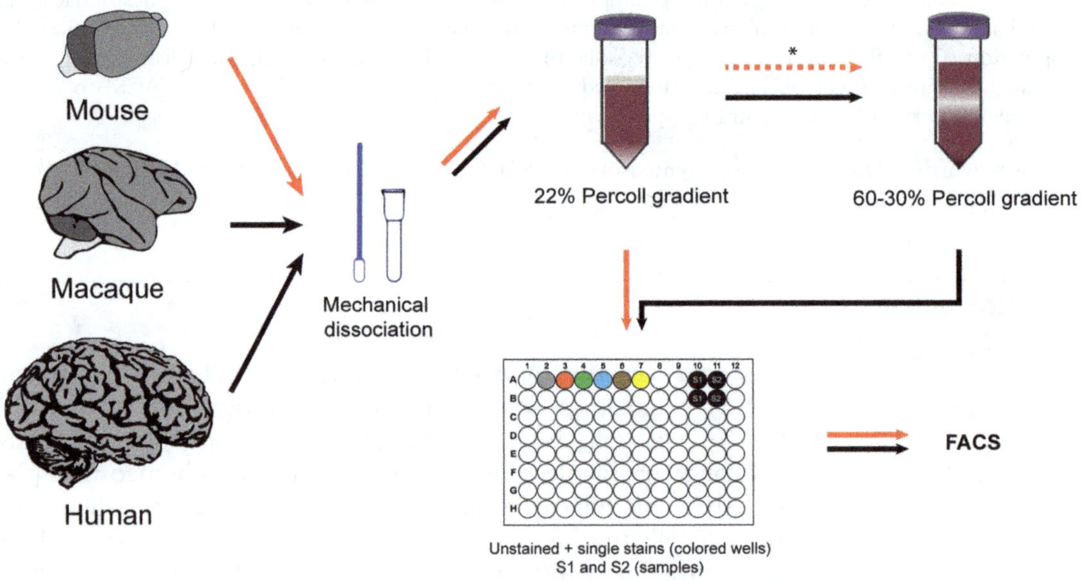

Fig. 1 Isolation protocol for microglia and immune infiltrates of the CNS. **Step 1**: mince brain tissue and dissociate with a glass tissue homogenizer until a homogeneous suspension is obtained. **Step 2**: myelin and cell debris are removed by Percoll gradient centrifugation. For small amounts of starting tissue, a single Percoll gradient is used (22 %) and the resulting pellet is used for the next step. For larger amounts and myelin-rich starting tissue, a second Percoll gradient separation is applied (60–30 %). In that case, the interphase between the two Percoll layers is used. **Step 3**: resulting cell suspension is blocked to reduce nonspecific antibody binding, then stained for the desired membrane markers. The cell suspension is then filtered in a FACS tube and FACS sorted (Beckman Coulter MoFlo Astrios/XDP). * Optional: for functional assays perform the 60–30 % Percoll gradient separation and continue from there

2 Samples

The origin and condition of the tissue sample is crucial for the end result of the isolation protocol. We have applied this optimized protocol to the following:

Mouse

Preferably, mice are perfused with 0.9% physiological saline solution prior to removal of CNS tissue to avoid contamination of CNS-immune cells with blood immune cells. Microglia have been successfully isolated from brain and spinal cord of several experimental conditions and molecular backgrounds, such as aged mice [11] and aging models (*mTerc*$^{-/-}$; *Ercc1*$^{\Delta/-}$) [12, 13], EAE (experimental autoimmune encephalomyelitis) [14], GL261 glioma injected brains, and Alzheimer's disease models (*APP23*, *5×FAD*).

Human and nonhuman primate samples

Human and nonhuman primate (Rhesus macaque; *Macaca mulatta*) brain samples have been collected under the course of full body autopsies. Donor age (increased cell-death and auto fluorescence with age), neuropathological condition (Alzheimer, Parkinson, and multiple sclerosis), CSF pH (pH ≤ 6.5 results in poor RNA quality) and *post mortem* interval (up to 24 h) varied between these samples, which affected cell yields. Microglia have also been successfully isolated from surgical biopsies collected after tumor resection (glioma) or temporal lobectomy of epilepsy surgeries.

3 Materials and Solutions

3.1 Materials

1. 50 and 15 mL tubes.
2. 5, 10, and 25 mL pipettes.
3. 1 mL, 200 μL, 20 μL, and 10 μL pipettes and tips.
4. 800 mL beaker glass with 106 and 300 μm sieve on top.
5. 70 μm cell-strainer.
6. Round bottom 96-wells microplate.
7. 5 mL polystyrene round-bottom tube with cell-strainer cap 12 × 75 mm style, referred to as "FACS tube".
8. 1.7 mL siliconized Eppendorf tubes.
9. 5 cm^3 or 15 cm^3 glass homogenizers.
10. Centrifuge with controllable acceleration and brake.

3.2 Solutions

1. **Isolation medium with phenol red (iMed⁺)** (this medium is not suitable for FACS, due to phenol red interference): 500 mL of HBSS (1×) with phenol red; 7.5 mL HEPES 1 M (f.c. 15 mM); 6.5 mL glucose 45% (f.c. 0.6%).
2. **Isolation medium without phenol red (iMed⁻)**: 50 mL of HBSS (1×) without phenol red; 750 μL HEPES 1 M (f.c. 15 mM); 650 μL glucose 45% (f.c. 0.6%); 100 μL 0.5 M EDTA pH 8.0 (f.c. 1 mM).
3. **Myelin gradient buffer**: prepare 1.5 L of $NaH_2PO_4 \cdot H_2O$ (0.78 g/L; f.c. 5.6 mM), solution 1. Prepare 1.5 L of Na_2HPO_4 $2H_2O$ (3.56 g/L; f.c. 20 mM), solution 2. Adjust solution 1 to pH 7.4 with solution 2. Measure the final volume and add: 8 g/L NaCl (f.c. 140 mM); 0.4 g/L KCl (f.c. 5.4 mM); 2 g/L glucose (f.c. 11 mM). Autoclave and keep sterile at 4 °C.
4. **22% Percoll gradient solution**: 110 mL Percoll; 12 mL NaCl 1.5 M; 378 mL myelin gradient buffer.
5. **100%-60%-30% Percoll solution**: prepare 100 % Percoll solution by mixing 27 mL Percoll with 3 mL 10x HBSS. For 60 % Percoll solution mix 18 mL 100% Percoll with 12 mL PBS; for 30 % Percoll solution mix 9 mL 100% Percoll with 21 mL PBS.
6. Virkon®S.
7. DAPI (200 μg/mL).
8. RNAlater.
9. RLT plus.

4 Methods

The whole procedure is conducted on ice and all centrifugation steps are performed at 4 °C. When dealing with primate samples, **steps 1–5** are carried out in a laminar flow due to potential biohazard risk. Waste is collected in 1% Virkon®S solution, stored for 24 h and autoclaved.

4.1 Preparation of a Single-Cell Brain Tissue Homogenate

1. Weigh tissue, place it in a petri dish with iMed⁺ and cut it into 2 mm³ pieces with a scalpel.
2. Transfer the minced tissue to a glass tissue homogenizer with iMed⁺ and homogenize until a uniform solution is obtained. When using a 5 cm³ glass tissue homogenizer, transfer up to 1 g of tissue each time, if a 15 cm³ glass tissue homogenizer is used, portions of 4 g can be transferred. Repeat the procedure until all tissue is homogenized (*see* **Note 1**).
3. For small amounts of tissue, use a pre-wetted (with 1 mL of iMed⁺) 70 μm cell-strainer on top of a 50 mL tube and filter the tissue homogenate. For larger amounts of tissue, put

106 μm and 300 μm sieves on top of an 800 mL beaker glass and filter the solution.

4. For large (primate) samples, divide the tissue homogenate over several 50 mL tubes, no more than 1.5 g starting material per 50 mL tube (for example: 7.5 g of tissue results in five tubes).
5. Rinse glass homogenizer and beaker glass with extra iMed$^+$ and add to the tissue homogenate after passing it through the sieve.
6. Centrifuge at $220 \times g$, 10 min (brake and acceleration: 9).
7. Carefully remove supernatant by pipetting.
8. Resuspend the cell pellet in 1 mL of 22% Percoll solution. Add 19 mL 22% Percoll solution to the 50 mL tube and mix well (or add 10 mL when using 15 mL tubes).
9. Carefully (without mixing) place 3 mL of PBS on top of the 22% Percoll solution.
10. Separate cells and myelin by centrifugation: 20 min, $950 \times g$ (acceleration 4; brake 0).
11. Carefully remove the myelin layer by pouring it off (or pipetting). Leave the cell pellet undisturbed. For human and non-human primate samples or functional assays that require vital cells (mouse; i.e. chemotaxis and phagocytosis), continue with **step 12**, otherwise continue with **step 20**.
12. Resuspend the cell pellet in 1 mL 60% Percoll using 1 mL pipette tip.
13. Add 14 mL of 60% Percoll solution (per 50 mL tube) to the suspension and homogenize.
14. Carefully place 14 mL of 30% Percoll on top of the 60% Percoll layer.
15. Carefully layer 3 mL PBS on top of the 30% Percoll. Centrifuge for 25 min, $800 \times g$ (acceleration 4; brake 0).
16. Collect the 60–30% interphase with a pre-wetted (with 1 mL iMed$^+$) glass pipette and transfer to a 50 mL tube containing iMed$^+$.
17. Add two volumes of iMed + equivalent to the collected cell-rich interphase.
18. Pellet cells by centrifugation: $600 \times g$, 10 min (brake and acceleration: 9).
19. Remove as much medium as possible (optional: place tube upside down).
20. Resuspend cell pellet in 100 μL iMed$^-$ (the cells can be used for functional assays).
21. To prevent aspecific binding of antibodies perform a blocking step. Incubate samples for 15 min on ice with the following blocking solution (Table 1):

Table 1
Blocking reagents

Sample origin	Blocking reagent	Supplier	Amount
Human/macaque	FcR-blocking	eBioscience	10/100 μL cell suspension
Mouse	Anti-mouse CD16/CD32	eBioscience	1/100 μL cell suspension

4.2 Settings of FACS Sorting Machine

In order to facilitate fluorochrome compensation and settings of the FACS machine, unstained and single stained reference samples should be made. A small volume of the sample(s) can be used for such purpose (further referred to as FACS setting solution), but keep in mind some of the markers are only lowly expressed in the brain. Preferably, beads can be used, or in case of mouse samples, splenocytes can be used for the settings (*see* **Note 2**). If a FACS setting solution is used, continue with **step 22**.

22. Transfer 5 μL of the sample to a separate tube for the settings. In case of multiple samples, take 5 μL of each sample and pool.
23. For primate samples fill the tube up to 300 μL with iMed$^-$, mouse samples up to 600 μL with iMed$^-$.
24. In a 96-well microplate, pipet 3 × 100 μL of FACS setting solution in 3 wells (unstained, CD11b PE single stain, CD45 FITC single stain) in case of primate samples; or 6 × 100 μL of FACS setting solution in 6 wells (unstained, CD11b PE single stain, CD45 FITC single stain; Ly-6C APC single stain, Ly-6G APC/Cy7 single stain, CD3 PE/Cy7 single stain) for mouse samples.

4.3 Antibody Incubation Procedure

25. Add antibodies to the single stains in the 96-well microplate as indicated in Table 2 below, keep on ice for 20–30 min, in the dark.
26. Prepare and add antibody mix to the samples (human: 1,2; macaque: 1,3; mouse: 4–8) in the falcon tubes as indicated in Table 2 below, keep on ice for 20–30 min, in the dark.
27. After incubation, divide the sample solution over several wells (100 μL in each well of a 96 well microplate). Wash the tube with an extra 100 μL of iMed$^-$ and pipet in a separate well. Add 100 μL of iMed$^-$ to all wells (single stains and samples).
28. Spin the cells down for 3 min at 300 × *g*.
29. Remove supernatant and add 100 μL of iMed$^-$ to each well.
30. Transfer each single stain to an individual FACS tube by filtering it through the pre-wetted (50–100 μL of iMed$^-$) filter.
31. Combine each divided sample into an individual pre-wetted (50–100 μL of iMed$^-$) FACS tube.

Table 2
Antibody dilution

Sample origin	Antibody	Clone	Isotype	Supplier	Dilution
1. Human/macaque	CD11b PE	ICRF44	Mouse IgG1, κ	Biolegend	1:25
2. Human	CD45 FITC	HI30	Mouse IgG1	Biolegend	1:25
3. Macaque	CD45 FITC	MB4-6D6	Mouse IgG1	Miltenyi Biotec	1:25
4. Mouse	CD11b PE	M1/70	Rat IgG2b, κ	eBioscience	1:170
5. Mouse	CD45 FITC	30-F11	Rat IgG2b, κ	eBioscience	1:250
6. Mouse	Ly-6C APC	HK1.4	Rat IgG2c, κ	Biolegend	1:130
7. Mouse	Ly-6G APC-Cy7	1A8	Rat IgG2a, κ	Biolegend	1:100
8. Mouse	CD3 PE/Cy7	17A2	Rat IgG2b, κ	Biolegend	1:100

32. Collect the remaining cells with iMed$^-$ (100–150 μL) from the 96 well microplate and add it to the corresponding FACS tubes.

4.4 FACS Isolation Myeloid Cells

33. 1–2 min before starting the FACS procedure add 0.5 μL of DAPI.
34. First, gate on all the events/cells (SSC^{height} vs FSC^{height}; to gate out cell debris), second gate on singlets (first gate in SSC^{width} vs FSC^{height} followed by FSC^{width} vs FSC^{height}) (single cells 1 and 2; Fig. 2).
35. Select the live, single cells by gating against DAPI (DAPI vs FSC^{height}).
36. For primate samples, plot for SSC^{height} vs a fluorochrome that is not in the panel (for example PE/Cy7 for primate samples) and gate for non-autofluorescent cells.
37. Then plot for CD11b vs CD45, the CD11b^{pos} CD45^{int} cells are the microglia. In case mouse samples are used, the microglia gate 1 can be plotted for SSC^{height} vs Ly-6C, as microglia are Ly-6C^{neg}. A pure microglia population can be sorted (CD11b^{pos} CD45^{int} Ly-6C^{neg}; Fig. 2).
38. In the CD11b vs CD45 plot, the CD11b^{high}CD45$^{int-high}$ cells (myeloid gate) are the infiltrates, consisting of macrophages and neutrophils that can be separated in mouse samples by gating for Ly-6G and Ly-6C (macrophages are Ly-6C^{pos} Ly-6G^{neg} and neutrophils are Ly-6C^{int} Ly-6G^{pos}).
39. In mouse samples, the CD45^{high} CD11b^{neg} fraction (lymphoid gate) in the CD11b vs CD45 plot can be plotted for SSC^{height} vs CD3 and a T-lymphocyte population can be sorted.

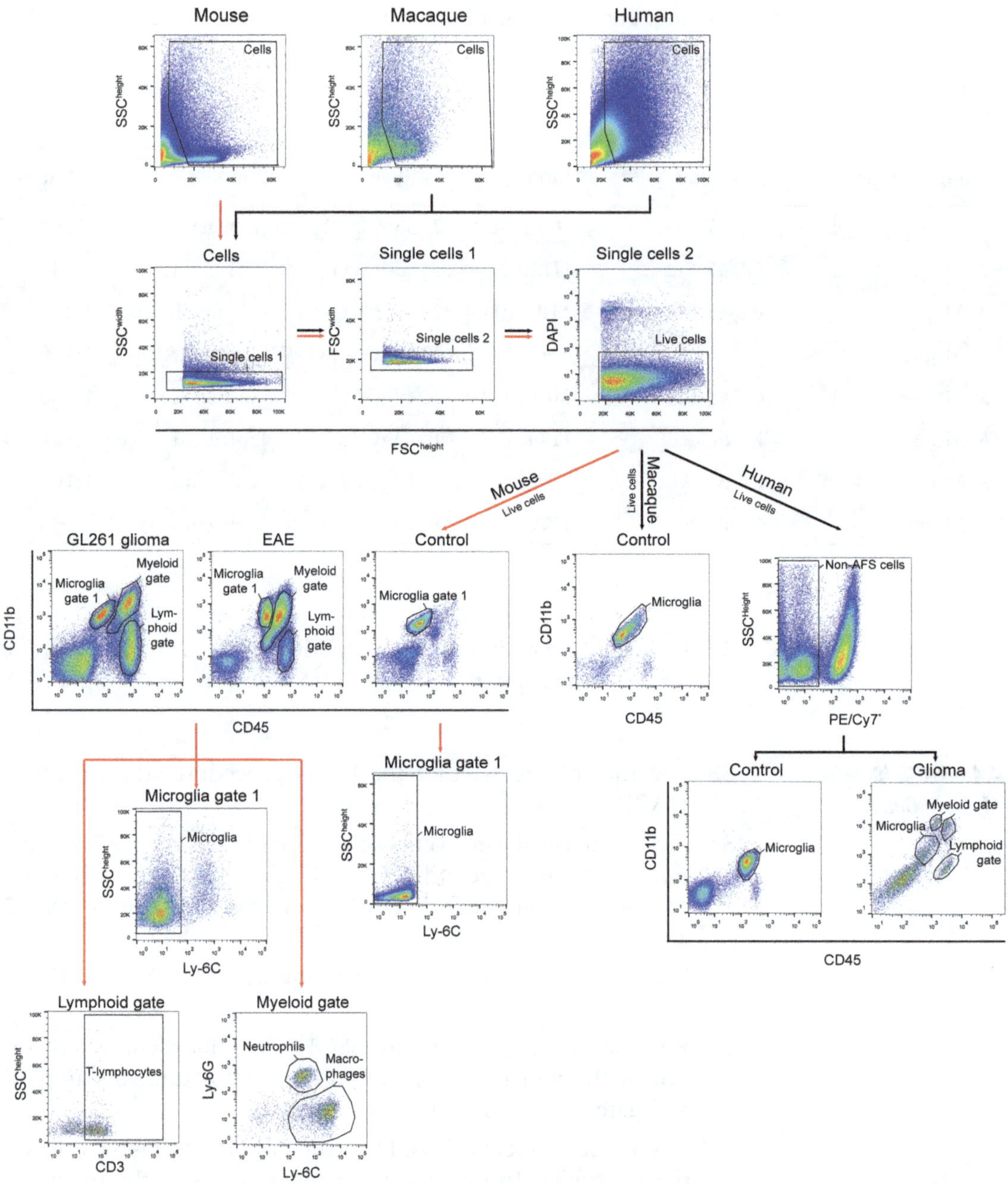

Fig. 2 FACS sorting strategy. To isolate pure populations of microglia and different immune infiltrates (macrophages, neutrophils, and T-lymphocytes), cells are first separated from cell debris and the remaining myelin by a gate in the SSC^{height} vs FSC^{height}. Single cells are selected in the SSC^{width} vs FSC^{height} followed by FSC^{width} vs FSC^{height} gates (single cells 1 and 2 gate). To obtain high quality RNA/DNA samples, live cells can be gated as $DAPI^{neg}$ (DAPI vs FSC^{height}). Depending on the experimental condition in mice, three well identifiable cell populations can be distinguished using CD11b vs CD45 plotting. From the microglia gate 1, microglia can be identified as Ly-$6C^{neg}$ when plotting for SSC^{height} vs Ly-6C. The myeloid gate contains two main populations when plotting for Ly-6G vs Ly-6C; macrophages are Ly-$6C^{pos}$ Ly-$6G^{neg}$ and neutrophils Ly-$6C^{int}$ Ly-$6G^{pos}$. T-lymphocytes ($CD3^{+}$) can be sorted when gating for SSC^{height} vs CD3 in the lymphoid gate. For the primate samples, after the live cells gate, the autofluorescent cells should be removed by gating on the non-autofluorescent (AFS) cells (SSC^{height} vs a fluorochrome that is not used, preferably APC or PE/Cy7). This has to be performed for human samples, but is not obligatory for macaque due to less autofluorescence. In the CD11b vs CD45 plot, microglia can be identified as $CD11b^{pos}$ $CD45^{int}$

40. During sorting, cells should be collected in siliconized tubes filled with the following, depending on desired downstream application:
    - 350 μL RNAlater, in case of RNA/DNA isolation for gene expression profiling.
    - 350 μL iMed^{-}, for other applications such as protein isolation and chromatin immunoprecipitation.
41. Collection of cells by centrifugation will depend on downstream application. i.e., for RNA/DNA isolation purposes, centrifuge 10 min, 5000 RCF; carefully remove RNA later and lyse (invisible) cell pellet in 350 μL RLTplus and store at −80 °C.
42. If cells are collected in iMed^{-}, centrifuge for 10 min at 500 RCF, remove supernatant and resuspend pellet in the appropriate buffer.

5 Notes

1. It is advised to use a 5 cm^3 glass tissue homogenizer for low myelin content samples (i.e., mouse brain, spinal cord, glioma tissue) and a 15 cm^3 glass tissue homogenizer for higher amounts of starting material or samples with high myelin content (primates).
2. Mouse splenocyte isolation: conduct **steps 1–7** as described above. Resuspend the pellet in 1 mL of lysis buffer (ammonium chloride 155 mmol/L, potassium bicarbonate 10 mmol/L, sodium edetate 0.1 mmol/L) to remove red blood cells and incubate on ice for 5 min. Fill to 15 mL with iMed + and perform **step 7** again. Carefully pour off (or pipet) supernatant and resuspend pellet in 1 mL of iMed−. Use this cell suspension for the calibration and settings of FACS sorting machine and continue with **step 24**.

References

1. Hoeffel G, Chen J, Lavin Y et al (2015) C-Myb(+) erythro-myeloid progenitor-derived fetal monocytes give rise to adult tissue-resident macrophages. Immunity 42:665–678
2. Aloisi F (2001) Immune function of microglia. Glia 36:165–179
3. Ransohoff RM, Perry VH (2009) Microglial physiology: unique stimuli, specialized responses. Annu Rev Immunol 27:119–145
4. Prinz M, Tay TL, Wolf Y et al (2014) Microglia: unique and common features with other tissue macrophages. Acta Neuropathol 128:319–331
5. Gosselin D, Link VM, Romanoski CE et al (2014) Environment drives selection and function of enhancers controlling tissue-specific macrophage identities. Cell 159:1327–1340
6. Lavin Y, Winter D, Blecher-Gonen R et al (2014) Tissue-resident macrophage enhancer landscapes are shaped by the local microenvironment. Cell 159:1312–1326
7. McMenamin PG, Wealthall RJ, Deverall M et al (2003) Macrophages and dendritic cells in the rat meninges and choroid plexus: three-dimensional localisation by environmental scanning electron microscopy and confocal microscopy. Cell Tissue Res 313:259–269
8. Chinnery HR, Ruitenberg MJ, McMenamin PG (2010) Novel characterization of

monocyte-derived cell populations in the meninges and choroid plexus and their rates of replenishment in bone marrow chimeric mice. J Neuropathol Exp Neurol 69: 896–909

9. Brendecke SM, Prinz M (2015) Do not judge a cell by its cover-diversity of CNS resident, adjoining and infiltrating myeloid cells in inflammation. Semin Immunopathol 37: 591–605
10. Olah M, Raj D, Brouwer N et al (2012) An optimized protocol for the acute isolation of human microglia from autopsy brain samples. Glia 60:96–111
11. Holtman IR, Raj DD, Miller JA et al (2015) Induction of a common microglia gene expression signature by aging and neurodegenerative conditions: a co-expression meta-analysis. Acta Neuropathol Commun 3:31
12. Raj DDA, Moser J, van der Pol SMA et al (2015) Enhanced microglial pro-inflammatory response to lipopolysaccharide correlates with brain infiltration and blood–brain barrier dysregulation in a mouse model of telomere shortening. Aging Cell 14:1003–1013
13. Raj DDA, Jaarsma D, Holtman IR et al (2014) Priming of microglia in a DNA-repair deficient model of accelerated aging. Neurobiol Aging 35:2147–2160
14. Vainchtein ID, Vinet J, Brouwer N et al (2014) In acute experimental autoimmune encephalomyelitis, infiltrating macrophages are immune activated, whereas microglia remain immune suppressed. Glia 62:1724–1735

Chapter 24

Investigating the Lymphatic Drainage of the Brain: Essential Skills and Tools

Nazira J. Albargothy, Matthew MacGregor Sharp, Maureen Gatherer, Alan Morris, Roy O. Weller, Cheryl Hawkes, and Roxana O. Carare

Abstract

In this chapter we describe in detail the surgical and imaging techniques employed for the study of the anatomical routes of drainage of cerebrospinal fluid (CSF) and interstitial fluid (ISF) from the brain. The types of tracers, sites of injection, and volumes injected are crucial. For example, when testing the drainage of ISF from the parenchyma, volumes larger than 0.5 μL result in spillage of ISF into the ventricular CSF.

Key words Mouse brain, Perivascular lymphatic drainage, Alzheimer's disease, Interstitial fluid, Cerebrospinal fluid, Solute clearance, Rodent perfusion, Intraparenchymal stereotactic injections, Cisterna magna injections

1 Introduction

Apart from blood, there are two major extracellular fluids associated with the CNS: cerebrospinal fluid (CSF) and interstitial fluid (ISF). The pathways of communication between the CSF and ISF or between ISF and the immune system are still unclear. We have demonstrated in rodents that (1) CSF drains alongside olfactory nerves into the nasal mucosa [1] and (2) solutes drain from the ISF along basement membranes of capillaries and arteries towards the surface of the brain [2]. Previous work suggests that ISF reaches deep cervical lymph nodes, but the exact route is not known [3]. Recent experimental work has demonstrated a "glymphatic" pathway whereby CSF and ISF equilibrate and the anatomical route is along the pial-glial basement membranes [4, 5].

In this chapter we describe several well-established surgical and imaging techniques developed and optimized at the University of Southampton by Professor Dr Roxana O. Carare and her research team. These techniques are evident in articles describing the study of extracellular fluid movement within mouse cerebral tissue [2,

Björn E. Clausen and Jon D. Laman (eds.), *Inflammation: Methods and Protocols*, Methods in Molecular Biology, vol. 1559, DOI 10.1007/978-1-4939-6786-5_24, © Springer Science+Business Media LLC 2017

5–21]. Briefly, intraparenchymal or intracisternal injections of tracers are performed on mice. The mice are then fixed by perfusion and their brains removed. Brains are then processed according to protocols optimized for protein identification (immunohistochemistry), tracer movement (fluorescent microscopy) and ultrastructural tracer position (Floating 3,3′diaminobenzidine (DAB) immunohistochemistry with electron microscopy). When combined these techniques provide a very powerful set of tools for advancing knowledge of the morphology and physiology of the lymphatic drainage of the brain. This is essential for understanding how soluble biomarker proteins reach the CSF and how the immune system reacts in neuroimmunological conditions and with increasing age [22].

2 Materials

A number of materials and reagents are required throughout the surgical and tissue processing techniques described in this chapter. Reagents that must be prepared prior to performing these techniques include fixative, appropriately diluted tracers, and anesthetic.

2.1 Fluorescent Tracers for Parenchymal and ntracisternal Injection

1. 10 mM 10 kDa Dextran Texas Red: Dissolve 5 mg of dextran in 100 μL of filtered ice-cold 0.01 M phosphate buffered saline (PBS), pH 7.2. Vortex (5 s) and aliquot 10 μL into ten Eppendorf tubes. Centrifuge for 5 min. Wrap aliquots in aluminum foil and store at −20 °C (*see* **Note 1**).
2. 100 μL human amyloid-beta (1–40) HiLyte Fluor 555: Add 50 μL of filtered 1% NH_4OH to 0.1 mg of Amyloid-beta (1–40) HiLyte Fluor 555 (Cambridge Bioscience). Vortex for 30 s. Add 52.6 μL of filtered 0.01 M PBS, pH 7.2. Vortex for 30 s. Pipette 10 μL into five separate Eppendorf tubes to produce stock 200 μL aliquots. Store on dry ice. Add 52.6 μL of filtered 0.01 M PBS, pH 7.2 to the remaining solution. Vortex for 5 s. Decanter into 10 μL aliquots to produce 100 μL solutions. Wrap all aliquots in aluminum foil and immediately store at −80 °C (*see* **Note 2**).

2.2 Induction of Anesthesia for Surgery

1. Experimental mice (*see* **Note 3**).
2. Scales.
3. Standard isoflurane anesthesia system.

2.3 Stereotactic Injection of Tracers into Mouse Hippocampus

1. Stereotaxic frame with nosepiece anesthesia attachment.
2. Dissection microscope.
3. Inspection light (ideally gooseneck cold LED) (*see* **Note 4**).
4. Rodent temperature controller system.

5. Hair clippers (Wella/Contura).
6. Micromotor drill with 0.7 mm burr.
7. Lacri-lube (ocular lubricant).
8. 1–5 μL Hirschmann microcapillary pipette with attached injection syringe (Fig. 5).
9. Pipette puller (*see* **Note 5**).
10. Dissection tools (sterile surgical scalpel (size 10A), tough cut scissors, forceps tip width 2.5 mm).
11. 0.9% saline.
12. Vaseline.
13. Paper towels.
14. Cotton buds.
15. Dust Off.
16. Pentobarbitone: 1:10 in 0.9% saline.

2.4 Injection of Tracers into Mouse Cisterna Magna

1. Stereotaxic frame with nosepiece anesthesia attachment.
2. Dissection microscope.
3. Inspection light (ideally gooseneck cold LED).
4. Rodent temperature controller system.
5. Hair clippers (Wella/Contura).
6. Micromotor drill with 0.7 mm burr.
7. Lacri-lube (ocular lubricant).
8. 1–5 μL Hirschmann microcapillary pipette with attached injection syringe (Fig. 5).
9. Pipette puller (*see* **Note 5**).
10. Dissection tools (sterile surgical scalpel (size 10A), tough cut scissors, forceps tip width 2.5 mm, length 12 cm and 2× curved dissection forceps).
11. 0.9% saline.
12. Vaseline.
13. Paper towels.
14. Cotton buds.
15. Dust Off.
16. Pentobarbitone: 1:10 in 0.9% saline.

2.5 Perfusion Fixation

2.5.1 Buffers

1. 0.2 M Piperazine-*N*,*N*′-bis-2-ethanesulfonic acid (PIPES) buffer, pH 7.2: Mix 60.48 g PIPES with 900 mL of distilled water. Add 10 M sodium hydroxide dropwise to bring the pH up to 7.2. Make up to 1 L with distilled water to produce a 0.2 M solution of PIPES buffer, pH 7.2. Store at 4 °C (*see* **Note 6**).

2. 0.01 M phosphate buffered saline (PBS), pH 7.2: Dissolve 50 PBS tablets (Sigma-Aldrich) in 1 L of distilled water to make 10× stock. Dilute 1:10 in distilled water for use. Store stock at room temperature.

2.5.2 Fixatives

1. 4% paraformaldehyde in 0.01 M PBS, pH 7.2: Mix 4 g of paraformaldehyde with 20 mL distilled water. Heat to 60 °C on a hotplate stirrer, add 2–4 drops of 1 M NaOH and stir until solution clears (*see* **Note 7**). Make up to 50 mL with distilled water, add 50 mL of 0.02 M PBS and adjust pH to 7.2 using NaOH or HCL. Store at 4 °C (*see* **Note 8**).
2. 3.4% formaldehyde plus 3% glutaraldehyde in 0.1 M PIPES buffer, pH 7.2: Mix 4 g of paraformaldehyde with 20 mL of distilled water. Heat to 60 °C on a hotplate stirrer, add 2–4 drops of 1 M NaOH and stir until the solution clears (*see* **Note 7**). Cool slightly and add 12 mL of 25% EM grade glutaraldehyde. Make up to 50 mL with distilled water and add 50 mL of 0.2 M PIPES buffer, pH 7.2. Store at 4 °C.

2.5.3 Perfusion

1. Syringe pump.
2. Dissection instruments (straight blunt scissors, standard pattern, gently curved blunt serrated larger finger loops, haemostat and small forceps).
3. 27 G × 0.38″ × 12″ butterfly needles.
4. 26 G ½″ × 0.45 × 13 mm needles.
5. 2 × 20 mL syringes.
6. 15 mL tubes.
7. Perfusion platform.

2.6 Tissue Processing

Tissue processing for immunohistochemistry and fluorescent/confocal microscopy can be performed on wax embedded, fresh (unfixed) and fixed frozen tissue. The materials listed here are for protocols optimized for tissue and antigen preservation in fixed frozen tissue. Processing for electron microscopy is performed on fixed tissue (Fig. 1).

2.6.1 Immunohistochemistry

The following materials are required for the processing of fixed frozen tissue with optimum tissue and antigen preservation.

1. 30% sucrose: Dissolve 30 g of sucrose in 100 mL of distilled water. Store at 4 °C.
2. OCT cryo-embedding media.
3. Base molds.
4. Liquid nitrogen.
5. Cryostat and associated microtomy equipment.

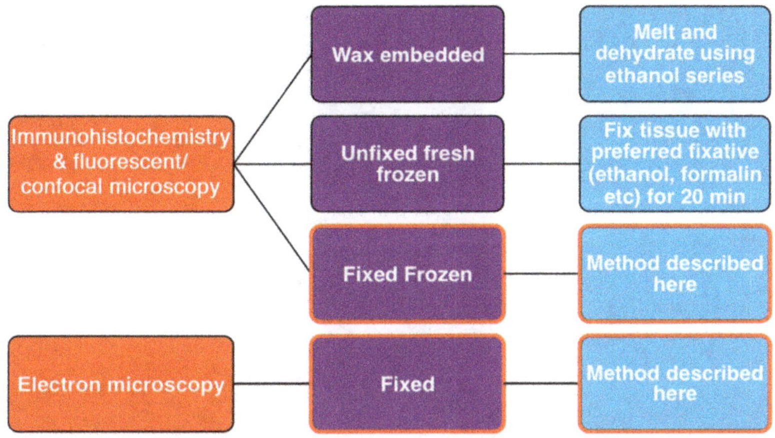

Fig. 1 Overview of tissue processing types. *Boxes highlighted in red* are relevant to the protocols described in this chapter

6. Superfrost slides.
7. Slide staining rack.
8. 0.01 M PBS, pH 7.2.
9. 3 % hydrogen peroxide.
10. Blocking serum (Fig. 2) (*see* **Note 9**).
11. Primary antibody (Fig. 2) (*see* **Note 9**).
12. Secondary antibody.
13. ABC vector.
14. 0.2 M sodium acetate: Dissolve 1.64 g of sodium acetate in 100 mL of deionized water. Adjust to pH 6.0 using 20 % acetic acid.
15. 0.1 M sodium acetate: Dilute 50 mL of 0.2 M sodium acetate in 50 mL of deionized water.
16. 2.5 g nickel ammonium sulfate.
17. 200 mg D-glucose.
18. 40 mg ammonium chloride.
19. 1.5 mg glucose oxidase (store at −18 °C until ready to use).
20. 60 mg DAB.
21. 1 in 5 diluted Harris hematoxylin.
22. Ethanol series in distilled water (50, 70, 95, 100 %).
23. Xylene.
24. DPX mounting medium.

Protein of interest	Serum	Primary antibody	Secondary antibody
Collagen IV	Goat	Polyclonal rabbit anti-collagen IV Dilution ratio: 1 : 400	Goat anti-rabbit IgG
Smooth muscle actin	Goat	Polyclonal rabbit anti-alpha smooth muscle actin Dilution ratio: 1 : 200	Goat anti-rabbit IgG

Fig. 2 Common antibodies used for immunohistochemistry. The two antibodies listed here are particularly useful for identifying cerebral blood vessels

Protein of interest	Serum	Primary antibody	Secondary antibody
Collagen IV	Goat	Polyclonal rabbit anti-collagen IV Dilution ratio: 1 : 400	Goat anti-rabbit alexaflour488 conjugate
Smooth muscle actin	Goat / Donkey / Horse	Mouse monoclonal anti-alpha smooth mucle actin (FITC) Dilution ratio: 1 : 200	Not required
Smooth muscle actin	Goat	Polyclonal rabbit anti-alpha smooth muscle actin Dilution ratio: 1 : 200	Goat anti-rabbit alexaflour488 conjugate

Fig. 3 Common antibodies used for fluorescent/confocal microscopy. The three antibodies listed here are particularly useful for identifying cerebral blood vessels

2.6.2 Fluorescence/Confocal Microscopy

The following materials are required for the processing of fixed frozen tissue.

1. Cryostat and associated microtomy equipment.
2. Superfrost slides.
3. Slide staining rack.
4. 0.01 M PBS, pH 7.2.
5. Blocking serum (Fig. 3) (*see* **Note 9**).

6. Primary antibody (Fig. 3) (*see* **Note 9**).
7. Secondary antibody (Fig. 3).
8. Mowiol mounting medium.

2.6.3 Floating DAB Immunohistochemistry for Transmission Electron Microscopy

The following materials are required for the processing of perfusion fixed tissue.

Human Amyloid-Beta (1–40) HiLyte Fluor 555 Fibril Test

1. Human amyloid-beta (1–40) HiLyte Fluor 555.
2. Thioflavin.
3. Formbar coated EM grid.
4. Oven (set at 37 °C).

Vibratome Slicing

1. Vibratome.
2. 0.01 M PBS, pH 7.2.
3. 12-well cell culture plate.
4. Small paintbrush.
5. Superglue.
6. Dissecting blades.

Floating DAB Immunohistochemistry

1. 24-well cell culture plate.
2. Shaker.
3. Parafilm.
4. 0.01 M PBS, pH 7.2.
5. 0.3% hydrogen peroxide: add 10 mL of 30% hydrogen peroxide to 90 mL of 0.01 M PBS, pH 7.2.
6. 70% formic acid.
7. 0.1% Triton X-100 in 0.01 M PBS, pH 7.2.
8. Blocking serum: 5% goat serum with 5% fetal bovine serum in 0.01 M PBS, pH 7.2.
9. Mouse monoclonal anti-Aβ40 (4G8) (BioLegend): dilute antibody 1:100 in 0.01% Triton in 0.01 M PBS, pH 7.2. Wrap with parafilm to prevent evaporation and store at 4 °C.
10. Horse anti-mouse biotinylated IgG: dilute antibody 1:400 in 0.01% Triton in 0.01 M PBS, pH 7.2.
11. ABC vector.
12. Deionized water.
13. 0.1 M sodium acetate.
14. 20% acetic acid.
15. 2.5 g nickel ammonium sulfate.

16. 200 mg D-glucose.
17. 40 mg ammonium chloride.
18. 1.5 mg glucose oxidase (store at −18 °C until ready to use).
19. 60 mg DAB.

Tissue Processing for Electron Microscopy

1. Glass vials and rotator.
2. PIPES buffer, pH 7.2.
3. 2% aqueous osmium tetroxide: Dissolve 1 g osmium tetroxide in 50 mL distilled water to produce 2% stock. Store in triple containment at 4 °C (*see* **Note 10**).
4. 2% uranyl acetate in 70% ethanol: Dissolve 2 g uranyl acetate in 50 mL of 70% ethanol. Store at 4 °C (*see* **Note 11**).
5. Graded ethanol series in distilled water (30, 50, 95, and 100%).
6. Acetonitrile.
7. TAAB resin: Mix 49 g TAAB hardener component with 49 g TAAB resin component (TAAB Laboratories). Mix well. Add 2.5 mL of TAAB accelerator and mix well. Store at −18 °C (*see* **Note 12**).
8. Flat molded embedding capsules (TAAB Laboratories) (*see* **Note 13**).
9. Capsule rack.
10. Oven (set to 60 °C).
11. Ultramicrotome and associated microtomy equipment.
12. Formbar coated 200 mesh copper/palladium grids.
13. Square 200 mesh copper/palladium grids.
14. Transmission electron microscope.

3 Methods

3.1 Induction of Anesthesia for Surgery

1. Set oxygen flow meter to 1.7 L/min.
2. Switch airflow valve to direct isoflurane and oxygen to the induction chamber.
3. Weigh mouse and place in the induction chamber.
4. Set isoflurane vaporizer to level four to induce anesthesia.
5. Monitor the level of anesthesia by using the toe pinch response; surgical plane is reached when the mouse does not respond to toe pinch.
6. Switch airflow valve to redirect isoflurane and oxygen to the stereotaxic frame.
7. Transfer mouse from induction chamber to the stereotaxic frame isoflurane mask.

3.2 Stereotaxic Injection of Tracers into Mouse Hippocampus

This technique allows for the injection of small amounts of tracers into mouse brain parenchyma at a controlled and physiologically relevant rate (0.5 μL/2.5 min). After injection, the capillary tip is left in situ for 2 min to allow for bolus diffusion. A further 5 min is then given for perivascular drainage. All procedures are performed using a dissection microscope (Fig. 4).

1. Position anesthetized mouse on to a heated pad on the stereotaxic frame using mouthpiece and ear bars. The head needs to be secure and not move when pressure is applied to the scalp (*see* **Note 14**).
2. Cover rectal probe in Vaseline and insert into mouse. Regulate temperature at 37 °C.
3. Apply Lacrilube to mouse eyes (*see* **Note 15**).
4. Make an incision down the midline of the scalp to expose the skull.
5. Clean the surface of the skull using PBS and cotton buds. Air-dry with Dust Off.
6. Front load the microcapillary pipette with tracer using a 1 mL Termo syringe attached to the pipette by narrow gauge tubing (Fig. 5). Attach on to stereotaxic frame using the injection pipette holder (*see* **Note 16**).

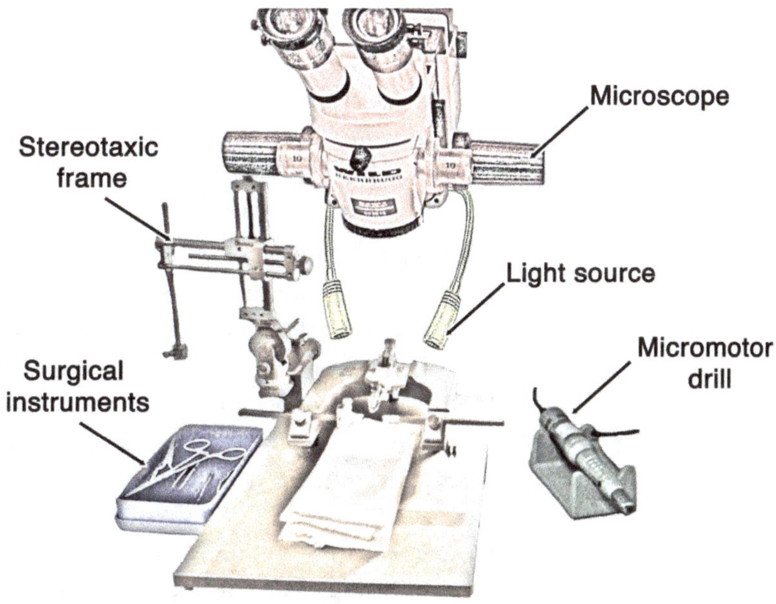

Fig. 4 Recommended equipment arrangement for stereotaxic surgeries. All procedures are performed using a dissecting microscope and an adequate cold LED light source. All required instruments/reagents should be readily accessible

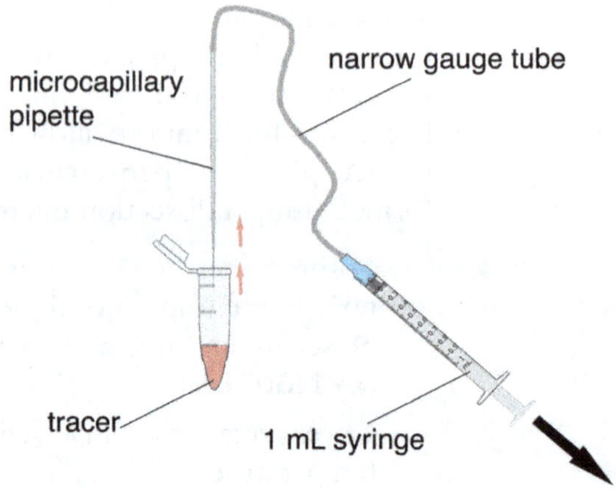

Fig. 5 Microcapillary pipette loading. A 1 mL syringe should be set to the 0.0 mL mark and fixed to a fine tube connected to the pipette. To load the pipette, the syringe needs to be pulled very gently until the tracer begins to move into the capillary. When the desired volume of tracer is loaded, the syringe must be pushed slightly to produce negative flow and then disconnected from the tube to take away pressure from the system

7. Use the stereotaxic *XYZ* controls to maneuver the microcapillary pipette so that the tip is located over Bregma (the point where the sagittal and coronal sutures intersect) (Fig. 6).
8. Adjust *XY* so that the pipette tip is positioned at the hippocampus (ML = −1.5 mm, AP = −2.0 mm) (Fig. 7) (*see* **Note 17**).
9. Mark the top of the skull underneath the pipette tip with a fine marker pen.
10. Adjust *Z*-axis to lift the tip away from the skull.
11. Use a fine drill at medium to high speed to gently shave away the skull previously marked by the pen. Stop when the dura mater becomes visible.
12. Clean the surgery area using PBS, pH 7.2 and cotton buds.
13. Gently adjust the *Z*-axis to lower the pipette tip until it touches the dura and then lower into the hippocampus (DV = 1.7 mm).
14. Slowly press the plunger of the syringe to inject 0.5 μL of tracer over 2.5 min.
15. Leave pipette tip in situ for 2 min to prevent reflux and then slowly remove it from the brain using the *Z*-axis stereotaxic control.
16. After another 3 min inject pentobarbitone intraperitoneally (200 mg/kg), using a 1 mL syringe and a 26 G ½″ × 0.45 × 13 mm needle.
17. Wait for 1 min and then transfer mouse on to perfusion mat. Prepare mouse for perfusion and start the flushing procedure.

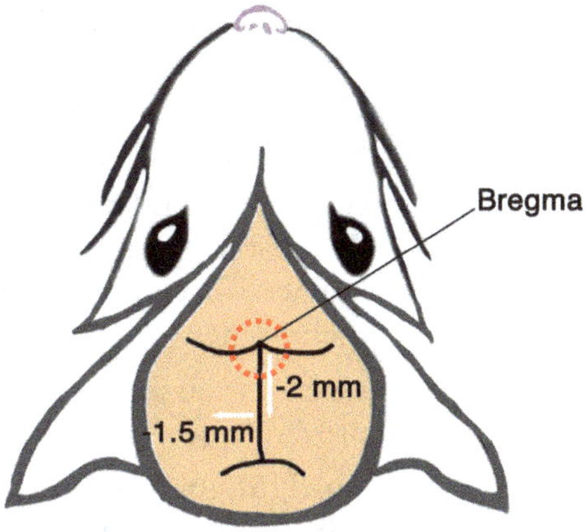

Fig. 6 Diagram showing the location of bregma and XY hippocampal stereotaxic coordinates on mouse brain. The *red dashed circle* indicates the point at which the sagittal and coronal sutures intersect

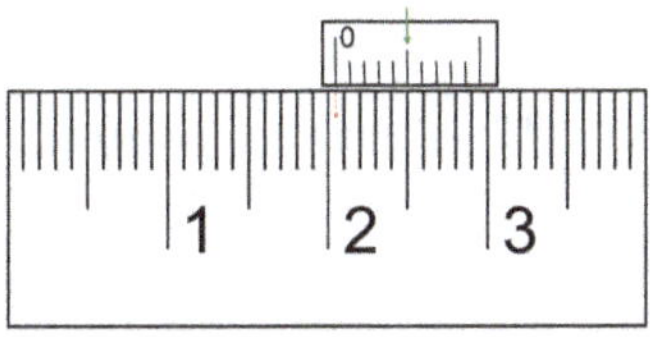

Fig. 7 Linear Vernier scale measurement. The large main scale (*bottom*) and smaller vernier scale (*top*) have been set to 20.5 mm. The *red dotted line* is aligned with 0 on the vernier scale but does not line up with any division on the main scale. The *green arrow* indicates the 0.5 division, which unlike any other mark, lines up directly with one of the main scale divisions

This should be timed to start when the 5 min perivascular drainage time has been reached.

3.3 Injection of Tracers into Mouse Cisterna Magna

Tracers are injected into mouse cisterna magna at a controlled rate of 0.2 μL/min. For good image analysis it is recommended to inject between 1 and 2 μL of tracer allowing for a 30 min drainage time. All procedures are performed using a dissection microscope.

1. Position anesthetized mouse on to a heated pad on the stereotaxic frame using mouthpiece and ear bars. The head needs to be secure and not move when pressure is applied to the scalp (*see* **Note 14**).
2. Cover rectal probe in Vaseline and insert into mouse. Regulate temperature at 37 °C.
3. Apply Lacrilube to mouse eyes (*see* **Note 15**).
4. Use hair clippers to shave scalp.

5. Using a size 10 sterile surgical scalpel, perform a sagittal incision of the skin inferior to the occiput. Clean the area using PBS, pH 7.2 and cotton buds.
6. Bluntly separate subcutaneous tissue and muscles (m. biventer cervicis and m. rectus capitis dorsalis major) using 2× curved dissection forceps. The dura mater of the cisterna magna (Atlanto-occipital membrane) will appear as a shiny elastic membrane.
7. Gently swab a thin layer of Vaseline or glycerol on the dura to prevent tracer reflux.
8. Readjust the position of the mouse so that the head forms a 135° angle with the body.
9. Front load the microcapillary pipette with tracer using a 1 mL Termumo syringe attached to the pipette by narrow gauge tubing (*see* **Note 16**) (Fig. 5).
10. Pierce the dura mater lateral to the arteria dorsalis spinalis with the injection pipette. Inject 1–2 μL at a rate of 0.2 μL/min (*see* **Note 18**).
11. After injection leave the capillary pipette in situ for 2 min to prevent reflux and then gently retract it away from the dura.
12. Leave mouse in situ for 28 min.
13. Inject pentobarbitone intraperitoneally (200 mg/kg), using a 1 mL syringe and a 26 G ½″ × 0.45 × 13 mm needle.
14. Wait for 1 min and then transfer the mouse on to the perfusion mat. Prepare mouse for perfusion and start the flushing procedure. This should be timed to start by the time the 30 min drainage time has elapsed.

3.4 Perfusion Fixation

Good fixation can be achieved by perfusing the mouse at a rate of 5 mL/min.

1. Front load 2 × 25 mL syringes with 25 mL of fixative or buffer.
2. Attach the syringe that contains buffer on to the perfusion pump. Attach a 27 G × 0.38″ × 12″ butterfly needle to the syringe (Fig. 8).
3. Clear any trapped air by starting the pump. Stop when a fine stream of solution is forced out of the butterfly needle.
4. Position mouse on to perfusion bed and pin into position via all four limbs using 4 × 26 G ½″ × 0.45 × 13 mm needles.
5. Expose the heart by dissection into the thoracic cavity. Use clamped forceps to maneuver cut regions of ribcage away from the perfusion site.

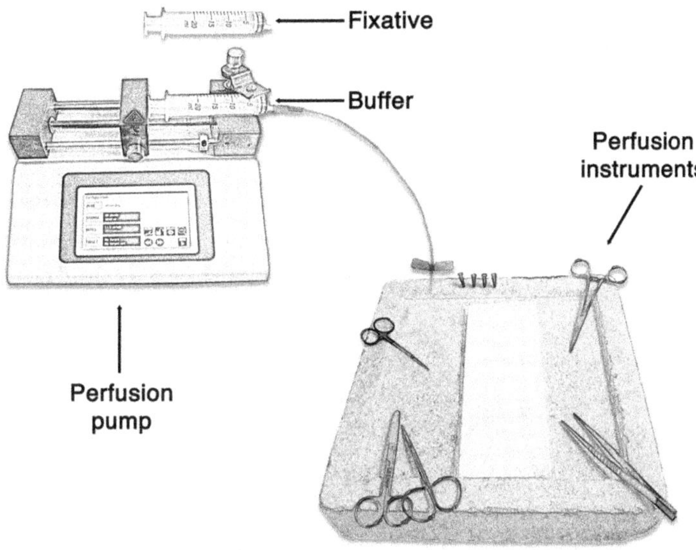

Fig. 8 Diagram showing a simple equipment setup for perfusion fixation

6. Insert butterfly needle into the left ventricle.
7. Using fine scissors gently cut into the right atrium.
8. Start the perfusion pump. Stop when the liver becomes clear of blood.
9. Change the syringes and restart pump. Stop when syringe is empty. Movement of the tail and contraction of muscles will indicate good fixation.
10. Decapitate mouse, dissect brain and store in fresh fixative.

3.5 Brain Dissection

1. Decapitate the mouse using straight blunt scissors.
2. Expose the skull using gently curved scissors. Perform a midline incision along the neck towards the top of the head and trim away any muscle covering the skull.
3. Gently peel away the top of the skull and underlying dura mater from the brain.
4. Lift the brain slightly away from the skull and cut the blood vessels posterior to the Circle of Willis.
5. Using closed scissors gently maneuver the brain and olfactory bulbs away from the skull.
6. Store the brain in fresh 4% paraformaldehyde in 0.01 M PBS, pH 7.2 for immunohistochemistry or 3.4% formaldehyde plus 3% glutaraldehyde in 0.1 M PIPES buffer, pH 7.2 for electron microscopy.

3.6 Immunohistochemistry and Visualization of Proteins of Interest

The method described below has been optimized for tissue fixation and antigen preservation. The steps can be applied to a large number of antibodies (*see* **Note 9**). This technique is particularly useful when trying to ascertain changes in the protein composition of drainage pathways.

1. Transfer a freshly perfused mouse brain into 30 % sucrose: 6 h.
2. Separate the cerebellum and brain stem from the cerebral hemispheres by slicing though the midbrain.
3. Place brain into a base mold with the frontal lobes facing upwards and cover with OCT cryo-embedding media.
4. Lower mold into liquid nitrogen to snap-freeze the tissue. Store at −80 °C until ready to section.
5. Transfer the frozen tissue block onto the cryostat and cut 14 μm thick sections.
6. Transfer sections onto superfrost slides.
7. Allow tissue to adhere to the slides by leaving to air-dry for 15 min.
8. Position slides on a staining rack.
9. Remove any remaining OCT by washing slides with 0.01 M PBS, pH 7.2: 3 × 5 min.
10. Quench any intrinsic peroxidase activity by incubating slides with 3 % hydrogen peroxide: 15 min.
11. Wash with 0.01 M PBS, pH 7.2: 3 × 10 min.
12. Block unspecific antibody binding by incubating in blocking serum: 30 min.
13. Tap off excess serum.
14. Wick away any remaining serum around the brain section.
15. Incubate in primary antibody (250 μL per slide) at 4 °C in a moist chamber: overnight (*see* **Note 19**).
16. Drain excess solution from tray.
17. Wash with 0.01 M PBS, pH 7.2: 3 × 10 min.
18. Incubate with secondary antibody at room temperature: 1 h (Fig. 2).
19. During **step 18** prepare the ABC vector: Dilute reagent A in 0.1 M PBS, pH 7.2 in 0.1 % Triton and vortex briefly. Repeat for reagent B. Add equal volumes of reagent A to reagent B to a final concentration of 1 in 200. Store at 4 °C.
20. Wash with 0.01 M PBS, pH 7.2: 3 × 10 min.
21. Tap off excess PBS.
22. Wick away any remaining PBS around the brain section.
23. Incubate in the ABC vector at room temperature: 1 h.
24. Wash with 0.01 M PBS, pH 7.2: 2 × 5 min.

25. Wash with 0.1 M sodium acetate: 2 × 10 min.
26. During **step 25** prepare DAB reagents: Add 2.5 g nickel ammonium sulfate, 200 mg D-glucose, 40 mg ammonium chloride, and 1.5 mg glucose oxidase to 50 mL of 0.2 M sodium acetate. Mix using a magnetic stirrer (solution A). Dissolve 60 mg of DAB in 50 mL of distilled water. Mix using a magnetic stirrer (solution B).
27. Mix solution A with solution B just before use (DAB staining solution).
28. Incubate with DAB staining solution to reveal color of antibody staining: 5 min.
29. Wash with 0.01 M PBS, pH 7.2: 2 × 5 min (*see* **Notes 20** and **21**).
30. Nuclear counter staining (optional)
    (a) Add 1 in 5 diluted Harris hematoxylin to sections: 2 min (*see* **Note 22**).
    (b) Rinse slides in running tap water: 5 min (Fig. 9).
31. Dehydrate in five changes of ethanol (50, 70, 95, 100, and 100%): 1 min each.
32. Clear in xylene: 5 min.
33. Clear in xylene: 2 × 2 min.
34. Mount slides with DPX mounting solution and store at room temperature (*see* **Note 23**).
35. View antibody staining using light microscopy.

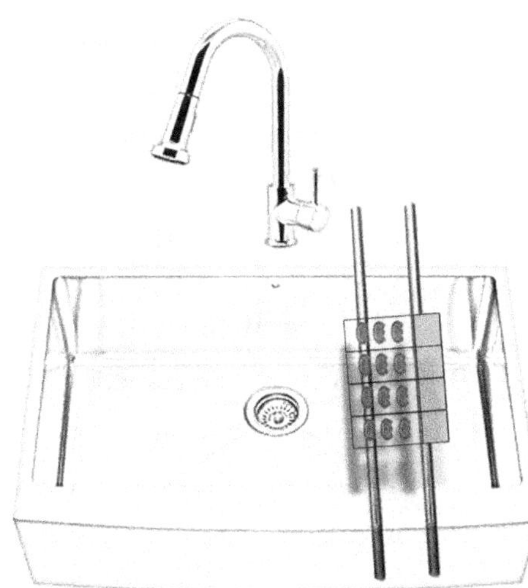

Fig. 9 Diagram showing a common setup for the optional Harris hematoxylin nuclear counterstaining. Slides are positioned adjacent to one another with no gaps in between them on supporting rods over a sink. After staining with Harris hematoxylin the slides are washed for 5 min with running tap water

3.7 Fluorescence/Confocal Microscopy

The method described below has been optimized for the visualization of fluorescent tracers after parenchymal or cisternal injection. In most cases, a combination of antibodies specific to components of the drainage pathways (collagen, smooth muscle, etc.) are used injunction with injectable fluorescence tracers (e.g., amyloid-beta (1–40) HiLyte Fluor 555).

1. Transfer a freshly perfused mouse brain into 30% sucrose: 6 h.
2. Separate the cerebellum and brain stem from the cerebral hemispheres by slicing though the midbrain.
3. Place brain into a base mold with the frontal lobes facing upwards and cover with OCT cryo-embedding media.
4. Lower mold into liquid nitrogen to snap-freeze the tissue. Store at −80 °C until ready to section.
5. Transfer the frozen tissue block onto the cryostat and cut 14 μm thick sections.
6. Transfer sections onto superfrost slides.
7. Allow tissue to adhere to the slides by leaving to air-dry for 15 min.
8. Position slides on a staining rack.
9. Remove any remaining OCT by washing slides with 0.01 M PBS, pH 7.2: 3 × 5 min.
10. Block unspecific antibody binding by incubating in blocking serum: 30 min.
11. Tap off excess serum.
12. Wick away any remaining serum around the brain section.
13. Incubate in primary antibody (250 μL per slide) at 4 °C in a moist chamber: overnight (Fig. 3) (*see* **Note 19**).
14. Drain excess solution from tray.
15. Wash with 0.01 M PBS, pH 7.2: 3 × 10 min.
16. Incubate with secondary antibody at room temperature: 1 h (Fig. 3).
17. Wash with 0.01 M PBS, pH 7.2: 3 × 10 min.
18. Tap off excess PBS.
19. Wick away any remaining PBS around the brain section.
20. Mount slides with Mowiol mounting medium.
21. Air-dry at 4 °C: overnight.
22. View antibody staining using fluorescent/confocal microscopy.

3.8 Floating DAB Immunohistochemistry and Identification of Human Amyloid-Beta (1–40) HiLyte Fluor 555 by Transmission Electron Microscopy

The following method enables the identification of human amyloid-beta (1–40) HiLyte Fluor 555 after stereotaxic injection into mouse brain. The method consists of four parts: confirming fibrillar properties of the injected amyloid beta, vibratome slicing, DAB immunostaining of human amyloid-beta (1–40) HiLyte Fluor 555, and tissue processing for transmission electron microscopy.

3.8.1 Fibrillar Properties of Amyloid Beta

We have shown that only solutes from the ISF drain along intramural perivascular lymphatic drainage pathways. It is therefore essential that only non-fibrillar soluble forms of amyloid-beta (1–40) HiLyte Fluor 555 are used. The steps outlined below enable this to be confirmed (Fig. 10).

1. Put a small drop of the amyloid-beta (1–40) HiLyte Fluor 555 used previously in surgery onto a Formbar coated EM grid.
2. Air-dry: 5 min.
3. Add a small drop of Thioflavin.

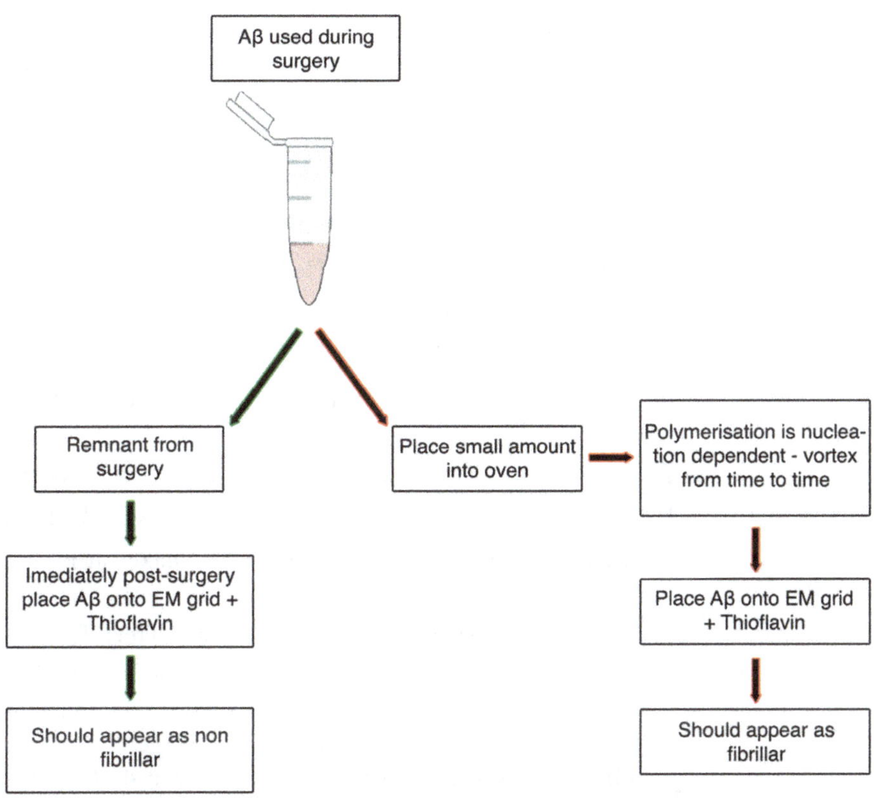

Fig. 10 Confirming fibrillar properties of amyloid beta. The diagram depicts a simple procedure to test the fibrillar properties of the amyloid-beta (Aβ) used during surgery

4. No fibrils should be observed using transmission electron microscopy.
5. Put a small amount of the amyloid-beta (1–40) HiLyte Fluor 555 used previously in surgery in a oven set to 37 °C and vortex intermittently: 24 h.
6. Put a small drop onto a Formbar coated EM grid.
7. Observe using a transmission electron microscope. Fibrils should be observed.

3.8.2 Vibratome Sectioning

1. Separate the cerebellum and brain stem from the cerebral hemispheres by slicing though the midbrain.
2. Use a small amount of superglue to stick the brain onto the mounting plate with the frontal lobes facing upwards.
3. Attach the mounting plate to the vibratome.
4. Fill the water bath with 0.01 M PBS, pH 7.2 to cover the brain.
5. Slice the brain into 50 μm coronal sections (*see* **Note 24**).
6. Use a fine paintbrush to collect sections and transfer them to a 12-well cell culture plate containing 0.01 M PBS, pH 7.2.

3.8.3 DAB Immunostaining

The method below details a series of steps in which a small paintbrush is used to float vibratome tissue sections between different solutions within wells of a 24-well cell culture plate. Each washing step requires the use of a different well.

1. Wash with 0.01 M PBS, pH 7.2 on a shaker: 3 × 10 min.
2. Quench any intrinsic peroxidase activity by incubating sections with 0.3 % hydrogen peroxide on a shaker: 30 min.
3. Wash with 0.01 M PBS, pH 7.2 on a shaker: 3 × 10 min.
4. Incubate with 70 % formic acid: 30 s (*see* **Note 25**).
5. Wash with 0.01 M PBS, pH 7.2 on a shaker: 3 × 10 min.
6. Block unspecific antibody binding by incubating in blocking serum: 1 h.
7. Incubate in primary antibody on a shaker at 4 °C: 48 h.
8. Wash with 0.01 M PBS, pH 7.2 on a shaker: 3 × 10 min.
9. Incubate in secondary antibody on a shaker at room temperature. Allow for 1000 μL per well: 2 h.
10. Wash with 0.01 M PBS, pH 7.2 on a shaker: 3 × 10 min.
11. During **step 10** prepare the ABC vector: Dilute reagent A in 0.1 M PBS, pH 7.2 in 0.1 % Triton and vortex briefly. Repeat for reagent B. Add equal volumes of reagent A to reagent B to a final concentration of 1 in 200. Store at 4 °C.

12. Incubate in the ABC vector on shaker at room temperature: 30 min.
13. Wash with 0.01 M PBS, pH 7.2: 3 × 10 min.
14. Wash with 0.1 M sodium acetate: 3 × 5 min.
15. During **step 14** prepare DAB reagents: Add 2.5 g nickel ammonium sulfate, 200 mg D-glucose, 40 mg ammonium chloride, and 1.5 mg glucose oxidase to 50 mL of 0.2 M sodium acetate. Mix using a magnetic stirrer (solution A). Dissolve 60 mg of DAB in 50 mL of distilled water. Mix using a magnetic stirrer (solution B).
16. Mix solution A with solution B just before use (DAB staining solution).
17. Incubate with DAB staining solution to reveal color of antibody staining: 2 min (*see* **Note 20**).
18. Wash with 0.1 M sodium acetate: 3 × 10 min.
19. Dissect regions of interest and cut into 1 mm^3 sections and transfer into glass vials containing PIPES buffer, pH 7.2. Start to process for transmission electron microscopy within 10 min of the final wash with 0.1 M sodium acetate.

3.8.4 Tissue Processing for Transmission Electron Microscopy

The following steps should be performed at room temperature in a fume hood. Use pipettes to remove/apply each solution. Dispose of used chemicals according to local health and safety guidelines. It is best to use a rotator during the processing to maximum chemical infiltration.

1. Wash in 0.1 M PIPES buffer, pH 7.2: 3 × 5 min.
2. Post fix in 1 % osmium in 0.1 M PIPES buffer, pH 7.2: 1 h (*see* **Notes 10** and **26**).
3. Wash in PIPES buffer, pH 7.2: 3 × 10 min.
4. Dehydrate in 30 % ethanol: 5 min.
5. Dehydrate in 50 % ethanol: 20 min.
6. Stain in 1 % uranyl acetate in 70 % ethanol: 40 min (*see* **Note 11**).
7. Dehydrate in 70 % ethanol: 20 min.
8. Dehydrate in 95 % ethanol: Overnight.
9. Dehydrate in absolute ethanol: 3 × 15 min.
10. Infiltrate with acetonitrile: 10 min.
11. Infiltrate with 50:50 acetonitrile:TAAB Resin: Overnight.
12. Infiltrate with fresh TAAB resin: 6 h.
13. Embed in fresh TAAB resin and polymerize at 60 °C: 16 h (*see* **Notes 12** and **13**).

4 Notes

1. The injectable dextran (Texas red, lysine fixable) is also available at a lower molecular weight of 3 kDa. However, the maximum solubility in aqueous buffer for this dextran is 100 mg/mL, in contrast to the 10 kDa dextran where it is 50 mg/mL. This is due to the decrease in solubility with an increase in the molecular weight.
2. Both dextran and amyloid beta are sensitive to changes in temperature. Amyloid beta will quickly form insoluble oligomers if exposed to several freeze-thaw cycles. It is therefore best to transfer the tracers from storage to ice at −18 °C only when ready to load the capillary pipette. Do not refreeze any unused tracer.
3. The procedures here can be applied to most strains of experimental mice. All animal procedures must be approved by and carried out in accordance with the Institutional committees for ethical use of experimental animals.
4. The light source required to illuminate the skull. Cold type LEDs are best, as they do not emit heat.
5. For minimal tissue damage, the capillary pipette should be pulled to a diameter of <50 μm. A Sutter P97 Flaming Brown Pipette puller is recommended.
6. It is easier to produce a larger quantity of buffer and decanter into 100 mL volumes. These can be frozen for long-term storage.
7. Fixatives are hazardous and toxic by inhalation and ingestion. All procedures should be performed in a fume hood wearing appropriate PPE.
8. 4% paraformaldehyde in 0.01 M PBS, pH 7.2 should be made fresh and stored for a maximum of 5 days at 4 °C. After 5 days aldehyde groups begin to form crosslinks reducing its effectiveness as a fixative for immunohistochemistry.
9. The type of serum and primary antibody used depends on the species in which the secondary antibody was raised and the protein of interest (one which is being localized). All antibodies are diluted in 0.01 M PBS–0.1% Triton X-100.
10. Osmium tetroxide is used as a secondary fixative; it stabilizes lipid membranes by reacting with unsaturated acyl chains. Osmium is volatile and should be handled in a fume hood wearing appropriate PPE. Dispose of osmium solutions by following local health and safety guidelines.
11. Uranyl acetate further enhances tissue contrast by reacting with nucleic acids. It is a derivative of depleted uranium and

should be handled in a fume hood wearing appropriate PPE. Dispose of uranyl acetate solutions by following local health and safety guidelines.

12. Before use allow the resin to reach room temperature before removing the lid of the container. This avoids water condensing on the surface of the resin.
13. A large variety of tissue embedding capsules are available for electron microscopy. We find that flat-bottomed embedding capsules allow optimal orientation of the tissue.
14. Initially, the process for securing the mouse's head to the stereotaxic frame can be challenging for someone performing the procedure for the first time. It is important that the mouse is prone with the head secured straight. This ensures accuracy when adjusting stereotaxic coordinates. There will also be variations in the height of the mouthpiece and ear bar settings between age and strain of mouse. Nevertheless, with a little patience and practice one can become very proficient at using the stereotaxic frame.
15. Rodents do not close their eyes while under anesthesia. To avoid eye dryness and/or cataract formation, Lacrilube (or other suitable) eye ointment should be used.
16. Front loading the microcapillary pipette can be tricky. The setup we have suggested here allows for the pipette tip to be dipped into the tracer. The attached 1 mL syringe is then pulled back to load the microcapillary pipette. When the desired volume of tracer is loaded, the syringe can be detached from the tubing to stop any further loading (Fig. 1).
17. This procedure is not limited to hippocampal injections and can easily be applied for different stereotaxic coordinates.
18. Be gentle when using the injection pipette to pierce the dura mater to avoid making contact with the cerebellum or brain stem.
19. Place damp paper towels in slide rack and cover to prevent tissue from drying out.
20. During this step check the staining has worked using a light microscope. For increased contrast repeat DAB staining.
21. DAB is mutagenic. Dispose of by mixing with an excess solution of acid permanganate overnight in a fume hood. Neutralize with sodium hydroxide and then filter. Dried filter paper can be disposed of as general laboratory waste.
22. An increase in contrast can be obtained by increasing the staining time in Harris hematoxylin (nuclei will appear more purple in color). To reduce contrast wash slides in acid alcohol (1% hydrochloric acid in 70% alcohol) for 10 s and then repeat stain in Harris hematoxylin for a shorter time period.

23. To mount slides evenly place a drop of DPX onto the coverslip and gently lower the slide onto the coverslip at a slight angle. Remove remaining bubbles by applying gentle pressure onto the coverslip.
24. A thickness of 50 μm gives reasonable morphology and sufficient antibody penetration.
25. Formic acid is corrosive. Handle in a fume hood with appropriate PPE.
26. Osmium tetroxide reacts with DAB to produce areas of increased contrast. It enables areas of specific DAB—amyloid-beta (1–40) HiLyte Fluor 555 staining to be visualized by transmission electron microscopy.

References

1. Kida S, Pantazis A, Weller RO (1993) CSF drains directly from the subarachnoid space into nasal lymphatics in the rat. Anatomy, histology and immunological significance. Neuropathol Appl Neurobiol 19(6):480–488
2. Carare RO, Bernardes-Silva M, Newman TA, Page AM, Nicoll JA, Perry VH, Weller RO (2008) Solutes, but not cells, drain from the brain parenchyma along basement membranes of capillaries and arteries: significance for cerebral amyloid angiopathy and neuroimmunology. Neuropathol Appl Neurobiol 34(2):131–144
3. Cserr HF, Ostrach LH (1974) Bulk flow of interstitial fluid after intracranial injection of blue dextran 2000. Exp Neurol 45(1):50–60
4. Iliff JJ, Wang M, Liao Y, Plogg BA, Peng W, Gundersen GA, Benveniste H, Vates GE, Deane R, Goldman SA, Nagelhus EA, Nedergaard M (2012) A paravascular pathway facilitates CSF flow through the brain parenchyma and the clearance of interstitial solutes, including amyloid beta. Sci Transl Med 4(147):147ra111
5. Morris AWJ, Sharp MM, Albargothy NJ, Fernandes R, Hawkes CA, Verma A, Weller RO, Carare RO (2016) Vascular basement membranes as pathways for the passage of fluid into and out of the brain. Acta Neuropathol 131(5):725–736
6. Zekonyte J, Sakai K, Nicoll JA, Weller RO, Carare RO (2016) Quantification of molecular interactions between ApoE, amyloid-beta (Abeta) and laminin: relevance to accumulation of Abeta in Alzheimer's disease. Biochim Biophys Acta 1862(5):1047–1053
7. Weller RO, Hawkes CA, Carare RO (2016) Lymphatic drainage of the brain and CSF: relevance to neuroimmunology and Alzheimer's disease. Neurol Psychiatry Brain Res 22(1):24
8. Weller RO, Carare RO, Hawkes CA, Galea I (2016) Chapter 19—Pathophysiology of lymphatic drainage of the central nervous system: implications for the pathophysiology of multiple sclerosis. In: Minagar A (ed) Multiple sclerosis. Academic, San Diego, pp 479–501
9. Nizari S, Carare RO, Hawkes CA (2016) Increased Abeta pathology in aged Tg2576 mice born to mothers fed a high fat diet. Sci Rep 6:21981
10. Keable A, Fenna K, Yuen HM, Johnston DA, Smyth NR, Smith C, Al-Shahi Salman R, Samarasekera N, Nicoll JA, Attems J, Kalaria RN, Weller RO, Carare RO (2016) Deposition of amyloid beta in the walls of human leptomeningeal arteries in relation to perivascular drainage pathways in cerebral amyloid angiopathy. Biochim Biophys Acta 1862(5): 1037–1046
11. Bakker EN, Bacskai BJ, Arbel-Ornath M, Aldea R, Bedussi B, Morris AW, Weller RO, Carare RO (2016) Lymphatic clearance of the brain: perivascular, paravascular and significance for neurodegenerative diseases. Cell Mol Neurobiol 36(2):181–194
12. Weller RO, Hawkes CA, Kalaria RN, Werring DJ, Carare RO (2015) White matter changes in dementia: role of impaired drainage of interstitial fluid. Brain Pathol 25(1):63–78
13. Weller RO, Hawkes CA, Carare RO, Hardy J (2015) Does the difference between PART and Alzheimer's disease lie in the age-related changes in cerebral arteries that trigger the accumulation of Abeta and propagation of tau? Acta Neuropathol 129(5):763–766

14. Tarasoff-Conway JM, Carare RO, Osorio RS, Glodzik L, Butler T, Fieremans E, Axel L, Rusinek H, Nicholson C, Zlokovic BV, Frangione B, Blennow K, Menard J, Zetterberg H, Wisniewski T, de Leon MJ (2015) Clearance systems in the brain-implications for Alzheimer disease. Nat Rev Neurol 11(8):457–470
15. Hawkes CA, Gentleman SM, Nicoll JA, Carare RO (2015) Prenatal high-fat diet alters the cerebrovasculature and clearance of beta-amyloid in adult offspring. J Pathol 235(4):619–631
16. Morris AW, Carare RO, Schreiber S, Hawkes CA (2014) The cerebrovascular basement membrane: role in the clearance of beta-amyloid and cerebral amyloid angiopathy. Front Aging Neurosci 6:251
17. Hawkes CA, Jayakody N, Johnston DA, Bechmann I, Carare RO (2014) Failure of perivascular drainage of beta-amyloid in cerebral amyloid angiopathy. Brain Pathol 24(4):396–403
18. Bueche CZ, Hawkes C, Garz C, Vielhaber S, Attems J, Knight RT, Reymann K, Heinze HJ, Carare RO, Schreiber S (2014) Hypertension drives parenchymal beta-amyloid accumulation in the brain parenchyma. Ann Clin Transl Neurol 1(2):124–129
19. Hawkes CA, Gatherer M, Sharp MM, Dorr A, Yuen HM, Kalaria R, Weller RO, Carare RO (2013) Regional differences in the morphological and functional effects of aging on cerebral basement membranes and perivascular drainage of amyloid-beta from the mouse brain. Aging Cell 12(2):224–236
20. Carare RO, Teeling JL, Hawkes CA, Puntener U, Weller RO, Nicoll JA, Perry VH (2013) Immune complex formation impairs the elimination of solutes from the brain: implications for immunotherapy in Alzheimer's disease. Acta Neuropathol Commun 1:48
21. Weller RO, Galea I, Carare RO, Minagar A (2010) Pathophysiology of the lymphatic drainage of the central nervous system: implications for pathogenesis and therapy of multiple sclerosis. Pathophysiology 17(4):295–306
22. Laman JD, Weller RO (2013) Drainage of cells and soluble antigen from the CNS to regional lymph nodes. J Neuroimmune Pharmacol 8(4):840–856

Chapter 25

Quantitative Assessment of Cerebral Basement Membranes Using Electron Microscopy

Matthew MacGregor Sharp, Anton Page, Alan Morris, Roy O. Weller, and Roxana O. Carare

Abstract

In this chapter we describe in detail the tissue processing techniques we employ for the study of cerebral tissue by transmission electron microscopy (TEM). In particular, we explain a technique that enables quantification of changes in cerebral basement membranes at the ultrastructural level. This is significant, as age related pathological conditions affecting the brain are often accompanied by ultrastructural changes in the cerebral vasculature.

Briefly, experimental mice are fixed by perfusion and their brains removed. Brains are then vibratomed into 100 μm slices with regions of interest microdissected and processed for TEM following a protocol optimized for the preservation of cerebral tissue. Changes in the thickness of cerebral basement membranes are then quantified using novel software. Some prior knowledge of general TEM specimen preparation and sectioning will be useful when performing this protocol.

Key words Transmission electron microscopy, Basement membrane, Tissue processing, Microtomy, Ultra-thin sectioning, Fixation, Dehydration, Resin embedding, Electron micrograph

1 Introduction

The basement membrane (BM) is an essential component of the blood vessels, acting as a pathway for the movement of fluids into and out of the brain [1–3]. Solutes drain from the interstitial fluid along BM of capillaries and arteries towards the surface of the brain, a route described as the intramural perivascular drainage pathway [3]. Cerebral spinal fluid penetrates the brain along pial-glial BM (gylmphatic pathway) [2].

BMs are dynamic 50–100 nm thick ubiquitous extracellular protein matrices of collagen type IV, laminin, entactin/nidogen and proteoglycans such as fibronectin and perlecan that are produced by epithelial, endothelial and mesenchymal cells [4–6]. Proteins are arranged into a trilaminar structure [7] with networks of collagen type IV and laminin interconnected by entactin/nidogen

Björn E. Clausen and Jon D. Laman (eds.), *Inflammation: Methods and Protocols*, Methods in Molecular Biology, vol. 1559, DOI 10.1007/978-1-4939-6786-5_25, © Springer Science+Business Media LLC 2017

and perlecan. Collagen type IV and laminin are critical for BM stability while entactin/nidogen and perlecan increase stability and influence structural integrity [8]. This enables blood vessels to withstand high sheer forces and accommodate changes in blood volume in the peripheral circulation [4].

BMs are capable of self-remodeling [6] and change with age; they thicken and show alterations in chemical composition. Age associated changes in levels of perlecan; fibronectin and laminin have been demonstrated in mouse brain capillaries and in TGF β-1 transgenic mice that accumulate Aβ (amyloid beta) proteins in the walls of arteries, without overexpression of Aβ [9, 10]. Increases in collagen type IV and BM thickening have been reported in aged human brains. Furthermore, more substantial increases in collagen type IV have been observed in cerebral vessels of brains affected by Alzheimer's disease [11].

Histochemistry and confocal microscopy are widely used techniques to access changes in BM composition. Proteomics, a relatively recent scientific field, can produce a global profile of BM proteins. In this chapter we describe a technique using quantitative electron microscopy that enables correlation between BM composition and BM ultrastructure. This technique allows for the quantitative assessment of basement membrane ultrastructure by measuring BM thickness [12].

2 Materials

2.1 Perfusion Fixation

2.1.1 Induction of Terminal Anesthesia

1. Experimental mice (*see* **Note 1**).
2. Scales.
3. Standard isoflurane anesthesia system.
4. Pentobarbitone (1:10 in 0.9% saline).

2.1.2 Buffers

1. 0.2 M piperazine-*N*,*N*′-bis-2-ethanesulfonic acid (PIPES) buffer, pH 7.2: Mix 60.48 g PIPES with 900 mL of distilled water. Add 10 M sodium hydroxide dropwise to bring the pH up to 7.2. Make up to 1 L with distilled water to produce a 0.2 M solution of PIPES buffer, pH 7.2. Store at 4 °C (*see* **Note 2**).

2.1.3 Fixatives

1. 3.4% formaldehyde plus 3% glutaraldehyde in 0.1 M PIPES buffer, pH 7.2: Mix 4 g of paraformaldehyde with 20 mL of distilled water. Heat to 60 °C on a hotplate stirrer, add 2–4 drops of 1 M NaOH and stir until the solution clears (*see* **Note 3**). Cool slightly and add 12 mL of 25% EM grade glutaraldehyde. Make up to 50 mL with distilled water and add 50 mL of 0.2 M PIPES buffer, pH 7.2. Store at 4 °C.

2.1.4 Perfusion

1. Syringe pump.
2. Dissection instruments (straight blunt scissors, standard pattern, gently curved blunt serrated larger finger loops, hemostat, and small forceps).
3. 27 G × 0.38″ × 12″ butterfly needles.
4. 26 G ½″ × 0.45 × 13 mm needles.
5. 2 × 20 mL syringes.
6. 15 mL tubes.
7. Perfusion platform.

2.2 Tissue Preparation for Transmission Electron Microscopy

2.2.1 Vibratome Slicing

1. Vibratome.
2. PIPES buffer, pH 7.2.
3. 12-well cell culture plate.
4. Small paintbrush.
5. Superglue.
6. Dissecting blades.
7. 3.4% formaldehyde plus 3% glutaraldehyde in 0.1 M PIPES buffer, pH 7.2.

2.2.2 Tissue Dissection

1. Dissecting microscope.
2. Dental wax.
3. 3.4% formaldehyde plus 3% glutaraldehyde in 0.1 M PIPES buffer, pH 7.2.
4. Dissection blade.
5. Small paintbrush.
6. Small glass vials.

2.2.3 Tissue Processing

Heavy Metal Stains

1. 2% aqueous osmium tetroxide: Dissolve 1 g osmium tetroxide in 50 mL distilled water to produce 2% stock. Store in triple containment at 4 °C (*see* **Note 4**).
2. 1% uranyl acetate in 70% ethanol: Dissolve 0.5 g uranyl acetate in 50 mL ethanol. Store at 4 °C (*see* **Note 5**).

Tissue Dehydration

1. Glass vials and rotator.
2. Graded ethanol series (30, 50, 95, and 100%).
3. Acetonitrile.

Tissue Embedding

1. TAAB resin: Mix 49 g TAAB hardener component with 49 g TAAB resin component (TAAB Laboratories). Mix well. ADD 2.5 mL of TAAB accelerator and mix well. Store at −18 °C (*see* **Note 6**).
2. Flat molded embedding capsules (TAAB Laboratories) (*see* **Note 7**).

3. Capsule rack.
4. Oven (set to 60 °C).

2.3 Electron Microscopy

1. Ultramicrotome and associated microtomy equipment.
2. 1 % v/v toluidine blue in 1 % w/v borax: Mix 2 g toluidine blue powder with 2 g borax in 200 mL of distilled water. Swirl gently and leave overnight. Filter before use.
3. Reynold's lead stain: Mix 1.33 g lead nitrate with 1.76 g trisodium citrate in 30 mL of distilled water. Shake intermittently for 30 min. Add 8 mL sodium hydroxide and make up to 50 mL with distilled water. Decant into 1 mL volumes and store at 4 °C.
4. Square 200 mesh copper/palladium grids.
5. 90 × 15 mm sterile disposable petri dish.
6. Parafilm.
7. Transmission electron microscope.
8. Digital imaging EMSIS software (formerly iTEM software, Universal TEM Imaging platform, Soft Imaging System, Münster, Germany) or suitable image analysis software.

3 Methods

3.1 Induction of Terminal Anesthesia

1. Set oxygen flow meter to 1.7 L/min.
2. Switch airflow valve to direct isoflurane and oxygen to the induction chamber.
3. Weigh mouse and place in the induction chamber.
4. Set isoflurane vaporizer to level four to induce anesthesia.
5. Monitor the level of anesthesia by using the toe pinch response; surgical plane is reached when the mouse does not respond to toe pinch.
6. Inject pentobarbitone intraperitoneally (200 mg/kg), using a 1 mL syringe and a 26 G ½″ × 0.45 × 13 mm needle.
7. Wait for 1 min and then transfer the mouse onto the perfusion mat.

3.2 Perfusion Fixation

Good fixation can be achieved by perfusing the mouse at a rate of 5 mL/min (*see* **Note 8**).

1. Front load 2 × 25 mL syringes with 25 mL of PIPES buffer, pH 7.2 or 3.4 % formaldehyde plus 3 % glutaraldehyde in 0.1 M PIPES buffer, pH 7.2.
2. Attach the syringe containing PIPES buffer, pH 7.2 onto the perfusion pump. Attach a 27 G × 0.38″ × 12″ butterfly needle to the syringe.

3. Clear any trapped air by starting the pump. Stop when a fine stream of solution is forced out of the butterfly needle.
4. Position mouse onto the perfusion mat and pin into position by all four limbs using 4×6 G ½″×0.45×13 mm needles.
5. Expose the heart by dissection into the thoracic cavity. Use clamped forceps to maneuver cut regions of the ribcage away from the perfusion site.
6. Insert butterfly needle into the left ventricle.
7. Using fine scissors gently cut into the right atrium.
8. Start the perfusion pump. Stop when the liver becomes clear of blood.
9. Change the syringes and restart pump. Stop when the syringe is empty (*see* **Note 9**).

3.3 Brain Dissection

1. Decapitate the mouse using straight blunt scissors.
2. Expose the skull using gently curved scissors. Perform a midline incision along the neck towards the top of the head and trim away any muscle covering the skull.
3. Gently peel away the top of the skull and underlying dura mater from the brain.
4. Lift the brain slightly away from the skull and cut the blood vessels posterior to the Circle of Willis.
5. Using closed scissors gently maneuver the brain and olfactory bulbs away from the skull.
6. Store the brain in fresh 3.4% formaldehyde plus 3% glutaraldehyde in 0.1 M PIPES buffer, pH 7.2 for electron microscopy.

3.4 Vibratome Slicing and Microdissection

1. Separate the cerebellum and brain stem from the cerebral hemispheres by slicing though the midbrain.
2. Use a small amount of superglue to stick the brain onto the mounting plate with the frontal lobes facing upwards.
3. Attach the mounting plate to the vibratome.
4. Fill the water bath with PIPES buffer, pH 7.2 to cover the brain.
5. Slice the brain into 100 μm coronal sections.
6. Use a fine paintbrush to collect sections and transfer them to a 12-well cell culture plate containing fixative.
7. Under a dissecting microscope use the fine paintbrush to transfer a coronal slice from the 12 well culture plate onto a piece of dental wax (*see* **Note 10**).
8. Dissect regions of interest and cut into 1 mm^3 sections: Store in glass vials containing fresh fixative at 4 °C.

3.5 Tissue Processing for Transmission Electron Microscopy

The following steps should be performed at room temperature in a fume hood. Use pipettes to remove/apply each solution. Dispose of used chemicals according to local health and safety guidelines. It is best to use a rotator during the processing to maximum chemical infiltration.

1. Wash in 0.1 M PIPES buffer, pH 7.2: 2 × 10 min.
2. Post fix in 1 % osmium in 0.1 M PIPES buffer, pH 7.2: 1 h.
3. Wash in PIPES buffer, pH 7.2: 2 × 10 min.
4. Dehydrate in 30 % ethanol: 10 min.
5. Dehydrate in 50 % ethanol: 10 min.
6. Stain in 1 % uranyl acetate in 70 % ethanol: 30 min.
7. Dehydrate in 95 % ethanol: 10 min.
8. Dehydrate in absolute ethanol: 2 × 15 min.
9. Infiltrate with acetonitrile: 10 min.
10. Infiltrate with 50:50 acetonitrile–TAAB resin: Overnight.
11. Infiltrate with fresh TAAB resin: 6 h.
12. Embed in fresh TAAB resin and polymerize at 60 °C: 16 h (*see* **Note 11**).

3.6 Tissue Sectioning for Electron Microscopy

1. Trim tissue blocks and shape into a trapezoid containing tissue.
2. Cut semi-thin 0.5 μm sections using an ultramicrotome.
3. Mount sections on glass slides and dry on a hotplate.
4. Stain sections with 1 % v/v toluidine blue in 1 % w/v borax: Drop a small amount of 1 % v/v toluidine blue in 1 % w/v borax onto the slide. Wait for a green fringe to appear around the edge of the stain. Remove slide form hotplate and wash immediately with warm running tap water. Blot-dry.
5. Identify areas of interest in the semi-thin sections. Trim the tissue block and cut ultrathin 80 nm sections (Fig. 1).
6. Collect 80 nm sections onto copper grids and allow to air-dry (*see* **Note 12**).
7. Counter stain tissue sections with Reynold's lead stain: Add a few sodium hydroxide pellets and a square of parafilm to a petri dish. Put a small drop of Reynold's lead stain onto the parafilm. Float grids with section side down on the Reynold's lead stain and seal the petri dish. After 5 min wash grids in distilled water three times and allow to air-dry.

3.7 Quantifying Basement Membrane Thickness by Electron Microscopy

1. Using the transmission electron microscope, scan the grid in a methodical manner from top left to bottom right.
2. Identify capillaries in transverse section with visible and well-defined BM and take a reference image at a magnification of ×9000 (Fig. 1a).

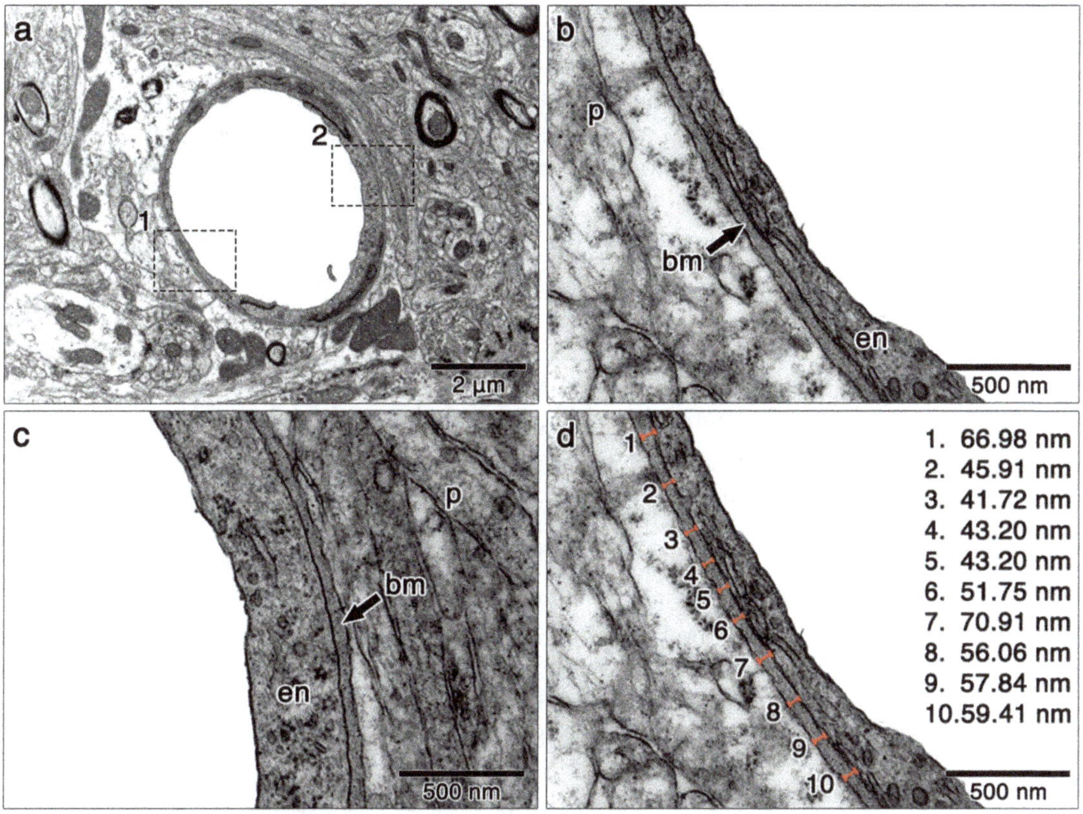

Fig. 1 Quantifying cerebral BM thickness by TEM. (**a**) Capillary in transverse section with visible and well-defined BM. TEM original magnification ×9000. (**b** and **c**) High powered electron micrographs of *boxes 1* (**b**) and *2* (**c**) seen in (**a**). The BM (*arrows*) can be seen separating the endothelium (*en*) from the surrounding parenchyma (*p*). TEM original magnification ×50,000. (**d**) To quantify BM thickness ten perpendicular measurement bars (*red bars*) are used to measure the distance between the inside and outside edge of the BM. TEM original magnification ×50,000

3. Take two higher powered images at a magnification of ×50,000 of the BM at opposite sides of the capillary (Fig. 1b, c).
4. Use perpendicular measurement bars to measure the distance between the inside and outside edges of the BM. Repeat this ten times for each high-powered micrograph for each capillary (Fig. 1d). Avoid measuring areas where the BM has been expanded by the presence of a pericyte.
5. Statistically analyze the measurements using a one-way ANOVA test, with Bonferroni correction for multiple comparisons (significance set at $p < 0.05$).

4 Notes

1. The procedures here can be applied to most strains of experimental mice. All animal procedures must be approved by and carried out in accordance with the Institutional committees for ethical use of experimental animals.
2. It is easier to produce a larger quantity of buffer and decant it into 100 mL volumes. These can be frozen for long-term storage.
3. Fixatives are hazardous and toxic by inhalation and ingestion. All procedures should be performed in a fume hood wearing appropriate PPE.
4. Osmium tetroxide is used as a secondary fixative; it stabilizes lipid membranes by reacting with unsaturated acyl chains. Osmium is volatile and should be handled in a fume hood wearing appropriate PPE. Dispose of osmium solutions by following local health and safety guidelines.
5. Uranyl acetate further enhances tissue contrast by reacting with nucleic acids. It is a derivative of depleted uranium and should be handled in a fume hood wearing appropriate PPE. Dispose of uranyl acetate solutions by following local health and safety guidelines.
6. Before use allow the resin to reach room temperature before removing the lid of the container. This avoids water condensing on the surface of the resin.
7. A large variety of tissue embedding capsules are available for electron microscopy. We find that flat-bottomed embedding capsules allow optimal orientation of the tissue.
8. For good statistical analysis it is recommended to perfuse and analyze a minimum of seven mice.
9. Movement of the tail and contraction of the muscles will indicate good fixation.
10. To avoid tissue degradation, microdissect the coronal slice by transferring the coronal slice onto a small drop of fixative on the dental wax before dissecting into smaller 1 mm^3 sections.
11. It is essential to position the tissue flat against the bottom of the embedding capsule. A simple way is to fill the capsule with fresh resin, place the sample into the top of the capsule and allow it to sink to the bottom. The sample can then be orientated to the center of the capsule before polymerization of the resin.
12. A large variety of grids are available for electron microscopy. We find that square 200 mesh copper/palladium grids are ideal for this protocol (Agar Scientific).

References

1. Iliff JJ, Wang M, Liao Y, Plogg BA, Peng W, Gundersen GA, Benveniste H, Vates GE, Deane R, Goldman SA, Nagelhus EA, Nedergaard M (2012) A paravascular pathway facilitates CSF flow through the brain parenchyma and the clearance of interstitial solutes, including amyloid beta. Sci Transl Med 4(147):147ra111
2. Morris AWJ, Sharp MM, Albargothy NJ, Fernandes R, Hawkes CA, Verma A, Weller RO, Carare RO (2016) Vascular basement membranes as pathways for the passage of fluid into and out of the brain. Acta Neuropathol 131(5):725–736
3. Carare RO, Bernardes-Silva M, Newman TA, Page AM, Nicoll JA, Perry VH, Weller RO (2008) Solutes, but not cells, drain from the brain parenchyma along basement membranes of capillaries and arteries: significance for cerebral amyloid angiopathy and neuroimmunology. Neuropathol Appl Neurobiol 34(2):131–144
4. Timpl R, Brown JC (1996) Supramolecular assembly of basement membranes. Bioessays 18(2):123–132
5. Timpl R (1996) Macromolecular organization of basement membranes. Curr Opin Cell Biol 8(5):618–624
6. Yurchenco PD, Schittny JC (1990) Molecular architecture of basement membranes. FASEB J 4(6):1577–1590
7. Farkas E, Luiten PGM (2001) Cerebral microvascular pathology in aging and Alzheimer's disease. Prog Neurobiol 64(6):575–611
8. LeBleu VS, Macdonald B, Kalluri R (2007) Structure and function of basement membranes. Exp Biol Med (Maywood) 232(9):1121–1129
9. Hawkes CA, Hartig W, Kacza J, Schliebs R, Weller RO, Nicoll JA, Carare RO (2011) Perivascular drainage of solutes is impaired in the ageing mouse brain and in the presence of cerebral amyloid angiopathy. Acta Neuropathol 121(4):431–443
10. Wyss-Coray T, Lin C, Sanan DA, Mucke L, Masliah E (2000) Chronic overproduction of transforming growth factor-β1 by astrocytes promotes Alzheimer's disease-like microvascular degeneration in transgenic mice. Am J Pathol 156(1):139–150
11. Kalaria RN, Pax AB (1995) Increased collagen content of cerebral microvessels in Alzheimer's disease. Brain Res 705(1–2):349–352
12. Hawkes CA, Gatherer M, Sharp MM, Dorr A, Yuen HM, Kalaria R, Weller RO, Carare RO (2013) Regional differences in the morphological and functional effects of aging on cerebral basement membranes and perivascular drainage of amyloid-beta from the mouse brain. Aging Cell 12(2):224–236

Chapter 26

Microglial Activation by Genetically Targeted Conditional Neuronal Ablation in the Zebrafish

Nynke Oosterhof, Laura E. Kuil, and Tjakko J. van Ham

Abstract

In neurodegenerative diseases activation of immune cells is thought to play a major role. Microglia are the main immune cells of the central nervous system. When encountering disease related stimuli microglia adopt an activated phenotype that typically includes a rounded morphology. The exact role of microglia or other potentially infiltrating myeloid cells in different brain diseases is not fully understood. In this chapter we present techniques in zebrafish to induce degeneration of neurons, to activate the microglia, and to study activation phenotypes by immunohistochemistry and in vivo by fluorescence microscopic imaging.

Key words Zebrafish, Microglia, Macrophages, Brain, Phagocytosis, Neurodegeneration, Nitroreductase, Live imaging, Immunohistochemistry, Aging, Alzheimer's disease

1 Introduction

The immune system plays a major role in many brain diseases, including diseases involving neuronal death. Microglia are brain-resident macrophages that are thought to be involved in the maintenance of brain homeostasis and the defense against pathogens and phagocytosis of dead cells and debris [1–4]. Upon encountering for example pathogens, tissue damage or protein aggregates, microglia adopt a rounded activated phenotype [2]. However, the exact mechanisms regulating microglia function and activation are still unclear. One reason for this lack of knowledge regarding microglia function is the relative inaccessibility of mammals and in particular the mammalian central nervous system (CNS) for in vivo studies.

Zebrafish are highly suitable for in vivo imaging studies, due to their rapid development and transparency during embryonic and larval stages [5]. Within 5 days after fertilization many organs, such as the heart, central nervous system, and cell types have developed, including innate immune cells and microglia. The zebrafish CNS is highly similar to the mammalian CNS with regard to development, anatomy, and cell types. Zebrafish microglia show strong

Björn E. Clausen and Jon D. Laman (eds.), *Inflammation: Methods and Protocols*, Methods in Molecular Biology, vol. 1559,
DOI 10.1007/978-1-4939-6786-5_26, © Springer Science+Business Media LLC 2017

similarities with mammalian microglia in developmental ontogeny and function as they are highly effective in phagocytizing apoptotic neurons [6–9].

As in mammals, primitive yolk sac macrophages colonize the embryonic brain in zebrafish before their differentiation into microglia. Intriguingly, this process was already visualized in great detail almost a decade before this was elegantly shown by mouse lineage tracing studies [9, 10].

Here, we present techniques to study microglial activation responses to neurodegeneration using the zebrafish as a model organism. We previously established transgenic brain-specific expression of the bacterial gene *nsfB* encoding the enzyme nitroreductase (NTR) as a specific, dose-dependent and reversible technique to induce neuronal cell death in zebrafish larvae [6, 11]. NTR catalyzes the conversion of the prodrug metronidazole (MTZ) into a DNA-crosslinking agent that causes apoptosis in targeted cells. NTR-mediated neuronal ablation allows controlled onset and extent of neurodegeneration. This model helped us to identify a transient activation responses involving increased phagocytosis by microglia and as well as an increase in numbers which is followed by resolution involving apoptosis of microglia by in vivo imaging and immunohistochemistry [7]. Since MTZ effectively crosses the blood-brain barrier, this technique can also be applied to adult zebrafish [12]. In this chapter, we describe how to use NTR-mediated neurodegeneration and monitor microglia activation with high resolution in vivo and in fixed tissue in larval and adult zebrafish. The system is versatile as expression can be directed to virtually any cell type and therefore these protocols will also be applicable to other neuronal or glial cell types or populations of interest using different promoters.

2 Materials

2.1 Imaging Microglial Activation in Response to Neuronal Ablation (Larvae)

2.1.1 Induction of Neuronal Cell Death

1. Zebrafish: tg(*NeuroG4*-mCherry, UAS-E1b:*nsfB*-mCherry, *Mpeg1*-GFP) [6, 7, 13–15].
2. Standard zebrafish supplies (28–28.5 °C incubator, 9 cm petri dishes, breeding tanks, automated fish circulation system).
3. 60× E3 stock solution, dissolve 34.4 g NaCl, 1.52 g KCl, 5.8 g $CaCl_2$, and 9.8 g $MgSO_4$ in 2 L ddH_2O. Adjust the pH to 7.2 with NaOH tablets and autoclave.
4. 1 M HEPES stock solution, dissolve 238.30 g HEPES in 1 L dd$H_2$0. Adjust the pH to 7.3 with NaOH tablets and autoclave.
5. Buffered 1× E3 medium, Add 16.6 mL 60× E3 stock solution and 20 mL 1 M HEPES stock solution to 1 L ddH_2O.
6. 3%1-phenyl 2-thiourea (PTU) stock solution (1000×), dissolve 300 mg PTU in 10 mL dimethylsulfoxide (DMSO).

7. 1 M metronidazole (MTZ) stock solution, dissolve 1.71 g MTZ in 10 mL DMSO (*see* **Note 1**).
8. 6-well or 12-well plate.
9. Fluorescence dissection microscope (e.g., Leica M165V).

2.1.2 Live Imaging and Immunohistochemistry of Microglial Activation (See Note 2)

1. 10× stock tricaine methanesulfonate solution (MS222; Sigma): add 0.16 g MS222 to 100 mL buffered 1× E3 medium and adjust the pH to 7.3 with NaOH (*see* **Note 3**). Final concentration = 0.16%.
2. 10× PBS stock solution: dissolve 80 g NaCl, 2 g KCl, 14.4 g Na_2HPO_4, 2.4 g KH_2PO_4 in 800 mL ddH_2O. Adjust pH to 7.4. Adjust volume to 1 L with additional distilled H_2O. Sterilize by autoclaving.
3. 1.8% low melting point (LMP) agarose (BDH Prolabo): dissolve 1.8 g of LMP agarose in 100 mL buffered 1× E3 medium. Heat in a microwave until it is completely dissolved (*see* **Note 4**).
4. 4% paraformaldehyde (PFA) in PBS.
5. 1× PBS-T (0.4% Triton X-100): add 2 mL Triton X-100 (Sigma) to 500 mL 1× PBS.
6. MeOH series in PBS (100%, 75%, 50%, 25%).
7. 10 mg/mL proteinase K stock solution (=1000 × solution).
8. Blocking solution: 1% BSA (0.01 g/mL), 1% DMSO (10 μL/mL) in PBS-T.
9. 1st antibody solution: 5% BSA (0.05 g/mL) in PBS-T.
10. 2nd antibody solution: 2% BSA (0.02 g/mL) in PBS-T.
11. Plastic Pasteur pipettes.
12. Glass bottom imaging dishes (MatTek).
13. 1.5 mL microcentrifuge tubes.
14. Tools to position larvae (e.g., gel loading tips).
15. Inverted confocal microscope (*see* **Note 5**).

2.2 Imaging Microglial Activation in Response to Neuronal Ablation (Adult Zebrafish)

2.2.1 Induction of Neuronal Cell Death in the Adult Zebrafish Brain

1. Adult zebrafish: tg(*NeuroG4*-mCherry, UAS:*nsfB*-mCherry, *mpeg1*-GFP) [6, 7, 13–15].
2. Standard zebrafish supplies (28–28.5 °C incubator, petri dishes, breeding tanks, circulation system).
3. Dimethyl sulfoxide (DMSO).
4. Metronidazole (MTZ).

2.2.2 Isolation of Fixed Complete Zebrafish Brain

1. Ice water.
2. Dissection microscope (e.g., Olympus SZX16, Leica M165V).

3. Scalpel.
4. 2× forceps (Dumont #5).
5. Spring scissors – 8 mm blades (F.S.T).
6. 1× PBS solution (pH 7.4).
7. MeOH series in PBS (100%, 75%, 50%, 25%).
8. 4% PFA in PBS.
9. 1.5 mL microcentrifuge tubes.

2.2.3 Sectioning of Zebrafish Brains for Immunofluorescence Staining

1. MeOH series in PBS (100%, 75%, 50%, and 25%).
2. 4% Low-melting point agarose in PBS: Place the required amount of PBS in a 50 mL tube, add the required amount of low-melting point agarose and shake briefly until the solution is homogeneous. Place the tube in a beaker containing water and heat it in a microwave until all agarose is dissolved (*see* **Note 6**).
3. 1× PBS solution.
4. Plastic Pasteur pipette.
5. Embedding base molds.
6. Scalpel.
7. Low-viscosity cyanoacrylate-based instant adhesive.
8. 4% PFA in PBS.
9. Vibratome (HM650V; Thermo Scientific).
10. 48-well plate.

2.2.4 Immuno-fluorescence Staining of Zebrafish Brain Sections

1. Goat serum (Dako).
2. 1× PBS-T (0.5% triton X-100): add 2.5 mL Triton X-100 (Sigma) to 500 mL 1× PBS.
3. Blocking buffer: Dissolve 1.5 g bovine serum albumin (BSA) in 50 mL PBST.
4. Antibody solution: Dissolve 2.5 g BSA in 50 mL PBST.
5. 1× PBS.
6. Microscope slides.
7. Vectashield mounting medium H1000.
8. Glass cover slips.
9. Parafilm.

3 Methods

3.1 Imaging Microglial Activation in Response to Neuronal Ablation (Larvae)

3.1.1 Induction of Neurodegeneration in Zebrafish Larvae

1. Day -1: Cross adult zebrafish tg(NeuroG4-mCherry; UAS:nsfB-mCherry; Mpeg1-GFP).
2. Day 0: Collect the eggs in buffered 1x E3 medium in a 9 cm petri dish and raise the embryos in a 28–28.5 °C incubator.
3. At 1 day post fertilization (dpf) replace medium by buffered 1× E3 medium containing 0.003% PTU (1:1000 dilution from 3% PTU stock solution) (*see* **Note 7**).
4. Screen embryos for bright mCherry signal on a fluorescence dissection microscope. Place the transgenic larvae in a new petri dish. (*see* **Note 8**).
5. At 3 dpf or later screen the larvae for *Mpeg1*-GFP expression (*see* **Note 9**).
6. Place the larvae in a 6-well or 12-well plate and replace the larval medium with buffered 1× E3 medium containing 0.003% PTU and 2 mM MTZ to induce neuronal cell ablation. Treatment with 2 mM MTZ for 16 h results in extensive neuronal cell ablation accompanied by microglia activation (*see* **Note 10**).
7. Wash larvae at least 3× with buffered 1× E3 medium containing 0.003% PTU (*see* **Note 11**).
8. The larvae can be subjected to live imaging or fixation for later staining at the desired time point.

3.1.2 Live Imaging Zebrafish Larvae

1. For live imaging anesthetize the larvae with 0.016% MS-222 in buffered E3 medium and place them in a glass bottom imaging dish (inverted confocal microscope) or in a 6 mm petri dish (upright confocal microscope) and place the dish under a dissection microscope.
2. Place 1.8% low melting point agarose on top of the larvae (*see* **Note 12**).
3. For inverted confocal microscope: Quickly position the larvae upside down with their "nose" facing the glass bottom before agarose solidifies (Fig. 1a) (*see* **Note 13**).
4. For upright confocal microscope: Position the larvae with their "nose" touching the surface on top of the LMP agarose drop (Fig. 1b) (*see* **Note 14**).
5. When the agarose has solidified fill the imaging dish with buffered 1× E3 medium containing 0.016% MS-222 to prevent drying of the sample (*see* **Note 15**).
6. Continue with imaging. Use appropriate laser wavelength (e.g., 488 nm to detect GFP and 543, 561 or 594 nm to detect mCherry). If possible, it is recommended to use the brightfield channel to include information about the imaging position (Fig. 2a) (*see* **Note 16**).

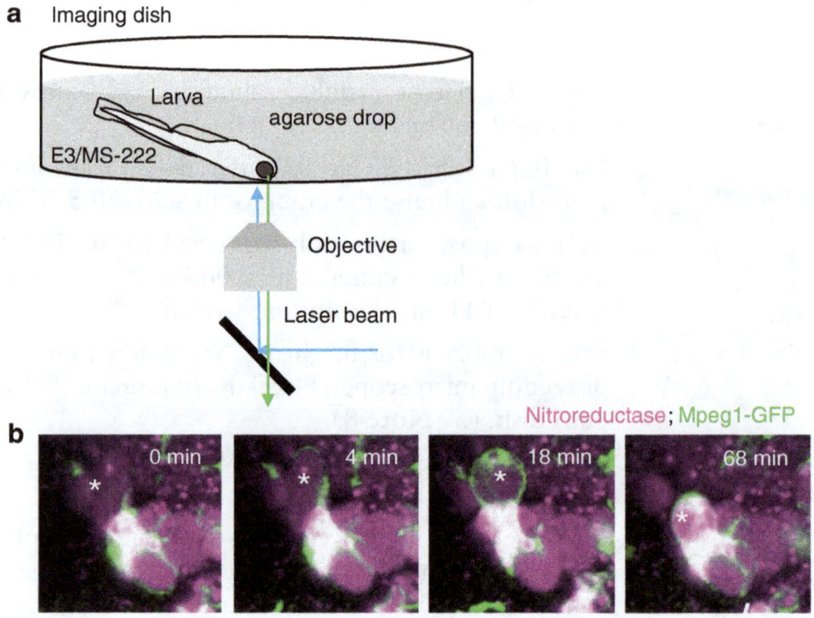

Fig. 1 Live imaging in larval zebrafish. (a) Position of larva in imaging dish for imaging with an inverted confocal microscope. (b) In vivo stills showing a GFP-expressing microglia (in *green*) engulfing an apoptotic neuron (in *magenta*, marked with *asterisks*). Scale bar = 10 μm

3.1.3 Immunohistochemistry Larvae

Prior to fixation anesthetize the larvae with 1× MS-222 and once they are anesthetized transfer them to a 1.5 mL micro centrifuge tube using a plastic Pasteur pipette or a cut 1 mL tip. It is recommended to perform all washing and incubation steps on a roller mixer unless stated otherwise (*see* **Note 17**). NB: All steps are performed at room temperature (RT) in volumes of 1 mL unless stated otherwise.

1. Euthanize the larvae with an overdose of MS-222 and transfer the larvae to 1.5 mL microcentrifuge tubes (*see* **Note 18**).
2. Briefly centrifuge the larvae in microcentrifuge tubes to collect them in the bottom of the tube and remove the medium.
3. Add 4 % PFA and invert the microcentrifuge tubes five times to expose all the larvae to the PFA solution.
4. Incubate the larvae at 4 °C in 4 % PFA for at least 16 h (*see* **Note 19**).
5. Wash the larvae at least twice with PBS-T for 5 min.
6. Perform stepwise dehydration with a methanol (MeOH) series (25 %, 50 %, 75 %, 100 %) 5 min per step.
7. Store the larvae at −20 °C for at least 24 h. Larvae can be stored for a few months at −20 °C at this point (*see* **Note 20**).
8. Perform stepwise rehydration with a MeOH series (75, 50, 25, and 0 %), 5 min per step.

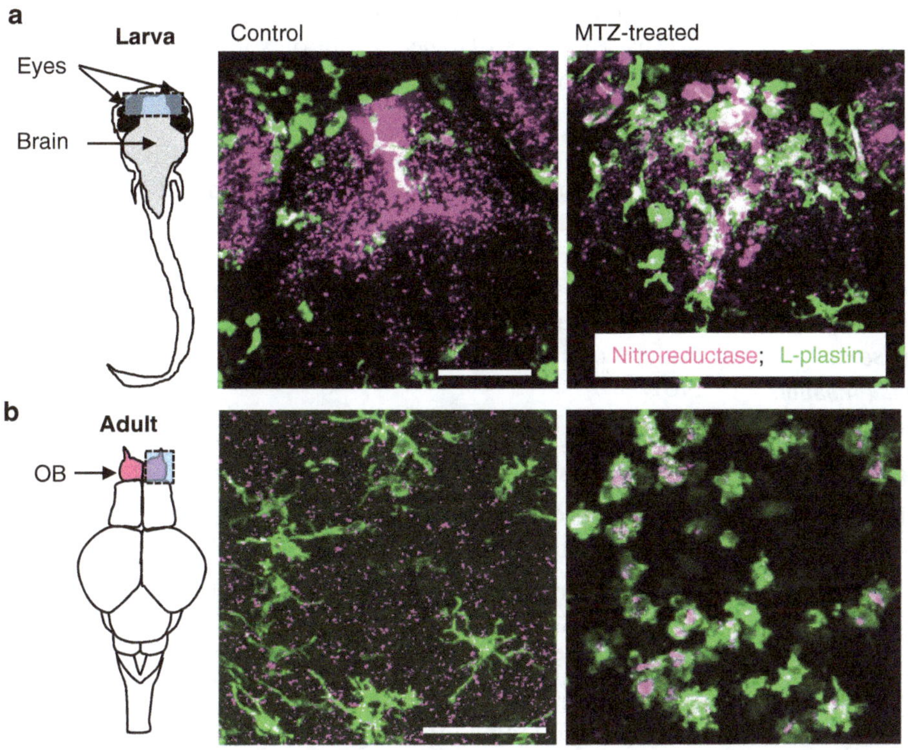

Fig. 2 Immunostaining of zebrafish larvae and adult brains. (a) Activated microglia (in *green* L-plastin+) in 6 dpf larvae at 1 day post-treatment (dpt) with 2 mM MTZ for 16 h. Phagocytosed neurons are visible as bright mCherry-positive dots (in *magenta*). (b) Immunostaining in adult zebrafish brain olfactory bulbs after treatment with 5 mM MTZ for 48 h. Microglia are shown in *green*, apoptotic, engulfed neurons are shown in *magenta*. Scale bar = 50 μm

9. Remove the PBST and incubate the larvae in 10 μg/mL proteinase K in PBS-T for 40 min.
10. Remove the 10 μg/mL proteinase K solution and incubate the larvae in 4 % PFA for 20 min.
11. Wash larvae at least twice with PBST for 5 min.
12. Remove the PBST and incubate the larvae in the blocking solution for 2 h.
13. Remove the blocking solution and incubate the larvae with 400 μL primary antibody solution containing 1:500 rabbit L-plastin (gift from Yi Feng, University of Edinburgh) at 4 °C on a shaker for at least 16 h (alternative incubation times may be required depending on the antibody) (*see* **Note 21**).
14. Wash the larvae at least 10× with PBS-T for 30 min.

15. Remove the PBS-T and incubate the larvae in 400 μL secondary Alexa 488 labeled antibody solution (DyLight Alexa 488, 1:250) with 1:10.000 Hoechst on a shaker at 4 °C for at least 16 h (*see* **Note 21**).
16. Wash the larvae at least six times with PBS-T for 10–15 min and continue for imaging (see mounting live imaging larvae) (*see* **Note 13**).

3.2 Imaging Microglial Activation in Response to Neuronal Ablation (Adult Zebrafish)

NB: During the entire experiment zebrafish can be fed according to the regular feeding regimen. Artemia or other live food is preferred since this causes less contamination of the water (*see* **Note 22**).

3.2.1 Metronidazole Treatment Adult Fish

1. Dissolve 0.642 g MTZ in 3.5 mL DMSO to obtain a 1 M 1000× stock solution and shake thoroughly (*see* **Note 23**).
2. Fill a breeding tank with 750 mL water tapped from the aquarium water circulation system.
3. Transfer the dissolved MTZ to the breeding tank containing 750 mL fish water, resulting in a 5 mM MTZ solution (*see* **Note 24**).
4. Transfer up to a maximum of three adult zebrafish to the breeding tank containing 5 mM MTZ (*see* **Note 25**).
5. Place the breeding tank containing the fish in an incubator of 28–28.5 °C for 24 h (*see* **Note 26**).
6. After the first 24 h of the experiment repeat **step 30–34** once.

3.2.2 Isolation of Fixed Complete Zebrafish Brain

1. Euthanize the adult zebrafish on ice water.
2. Sever the head just behind the gills using a scalpel.
3. Place the head under a dissection microscope.
4. Remove the gills, jaws and remaining tissues until only the skull and eyes are left using forceps.
5. Place the skull containing the brain, eyes attached, in 4% PFA at 4 °C for at least 20 h (*see* **Note 27**).
6. Wash the skulls containing the brains at least 3× with 1× PBS for 5 min at room temperature.
7. Place the skulls containing the brains with the ventral side facing upwards and carefully cut the optic nerves (white bands connecting the eyes to the head) with the scissors and remove the eyes.
8. Split the caudal half of the skull base in two equal parts with the break line in the rostral to caudal direction (*see* **Note 28**).
9. Carefully remove the frontal part of the skull base (*see* **Note 29**).
10. Remove the skull from the brain by pushing the caudal parts of the skull base apart.

11. Collect the brains in 1.5 mL micro centrifuge tubes (*see* **Note 30**).
12. Perform stepwise dehydration with a methanol (MeOH) series (25 %, 50 %, 75 %, and 100 %) 5 min per step at RT.
13. The brains can be stored at −20 °C for several weeks to months. For direct use, store them at −20 °C for at least 16 h.

3.2.3 Sectioning of Zebrafish Brains for Immunofluorescence Staining

1. Rehydrate the zebrafish brains in a methanol (MeOH) dilution series by subsequently incubating brains in 75% MeOH, 50% MeOH, 25% MeOH and 0% MeOH in 1× PBS at RT (*see* **Note 31**).
2. Wash the brains once with 1× PBS to remove methanol traces.
3. Use the plastic Pasteur pipette to fill an embedding base mold with 4% LMP agarose (*see* **Note 32**).
4. Place the zebrafish brain in the LMP agarose and position it in the desired orientation (*see* **Note 33**).
5. Wait until the agarose gel has solidified (*see* **Note 6**).
6. Remove the gel from the embedding base mold and cut it into a cube (using the scalpel) with at least 2 mm agarose on each side of the brain. Do not cut the agarose at the ventral side of the brain (*see* **Note 34**).
7. Use the vibratome to cut 80 μm sections of the desired area.
8. For immunofluorescence staining transfer the brain sections to a 48-well plate containing 1× PBS (*see* **Note 35**).

*3.2.4 Immuno-fluorescence Staining of Zebrafish Brain Sections (See **Note 36**)*

1. Remove the PBS from the wells containing brain sections, add ~ 300 μL blocking buffer and incubate at room temperature on a shaker for 75 min.
2. Remove the blocking solution, add ~300 μL antibody solution 1 containing the primary L-plastin antibody (L-plastin, Rabbit, 1:1000, gift from Yi Feng, University of Edinburgh) and incubate at 4 °C on a shaker for at least 16 h.
3. Remove antibody solution and was at least 6× with PBST for 20 min.
4. Remove PBST, add ~300 μL blocking buffer containing the secondary antibody (e.g., Dylight α-Rabbit 488, 1:500) and incubate at 4 °C on a shaker for at least 16 h.
5. Remove antibody solution and wash at least 5× with 1× PBS for 20 min.
6. Transfer the brain sections to a microscope slide (*see* **Note 37**).
7. Place small strips of Parafilm on either side of the brain sections and place 1–2 drops of Vectashield mounting medium on the brain sections. Cover with a cover glass and continue to imaging procedure (Fig. 2b) (*see* **Note 38**).

4 Notes

1. Dissolved MTZ can be stored at −20 °C (preferably in aliquots).
2. Apoptotic cells can be labeled in vivo by combining imaging with secA5-YFP transgenic animals or in fixed tissue by TUNEL staining (Click-it Alexa Fluor 647 kit; Invitrogen) [16].
3. 10× MS-222 stock solution can be stored at −20 °C. 10× MS-222 stock solution can be kept protected from light at 4 °C or room temperature for a few weeks.
4. In order to prevent setting of the gel, the 1.8% LMP agarose solution can be kept at 55 °C.
5. We used a Zeiss LSM700, Zeiss LSM780, and Zeiss MPL for image acquisition. For imaging GFP a laser of 488 nm is necessary and for imaging of mCherry laser lines of 543, 555, 561, or 594 can be used. We used a 40× water lens with a numerical aperture (NA) of 1.2 for most of the image acquisition. In addition to a relatively high NA, this lens has a long working distance, which is ideal for making high quality images throughout the entire larval brain. It is possible to increase the quality of images by using lenses with a higher NA, however, these lenses usually have a shorter working distance, that do not allow imaging of the entire brain.
6. It is recommended to make the 4% LMP agarose solution when the brains have been rehydrated. In order to prevent premature setting of the gel, it is recommended to dissolve the agarose while the tube is placed in water and to keep it in the water while pipetting out the solution. Make sure there are no bubbles in the low melting point agarose transferred to the embedding base mold. This can make it more difficult to properly section tissue.
7. PTU prevents pigment formation [17]. As soon as the PTU is removed from the medium, pigment formation will occur. Therefore it is important to keep the PTU in the medium during the course of the experiment. An alternative to using PTU would be the use of fish without pigment formation (e.g., Casper, [18]).
8. In case a line in which cell type-specific expression is accomplished by the use of the Gal4/UAS system in which the Gal4 driver as well as the NTR are labeled with mCherry, it is recommended to use the GFP filter for the selection of NTR/mCherry-positive larvae if possible. Only the larvae with the highest mCherry expression will show a red central nervous system while using the GFP filter. This reduces the number of NTR-negative larvae in the experiment that seem positive.

Use a plastic Pasteur pipette or a 1 mL Gilson pipette with the tip cut off (0.5 cm) to transfer the positive larvae to a new petri dish. The brightest mCherry larvae are positive for both the neuronal gal4 driver and the UAS:NTR-mCherry construct.

9. From 2 to 3dpf onwards *Mpeg1*-GFP can be clearly observed. At 3 dpf the larvae have hatched and will be able to swim around. To sedate the larvae add some flaked ice to the petri dishes and allow the ice to melt, while swirling the dish. Swirling will cause the sedated larvae to accumulate in the center of the dish.
10. Make sure the larvae are treated in the 28–28.5 °C incubator since lower temperatures may cause a weaker microglia response. The amount of induced cell death is dose and time dependent. Therefore one can choose to treat the larvae over a longer time period with a lower concentration or conversely to induce the same amount of cell death but over variable time periods (for more information see van Ham et al., 2012). Treatment with MTZ will work as soon as NTR is expressed.
11. The MTZ or DMSO containing solution is removed at the desired time point and the larvae are washed twice for 10 min with fresh HEPES buffered E3 containing 0.003% PTU to remove the MTZ. We put 10–15 larvae per well in a 6-well plate.
12. When applying the 1.8% LMP agarose make sure the agarose has cooled to around 30 °C as higher temperatures may damage/kill larvae.
13. It is crucial to mount the larva as close as possible to the cover glass, to reduce the distance to the lens as high magnification objectives tend to have low working distance. Make sure the larva is positioned correctly before the agarose completely polymerizes. While the agarose is polymerizing keep the larva in place with a thin pipette tip or needle. We use Seque/Pro™ Capillary Pipet Tips from Roche.
14. For in vivo imaging using an upright microscope it is necessary to use a ceramic/dipping lens. To assure proper positioning of the larvae for imaging with an upright microscope it is also possible to mount them as described for the inverted microscope. Then the LMP agarose containing the larva can be taken out of the glass bottom dish and placed upside down in a droplet of LMP agarose in a 6 cm petri dish. Make sure to use sufficient LMP agarose to prevent detachment of the agarose from the petri dish, as this will cause the larva to move out of focus during the imaging (Fig. 1a).
15. Make sure to add the buffered 1x E3 medium with 0.016% MS-222 very carefully. The agarose detaches easily from the bottom of the dish. Addition of E3 medium is necessary to prevent shrinking of the agarose due to dehydration. Also the larva needs to stay anesthetized during the imaging.

16. When a water lens is used for long-term imaging, use Immersol instead of water as to avoid evaporation. It is crucial to put sufficient buffered 1× E3 medium in the imaging dish and to keep the lid on the dish to prevent evaporation and subsequent drying of the LMP agarose.
17. Put the 1.5 mL tubes in a 50 mL tube to place them on a roller mixer.
18. To assure equal antibody labeling in all larvae do not stain more than 20 larvae in a 1.5 mL tube.
19. Instead of overnight incubation at 4 °C, 3 h at room temperature is also sufficient.
20. Fluorescence of mCherry is retained after immunohistochemistry, however when samples are stored for longer time periods (multiple months) mCherry fluorescence will fade.
21. In case incubation on a roller mixer is preferred, use at least 400 μL, preferably more, antibody solution. Less solution may cause insufficient labeling due to larvae sticking to the walls of the tube diminisheing contact with the antibody solution.
22. Depending on the ablated brain area or cell type, fish may show impaired feeding behavior.
23. The solution should turn slightly yellow.
24. After transferring the MTZ solution to the water, take care to mix the MTZ solution with water to obtain a completely transparent homogeneous solution. The mixing can be done by stirring the solution with a plastic Pasteur pipette.
25. We have performed these experiments in adult male and female fish of an age ranging from 3 to 9 months.
26. It is important to keep the fish at a temperature of at least 28 °C. Lower temperatures may lead to a weaker microglia response to neuronal cell death.
27. PFA fixation within the skull facilitates the isolation of the brains and reduces the chance of damaging and losing brain tissue during dissection.
28. This is most easily done by pushing one arm of the forceps in between the brain and the caudal half of the skull base in the rostral to caudal direction. Subsequently squeezing of the forceps will result in a break line in the caudal part of the skull base. Then take out the forceps. Take care not to remove these parts of the skull base.
29. After the frontal part of the skull base has been removed the telencephalon and olfactory bulb should be exposed. This step is important, because otherwise the chance of losing (part of) the olfactory bulb is relatively high. Especially in the model described in this chapter, the effects are most pronounced in

the olfactory bulb. Therefore it is important to preserve this part during the procedure.

30. It is possible to put multiple brains into a single microcentrifuge tube.
31. In order to assure optimal rehydration, the microcentrifuge tubes containing the brains can be put in a 50 mL tube during incubation and placed on a roller mixer.
32. For horizontal sections, position the brain with the dorsal side facing upward and the ventral side facing downward. For sectioning it is most convenient to place the brain as close to the surface as possible. The deeper the brain has sunk, the more agarose has to be cut before actual sectioning of the brain.
33. To speed up solidification of the gel, place the embedding base mold containing the brain on ice. Make sure to check regularly whether the brain is still in the desired position and correct when necessary. Sometimes during the solidification of the gel, the tissue sinks or tilts. This can be easily corrected as long as the gel has not completely solidified yet.
34. It is crucial that the ventral part is completely flat for optimal adhesion to the surface of the magnetic platform during the sectioning. Otherwise the agarose cube may detach. Also the position of the brain may change if the ventral part of the agarose tube is not properly cut.
35. An easy way to transfer the brain sections to a 48-well plate is to catch the sections on a microscope slide and then to use PBS to flush them into the desired well in the 48-well plate. It is possible to place multiple sections per well. 12-well plates can be used as well; however, much more antibody will then be required.
36. All incubation and washing steps should be performed on a shaker.
37. One way to transfer the sections to the microscope slide is to first place a drop of PBS on the microscope slide and then scoop the sections out of the 48-well plate using a 200 μL pipette tip. Then hold the tip in the drop of PBS. The brain section will detach. Then remove excess PBS.
38. These slides can be stored at 4 °C for several months.

Acknowledgments

This work was sponsored by ZonMW [VENI grant number 016.136.150], a Marie Curie Career Integration Grant [Saving Dying Neurons, 322368], and an Alzheimer Nederland fellowship [grant number WE.15-2012-01] to T.J.v.H..

References

1. Tremblay ME, Stevens B, Sierra A, Wake H, Bessis A, Nimmerjahn A (2011) The role of microglia in the healthy brain. J Neurosci 31(45):16064–16069. doi:10.1523/JNEUROSCI.4158-11.2011, doi:31/45/16064 [pii]
2. Kettenmann H, Hanisch U-K, Noda M, Verkhratsky A (2011) Physiology of microglia. Physiol Rev 91(2):461–553. doi:10.1152/physrev.00011.2010
3. Hanisch UK, Kettenmann H (2007) Microglia: active sensor and versatile effector cells in the normal and pathologic brain. Nat Neurosci 10(11):1387–1394. doi:10.1038/nn1997, doi:nn1997 [pii]
4. Prinz M, Priller J, Sisodia SS, Ransohoff RM (2011) Heterogeneity of CNS myeloid cells and their roles in neurodegeneration. Nat Neurosci 14(10):1227–1235. doi:10.1038/nn.2923, doi:nn.2923 [pii]
5. Oosterhof N, Boddeke E, van Ham TJ (2015) Immune cell dynamics in the CNS: Learning from the zebrafish. Glia 63(5):719–735. doi:10.1002/glia.22780
6. van Ham TJ, Kokel D, Peterson RT (2012) Apoptotic cells are cleared by directional migration and elmo1- dependent macrophage engulfment. Curr Biol 22(9):830–836. doi:10.1016/j.cub.2012.03.027, doi:S0960-9822(12)00314-4 [pii]
7. Van Ham TJ, Brady CA, Kalicharan RD, Oosterhof N, Kuipers J, Veenstra-Algra A, Sjollema KA, Peterson RT, Kampinga HH, Giepmans BN (2014) Intravital correlated microscopy reveals differential macrophage and microglial dynamics during resolution of neuroinflammation. Dis Model Mech 7(7):857–869. doi:10.1242/dmm.014886, doi:7/7/857 [pii]
8. Peri F, Nusslein-Volhard C (2008) Live imaging of neuronal degradation by microglia reveals a role for v0-ATPase a1 in phagosomal fusion in vivo. Cell 133(5):916–927. doi:10.1016/j.cell.2008.04.037, doi:S0092-8674(08)00611-9 [pii]
9. Herbomel P, Thisse B, Thisse C (2001) Zebrafish early macrophages colonize cephalic mesenchyme and developing brain, retina, and epidermis through a M-CSF receptor-dependent invasive process. Dev Biol 238(2):274–288. doi:10.1006/dbio.2001.0393, doi:S0012-1606(01)90393-8 [pii]
10. Ginhoux F, Greter M, Leboeuf M, Nandi S, See P, Gokhan S, Mehler MF, Conway SJ, Ng LG, Stanley ER, Samokhvalov IM, Merad M (2010) Fate mapping analysis reveals that adult microglia derive from primitive macrophages. Science 330(6005):841–845. doi:10.1126/science.1194637, doi:science.1194637 [pii]
11. Curado S, Anderson RM, Jungblut B, Mumm J, Schroeter E, Stainier DY (2007) Conditional targeted cell ablation in zebrafish: a new tool for regeneration studies. Dev Dyn 236(4):1025–1035. doi:10.1002/dvdy.21100
12. Oosterhof N, Holtman IR, Kuil LE, van der Linde HC, Boddeke EW, Eggen BJ, van Ham TJ (2016) Identification of a conserved and acute neurodegeneration-specific microglial transcriptome in the zebrafish. Glia 65(1):138–149. doi:10.1002/glia.23083
13. Distel M, Wullimann MF, Koster RW (2009) Optimized Gal4 genetics for permanent gene expression mapping in zebrafish. Proc Natl Acad Sci U S A 106(32):13365–13370. doi:10.1073/pnas.0903060106, doi:0903060106 [pii]
14. Ellett F, Pase L, Hayman JW, Andrianopoulos A, Lieschke GJ (2011) mpeg1 promoter transgenes direct macrophage-lineage expression in zebrafish. Blood 117(4):e49–e56. doi:10.1182/blood-2010-10-314120, doi:blood-2010-10-314120 [pii]
15. Davison JM, Akitake CM, Goll MG, Rhee JM, Gosse N, Baier H, Halpern ME, Leach SD, Parsons MJ (2007) Transactivation from Gal4-VP16 transgenic insertions for tissue-specific cell labeling and ablation in zebrafish. Dev Biol 304(2):811–824. doi:10.1016/j.ydbio.2007.01.033, doi:S0012-1606(07)00080-2 [pii]
16. van Ham TJ, Mapes J, Kokel D, Peterson RT (2010) Live imaging of apoptotic cells in zebrafish. FASEB J 24(11):4336–4342. doi:10.1096/fj.10-161018, doi:fj.10-161018 [pii]
17. Karlsson J, von Hofsten J, Olsson PE (2001) Generating transparent zebrafish: a refined method to improve detection of gene expression during embryonic development. Mar Biotechnol (NY) 3(6):522–527. doi:10.1007/s1012601-0053-4
18. White RM, Sessa A, Burke C, Bowman T, LeBlanc J, Ceol C, Bourque C, Dovey M, Goessling W, Burns CE, Zon LI (2008) Transparent adult zebrafish as a tool for in vivo transplantation analysis. Cell Stem Cell 2(2):183–189. doi:10.1016/j.stem.2007.11.002, doi:S1934-5909(07)00275-5 [pii]

Chapter 27

Experimental Arthritis Mouse Models Driven by Adaptive and/or Innate Inflammation

W. Razawy, C.H. Alves, M. Molendijk, P.S. Asmawidjaja, A.M.C. Mus, and E. Lubberts

Abstract

Rheumatoid arthritis (RA) is a chronic systemic autoimmune disease mainly affecting synovial joints. The clinical presentation of RA shows the heterogeneity of this disease with its underlying complex interactions between the innate and adaptive immune system and flare-ups of disease. Different disease models such as collagen induced arthritis, antigen induced arthritis, and *Streptococcal* cell wall induced arthritis can be exploited to investigate different aspects of the pathogenesis of arthritis. The disease can be monitored macroscopically over time via scoring systems. For histological examination, paraffin embedded knee sections can be used for hematoxylin and eosin staining to visualize cellular infiltration as well as for tartrate-resistant acid phosphatase (TRAP) staining to identify osteoclast-like cells. Cellular infiltration of the synovium by different myeloid cells such as tissue resident macrophages, dendritic cells and neutrophils can be monitored using flow cytometry. Here, we describe the methods for inducing the different mouse models for arthritis, including scoring systems per model, histological and flow cytometric analysis.

Key words Antigen induced arthritis, Cellular infiltration, Collagen induced arthritis, Flow cytometry, Histology, *Streptococcal* cell wall, Synovium

1 Introduction

Rheumatoid arthritis (RA) is a chronic systemic autoimmune disease mainly affecting synovial joints. This disease affects ~1 % of the population worldwide, most commonly middle-aged women. Although RA disease etiology is still largely unknown, genetic susceptibility, auto-antibody formation, and environmental factors such as smoking are major RA risk factors [1–3]. In early disease, pro-inflammatory cells migrate to the synovium and induce a chronic inflammation. As the disease progresses, synovial hyperplasia, angiogenesis, and pannus tissue formation will be induced. Without proper treatment, these processes will ultimately lead to irreversible joint destruction.

Björn E. Clausen and Jon D. Laman (eds.), *Inflammation: Methods and Protocols*, Methods in Molecular Biology, vol. 1559, DOI 10.1007/978-1-4939-6786-5_27,

Pro-inflammatory cytokines play a central role in RA. Regulation of the cytokine imbalance might represent a solid way to control this disease. The pro-inflammatory cytokines tumor necrosis factor α (TNFα) and interleukin-6 (IL-6) play a crucial role in the pathogenesis of arthritis, driving enhanced production of cytokines, chemokines, and degradative enzymes [1, 2]. The efficacy of blocking TNFalpha and IL-6 activity was shown in clinical studies. In addition, early in the disease process inflammatory T cells and their cytokines are present in the joint synovium and contribute to the progression of an early synovial inflammation towards a persistent and chronic arthritis, indicating that inflammatory T cells and their cytokines play a central role in the pathogenesis of RA [2, 4–6].

Rheumatoid arthritis is a complex and heterogeneous disease with interactions between the innate and adaptive immune system and flare-ups of disease. Currently there is no animal model that represents all the features of rheumatoid arthritis. However, there are several mouse models that can be exploited to investigate different aspects of the pathogenesis of arthritis. The collagen induced arthritis (CIA) model is an autoimmune model in which autoreactive T cells and auto-antibodies can be detected. TNFα, IL-1, and IL-6 are key cytokines in CIA. An advantage of CIA is the ability to examine pathological processes leading to disease prior to the occurrence of symptoms. Antigen induced arthritis (AIA) is a second (non-autoimmune) model in which joint inflammation is driven by T cells. This model provides the opportunity to investigate reoccurrences or flare-ups of arthritis. The role of the innate immune system can be investigated using the *Streptococcal* cell wall (SCW) induced model. This acute joint inflammation is strongly TLR2/NOD2 driven and mediated by myeloid-derived pro-inflammatory cytokines. The acute inflammation can turn into a chronic disease with involvement of T cells and their cytokines by repeated local injections of SCW without using adjuvants such as Complete Freund's Adjuvant (CFA). In the chronic phase of SCW induced arthritis, destruction of bone and cartilage is observed.

Studies of the abovementioned arthritis models have been a major contribution to our increasing scientific knowledge of arthritis pathogenesis. For example, IL-17 receptor A (IL-17RA) knockout mice are completely resistant to the induction of CIA and blocking IL-17RA results in reduced AIA score [7]. In addition, Th17 cells, which are known to produce IL-17A, play an important role in the pathogenesis of arthritis [8]. Another important cytokine in the pathogenesis of arthritis is IL-23. This was shown by the resistance of IL-23 knockout mice to develop CIA and full blown AIA [7–9]. As IL-23 receptor has been shown to be present on T cells, monocytes, and dendritic cells (DCs), IL-23 can exert its pro-inflammatory effects not only on T cells, but also on different myeloid cells [10, 11].

In this chapter the induction of collagen induced arthritis (CIA), antigen induced arthritis (AIA), and *Streptococcal* cell wall (SCW) induced arthritis is explained. Scoring systems and methods for measuring outcomes macroscopically and histologically are described. Furthermore, the focus is on the flow cytometric analysis of cells from the myeloid lineage, isolated from mouse synovial tissue.

2 Materials

2.1 Collagen Induced Arthritis

1. 8–12-week-old C57BL/6JOlaHsd ($H2^b$) for both genders or male DBA/1 ($H2^q$) mice.
2. 2 and 5 ml syringes.
3. 25 G and 30 G needles.
4. Supplemented Complete Freund's Adjuvant (CFA): Dissolve 100 mg *Mycobacterium tuberculosis* (Mt) H37Ra in 1 ml Incomplete Freund's Adjuvant (IFA). Add 500 μl of the Mt/IFA solution to 10 ml CFA. Divide the supplemented CFA over two 10 ml glass vials.
5. Immunization emulsion: Dissolve 10 mg of chicken type II collagen (for C57BL/6 mice) or bovine type II collagen (for DBA/1 mice) in 1 ml 0.1 M acetic acid during 16 h in the dark at 4 °C. Dilute the collagen solution by adding 4 ml of NaCl (0.9% NaCl in sterile H_2O) to reach a concentration of 2 mg/ml. Push the collagen solution vigorously through a 5 ml syringe with a 30 G needle into the glass vial containing 5 ml supplemented CFA (*see* Subheading 2.1, **item 4**) to get a final concentration of 1 mg/ml collagen. Mix vigorously using a 2 ml syringe to make the emulsion (*see* **Note 1**).
6. Boost emulsion for DBA/1 mice: Dissolve 10 mg of bovine type II collagen in 1 ml 0.1 M acetic acid overnight in the dark at 4 °C. Add 9 ml of NaCl (0.9% in sterile H_2O) to the dissolved collagen to bring the concentration of the collagen type II to 1 mg/ml. The total volume is 10 ml (*see* **Note 2**).
7. Isoflurane system: Isoflurane vaporizer, supply gas regulator, flowmeter, induction chamber, connection tubing and valves, face mask or intubation supply.

2.2 Antigen Induced Arthritis

2.2.1 Immunization

1. 8–12-week-old mice from both genders (*see* **Note 3**).
2. 10× NaCl stock: 9% NaCl in sterile H_2O.
3. Isoflurane system: Isoflurane vaporizer, supply gas regulator, flowmeter, induction chamber, connection tubing and valves, face mask or intubation supply.
4. 70% ethanol (i.a. injections).

5. 5×5 cm bandage gauze (i.a. injections).
6. Caliper device (i.a. injections).
7. Fine scissors (i.a. injections).
8. Dressing forceps (i.a. injections).
9. Methylated bovine serum albumin (mBSA) stock solution (40 mg/ml): Dissolve 400 mg of mBSA in 9 ml sterile H_2O. You can speed-up the process by incubating the solution in a 37 °C heated water bath. If the solution is completely dissolved, add 1 ml of 10× NaCl to bring concentration to 40 mg/ml. The solution can be aliquoted in portions of 1.1 ml and stored at −80 °C.
10. Supplemented Complete Freund's Adjuvant (CFA), H37Ra: Resuspend 100 mg of *Mycobacterium tuberculosis* (Mt) H37Ra in 1 ml of Incomplete Freund's Adjuvant (IFA). Mix 400 μl (40 mg) dissolved Mt with 10 ml of CFA. Divide this mixture into two 10 ml glass vials, each containing 5 ml of supplemented CFA.
11. Immunization emulsion: Dilute 1 ml of the mBSA stock solution (*see* Subheading 2.2.1, **item 9**) with 4 ml 1× NaCl to achieve 8 mg/ml. Transfer this into the glass vial containing 5 ml supplemented CFA (*see* Subheading 2.2.1, **item 10**) using a 5 ml syringe with a 30 G needle. The final concentration of mBSA is 4 mg/ml. The emulsion must be prepared by pressing the syringe firmly in order to homogenize. After this, mix vigorously by using a 2 ml syringe until the mixture turns into a stiff and white emulsion (*see* **Note 1**).
12. 25G needle.

2.2.2 Intra-articular (i.a.) injection

1. 10 mg/ml mBSA: Dilute the mBSA stock solution (*see* Subheading 2.2.1, **item 9**) to 10 mg/ml by adding 3 ml of 1× NaCl to 1 ml of the stock solution. The mBSA can be aliquoted in portions of 0.5 ml and stored at −80 °C.
2. 50 μl Hamilton glass syringe.
3. 30 G needle.

2.3 Streptococcal Cell Wall Induced Arthritis

1. 8–12-week-old mice from both genders (*see* **Note 3**).
2. 10× NaCl: 9% NaCl in sterile H_2O.
3. Sterile H_2O.
4. SCW PGPS 100P: prepare at a concentration of 4.17 mg/ml in 1× NaCl (*see* **Note 4**).
5. Isoflurane system: Isoflurane vaporizer, supply gas regulator, flowmeter, induction chamber, connection tubing and valves, face mask or intubation supply.
6. 70% ethanol.

7. Caliper device.
8. 5 × 5 cm bandage gauze.
9. 50 μl Hamilton glass syringe.
10. 30 G needle.

2.4 Histology: Mouse Knees

The most common way to process paws for joint morphology, is to embed them in paraffin. The removal of calcium deposits is essential for a good embedding procedure. Decalcification is usually carried out between the fixation and processing steps. A variety of agents or techniques have been developed to decalcify tissues, each with advantages and disadvantages. Consideration must be given to the type of investigation being carried out. Immersion in solutions containing mineral acids, organic acids, or chelating agents such as ethylenediaminetetracetic acid (EDTA) are the predominant methods used. Chelating agents, such as EDTA, work by capturing the calcium ions from the surface of the apatite crystal, slowly reducing its size. Because the process is very slow but gentle, this reagent is not suitable for urgent specimens but more appropriate for research applications where very high quality morphology is required or particular molecular elements must be preserved [12, 13] (*see* **Note 5**).

Strong mineral acids as nitric and hydrochloric acids are used with dense cortical bone, because they are able to remove large quantities of calcium in a short time period. As these strong acids damage cellular morphology, they are not recommended for delicate tissues as bone marrow. Weak organic acids such as acetic or formic acid are more suitable for use in bone marrow or soft tissues. Formic acid at a 10% concentration is commonly used.

2.4.1 Preparation of Knees and Hematoxylin and Eosin Staining

1. 10% formalin.
2. 10% formic acid.
3. Absolute ethanol.
4. 95% ethanol.
5. 70% ethanol.
6. Xylene.
7. Phosphate buffered saline (PBS; 2.6 mM KH_2PO_4, 26 mM Na_2HPO_4, 145 mM NaCl, pH 7.2).
8. Paraffin.
9. Scissors and forceps.
10. Histology cassettes.
11. Molds.
12. Embedding station.
13. Microtome.

14. Water bath.
15. Slides.
16. Cover slides.
17. Hematoxylin.
18. Eosin.
19. Mounting medium.
20. Light microscope.

2.4.2 Tartrate-Resistant Acid Phosphatase Staining

TRAP staining is performed by a leukocyte acid phosphatase kit from Sigma Chemical Co.

1. 12.5 mg/ml naphthol As-Bi phosphoric acid solution.
2. 7.0 mg/ml Fast Garnet GBC Base solution in 0.4 M hydrochloric acid with stabilizer.
3. Acetate solution: 2.5 M acetate buffer, pH 5.2 ± 0.1.
4. 0.335 M L(+)-tartrate buffer, pH 4.9 ± 0.1.
5. Sodium nitrite solution: 0.1 M sodium nitrite.
6. 6.0 g/l hematoxylin, certified, 0.6 g/l sodium iodate, 52.8 g/l aluminum sulfate, and stabilizers.
7. Fixative solution: Prepare citrate solution: 18 mM citric acid, 9 mM sodium citrate, 12 mM sodium chloride and surfactant, pH 3.6 ± 0.1. Combine 25 ml citrate solution, 65 ml acetone, and 8 ml of 37% formaldehyde. Place in glass bottle and cap tightly.
8. Two staining jars.
9. Two 100 ml beakers.

2.5 Analysis of Synovial Cell Infiltration by Flow Cytometry

2.5.1 Preparation of Synovial Tissue

1. Standard laboratory equipment including 100-μm nylon cell strainers, FACS tubes, and 50 ml Falcon tubes.
2. RPMI 1640 without supplements.
3. Liberase TM Research grade (*collagenase* I and II): dissolve in sterile H_2O to obtain 500 μg/ml and aliquot in 1.5 ml microcentrifuge tubes.
4. 1 or 2 ml syringes.
5. Scissors.
6. 24-well plates.

2.5.2 Flow Cytometry

1. FACS buffer: PBS supplemented with 0.5% BSA and 0.05% sodium azide.
2. 2% paraformaldehyde (PFA) in PBS.
3. Antibodies as indicated in Table 2.

4. Brilliant stain buffer (BD buffer).
5. Anti-FcγRII and III (Fc block).
6. BD LSRII flow cytometer.

3 Methods

3.1 Collagen Induced Arthritis

The classical background for CIA induction is the DBA/1 strain. Observed disease incidence and severity in this strain is higher compared to C57BL/6 mice, since DBA/1 have the H2^{q} MHC haplotype required for CIA induction. For induction of CIA in the C57BL/6 or DBA/1 strain, mice are immunized intradermally (i.d.) with type II collagen (CII)/CFA emulsion to trigger an immune response. After 21 days, C57BL/6 mice are boosted again with the same emulsion subcutaneously (s.c in the back of the neck). DBA/1 mice are boosted intraperitoneally (i.p.) with the emulsion described under Subheading 2.1, **item 6**. Collagen induced arthritis phenotype is observed between days 26–30 after the first immunization.

3.1.1 Immunization

1. Put the mice under anesthesia using isoflurane.
2. Immunize mice with 100 μl CII emulsion by an i.d. injection using a 25 G needle at the base of the tail (*see* **Note 6**).
3. Place the mice on a heating pad and carefully monitor their recovery from the anesthesia (*see* **Note 7**).

3.1.2 Boost Injection

1. Inject DBA/1 mice i.p. with 100 μl of the 1 mg/ml of CII solution using a 25G needle.

   Between days 26–30 the onset of CIA will start randomly in the group of mice (*see* **Note 7**).
2. Score the mice every other day using the method described below.

3.1.3 CIA Scoring

Arthritis development must be scored macroscopically by two independent observers, without knowledge of the experimental groups. The maximum score using our scaling system is 8 per mouse (2 per paw). Mice are considered to have arthritis when significant changes in redness and/or swelling are noted in the digits or in other parts of the paws. Arthritis is scored visually using the following scale per paw: 0, non-inflamed; 1, mild inflammation; 1.5, marked inflammation; 2, severe inflammation (Fig. 1).

3.2 Antigen Induced Arthritis

In contrast to CIA where a systemic inflammation occurs affecting multiple joints, AIA can be induced locally. On day 0 mice are immunized with mBSA/supplemented CFA emulsion to trigger an immune response and 7 days after immunization, arthritis is induced in the knee by an i.a. injection of the mBSA protein. This

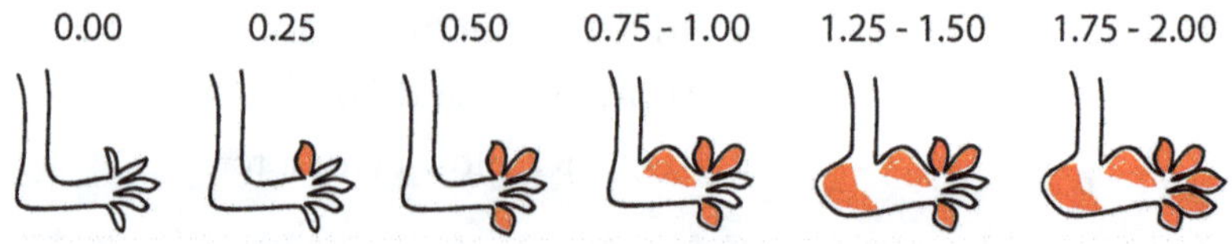

Fig. 1 Illustration of possible arthritis scores for the hind paw. In our scaling system the maximal score per paw is 2. One swollen and red finger has a score of 0.25, three fingers 0.5, all the five fingers are scored from 0.75 up to 1 depending on the severity. A swollen and red ankle or a swollen and red footpad counts 0.25–0.5 each depending on the severity. Swollen and red ankle and footpad are scored as 1. In this scale a score interval of 0.25–0.5 is dependent on the arthritis severity, defining the size and redness of the swollen area

inflammation occurs within a few days. After ~21 days, the inflammation is resolved (*see* **Note 8**).

3.2.1 Immunization

1. Put the mice under anesthesia using isoflurane.
2. Immunize the mice with 100 μl mBSA emulsion by an i.d. injection at the base of the tail using a 25 G needle.
3. Put the mice on a heating pad and carefully monitor their recovery from the anesthesia.

3.2.2 Intra-articular Injection (day 7)

1. Put the mice under anesthesia using isoflurane.
2. Lay the mice in a supine position.
3. Spray the knees with ethanol and smoothen the hair in the direction of growth with a bandage gauze.
4. Make a small cut in the skin above the knee, using a pair of fine scissors and forceps. This will heal within the next day.
5. Inject 6 μl (60 μg) of mBSA solution in the knee joints, using the Hamilton glass syringe with a 30 G needle. Bend the knee in a 20° position. When you are not so experienced, inject through the tendon, below the patella in the direction of the femur. This should go smoothly without scratching the bone. The needle should just go through the tendon while the patella is slightly lifted up. Inject the mBSA solution and remove the needle after about three seconds out of the knee joint.
6. Put the mice on a heating pad and carefully monitor their recovery from the anesthesia.

3.2.3 Caliper Measurement

1. Put the mice under anesthesia using isoflurane.
2. Spray the knees with ethanol and smoothen the hair in the direction of growth with a bandage gauze.
3. Measure the knee thickness at different time points (day 0, 1, 2, 4, 7, and 10 after i.a. injection) using a caliper device.

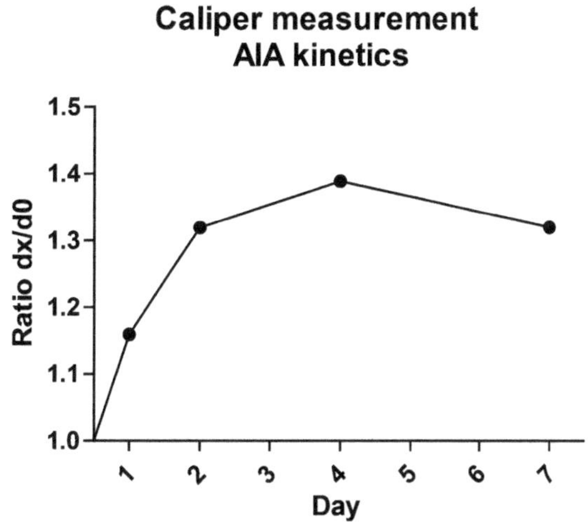

Fig. 2 Representative curve of AIA kinetics during 7 days of caliper measurements. At indicated time points, knee thickness of mBSA treated mice is measured using a caliper and divided by the values on day 0 (before injection) to determine the ratio of knee swelling. Peak of knee thickness is observed around day 4 after which knee thickness gradually normalizes

Measure knee joint thickness at the thickest part of the patella. All patellae should be measured 3 times by the same observer at each time point (Fig. 2).

4. Put the mice on a heating pad and carefully monitor their recovery from the anesthesia.

3.3 Streptococcal Cell Wall Induced Arthritis

In contrast to CIA where a systemic inflammation occurs affecting multiple joints, SCW induced arthritis can be induced locally. In the acute SCW arthritis model, synovitis is induced with a reversible damage to cartilage, but without bone erosion. However, chronic inflammation can be induced by repeating i.a. injections of SCW, leading to bone erosion and destruction of cartilage without the involvement of adjuvant such as CFA.

3.3.1 Intra-articular Injection

1. Put the mice under anesthesia using isoflurane.
2. Spray the knees with ethanol and smoothen the hair in the direction of growth with a bandage gauze.
3. Make a small cut in the skin above the knee, using a pair of fine scissors and forceps. This will heal within the next day.
4. Inject 6 μl (25 μg) of SCW solution in the knee joint, using the Hamilton glass syringe with a 30 G needle. Bend the knee in a 20° position. When you are not so experienced, inject through the tendon below the patella in the direction of the femur. This should go smoothly without scratching the bone. The needle should just go through the tendon while the patella is slightly lifted up. Remove the needle after about 3 s out of the knee joint.

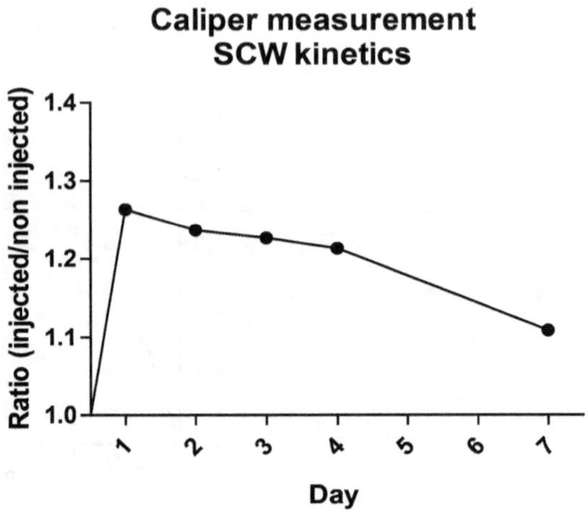

Fig. 3 Representative curve of SCW kinetics during 8 days of caliper measurements. At indicated time points, thickness of SCW injected knees is measured using a caliper and divided by the values of the non-injected knees. Peak of disease occurs around day 1–2 after which knee thickness gradually normalizes

5. Put the mice on a heating pad and carefully monitor their recovery from the anesthesia.

   Inflammation occurs within a few hours, with its maximum at day 1, and declines within a week to normal (*see* **Note 9**).

3.3.2 Caliper Measurement

1. Put the mice under anesthesia using isoflurane.
2. Spray the knees with ethanol and smoothen the hair in the direction of growth with a bandage gauze.
3. Measure knee thickness at different time points (days 0, 1, 2, 3, 4, and 7 after i.a. injection) using a caliper device. Measure knee joint thickness at the thickest part of the patella. All patellae should be measured three times by the same observer (Fig. 3).
4. Put the mice on a heating pad and carefully monitor their recovery from the anesthesia.

3.4 Histology: Mouse Knees

3.4.1 Fixation of Mouse Knees

1. Remove the skin from the paw.
2. Dissect the knee joint by cutting the femur 1 cm above the patellar tendon and the tibia 1.5 cm below the patellar tendon. The entire soft tissue should not be removed to prevent damage to the synovial capsule or destruction of the meniscus (*see* **Notes 10** and **11**).
3. Place the knee in a white embedding cassette in a flexed position at an angle of 120° and close properly (*see* **Note 12**).
4. Fix the knees in 10% formalin for a minimum of 72 h at room temperature. Make sure the knees are submerged in fixative.

5. After 3–6 days of fixation, the knees should be placed in 70% ethanol, either for immediate use or long-term storage.

3.4.2 Decalcification of Bone

1. Rinse tissue once in PBS.
2. Immerse tissue cassette in 10% formic acid for 3–6 days in a fume hood. The tissue cassettes should be submerged.
3. Wash tissue with distilled water twice for 8 h to remove the acid.
4. Store tissue in 70% ethanol.

3.4.3 Paraffin Infiltration

In this procedure, tissue is dehydrated through a series of graded ethanol baths to displace the water and then infiltrated with paraffin. The infiltrated tissues are then embedded into paraffin blocks. Once the tissue is embedded, it is stable for many years.

Dehydrate and embed the tissue in paraffin using a tissue processor machine, as follows (*see* **Note 13**):

1. 80% ethanol for 5 h at 45 °C.
2. 96% ethanol for 5 h at 45 °C.
3. 100% ethanol for 5 h at 45 °C.
4. 100% ethanol 5 h at 45 °C.
5. Xylene 5 h at 50 °C.
6. Xylene 5 h at 50 °C.
7. Xylene 5 h at 50 °C
8. Paraffin 5 h at 60 °C.
9. Paraffin 5 h at 60 °C.
10. Paraffin 5 h at 60 °C.
11. Paraffin 5 h at 60 °C.

3.4.4 Embedding Knees in Paraffin Blocks

1. The tissues processed into paraffin will have wax in the cassettes. Melt the wax away and place the entire cassette in 58 °C paraffin bath for 15 min in order to create smooth wax blocks.
2. Turn on the heat block to melt the paraffin one hour before adding the tissue cassettes.
3. Open the cassette to view tissue sample and choose a mold that best corresponds to the size of the tissue. A margin of at least 2 mm of paraffin surrounding all sides of the tissue gives the best cutting support. Discard the cassette lid.
4. Put a small amount of molten paraffin, dispensing from paraffin reservoir, into the mold.
5. Using warm forceps, transfer tissue into the mold. For coronal sections, place the patella facing down in the embedding mold; the tibia should be almost flat on the bottom of the mold and the femur directed upwards at a 60° angle from the bottom. It

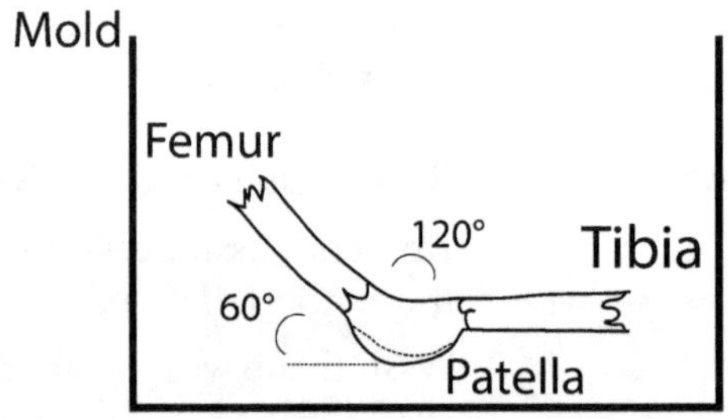

Fig. 4 Scheme of the embedding of the knee in the paraffin block. For coronal sections, place the patella facing down in the embedding mold, the tibia should be almost flat on the bottom of the mold and the femur directed upwards at a 60° angle from the bottom

is important that the joint is flat on the bottom to make sure that left and right side of the joint will be sectioned at the same depth (Fig. 4).

6. Transfer the mold to the cold plate, and press the tissue gently flat. Paraffin will solidify in a thin layer, which holds the tissue in position.
7. When the tissue is in the desired orientation, add the labeled tissue cassette on top of the mold as a backing and press firmly.
8. Add hot paraffin from the paraffin dispenser to the mold. Make sure there is enough paraffin to cover the surface of the plastic cassette.
9. Paraffin solidifies in 30 min. When the wax is completely cooled and hardened (30 min), pop the paraffin block out of the mold; the wax blocks should not stick. If the wax cracks or the tissues are not aligned well, melt the wax again and solidify (*see* **Notes 14** and **15**).

3.4.5 Sectioning Knees

1. Section the tissues using a microtome.
2. Turn on the water bath and make sure that the temperature is 35–37 °C (**step 6**).
3. Place the blocks to be sectioned on an ice block for 10 min.
4. Insert the block into the microtome chuck so the wax block faces the blade and is aligned in the vertical plane.
5. Set the dial to cut 20 μm sections in order to plane the block. Set the dial to cut 7 μm sections once the cutting goes smoothly.
6. Angle the blade at 5°. Continue sectioning until the desired tissue plane is obtained. Once the sections are in the desired tissue plane and the sectioning is going well, cut five sections and pick them up with forceps or a fine paint brush and float them on the surface of the 37 °C water bath (*see* **Note 16**). If the block is not ribboning well then it should be placed back on the ice block to cool off and firm up the wax.

7. Place the floating sections onto the surface of clean glass slides.
8. Place the slides with the paraffin sections on the warming block in a 65 °C oven for 20 min (so the wax just starts to melt) to bond the tissue to the glass. Slides can be stored at room temperature.

3.4.6 Hematoxylin and Eosin Staining

1. Deparaffinize sections by immerging the slides twice in xylene, 5 min each time.
2. Dehydrate in absolute ethanol for 5 min.
3. Incubate in 90% ethanol for 5 min
4. Incubate in 70% ethanol for 5 min.
5. Stain in Mayer's hematoxylin solution for 8 min.
6. Wash in running tap water for 10 min.
7. Counterstain in eosin Y solution for 30 s up to 1 min.
8. Wash briefly in 70% ethanol.
9. Dehydrate with 90% ethanol for 5 min.
10. Incubate in absolute ethanol for 5 min.
11. Wash twice in xylene for 5 min each time.
12. Mount coverslip to the tissue with xylene based mounting medium.

3.4.7 Tartrate-Resistant Acid Phosphatase Staining

Tartrate-resistant acid phosphatase (TRAP) is a histochemical marker of osteoclast-like cells. TRAP staining can be performed on EDTA decalcified joints.

1. Prewarm deionized water to 37 °C.
2. Bring fixative solution to room temperature (18–26 °C).
3. Fix slides by immersing them in fixative solution for 30 s.
4. Rinse slides thoroughly in deionized water. It is important to prevent drying of the slides.
5. Per 2 slides, add a mixture of 0.5 ml Fast Garnet GBC Base Solution and 0.5 ml Sodium Nitrite Solution Mix gently and let stand for 2 minutes.
6. Label two 100 ml beakers "A" and "B" and add the following reagents while mixing (Table 1). Beaker "A" serves as control.
7. Label two staining jars "A" and "B" and transfer solutions from the beakers into the appropriate staining jar.
8. Warm the solutions in the jars to 37 °C in water bath.
9. Add the slides to the staining jars (temperature should be 37 °C) and incubate 1 h in 37 °C water bath protected from light.

Table 1
Contents of beakers A and B

	Beakers A (ml)	Beakers B (ml)
Deionized water prewarmed to 37 °C	45	45
Diazotized fast garnet GBC solution from **step 5**	1.0	1.0
Naphthol AS-BI phosphate solution	0.5	0.5
Acetate solution	2.0	2.0
Tartrate solution		1.0

10. After 1 h, rinse slides thoroughly in deionized water, then counterstain for 2 min in hematoxylin solution.
11. Rinse the slides for several minutes in alkaline tap water to blue nuclei.
12. Air dry slides and evaluate microscopically. Cover slipping is not recommended since dye fades with time.

3.4.8 Histopathological Quantification

1. Assess the sections for joint inflammation (cell infiltrate) and bone and cartilage erosions. Score histopathological changes in the knee joints in the patella/femur region on three semi-serial sections of the joint, spaced 70 μm apart.
2. Use the following scoring system to determine the severity of inflammation: Use a scale of 0–3. 0 = no cellular infiltrate, 1 = mild cellularity, 2 = moderate cellularity, and 3 = maximal cellularity (Fig. 5).
3. Score the severity of bone and cartilage damage separately based on erosions using a scale from 0 to 3 (0 = no erosion, 1 = mild erosion, 2 = moderate erosion, and 3 = maximal erosion).
4. Score chondrocyte death: (0 = no cell death, 1 = mild cell death, 2 = moderate cell death, and 3 = maximal cell death).

3.5 Analysis of Synovial Cell Infiltration by Flow Cytometry

3.5.1 Preparation of Synovial Tissue

1. Sacrifice mice and take synovial tissue from the knee joints without disrupting bone marrow. Cut the patellae ligament with a fine scissor. Make an incision in the quadriceps to create space. Bend the knee and make an incision straight down at the medial side and one at the lateral side of the joint. Cut the synovium loose by cutting from both sides towards the femur (*see* **Note 17**).
2. Put synovium of both knees from one mouse in 2 ml RPMI medium in a 24-well plate.

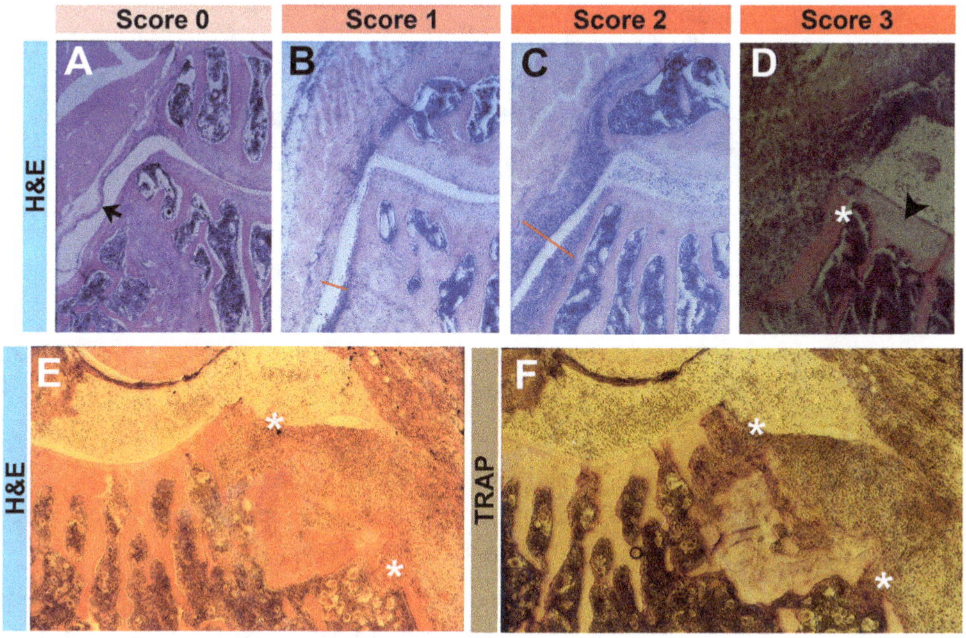

Fig. 5 Histology figures of CIA positive mice with no (**a**), mild (**b**), moderate (**c**), and severe (**d**) joint inflammation. (**e**+**f**) Serial sections of severe CIA showing focal bone erosion (**b**, **e**, **f**, *asterisk*) and osteoclast-like cell activity by TRAP staining (**f**). The synovial membrane (**a**, *arrow*) thickness is increased during disease due to influx of immune cells and high proliferation of synovial fibroblasts (**b** and **c**, *red bars*). In animals with severe inflammation chondrocyte death can be observed (*arrowhead*)

3. Process the synovium by cutting it into smaller pieces using scissors before proceeding.
4. Transfer the synovium and RPMI medium from the 24-well plate into a 50 ml tube and add another 3 ml RPMI to reach a total volume of 5 ml.
5. Add 50 μL Liberase and shake the tube gently a few times.
6. Incubate the 50 ml tube at 37 °C, 5% CO_2 for 1.5–2 h, depending on the size of the tissue.
7. Every 15–30 min, shake the tube by hand (do not vortex).
8. After incubation, remove excess tissue by adding the suspension on top of the cell strainer placed on a 50 ml tube and crushing the tissue through it with the plunge of a 2 ml syringe.
9. Wash the cell strainer well with medium and discard.
10. Centrifuge the cells at 380 G for 10 min.
11. Discard medium and resuspend cells in the remaining volume in the 50 ml tube. Transfer cells to U-bottom 96-well plates. The cells are ready to be used for analysis by flow cytometry.

Table 2
Antibodies used for flow cytometric analysis of synovial myeloid cells

Antibody	Label	Company	Clone
Ly-6G	PE-CF594	BD Horizon	1A8
MHCII	Pe.Cy7	eBioscience	M5/114.15.2
CD11b	ef450	eBioscience	M1/70
CD45	BV785	Biolegend	104
CD64	APC	Biolegend	X54-5/7.1
CD11c	Pe	Biolegend	N418

3.5.2 Flow Cytometric Analysis of Myeloid Cells

Centrifuge the cells at 280 G for 2.5 min unless stated otherwise. The indicated volumes of reagents are per well.

1. Centrifuge the cells in the 96-well plate and discard medium.
2. Wash the cells with 150 μl FACS buffer to remove medium.
3. Incubate the cells for 30 min with 25 μl Fc block at 4 °C.
4. Wash the cells with 150 μl FACS buffer.
5. Prepare the antibody mix in BD buffer and incubate the cells in 25 μl of the antibody mix (*see* **Note 18** and Table 2) for 30 min at 4 °C.
6. Wash the cells with 150 μl FACS buffer to remove the antibody mix.
7. Wash the cells with 150 μl PBS (*see* **Note 19**).
8. Fix the cells with 150 μl 2% PFA and incubate for 5 min at 4 °C in the dark.
9. Wash the cells with 150 μl PBS to remove the PFA.
10. (Optional) Wash the cells with 150 μl FACS buffer.
11. Take up the cells in 85 μl FACS buffer. The cells are ready to be measured (*see* **Note 20**).

3.5.3 Analysis of Synovial Myeloid Cells

In steady state, the mouse joint harbors a heterogeneous population of tissue resident macrophages with very small numbers of CD11b$^+$ DCs, eosinophils and neutrophils present [14]. However, in inflamed conditions the presence of the different cell populations in the joint with respect to each other is altered. For analyzing cell populations in the inflamed joints, gate on all cells (Fig. 6a). Exclude the doublets by plotting the forward scatter width (FSC-W) of fluorescence light against the height (FSC-H). Repeat the same procedure for the side scatter width and height (SSC-W against SSC-H) (Fig. 6b). As doublets are bigger and need more

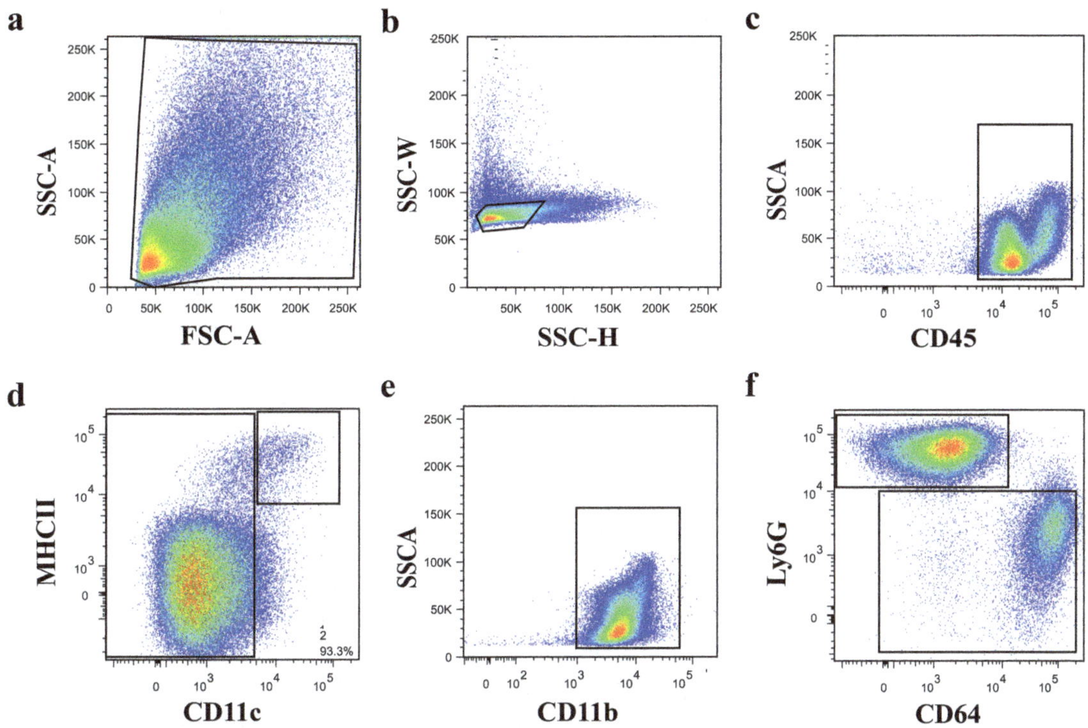

Fig. 6 Gating strategy for analysis of synovial myeloid cells. (**a**) Gating on total cells. (**b**) Doublet discrimination. (**c**) Identification of CD45⁺ cells. (**d**) Identification of DCs. (**e**) Identification of CD11b⁺ myeloid cells. (**f**) Excluding neutrophils and distinguishing CD64 high and intermediate cells. The CD64^{int} cells are identified as monocytes and F480⁺ CD64⁺ are macrophages

time to pass through the laser beam, they have a greater pulse width than single cells. The height correlates with the intensity of a cell's signal. Thus, disproportions between H and W in the forward and side scatter can be used to identify doublets.

Hematopoietic cells can be identified based on their expression of CD45 (Fig. 6c), which is a member of the protein tyrosine phosphatase family. The DCs are subsequently identified as CD11c⁺ MHCII⁺ cells (Fig. 6d). The remaining cells, which are mainly MHCII⁻, are CD11b⁺ myeloid cells (Fig. 6e). Monocytes and macrophages are highly plastic and can differentiate into different subsets in response to environmental changes (*see* **Note 21**). By gating on Ly6G⁺ cells, neutrophils can be identified (Fig. 6f). Neutrophils are necessary for synovial inflammation and are attracted to the synovium through chemokine-chemokine receptor interaction [15]. In contrast to resting peripheral blood neutrophils, which are relatively short-lived, primed and activated neutrophils have undergone molecular changes that extend their life span and alter their molecular properties. This allows them to carry out many functions that have been historically attributed to macrophages. Furthermore, activated neutrophils gain functions such as the synthesis of pro-inflammatory mediators (cytokines and chemokines) and the ability to present antigen to T cells. These characteristics equip tissue neutrophils with the capability to actively drive inflammatory processes (reviewed in [16]).

4 Notes

1. The emulsion should look white and have a stiff texture. This can be tested by dripping the emulsion in water: the emulsion should stay as a drop in the water.
2. For boost induction in C57BL/6 mice, the immunization emulsion, as described in Subheading 2.1, **item 5**, can be used. The mouse is injected s.c. with the immunization emulsion on the back.
3. Model is independent of the mouse strain.
4. It is recommended to determine the optimal concentration of the SCW for a proper induction of inflammation as this may differ per batch and supplier of SCW.
5. Decalcification using formic acid is less suitable for TRAP staining. When EDTA is used for decalcification, it is not possible to perform Safranin O staining. Hematoxylin and eosin staining is possible for both decalcification methods.
6. All solutions should be kept on ice.
7. Check the mice around day 18–21 for the onset of CIA (1–10% of the animals can develop CIA before the boost injection).
8. It is possible to induce reactivation of arthritis (flare-up), after the acute phase is resolved (about 21 days after the i.a. injection of mBSA), by locally injecting 2 μg of mBSA in the knee joint. This flare-up reaction is predominantly mediated by memory T cells.
9. It is also possible to induce chronic inflammation in the knee joint by repeating SCW injections on days 8, 15 and 22 after the first i.a. injection. In contrast to the first injection, which leads to a macrophage-mediated inflammation during the first week, repeating SCW i.a. injections will induce a T cell-mediated chronic inflammation.
10. Leaving too much soft tissue will lead to unnecessary extra time for the fixation and impairment of paraffin impregnation.
11. Bones should always be open at least on one side for better impregnation of the various chemicals and paraffin.
12. We aim for coronal sections where patella, femur and tibia can be found in the same section. If the joint is too flexed, the patella is positioned too proximal and will not be seen in the

first sections. If the knee is too straight, the patella is completely in front of the joint space and therefore will be cut before the first tibial/femoral sections are made. After fixation changing the angle is impossible without breaking the ligaments.

13. It is important not to keep the tissues in hot paraffin too long as they might become hard and brittle.
14. The tissue and paraffin attached to the cassette have formed a block, which is ready for sectioning.
15. Tissue blocks can be stored at room temperature for years.
16. If the specimens fragment when placed in the water bath, the water may be too hot.
17. Damaging blood vessels with the scissor must be avoided as this contaminates samples with blood cells, interfering with the analysis.
18. Before using antibodies, it is highly recommended to titrate the antibody for optimal results with flow cytometry. Since the amount of tissue obtained from the synovium itself is too low, antibodies can be titrated on newly harvested splenocytes.
19. It is recommended to use a live/dead marker for gating out the dead cells. Live/dead Aqua viability dye (diluted in PBS) can be used before fixation and incubated 30 min at 4 °C.
20. When synovium of both knees from one mouse is pooled and processed well, typically about 100–150,000 events can be measured by flow cytometry. The amount of events or cells measured depends on the severity of inflammation. The number of measured events in naïve/non-injected knees is therefore lower (50–100,000).
21. Further subdividing of the $CD64^{int}$ and $CD64^{high}$ cells can be done by including antibodies against Ly6C and F480. The $Ly6C^{+}$ $F480^{low}CD64^{int}$ cells are identified as monocytes and $F480^{+}$ $CD64^{+}$ are macrophages [14]. CD115 can be used as an additional marker for the identification of monocytes.

References

1. Klareskog L, Catrina AI, Paget S (2009) Rheumatoid arthritis. Lancet 373:659–672
2. McInnes IB, Schett G (2011) The pathogenesis of rheumatoid arthritis. N Engl J Med 365:2205–2219
3. Isaacs JD (2010) The changing face of rheumatoid arthritis: sustained remission for all? Nat Rev Immunol 10:605–611
4. Cope AP (2008) T cells in rheumatoid arthritis. Arthritis Res Ther 10(Suppl 1):S1
5. Lubberts E (2015) Role of T lymphocytes in the development of rheumatoid arthritis. Implications for treatment. Curr Pharm Des 21:142–146
6. Brennan FM, McInnes IB (2008) Evidence that cytokines play a role in rheumatoid arthritis. J Clin Invest 118:3537–3545
7. Corneth OB, Mus AM, Asmawidjaja PS et al (2014) Absence of interleukin-17 receptor a signaling prevents autoimmune inflammation of the joint and leads to a Th2-like phenotype in collagen-induced arthritis. Arthritis Rheumatol 66(2):340–349. doi:10.1002/art.38229

8. Murphy CA, Langrisch CL, Chen Y et al (2003) Divergent pro- and antiinflammatory roles for IL-23 and IL-12 in joint autoimmune inflammation. J Exp Med 198(12):1951–1957
9. Cornelissen F, Mus AM, Asmawidjaja PS et al (2009) Interleukin-23 is critical for full-blown expression of a non-autoimmune destructive arthritis and regulates interleukin-17A and RORgammat in gammadelta T cells. Arthritis Res Ther 11(6):R194. doi:10.1186/ar2893
10. Oppmann B, Lesley R, Blom B et al (2000) Novel p19 protein engages IL-12p40 to form a cytokine, IL-23, with biological activities similar as well as distinct from IL-12. Immunity 13(5):715–725
11. Parham C, Chirica M, Timans J et al (2002) A receptor for the heterodimeric cytokine IL-23 is composed of IL-12Rbeta1 and a novel cytokine receptor subunit, IL-23R. J Immunol 168(11):5699–5708
12. Vollmer RT (1983) Theory and practice of histological techniques - Bancroft, Jd, Stevens, A. JAMA 250(14):1909–1909
13. Callis G, Sterchi D (1998) Decalcification of bone: literature review and practical study of various decalcifying agents, methods, and their effects on bone histology. J Histotechnol 21(1):49–58
14. Misharin AV et al (2014) Nonclassical Ly6C(−) monocytes drive the development of inflammatory arthritis in mice. Cell Rep 9(2):591–604
15. Coelho FM et al (2008) The chemokine receptors CXCR1/CXCR2 modulate antigen-induced arthritis by regulating adhesion of neutrophils to the synovial microvasculature. Arthritis Rheum 58(8):2329–2337
16. Wright HL et al (2010) Neutrophil function in inflammation and inflammatory diseases. Rheumatology 49(9):1618–1631

Chapter 28

Pain Relief in Nonhuman Primate Models of Arthritis

Michel P.M. Vierboom, Elia Breedveld, Merei Keehnen, Rianne Klomp, and Jaco Bakker

Abstract

Animal models of rheumatoid arthritis are important in the elucidation of etiopathogenic mechanisms of the disease and for the development of promising new therapies. Species specificity of new biological compounds and their mode of action preclude safety and efficacy testing in rodent models of disease. Nonhuman primates (NHP) can fill this niche and provide the only relevant model. Over the last two decades models of collagen-induced arthritis (CIA) were developed in the rhesus monkey and the common marmoset. However, NHP are higher-order animals and complex sentient beings. So especially in models where pain is an intricate part of the disease, analgesia needs to be addressed because of ethical considerations. In our model, a morphine-based pain relief was used that does not interfere with the normal development of disease allowing us to evaluate important mechanistic aspects of the arthritis.

Key words Autoimmunity, Inflammatory arthritis, Nonhuman primates, NSAID, Pain relief, Refinement

1 Introduction

Rheumatoid arthritis (RA) is an immune mediated inflammatory disease that affects 1 % of people in the western countries. RA is characterized by chronic inflammation of synovial joints. A commonly used model for translational research into the (immune-) mechanisms that initiate or perpetuate inflammatory arthritis and the development of new therapeutics is collagen-induced arthritis (CIA). The species of choice are mice and rats [1, 2]. However, species specificity of new biological compounds sometimes precludes the use of rodent models. In some cases NHP provide models to fill this evolutionary gap. However, NHP are higher-order complex sentient beings and they may only be used for experimentation if there are no valid alternative ways to obtain essential information on new therapies or pathogenic mechanisms. Since NHP are complex sentient living beings it is a moral imperative that we relieve pain associated with the arthritis to the best of our ability.

Björn E. Clausen and Jon D. Laman (eds.), *Inflammation: Methods and Protocols*, Methods in Molecular Biology, vol. 1559, DOI 10.1007/978-1-4939-6786-5_28,

Over the past two decades we have developed CIA models in the rhesus monkey (*Macaca mulatta*) [3, 4] and the common marmoset (*Callithrix jacchus*) [5]. The protocol described here focuses on the rhesus monkey CIA model. For the ethical management of the experiment the animals are sedated twice a week and scored for the development of clinical signs with a clinical scoring (CS) system Table 1. In addition, all animals are inspected by the animal caretakers on a daily basis. Before the clinical onset of the disease the animals display behavioral signs of discomfort. This is the moment the veterinarian decides to start with the administration of analgesics.

- Morphine versus the use of paracetamol or NSAID.

The most common classes of compounds for pain relief are NSAID (nonsteroidal anti-inflammatory drugs), paracetamol, and opiates [6, 7]. NSAID are used for the treatment of pain (analgesic), fever (antipyretic) and inflammation. NSAID's target both COX-1 and COX-2 enzymes (also known as prostaglandin G/H or PGG/H synthase), thereby blocking the production of prostaglandins. NSAID are effective in the treatment of pain but have a robust impact on the inflammation. Paracetamol (acetaminophen) is a mild analgesic with minimal anti-inflammatory properties [8], while opiates like morphine and buprenorphine (Buprecare®) have a very strong analgesic action with limited anti-inflammatory properties.

Buprenorphine has been selected as an analgesic to treat the pain resulting from the development of CIA in NHP. Good results were obtained in the CIA model when buprenorphine was administered three times daily via intramuscular (i.m.) injection

Table 1
Clinical scoring table

Clinical score	Characteristics	Monitoring frequency	Maximal duration
0	No disease symptoms	Daily	End of experiment
0.5	Fever (>0.5 °C)	2× per week	12 weeks
1	Apathy, loss of appetite weight-loss	Daily 2× per week	10 weeks
2	Warm and tender joints, but without STS[a]	2× per week	6 weeks
3	Moderate STS but normal flexibility of affected joints	2× per week	4 weeks
4	Severe redness + STS of joints, with joint stiffness	2× per week	2 weeks
5	Humane endpoint: such severe disease that euthanasia is necessary	Daily	18 h

[a] *STS* = soft tissue swelling; requires sedation of the monkey

during periods of suspected pain. The duration of the analgesic effect is dependent on the dose administered [9]. It is 25–50× more potent than morphine [10]. It does not lead to physical dependence since there are minimal signs of withdrawal after discontinuation [11].

The treatment with buprenorphine is aimed at pain relief, restoring normal behavior including locomotion, and a normal eating pattern so that the animal can maintain a normal food supply. Treatment with Buprenorphine does not influence bodyweight [12, 13], which is used as a surrogate disease parameter. The loss of bodyweight is a direct consequence of the TNF-α produced during the inflammation resulting in a loss of appetite (cachectic syndrome). The use of buprenorphine for pain relief has been validated in our rhesus monkey model of CIA (>400 animals) without interfering in the development of the disease. This has allowed us to evaluate new anti-inflammatory therapies with significantly less discomfort to the monkey.

2 Materials

2.1 Animals

CIA-sensitive animals developing inflammatory arthritis. Indian origin rhesus monkeys (*Macaca mulatta*) purpose bred at the BPRC were selected for absence of the MHC class I resistance marker Mamu-B*001 as identified by genotyping ([14]). Historical data show that usage of rhesus monkeys from the BPRC colony that lack this marker give a CIA-incidence of ±95 % [14–16].

2.2 Disease-Inducing Agent

- Complete Freund's Adjuvant (263810, DIFCO;BD). CFA is a suspension of desiccated Mycobacterium butyricum in a mixture of paraffin oil and an emulsifying agent, mannide monooleate. Formulation per 10 mL ampule: mannide monooleate (1.5 mL), paraffin oil (8.5 mL), and Mycobacterium butyricum (5 mg).
- Chicken collagen type II ((Immunization Grade Lyophilized; MD Biosciences).
- 0.1 M acetic acid.

2.3 Pain Relief

- Buprenorphine (Buprecare®) [17]: Increasing doses of buprenorphine. The dose of the solution is 300 μg/mL.

3 Methods

3.1 Induction of CIA

CIA is induced by immunizing rhesus monkeys, sensitive to to the development of CIA, with chicken collagen type II dissolved in 0.1 M acetic acid (10 mg/mL) emulsified in an equal volume of CFA (*see* Subheading 2.2).

Table 2
Example of dose calculation sheet

PID[1]	Time	Weight (kg)	Dose (μg/kg)	Volume (mL)[2]
17	16.00	9.78	20	0.65
17	23.00	9.78	20	0.65
18	07.30	9.78	40	1.30
18	16.00	9.53	40	1.27
18	23.00	9.53	40	1.27
19	07.30	9.53	60	1.91
19	16.00	9.53	60	1.91
19	23.00	9.53	60	1.91
20	07.30	9.53	80	2.54
20	16.00	9.53	80	2.54
20	23.00	9.53	80	2.54
21	07.30	9.53	80	2.54

[1]Post induction day
[2]Formula to calculate the "Volume" = "Weight" × ("Dose"/300)

3.2 Preparation of CIA Inducing Agent

Chicken type II collagen (10 mg/vial,) is dissolved for 4 days at 4 °C in in 1 mL of 0.1 M acetic acid. On the day of induction an equal volume of the collagen solution (10 mg/mL) is emulsified in an equal volume of CFA under gentle stirring at 4 °C.

1 mL of this emulsion is injected into the dorsal skin as ten spots of 100 μL. These spots can develop into granulomatous lesions that may be irritating and painful. After 2–3 weeks the animals will start to develop clinical signs of arthritis (swelling of synovial joints) and signs of systemic inflammation, such as cachectic syndrome.

3.3 Administration of Pain Relief

Buprenorphine is administered three times per day (Table 2; intramuscularly with 26 G needles) because its analgesic effect lasts for ± 6–12 h ([10]; depending on the dose administered).

4 Notes

1. Important for the assessment of behavioral cues is that we know the normal behavior of the individual monkey before we induce the disease (day 0 behavior). For example, if a monkey has already a quiet behavior then tranquility is not an overt cue of pain for that monkey.

2. Protocol for pain assessment.

   When a monkey is found to be in pain we immediately start providing pain relief by intramuscular injection with buprenorphine.

   The animal caretaker inspects the monkeys for behavioral signs indicating pain. During the experiment the monkey is offered a piece of marshmallow or a grape, each morning, to see whether they have normal locomotion and if they put weight on hands and feet. If a monkey is hanging by its feet and hands at the bars of the cage we assume the animal has no pain.

   The most overt changes in behavior are:

   - The monkey shifts on its but through the cage over small distances to relieve weight from its feet/legs.
   - The monkey does not eat its food pellets. This might be a consequence of the inflammation-induced cachectic syndrome or pain in joints of hands and jaws preventing them from grabbing food or chewing the hard pellets.
   - The monkey is less mobile and sits quietly in the cage (less use of limbs), apathy.

3. Three times dosing per day. Treatment in the morning is administered early in the morning (±7.30) after animal behavior has been scored. The second dose is given late in the afternoon (±16.00) and the final dose is given late at night (±23.00). This dosing schedule should provide sufficient pain relief during day and night (for an example see Table 2).

4. Treatment doses increasing from 20 μg to 100 μg/kg. The dose volume administered is based on the last recorded weight (they are weighed twice per week; *see* Table 2 for an example). This is important because animals can lose up to 25% of their weight over a period of 3–4 weeks. When we do not observe a detectable improvement in behavior within 24 h after start of treatment the dose is increased from 20 to 40 μg/kg with an upper limit of 100 μg/kg. If the monkey does not respond to a dose of 100 μg/kg the pain is defined as untreatable and the animal will be sacrificed (humane endpoint; clinical score of 5; *see* Table 1).

5. Animals can be trained to receive i.m. injection of pain relief drugs without being sedated or brought to the front of the cage by squeezing.

6. Buprenorphine is injected into the thigh muscle (quadriceps femoris vastus lateralis).

7. Monkeys that receive pain relief are provided with a rubber mat to soften the impact on painful joints. If the monkey does not eat its pellets, the diet is supplemented with soft, small chopped fruit and vegetables.

8. The use of pain relief in nonhuman primates is mandatory for a model with serious discomfort as has been described in the

current protocol. The question arises why this type of pain relief is not used in rodent models of CIA. An important condition is that the analgesic treatment should not interfere with the inflammatory process. Anti-inflammatory effects have been described for all classes of analgesics. Both paracetamol [8] and buprenorphine [18] are commonly used as analgesics, while the impact on inflammation is limited. However, the analgesic potency of buprenorphine is far higher than that of paracetamol [11, 19]. NSAID, on the other hand, have a prominent anti-inflammatory effect and their analgesic potency is in part a consequence of the suppression of the inflammation. Their use is contraindicated when one wants to evaluate new anti-inflammatory or immunosuppressive compounds.

9. We have seen marked improvements after treatment with buprenorphine. In several cases (when the animal improved clinically) we reduced the dosage of buprenorphine. If treatment with a new compound is effective in mitigating disease resulting in the restoration of locomotion and eating habits and less administration of buprenorphine is required then the amount of buprenorphine the monkey received might be used as readout for the effect of a new treatment.
10. Is there a danger of addiction? Although buprenorphine is 25–50 times more potent than morphine one of its features is that no physical dependence has been observed even at the high dose we use for pain relief. There are no signs of withdrawal even after acute discontinuation of treatment [11]. On the other hand, the period the animals receive buprenorphine is limited and at the end of the experiments the animals are sacrificed for immunological and histopathological analysis.
11. Although side effects as respiratory suppression, nausea or constipation have been described for morphine and its derivatives, we have not observed any of these adverse effects in our large cohort of animals (>400 rhesus monkeys) engaged in CIA experiments, not even in cases where the highest dose was administered. Nonetheless, special attention should be given for these effects.

Acknowledgments

The animal caretakers of the BPRC are acknowledged for their commitment to the best care of the animals.

References

1. Brand DD, Kang AH, Rosloniec EF (2003) Immunopathogenesis of collagen arthritis. Springer Semin Immunopathol 25(1):3–18. doi:10.1007/s00281-003-0127-1
2. Holmdahl R, Bockermann R, Backlund J, Yamada H (2002) The molecular pathogenesis of collagen-induced arthritis in mice--a model for rheumatoid arthritis. Ageing Res Rev 1(1):135–147
3. Vierboom MPM, Breedveld E, 't Hart BA (2008) Preclinical evaluation of anti-rheumatic drugs in a non-human primate model of arthritic disease. Drug Discov Today Dis Model 5(2):89–95. doi:10.1016/j.ddmod.2008.06.003
4. Vierboom MP, Zavodny PJ, Chou CC, Tagat JR, Pugliese-Sivo C, Strizki J, Steensma RW, McCombie SW, Celebi-Paul L, Remarque E, Jonker M, Narula SK, 't Hart BA (2005) Inhibition of the development of collagen-induced arthritis in rhesus monkeys by a small molecular weight antagonist of CCR5. Arthritis Rheum 52(2):627–636. doi:10.1002/art.20850
5. Vierboom MP, Breedveld E, Kondova I, 't Hart BA (2010) Collagen-induced arthritis in common marmosets: a new nonhuman primate model for chronic arthritis. Arthritis Res Ther 12(5):R200. doi:10.1186/ar3172
6. Bandolier (2003) Acute pain. Bandolier extra February. Avalaible at http://www.ebandolier.com
7. Dulos J, Mihara K, Smeets R, Van Lierop M-J, De Groot D, Van Boxtel S, Dokter W (2008) Use of painkilling in the collagen-induced arthritis (CIA) model
8. Botting RM (2000) Mechanism of action of acetaminophen: is there a cyclooxygenase 3? Clin Infect Dis 31(Suppl 5):S202–S210. doi:10.1086/317520
9. Nunamaker EA, Halliday LC, Moody DE, Fang WB, Lindeblad M, Fortman JD (2013) Pharmacokinetics of 2 formulations of buprenorphine in macaques (Macaca mulatta and Macaca fascicularis). J Am Assoc Lab Anim Sci 52(1):48–56
10. Houde RW (1979) Analgesic effectiveness of the narcotic agonist-antagonists. Br J Clin Pharmacol 7(Suppl 3):297S–308S
11. Mello NK, Bree MP, Mendelson JH (1981) Buprenorphine self-administration by rhesus monkey. Pharmacol Biochem Behav 15(2):215–225
12. Mello NK, Bree MP, Lukas SE, Mendelson JH (1985) Buprenorphine effects on food-maintained responding in Macaque monkeys. Pharmacol Biochem Behav 23(6):1037–1044
13. Mysels DJ, Sullivan MA (2010) The relationship between opioid and sugar intake: review of evidence and clinical applications. J Opioid Manag 6(6):445–452
14. Doxiadis GG, de Groot N, Otting N, de Vos-Rouweler AJ, Bolijn MJ, Heijmans CM, de Groot NG, van der Wiel MK, Remarque EJ, Vangenot C, Nunes JM, Sanchez-Mazas A, Bontrop RE (2013) Haplotype diversity generated by ancient recombination-like events in the MHC of Indian rhesus macaques. Immunogenetics 65(8):569–584. doi:10.1007/s00251-013-0707-8
15. Bakker NP, van Erck MG, Otting N, Lardy NM, Noort RC, 't Hart BA, Jonker M, Bontrop RE (1992) Resistance to collagen-induced arthritis in a nonhuman primate species maps to the major histocompatibility complex class I region. J Exp Med 175(4):933–937
16. Otting N, Heijmans CM, Noort RC, de Groot NG, Doxiadis GG, van Rood JJ, Watkins DI, Bontrop RE (2005) Unparalleled complexity of the MHC class I region in rhesus macaques. Proc Natl Acad Sci U S A 102(5):1626–1631. doi:10.1073/pnas.0409084102
17. Animal-Care-Limited (2011) Buprecare product information sheet
18. Walker JS, Chandler AK, Wilson JL, Binder W, Day RO (1996) Effect of mu-opioids morphine and buprenorphine on the development of adjuvant arthritis in rats. Inflamm Res 45(11):557–563
19. Kidd BL, Langford RM, Wodehouse T (2007) Arthritis and pain. Current approaches in the treatment of arthritic pain. Arthritis Res Ther 9(3):214. doi:10.1186/ar2147

Chapter 29

Isolation and Characterization of Aortic Dendritic Cells and Lymphocytes in Atherosclerosis

Tae Jin Yun, Jun Seong Lee, Dahee Shim, Jae-Hoon Choi*, and Cheolho Cheong*

Abstract

Dendritic cells (DCs) are central to initiate antigen-specific immunity and tolerance. The in vivo development and distribution of DCs are now better understood even in nonlymphoid tissues [1]. Atherosclerosis is a chronic inflammatory disease of blood vessels and DCs are highly enriched in the intimal area of the aorta, which is predisposed to develop atherosclerosis. Previously, we were the first to show antigen presenting DCs and their subsets in the aorta [2, 3]. Here, we discuss several useful methods to characterize not only DCs but also other immune cells in steady state and atherosclerotic aorta. These comprise multiparameter flow cytometry strategies including intracellular staining and cell sorting, *en face* immunohistochemistry of DCs and regulatory T cells (Tregs), and Oil Red O staining of atherosclerotic lesions in the aorta.

Key words Atherosclerosis, Dendritic cells, CD11c, Aorta, Macrophage, Regulatory T cells (Tregs)

1 Introduction

In addition to their role in lipid uptake and systemic lipid metabolism [4, 5], DCs have been shown to be important in modulating immune responses in atherosclerosis in mouse models. For example, these studies have demonstrated an atherosclerosis-promoting role of T cell costimulatory and antigen-presenting molecules expressed on the surface of DCs (e.g., CD80, CD86, MHCI/II) [6, 7], an atheroprotective role of the DC maturation-signaling pathway through DC-specific elimination of Myd88 [8], and regulation of regulatory T cell (Treg) homeostasis by subsets of DCs, such as CCL17^{+} DCs and Flt3-dependent DCs [3, 9]. These observations suggest a critical role for DCs in the regulation of T cells and possibly atheroprotective Tregs [10].

The original version of this chapter was revised. The erratum to this chapter is available at: DOI 10.1007/978-1-4939-6786-5_31

* Contributed Equally.

Björn E. Clausen and Jon D. Laman (eds.), *Inflammation: Methods and Protocols*, Methods in Molecular Biology, vol. 1559, DOI 10.1007/978-1-4939-6786-5_29, © Springer Science+Business Media LLC 2017

However, it is very demanding to obtain enough aortic DCs to functionally address their characteristics. In this regard, many studies in the field of atherosclerosis have used preferentially bone marrow-derived or lymphoid DCs to uncover the mechanism behind observed atherosclerotic phenotypes. Of note, it is prudent to analyze the interplay of immune cells in healthy and diseased aorta to understand the initiation and progression of atherosclerosis. Here we summarize useful methods to analyze DCs and immune cells in healthy and diseased aorta.

The advent of genetically modified mouse models such as low-density lipoprotein receptor (*Ldlr*) or Apolipoprotein E (*ApoE*)-deficient mice has facilitated atherosclerosis studies in mice that closely recapitulate human disease [11, 12]. While cell type analysis in atherosclerotic lesions by immunohistochemistry has been informative, recent advances in flow cytometric analysis of aortic cell suspensions allowed monitoring various immune cell types simultaneously in the aorta [13]. However, *a*utofluorescent macrophages affect flow cytometric analysis of aortic cell suspensions especially in multiparameter flow cytometry. Therefore, it is critical to remove macrophages from the beginning to faithfully analyze other immune cells such as DCs and Tregs. To this end, the use of macrophage specific markers such as CD64 and MerTK in combination with CD11b or F4/80 is very helpful [14, 15]. In our protocol, FACS staining is optimized for 96 well formats to save antibody-related reagents and minimize cell loss. Of note, several cell surface markers are easily degraded via collagenase treatment. To overcome this issue, intracellular staining of CD4 is employed in our protocol [16]. To measure regulatory T cells in the aorta, CD4 and Foxp3 are simultaneously stained. Notably, the Foxp3 staining method (eBioscience) has been modified and optimized for aortic Treg measurement.

Traditionally, staining aortic immune cells *en face* has provided valuable information on their anatomical location and distribution. We previously reported that DCs are enriched in the intimal space of aortas while macrophages are enriched in adventitia [2, 3]. *En face* staining allows one to image both the intimal and adventitia sides of the aorta. Here, we describe a method to stain whole mount *en face* of aortic DCs and macrophages. To this aim, the basic protocol (TSA Protocol, Life Technologies) has been modified and optimized for the aorta. In atherosclerotic lesions, Oil Red O staining is a classical method to measure lesions and assess the severity of atherosclerosis in mouse models [17]. For a sound assessment of atherosclerotic lesions, it is critical to embed the aorta in the correct orientation for frozen section preparation. We illustrate this procedure in detail and show representative stainings of Oil Red O and CD11c$^+$ cells in the aorta. Finally, we also provide one example of functional analysis to differentiate DCs from macrophages. The classical feature of DCs is their lower phagocytic activity compared with macrophages [3]. In this protocol, aortic cell suspensions are incubated with fluorescent beads to assess phagocytic activity and then purified by fluorescence-activated cell sorting to observe the morphological characteristics of DCs and macrophages.

2 Materials

2.1 Mouse Aorta Isolation

2.1.1 Mouse Handling

1. C57BL/6 mouse.
2. 70% ethanol.
3. Surgical scissors (Fig. 1a).
4. Surgical forceps.
5. 10 ml syringe.
6. 24-gauge needle.
7. 1× PBS.
8. Surgical tray.

2.1.2 Aorta Isolation

1. Dissecting microscope.
2. Dissecting dish: heat-resistant glass dishes, black wax (Nasco, SA04451MH), hotplate stirrer (Fig. 1b, c, *see* **Note 1**).
3. Microdissection scissors.
4. Microdissection forceps.
5. Pin.

2.2 Flow Cytometry Analysis

2.2.1 Preparation of Single Cell Suspension

1. 1 ml Collagenase cocktail: 600 μl 1× HBSS, 100 μl Collagenase type I (Sigma-Aldrich, C0130, 10× stock: 6750 U/ml), 100 μl Collagenase type XI (Sigma-Aldrich, C7657, 10× stock: 187.5 U/ml), 100 μl Hyaluronidase type I-s (Sigma-Aldrich, H1115000, 10× stock: 900 U/ml), 100 μl DNase I (Sigma-Aldrich, 11284932001, 10× stock: 900 U/ml) (*see* **Note 2**).

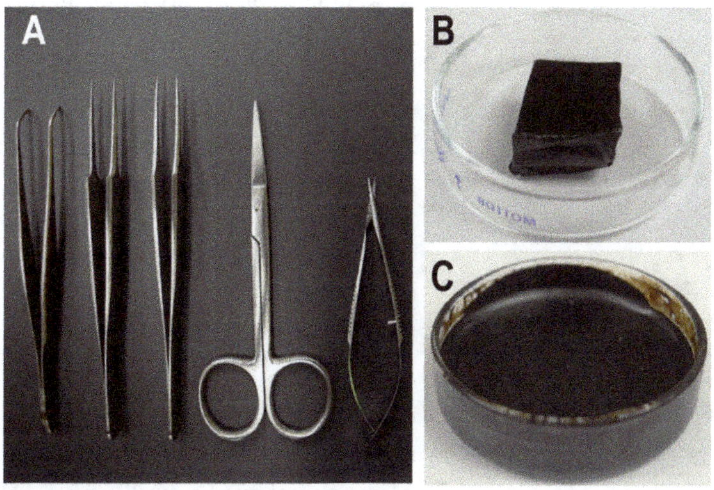

Fig. 1 Materials for mouse aorta isolation. (**a**) From *left* to *right*, angled surgical forceps with serrated tips, sharp-nose surgical forceps, microdissection forceps, surgical scissors, and microdissection scissors. (**b, c**) Dissecting dish preparation. Heat-resistant glass dish before (**b**) and after (**c**) black wax was applied

2. Rotator.
3. Collagenase digestion tube with cap (Falcon, 352063) (*see* **Note 3**).
4. Parafilm M.
5. 70-μm strainers.
6. 15 ml tube.
7. 500 ml wash media: 25 ml heat-inactivated FBS, 475 ml 1× RPMI-1640, 5 ml 100× antibiotic–antimycotic.
8. Swinging rotor.

2.2.2 Surface Staining

1. Fluorochrome-conjugated monoclonal antibodies (all from BioLegend): PE-CD45 (clone 30-F11), PerCP/Cy5.5-CD64 (clone X54-5/7.1), BV711-CD11b (clone M1/70), PeCy7-CD11c (clone N418), and A700-MHCII (clone M5/114.15.2).
2. FcBlock: culture supernatant from 2.4G2 hybridoma (ATCC, HB-197).
3. 500 ml FACS buffer: 10 ml heat-inactivated FBS, 490 ml 1× PBS with calcium/magnesium, 5 ml 100× antibiotic–antimycotic.
4. 96-well v-bottom plates.
5. Microtiter tubes.
6. 5 ml tubes.
7. Flow cytometry analyzer.

2.2.3 Intracellular Foxp3 Staining

1. Fluorochrome-conjugated monoclonal antibodies (all from BioLegend, unless noted otherwise): APC-CD45 (BD Biosciences, clone 30-F11), PerCP/Cy5.5-CD64 (clone X54-5/7.1), BV711-CD11b (clone M1/70), APC-e780-CD3 (eBioscience, clone 17A2), BV785-CD4 (clone RM4-5), and PE-Foxp3 (eBioscience, clone FJK-16s).
2. Foxp3 / Transcription Factor Staining Buffer Set (eBioscience, 00-5523-00).
3. Materials as described in Subheading 2.2.2, from **item 2** to 7.

2.3 Visualization in Aorta

2.3.1 Dendritic Cell Staining

1. 6-well plate.
2. 0.25% Triton X-100: 125 μl Triton X-100, 50 ml 1× PBS (*see* **Note 4**).
3. 1.5 ml tube.
4. 0.3% H_2O_2: 100 μl 30% H_2O_2, 10 ml 1× PBS (*see* **Note 5**).
5. Monoclonal antibody: Biotin-CD11c mAb (BioLegend, clone N418).
6. TSA kit, HRP-Streptavidin with Alexa Flour 555 (Invitrogen, T-30955).

7. Shaker.
8. DAPI.
9. Glass slides for cryosection.
10. 4% formaldehyde: 4 ml 10% formaldehyde, 6 ml 1× PBS.
11. 1× PBS.
12. Mounting solution.
13. Coverslip.
14. Transparent nail polish.
15. Scotch tape.

2.3.2 Oil Red O Staining (en face)

1. *Ldlr*$^{-/-}$ mouse or *ApoE*$^{-/-}$ mouse.
2. CHOW diet (TestDiet, 5015) or Western diet (TestDiet, AIN-76A).
3. Dissecting dish.
4. Distilled water.
5. Glass slides.
6. Pin.
7. 0.5% Oil Red O solution I: 0.5 g Oil Red O, 100 ml 100% propylene glycol (*see* **Note 6**).
8. 85% propylene glycol: 85 ml 100% propylene glycol, 15 ml distilled water.
9. Materials from Subheading 2.3.1, **items 10–15**.

2.3.3 Oil Red O Staining (Cryosection)

1. Razor blade.
2. Embedding mold.
3. OCT compound.
4. Cryostats.
5. Glass slides for cryosection.
6. Harris' hematoxylin (National Diagnostics, HS-400).
7. 0.5% Oil Red O solution II: 1 g Oil Red O, 100 ml 70% ethanol, 100 ml acetone (*see* **Note** 7).
8. 70% ethanol.
9. Materials from the Subheading 2.3.1, from **items 10** to **15**.
10. Mice and materials from Subheading 2.3.2, **items 1–4**.

2.3.4 Immunostaining (Cryosection)

1. TSA kit, HRP-Streptavidin with Alexa Flour 594 (Invitrogen, T-20935).
2. 0.3% H_2O_2: 100 µl 30% H_2O_2, 10 ml 1× PBS (*see* **Note 5**).
3. Monoclonal antibody: Biotin-CD11c mAb (BD Pharmigen, clone HL3).

4. DAPI.
5. Materials from the Subheading 2.3.1, from **items 10** to **15**.
6. Mouse and materials from the Subheading 2.3.2, from **items1** to **4**.
7. Materials from the Subheading 2.3.3, from **items 2** to **5**.

2.4 Bead Phagocytosis Assay

2.4.1 Bead Phagocytosis and Sorting

1. Fluoresbrite 1 μm bead (Polysciences, 15702).
2. Collagenase digestion tube with cap (Falcon, 352063).
3. 500 ml culture media: 25 ml sterile heat-inactivated FBS, 475 ml sterile 1× RPMI-1640, 5 ml sterile 100× antibiotic–antimycotic, 5 ml sterile 100× GlutaMAX, 5 ml sterile 100X MEM nonessential amino acids. Add sterile 0.5 ml 1000× 2-mercaptoethanol right before using culture media.
4. Fluorochrome-conjugated monoclonal antibodies (all from BioLegend, unless noted otherwise): APC-CD45 (BD Biosciences, clone 30-F11), PerCP/Cy5.5-CD64 (clone X54-5/7.1), BV711-CD11b (clone M1/70), PeCy7-CD11c (clone N418), and A700-MHCII (clone M5/114.15.2).
5. 15 ml tube.
6. Cell sorter.
7. 500 ml FACS buffer: 10 ml heat-inactivated FBS, 490 ml 1× PBS with calcium/magnesium, 5 ml 100× antibiotic–antimycotic.

2.4.2 Cytospin and Fixation

1. Glass slides for cryosection.
2. Shanon filter card.
3. Cytospin cytocentrifuge.
4. 4% formaldehyde: 4 ml 10% formaldehyde, 6 ml 1× PBS.
5. 1× PBS.
6. DAPI.
7. Mounting solution.
8. Coverslip.
9. Transparent nail polish.

3 Methods

3.1 Mouse Aorta Isolation

3.1.1 Mouse Handling

1. Prepare a 10 ml syringe filled with 10 ml of ice cold 1× PBS (per mouse). Attach a 24-gauge needle to the syringe.
2. Euthanize mouse with CO_2. As soon as the mouse stops breathing, bring it out of the CO_2 chamber.
3. Spray 70% ethanol onto the mouse and place it on a surgical tray under a light source.

4. Place mouse abdomen up and stretched with 24-gauge needles onto its four paws.
5. Locate and lift abdominal skin, insert scissors and make incisions from thoracic cavity to peritoneum. Avoid cutting blood vessels, which can cause bleeding.
6. Open the abdominal wall below the ribcage.
7. Lift the sternum with forceps and cut the diaphragm. The heart should be visible.
8. Locate right and left iliac blood vessels between peritoneum and hind legs and make incisions for blood drainage.
9. Insert the 10 ml syringe needle into the apex of the right ventricle and flush the blood out of the mouse for 2 min.
10. Cut away the entire ribcage to expose the heart and lungs.
11. Remove lungs, esophagus, and intestine with scissors.

3.1.2 Aorta Isolation

1. You should be able to see connective tissues along the spine. The aorta is located along the spine and surrounded by connective tissues.
2. Lift the heart and detach connective tissues all the way down to the bladder.
3. Flush the heart again through the right and left ventricles using a 10 ml syringe containing 10 ml of cold 1× PBS to clean out residual blood.
4. Place the aorta on the dissecting dish (*see* Fig. 1 for the preparation of dissection dish) with 1× cold PBS under a dissecting microscope.
5. Using microdissection scissors cut the heart horizontally and pin the heart with a needle (Fig. 2a).
6. Remove the fat and connective tissues surrounding aorta carefully, leaving intact the sinus, aortic arch and three arteries (Brachiocephalic, Left common carotid and Left subclavian artery) on aortic arch (Fig. 2b, c).
7. Cut along the lesser curvature side of aorta from aortic sinus to the end of descending aorta (Fig. 2d, e).
8. Cut distal ascending side of aorta where three arteries are located, from aortic sinus to the end of left subclavian artery (Fig. 2f, g).

3.2 FACS Analysis

3.2.1 Preparation of Single Cell Suspension

1. Prepare 1 ml collagenase cocktail.
2. Add 100 μl of collagenase cocktail into a collagenase digestion tube per one isolated aorta (Fig. 2h).
3. Cut the aorta into small pieces with surgical scissors to facilitate collagenase digestion and add additional 900 μl of collagenase cocktail to make 1 ml in total (Fig. 2h).

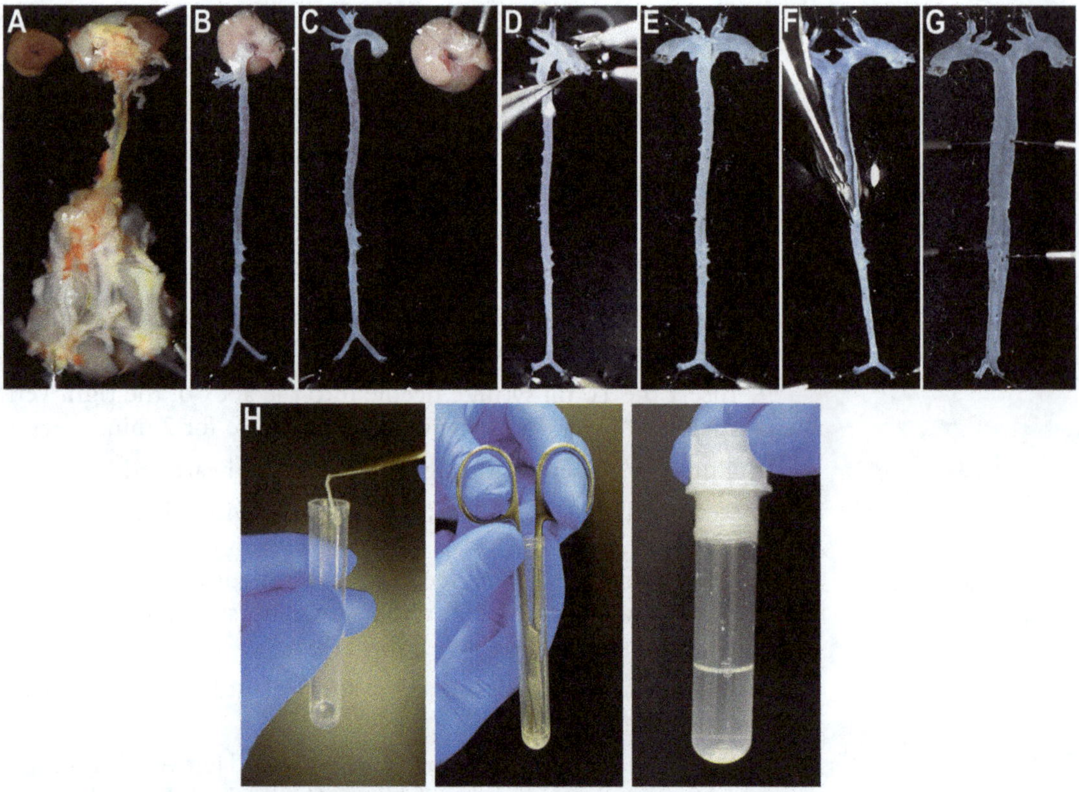

Fig. 2 Mouse aorta isolation under dissecting microscope. (**a**) Isolated tissues containing aorta and heart on dissecting dish with cold 1× PBS. Heart was cut in half horizontally and pinned on the dissection dish to facilitate locating aortic arch and three arteries. (**b, c**) Aorta was trimmed but aortic sinus is still inside the heart (**b**) and aortic sinus was separated intact from the heart (**c**). (**d–g**) Trimmed aorta was opened in Y shape. Distal ascending side of aorta where three arteries are located was cut (**d** and **e**) and lesser curvature side of aorta from aortic sinus to the end of descending aorta was cut (**f** and **g**). (**h**) Isolated aorta in a collagenase digestion tube was cut into small pieces with surgical scissors and filled with 1 ml of collagenase cocktail. The tube was closed with cap and tightly sealed with Parafilm

4. Close the tube with a cap and seal the cap tightly with Parafilm. Then, incubate at 37 °C for 40 min with rotation (Fig. 2h).
5. Remove the tube from incubator after 40 min and centrifuge the tubes briefly at 800 ×*g*.
6. Pipette the digested aorta up and down about 100 times and pass through 70-μm strainers into a 15 ml tube.
7. Wash the collagenase digestion tube with 1 ml of wash media to minimize cell loss and transfer the 1 ml into the 15 ml tube.
8. Centrifuge the 15 ml tube at 800 ×*g* for 5 min at 4 °C and aspirate supernatant (Use swinging rotor to maximize cell pellet).
9. Repeat **steps** 7 and **8**.

3.2.2 Surface Staining

1. Resuspend and incubate cells in 150 μl FcBlock at 4 °C for at least 20 min.
2. Prepare antibody cocktail in FACS buffer (anti-CD45, anti-CD64, anti-CD11b, anti-CD11c, and anti-MHCII mAb).
3. Transfer cells into one well of a 96-well v-bottom plate.
4. Centrifuge the plate at 800×*g*, 4 °C for 2 min and flick the plate in a quick single motion with sufficient force to discard supernatant (Do not aspirate).
5. Wash the cells in 100 μl of FACS buffer and repeat **step 4**.
6. Resuspend the cells in 30 μl of antibody cocktail at 4 °C in the dark for 30 min.
7. Add 100 μl of FACS buffer, resuspend the stained cells and repeat **step 4**.
8. Repeat **step 7**, twice.
9. Suspend the stained cells in 100 μl of FACS buffer and pass through 70-μm strainers into a microliter tube.
10. Place the microliter tube into a 5 ml tube used for flow cytometry analysis and read the cells on a flow cytometer (Fig. 3a).

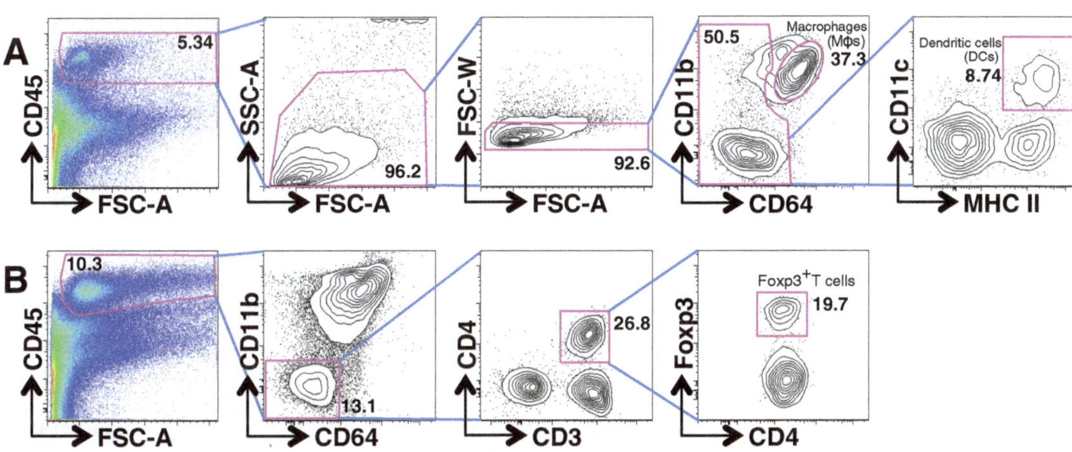

Fig. 3 Aortic lymphocytes gating strategy. (**a**) Aortic cells from C57BL/6 mouse were stained for CD45, CD64, CD11b, CD11c, and MHCII. Entire cells from one aorta were acquired. First CD45$^+$ lymphocytes were gated and plotted onto forward scatter (FSC) and side scatter (SSC). Cell doublets were excluded using FCS-A and FSC-W, and CD64$^+$ macrophage and CD64$^-$ non-macrophage cells were separated. Finally, CD64$^-$ non-macrophage cells were plotted onto CD11c and MHCII and CD11c$^+$ MHCII$^+$ aortic dendritic cells can be identified. (**b**) Aortic cells from *Ldlr*$^{-/-}$ mouse fed with western diet for 8 weeks were stained for CD45, CD64, CD11b, CD3, CD4, and Foxp3. Entire cells from one aorta were acquired. First, CD45$^+$ lymphocytes were gated and plotted onto forward scatter (FSC, not shown) and side scatter (SSC, not shown). Cell duplets were excluded using FCS-A and FSC-W (not shown). Second, CD64$^-$CD11b$^-$ cells were gated. Third, CD3$^+$CD4$^+$ cells were isolated and, finally, CD4$^+$Foxp3$^+$ cells can be identified. Data was analyzed using FlowJo software (TriStar)

3.2.3 Intracellular Foxp3 Staining

1. Resuspend and incubate cells in FcBlock at 4 °C for at least 20 min.
2. Prepare antibody cocktail in FACS buffer (anti-CD45, anti-CD64, anti-CD11b, and anti-CD3 mAb).
3. Transfer cells into one well of a 96-well v-bottom plate.
4. Centrifuge the plate at 800×*g*, 4 °C for 2 min and flick the plate in a quick single motion with sufficient force to discard supernatant (Do not aspirate).
5. Wash the cells in 100 μl of FACS buffer and repeat **step 4**.
6. Resuspend the cells in 30 μl of antibody cocktail for surface markers at 4 °C in the dark for 30 min.
7. Add 100 μl of FACS buffer, resuspend the stained cells, and repeat **step 4**.
8. Repeat **step 7**, twice.
9. Prepare fresh 1× Fixation/Permeabilization buffer (50 μl per sample/well, *see* **Note 8**).
10. Resuspend and fix the surface stained cells in 50 μl of 1× Fixation/Permeabilization buffer at 4 °C at least 7 h or overnight (Cover the plate if fixed overnight).
11. Centrifuge the plate at 800×*g* for 3 min and flick the plate in a quick single motion with sufficient force to discard buffer (Do not aspirate, *see* **Note 9**).
12. Prepare fresh 1× Permeabilization buffer (Total 340 μl per sample/well).
13. Prepare antibody cocktail in 1× Permeabilization buffer (anti-CD4 and anti-Foxp3 mAb).
14. Resuspend and wash the fixed cells in 100 μl of 1× Permeabilization buffer.
15. Centrifuge the plate at 800×*g* for 3 min and flick the plate in a quick single motion with sufficient force to discard buffer (Do not aspirate).
16. Repeat **steps 14** and **15**.
17. Resuspend and incubate the fixed cells in 40 μl of antibody cocktail for intracellular staining at 4 °C for 7 h.
18. Resuspend the stained cells in 100 μl of 1× Permeabilization buffer and repeat **step 15**.
19. Resuspend the stained cells in 100 μl of FACS buffer and repeat **step 15**.
20. Repeat **step 19**.
21. Resuspend the surface and intracellular stained cells in 100 μl of FACS buffer and pass through 70-μm strainers into a microliter tube.

22. Place the microliter tube into a 5 ml tube used for flow cytometry and analyze the cells on a flow cytometer (Fig. 3b).

3.3 Visualization in Aorta

3.3.1 Dendritic Cell Staining (en face)

1. Fix the isolated aorta (prepared from Subheading 3.1.2) in 4% formaldehyde in a 6-well plate at 4 °C, 40 min.
2. Wash the fixed aorta in 1× PBS in a 6-well plate on shaker for 10 min, three times.
3. Permeabilize the aorta in 0.25% Triton X-100 in 1.5 ml tube for 20 min with rotation at room temperature.
4. Repeat **step 2**.
5. Inactivate endogenous peroxidase by incubating the permeabilized aorta in 0.3% H_2O_2 in a 6-well plate at room temperature for 1 h.
6. Repeat **step 2**.
7. Block the aorta with 2% TSA blocking solution for 1 h with rotation at room temperature (*see* **Note 10**).
8. Repeat **step 2**.
9. Incubate the aorta with biotin-CD11c mAb (0.75 μg in 300 μl of 1% TSA blocking solution) in a 48-well plate at room temperature for 2 h on shaker.
10. Repeat **step 2**.
11. Incubate the aorta with streptavidin-HRP Ab (0.325 μg in 300 μl of 1% TSA blocking solution) at room temperature for 1 h on shaker.
12. Repeat **step 2**.
13. Label the aorta in 300 μl of TSA reaction mix (1 μl Alexa fluorochrome in 300 μl reaction buffer) in 48 well plates on shaker for 20 min.
14. Wash the fixed aorta in 1× PBS in a 6-well plate on shaker for 10 min.
15. Incubate the stained aorta with DAPI (1 μl in 5 ml 1× PBS) for 1 min.
16. Repeat **step 2** (*see* **Note 11**).
17. Place the aorta in a Y shape onto a coverslip under a dissecting microscope and close the coverslip with mounting solution and another coverslip. (CAUTION: DO NOT fold aorta, this will result in autofluorescence, poor images, and difficulty in distinguishing intima and adventitia).
18. Dry the slide in the dark and seal the coverslip with nail polish. Tape the sample onto a glass slide.
19. Examine intima and adventitia by fluorescence microscope (Fig. 4a–c).

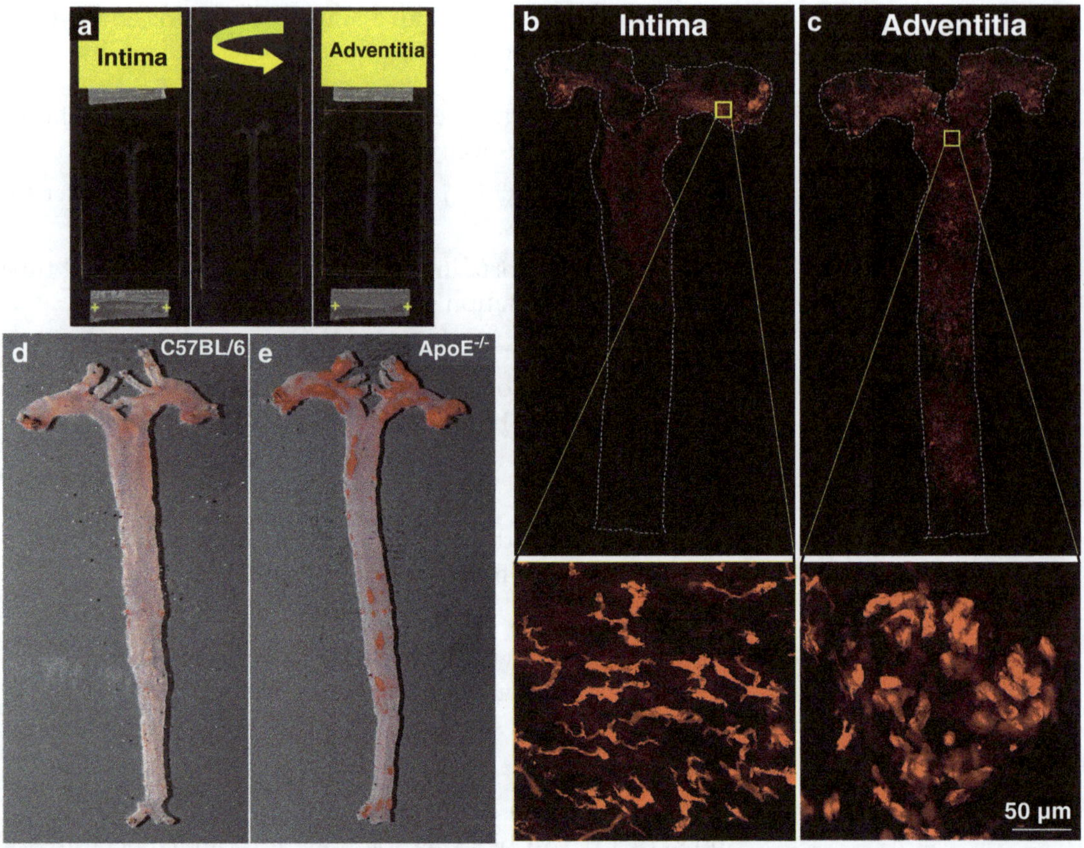

Fig. 4 Visualization of aortic CD11c+ cells and atherosclerotic lesions. (**a**) Fixed and stained aorta was mounted on coverslips. Intima can be examined by placing it on a glass slide with tape, and adventitia can be examined by flipping only the cotverslips. (**b** and **c**) Aorta from C57BL/6 mouse was isolated, fixed and stained for CD11c and labeled with TSA Alexa 555 kit. *White dotted line* indicates boundary of aorta and entire aorta image was taken by tile scanning. Alexa 555 positive cells can be observed in lesser curvature in intima (**b**) and throughout in adventitia (**c**). Inset image shows dendritic cell morphology in intima and non-dendritic cell morphology with no dendrites in adventitia. Images were examined using LSM 710 confocal microscope (Zeiss). (**d** and **e**) Aortas from C57BL/6 mouse and *ApoE*$^{-/-}$ mouse, both fed with CHOW diet and 300 days old, were fixed and stained for Oil Red O. Aorta from *ApoE*$^{-/-}$ mouse (E) shows atherosclerotic lesions which are not observed in aorta of C57BL/6 (**d**). Most of atherosclerotic lesions in *ApoE*$^{-/-}$ mouse are located in aortic sinus and aortic arch. Both images show the intima

3.3.2 Oil Red O Staining (en face)

1. Prepare *Ldlr*$^{-/-}$ mouse or *ApoE*$^{-/-}$ mouse fed with western diet for at least 6 weeks, or at least 200 days old *ApoE*$^{-/-}$ mouse fed with CHOW diet.
2. Place the aorta (prepared from Subheading 3.1.2) on the dissecting dish with ice cold 1× PBS under a dissecting microscope.
3. Pin the aorta in a Y shape so that the atherosclerosis lesions of intima are exposed.

4. Replace PBS with 4% formaldehyde and incubate at room temperature for 1 h.
5. Replace 4% formaldehyde with 1× PBS and wash for 1 h.
6. Replace PBS with 100% propylene glycol and incubate for 5 min.
7. Replace 100% propylene glycol with 0.5% Oil Red O solution I and incubate the aorta for 9 h at room temperature.
8. Replace 0.5% Oil Red O solution with 85% propylene glycol and wash the aorta for 10 min.
9. Replace 85% propylene glycol with 1× PBS and wash the aorta in 1× PBS at room temperature for 1 h.
10. Place the aorta in a Y shape onto a coverslip under a dissecting microscope and close the coverslip with mounting solution and another coverslip.
11. Dry the slide and seal the coverslip with nail polish. Tape the sample onto a glass slide.
12. Examine intima by microscope (Fig. 4d and e).

3.3.3 Oil Red O Staining (Cryosection)

1. Prepare *Ldlr*$^{-/-}$ mouse or *ApoE*$^{-/-}$ mouse fed with Western diet for at least 6 weeks, or at least 200-day-old *ApoE*$^{-/-}$ mouse fed with CHOW diet.
2. Follow the steps in Subheading 3.1.1 until **step 5** in Subheading 3.1.2.
3. Using a sharp razor blade cut along Line-a in the middle between the bottom of the heart and a plane of both bottom of right and left atria (Line-b). Line-a is also parallel with Line-c (Fig. 5a, *see* **Note 12**).
4. Pin the heart with a needle and remove the fat and connective tissues surrounding aorta carefully, leaving intact the aortic arch and three arteries (Brachiocephalic, Left common carotid and Left subclavian artery) on aortic arch. Please do not separate the heart and aorta.
5. Fix the heart and aorta in 4% formaldehyde at room temperature for 1 h (Fig. 5a).
6. Wash the fixed heart and aorta in 1× PBS at room temperature for 1 h (Fig. 5a).
7. Cut along Line-d to remove aorta but only leaving the aortic sinus (Fig. 5a).
8. Place the heart and aortic sinus in an embedding mold and fill with OCT compound at room temperature. Wait for 10 min (Fig. 5a).
9. If the sample floats to the surface, squeeze the tissue with forceps slightly to remove air bubbles.

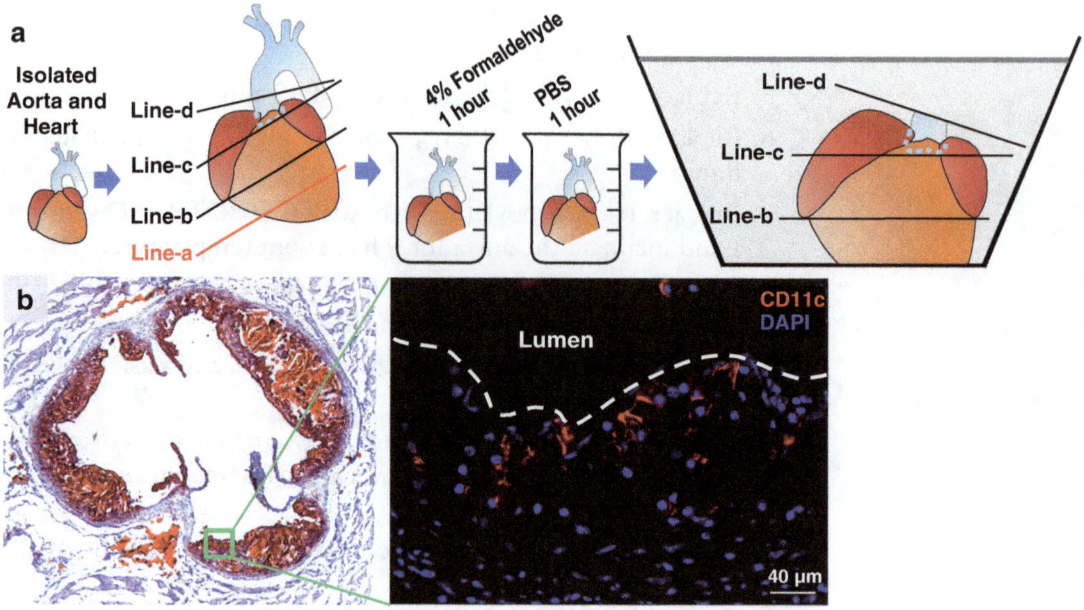

Fig. 5 Oil Red O staining and CD11c⁺ cell staining with frozen sections from atherosclerotic lesions in aortic sinus. (**a**) Isolated heart was cut along Line-a, which is located halfway between the bottom of the heart and a plane of both lower *right* and *left* atria (Line-b). Line-a must be parallel with Line-b, which results in also being parallel with Line-c. The trimmed heart was fixed and washed in 4 % formaldehyde and PBS, respectively. The fixed heart was cut along Line-d, which is parallel to both apex of *right* and *left* atria, and placed frozen in an embedding mold filled with OCT compound. (**b**) The cross section of aortic sinus with three sinus valves was stained with Oil Red O and Harris' hematoxylin. Atherosclerotic lesions are shown in *red* in sinus valves (*left*). Image in inset shows cells stained for CD11c by TSA staining kit (*right*) using Eclipse 50i microscope (Nikon)

10. Bring the embedding cassette to −80 °C for at least 4 h.
11. Start cryosection in 5 μm thickness.
12. Cut the frozen block until the heart is exposed and place it on a glass slide.
13. Examine the slide under the microscope if aortic sinus and valves are visible.
14. Prepare several slides with intact aortic sinus with all three leaflets of the valve.
15. Wash the slides with distilled water for 3 min.
16. Stain in Harris' hematoxylin for 30 s.
17. Aspirate hematoxylin and repeat **step 15**.
18. Apply 70 % ethanol for 2 s.
19. Aspirate 70 % ethanol and add 0.5 % Oil Red O solution II for 2 min.
20. Aspirate Oil Red O solution and wash with 70 % ethanol for 30 s.
21. Aspirate and wash with 70 % ethanol for 30 s again.

22. Aspirate 70% ethanol and stain in hematoxylin for 30 s.
23. Wash the slides with distilled water for 3 min.
24. Close the slides with mounting solution and coverslips.
25. Dry the slide and seal the coverslip with nail polish.
26. Examine by light microscopy (Fig. 5b Left).

3.3.4 Immunostaining (Cryosection)

1. Prepare aortic sinus slides according to the description in Subheading 3.3.3 up to **step 14**.
2. Dry the slides at 60 °C for 1 h.
3. Hydrate sections with PBS at room temperature for 5 min.
4. Block endogenous peroxidase activity with 0.3% H_2O_2 for 1 h.
5. Wash the slides twice with PBS for 5 min.
6. Block sections with 1% TSA blocking solution for 1 h.
7. Repeat **step 5**.
8. Stain sections with biotin-CD11c mAb (0.5 μg in 100 μl of 1% TSA blocking solution) at room temperature for 1 h.
9. Repeat **step 5**.
10. Incubate sections with streptavidin-HRP Ab (0.125 μg in 100 μl of 1% TSA blocking solution) at room temperature for 1 h.
11. Repeat **step 5**.
12. Label sections in 100 μl of TSA reaction mix (0.25 μl Alexa fluorochrome in 100 μl reaction buffer) for 20 min at room temperature. Avoid light.
13. Repeat **step 5.**
14. Incubate sections with DAPI (1 μl in 5 ml 1× PBS) for 1 min.
15. Repeat **step 5**.
16. Close the slides with mounting solution and coverslips.
17. Dry the slides in the dark and seal the coverslip with nail polish.
18. Examine by fluorescence microscopy (Fig. 5b Right).

3.4 Bead Phagocytosis Assay

3.4.1 Bead Phagocytosis and Sorting

1. Perform Subheadings 3.1 and 3.2.1 under sterile conditions in a cell culture hood (Centrifuge samples at 450×*g* in Subheading 3.2.1, instead of 800×*g*).
2. All procedures in this Subheading (3.4.1) should be carried out in sterile conditions in a culture hood.
3. Incubate the cells with beads (1 μl of beads/ml) in 1 ml of sterile culture media in a collagenase digestion tube at 37 °C in an incubator for 1 h (*see* **Note 13**).
4. Transfer the cells into a sterile 15 ml tube.

5. Add 1 ml of sterile culture media into the collagenase digestion tube to collect leftover cells, and transfer into the 15 ml tube.
6. Wash the cells with an additional 2 ml of sterile culture media by centrifuge at 450 × *g*, 4 °C for 5 min.
7. Aspirate supernatant and repeat **step 6**.
8. Resuspend and incubate cells in 300 μl of sterile FcBlock at 4 °C for at least 20 min.
9. Prepare antibody cocktail in culture media (anti-CD45, anti-CD64, anti-CD11b, anti-CD11c, and anti-MHCII mAb).
10. Repeat **step 6**.
11. Aspirate supernatant and stain the cells with 300 μl antibody cocktail at 4 °C for 30 min.
12. Repeat **step 6**.
13. Aspirate supernatant and repeat **step 6**.
14. Resuspend the stained cells in 500 μl culture media and pass through 70-μm strainers into an appropriate tube used for cell sorting.
15. Sort the aortic cells into two groups; $CD64^+CD11b^+$ macrophages and $CD11c^+MHCII^+$ dendritic cells.
16. Wash the sorted cells with 5 ml of sterile FACS buffer at 4 °C at 450 × *g* for 15 min.
17. Aspirate supernatant and repeat **step 16**.
18. Aspirate supernatant and resuspend cells in 100 μl of FACS buffer in the dark at 4 °C (*see* **Note 14**).

3.4.2 Cytospin and Fixation

1. Assemble a pre-coated slide and a filter card into one of the slots of a cytospin centrifuge.
2. Transfer 100 μl of FACS sorted sample into the assembled slot, and spin at 32 × *g* for 5 min.
3. Carefully separate the slide from the filter card not to damage the sample on the slide.
4. Dry the slide for 10 min in the dark at room temperature.
5. Prepare 4% formaldehyde and apply it carefully onto the sample on the slide to fix the cells in the dark at room temperature for 20 min.
6. Wash the slide with PBS for 5 min in the dark at room temperature.
7. Prepare diluted DAPI solution (1 μl in 5 ml of 1× PBS).
8. Aspirate 1× PBS from the slide and gently apply 100 μl diluted DAPI solution for 1 min.
9. Aspirate and repeat **step 6**, twice.

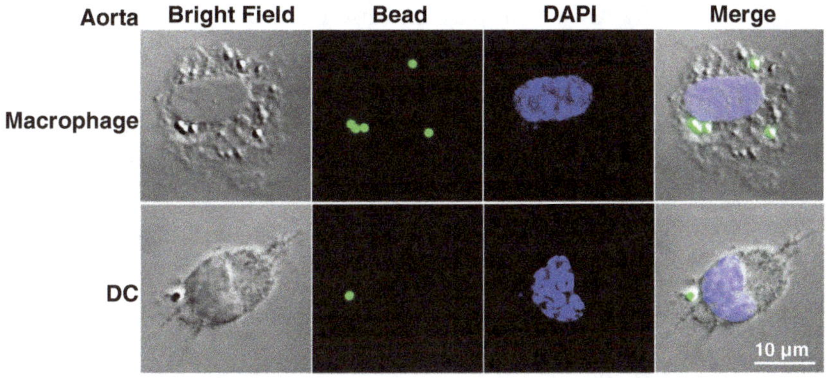

Fig. 6 Visualization of Bead phagocytosis in sorted and cytospin centrifuged aortic cells. Total aortic cells from a C57BL/6 mouse were incubated with Fluoresbrite 1-μm beads for phagocytosis, stained with antibodies (CD45, CD64, CD11b, CD11c and MHCII) for cell sorting and cytospin centrifugation (32 × *g*, 5 min). Aortic macrophages were gated from $CD45^{+}CD64^{+}CD11b^{+}$ cells and aortic dendritic cells (DC) were gated from $CD45^{+}$ $CD64^{-}CD11c^{+}MHCII^{+}$ cells. Cytospin slides were fixed and stained with DAPI. The images were examined using a LSM 710 confocal microscope (Zeiss)

10. Close the slide with mounting solution and coverslip.
11. Dry the slide in the dark and seal the coverslip with nail polish and examine by fluorescence microscopy (Fig. 6).

4 Notes

1. Put glass dishes on a hotplate stirrer. Cut black wax into small chunks and place into the glass dishes. Increase temperature of hotplate stirrer until the black wax starts melting. Once the black wax melts and spreads evenly, leave the glass dishes at room temperature to solidify. Be careful since the plates are very hot. Prepare dissecting dishes in fume hood as black wax produces an unpleasant odor when melted (*see* Fig. 1).
2. All 10X stock enzymes are sterilely reconstituted in 1× HBSS and aliquots are stored at −20 °C. Carefully check the original units of each enzyme from the company website.
3. All plastic tubes should be made of polypropylene to prevent the scarce number of aortic lymphocytes from adhering to the plasticware.
4. Always prepare and use fresh 0.25 % Triton X-100. Prepare the solution at least 1 h earlier since it takes time to dissolve Triton X-100 in PBS. Triton X-100 is viscous. Slowly release pipette plunger to allow the pipette tip to fill up with the correct volume. Discharge Triton X-100 and the pipette tip in PBS to recover full amount of Triton X-100.

5. Always prepare and use fresh 0.3 % H_2O_2.
6. Gently heat Oil Red O mixed propylene glycol in boiled water. Avoid overheating above 110 °C, which causes high background staining of Oil Red O. Filter the Oil Red O solution with 25 μm filter paper and store in the dark at room temperature.
7. Filter the Oil Red O solution with 25 μm filter paper right before use.
8. Fixation and permeabilization buffers should be diluted according to the manufacturer's instructions.
9. Fixed cells become slippery and pellets may seem less condensed even after centrifugation. Please make sure not to flick the 96-well plate more than once after centrifugation. If insufficient force was applied, please re-centrifuge the plate and flick again to minimize cell loss. If cell loss is still a concern, centrifuge the plate for 4–5 min at 800 × *g*. Aspiration of supernatant on a 96-well plate has a high risk of touching cell pellets, and is not recommended.
10. Buffers of the TSA kit should be prepared according to the manufacturer's instructions.
11. If the aorta still has high background fluorescent staining in TSA protocol, wash in PBS for longer until background decreases. Thus, it is critical to examine background fluorescence under a fluorescent microscope or confocal microscope before mounting.
12. Line-a and Line-b should be parallel, so that the three aortic valves can be visualized on the same cross section as Line-c.
13. During incubation, leave the cap loosely attached to the tube to allow gas exchange.
14. 1 % BSA containing PBS can replace FACS Buffer.

Acknowledgment

This work was supported by grants from National Research Foundation of Korea (GRN-2013S1A2A2035348) (JHC and CC) and Canadian Institutes of Health Research (CIHR, MOP-125933 and HIG-133050) (CC). CC holds a Chercheur-Boursier Junior of Fonds de recherche du Québec-Santé (FRQS)—Société québécoise d'hypertension artérielle (SQHA) and CIHR New Investigator Salary Award.

References

1. Steinman RM (2012) Decisions about dendritic cells: past, present, and future. Annu Rev Immunol 30:1–22
2. Choi JH, Do Y, Cheong C, Koh H, Boscardin SB, Oh YS, Bozzacco L, Trumpfheller C, Park CG, Steinman RM (2009) Identification of antigen-presenting dendritic cells in mouse aorta and cardiac valves. J Exp Med 206:497–505
3. Choi JH, Cheong C, Dandamudi DB, Park CG, Rodriguez A, Mehandru S, Velinzon K, Jung IH, Yoo JY, Oh GT, Steinman RM (2011) Flt3 signaling-dependent dendritic cells protect against atherosclerosis. Immunity 35:819–831
4. Paulson KE, Zhu SN, Chen M, Nurmohamed S, Jongstra-Bilen J, Cybulsky MI (2010) Resident intimal dendritic cells accumulate lipid and contribute to the initiation of atherosclerosis. Circ Res 106:383–390
5. Gautier EL, Huby T, Saint-Charles F, Ouzilleau B, Pirault J, Deswaerte V, Ginhoux F, Miller ER, Witztum JL, Chapman MJ, Lesnik P (2009) Conventional dendritic cells at the crossroads between immunity and cholesterol homeostasis in atherosclerosis. Circulation 119:2367–2375
6. Buono C, Pang H, Uchida Y, Libby P, Sharpe AH, Lichtman AH (2004) B7-1/B7-2 costimulation regulates plaque antigen-specific T-cell responses and atherogenesis in low-density lipoprotein receptor-deficient mice. Circulation 109:2009–2015
7. Sun J, Hartvigsen K, Chou MY, Zhang Y, Sukhova GK, Zhang J, Lopez-Ilasaca M, Diehl CJ, Yakov N, Harats D, George J, Witztum JL, Libby P, Ploegh H, Shi GP (2010) Deficiency of antigen-presenting cell invariant chain reduces atherosclerosis in mice. Circulation 122:808–820
8. Subramanian M, Thorp E, Hansson GK, Tabas I (2013) Treg-mediated suppression of atherosclerosis requires MYD88 signaling in DCs. J Clin Invest 123:179–188
9. Weber C, Meiler S, Doring Y, Koch M, Drechsler M, Megens RT, Rowinska Z, Bidzhekov K, Fecher C, Ribechini E, van Zandvoort MA, Binder CJ, Jelinek I, Hristov M, Boon L, Jung S, Korn T, Lutz MB, Forster I, Zenke M, Hieronymus T, Junt T, Zernecke A (2011) CCL17-expressing dendritic cells drive atherosclerosis by restraining regulatory T cell homeostasis in mice. J Clin Invest 121:2898–2910
10. Ait-Oufella H, Salomon BL, Potteaux S, Robertson AK, Gourdy P, Zoll J, Merval R, Esposito B, Cohen JL, Fisson S, Flavell RA, Hansson GK, Klatzmann D, Tedgui A, Mallat Z (2006) Natural regulatory T cells control the development of atherosclerosis in mice. Nat Med 12:178–180
11. Ishibashi S, Brown MS, Goldstein JL, Gerard RD, Hammer RE, Herz J (1993) Hypercholesterolemia in low density lipoprotein receptor knockout mice and its reversal by adenovirus-mediated gene delivery. J Clin Invest 92:883–893
12. Zhang SH, Reddick RL, Piedrahita JA, Maeda N (1992) Spontaneous hypercholesterolemia and arterial lesions in mice lacking apolipoprotein E. Science 258:468–471
13. Butcher MJ, Herre M, Ley K, Galkina E (2011) Flow cytometry analysis of immune cells within murine aortas. J Vis Exp pii:2848
14. Gautier EL, Shay T, Miller J, Greter M, Jakubzick C, Ivanov S, Helft J, Chow A, Elpek KG, Gordonov S, Mazloom AR, Ma'ayan A, Chua WJ, Hansen TH, Turley SJ, Merad M, Randolph GJ (2012) Gene-expression profiles and transcriptional regulatory pathways that underlie the identity and diversity of mouse tissue macrophages. Nat Immunol 13:1118–1128
15. Jakubzick C, Gautier EL, Gibbings SL, Sojka DK, Schlitzer A, Johnson TE, Ivanov S, Duan Q, Bala S, Condon T, van Rooijen N, Grainger JR, Belkaid Y, Ma'ayan A, Riches DW, Yokoyama WM, Ginhoux F, Henson PM, Randolph GJ (2013) Minimal differentiation of classical monocytes as they survey steady-state tissues and transport antigen to lymph nodes. Immunity 39:599–610
16. Cheong C, Choi JH (2012) Dendritic cells and regulatory T cells in atherosclerosis. Mol Cells 34:341–347
17. Paigen B, Morrow A, Holmes PA, Mitchell D, Williams RA (1987) Quantitative assessment of atherosclerotic lesions in mice. Atherosclerosis 68:231–240

Chapter 30

Assessment of Vascular Dysfunction and Inflammation Induced by Angiotensin II in Mice

Jeremy Lagrange, Sabine Kossmann, and Philip Wenzel

Abstract

Vascular inflammation in cardiovascular diseases is recognized to be linked with immune cell activation. Recruitment of immune cells into the vessel wall is an early step in angiotensin II-induced vascular dysfunction and arterial hypertension. Exploring the role of monocytes and macrophages in angiotensin II-induced hypertension and vascular inflammation in mouse models highlights the importance of these pathophysiological processes. Here we describe our routinely used protocols concerning angiotensin II-induced hypertension, assessment of blood pressure, vascular function, and immune cell infiltration.

Key words Inflammation, Vascular dysfunction, Endothelial dysfunction

1 Introduction

Chronic or acute vascular inflammation is well recognized to be part of the pathophysiology of cardiovascular diseases, most importantly hypertension and atherosclerosis [1, 2]. Vascular inflammation, endothelial dysfunction, and oxidative stress are also attributed to activated immune cells. One early step in vascular dysfunction and arterial hypertension is the recruitment of immune cells into the vessel wall [3]. T cells, dendritic cells and monocytes/macrophages are known to be activated in hypertension and diminishing the inflammatory response is well known to be beneficial in hypertension and other cardiovascular diseases [4, 5]. Myelomonocytic cells specifically express the major isoform of lysozyme, lysozyme M (LysM) [6]. $LysM^+$ cells have been shown to be involved in the pathogenesis of atherosclerosis [7–9]. Drechsler et al. showed in $ApoE^{-/-}$ mice under high-fat diet that neutrophils infiltrate arteries mainly during the early stage of atherosclerosis development. Rotzius et al. also found granulocytes in atherosclerotic lesions while neutrophils were located at sites of high monocyte density. Recently, our work highlighted the role of immune cells and inflammation in hypertension [5, 10–12]. We showed that

Björn E. Clausen and Jon D. Laman (eds.), *Inflammation: Methods and Protocols*, Methods in Molecular Biology, vol. 1559, DOI 10.1007/978-1-4939-6786-5_30, © Springer Science+Business Media LLC 2017

ablation of LysM+ monocytes from the circulation and macrophages from the vasculature attenuates angiotensin II (ATII)-induced arterial hypertension, vascular dysfunction, and oxidative stress. Interestingly, depletion of these cells resulted in strongly attenuated vascular fibrosis as well as medial hypertrophy, suggesting a direct effect of LysM+ cells on ATII-induced vascular remodeling. ATII signaling is essential for monocyte migration and mobilization involving the ATII receptor type 1 [13, 14].

The activation of the immune system is increasingly explored in animal models of hypertension (angiotensin II-induced hypertension, spontaneously hypertensive rats, salt dependent hypertension and others). In this chapter we share our routinely used protocols in the triggering of hypertension, assessment of blood pressure and vascular reactivity, and quantification of immune cells present in the vessel wall. Induction of hypertension and vascular inflammation in mice is possible via implantation of osmotic minipumps releasing angiotensin II at a defined dose and rate of delivery. Monitoring of blood pressure is performed by telemetry via carotid catheters or by tail cuff measurements. After 1 week of treatment vascular reactivity is explored in individual aortic rings in an organ bath by isometric tension measurement, while flow cytometric analysis of aortic lysates is able to discriminate the amount and type of immune cells that have migrated into the vascular wall.

2 Materials

2.1 Mouse Anesthesia and Surgery

1. Midazolam (Ratiopharm GmbH, Ulm, Germany).
2. Medetomidine (Pfizer Deutschland GmbH, Berlin, Germany).
3. Fentanyl (Janssen-Cilag GmbH, Neuss, Germany).
4. 1 ml syringe.
5. 26 G needle.
6. Alzane (Zoetis, Florham Park, NJ, USA).
7. Flumazenil (Hikma pharma, Gräfelfing, Germany).
8. Buprenorphine (RB Pharmaceuticals, Germany).
9. Braunol (B Braun, Melsungen, Germany).
10. Octeniderm (Schülke, Norderstedt, Germany).
11. Cotton swabs.
12. Bepanthen eye and nose ointment (Bayer, Leverkusen, Germany).
13. Deconex (Borer, Zuchwil, Switzerland).
14. Standard straight scissors.
15. Thin spring scissors.
16. Straight hemostat.

17. Curved hemostat.
18. Straight 0.3 × 0.25 mm forceps.
19. Curved 0.3 × 0.25 mm forceps.
20. Shaving razor.
21. 7-0 prolene suture (Ethicon, Inc. Somerville, USA).

2.2 Angiotensin II Pump

1. Mini-osmotic pumps (model 1007D, ALZET, Cupertino, CA).
2. Angiotensin II human (Sigma-Aldrich, St. Louis MO, USA).

2.3 Blood Pressure Recordings

1. Mice carotid catheters, TA-PA11C10 (Data Sciences International, St. Paul, MN, USA).
2. Ponemah 6.00 data acquisition and analysis software or Dataquest A.R.T. software (Data Sciences International, St. Paul, MN, USA).
3. Leica stereo microscope M50 (Leica Microsystem, Wetzlar, Germany).
4. 26 G needle with a 90° bend point.

2.4 Organ Bath

1. MSZ5000-T-IL-TL stereomicroscope (A.KRÜSS Optronic, Hamburg, Germany).
2. Krebs-Henseleit (KH) buffer (freshly prepared), for 1 l dissolve in 0.8 l of distillated water 5.782 g NaCl, 0.35 g KCl, 0.366 g $CaCl_2$, 0.296 g $MgSO_4$, 0.14 g K_2HPO_4, 2.2 g $C_6H_{12}O_6$, 2.1 g $NaHCO_3$, 5.201 g HEPES. Adjust pH to 7.35, complete the volume to 1 l, and keep at 4 °C on ice.
3. Organ bath (OB) buffer (freshly prepared), for 5 l dissolve in 4.8 l of distillated water, 28.91 g NaCl, 1.75 g KCl, 1.835 g $CaCl_2$, 1.48 g $MgSO_4$, 0.7 g K_2HPO_4, 11.0 g $C_6H_{12}O_6$, 10.5 g $NaHCO_3$, indomethacin 15 ml (15 ml water + 17.875 mg indomethacin + 5 drops sodium hydroxide 1 N (1 $mol{\cdot}l^{-1}$)). Adjust pH to 7.35 and complete the volume to 5 l.
4. Organ baths and Transducers of Radnoti (ADInstruments, Oxford, UK).
5. Octal Bridge Amplifier and 8/30 Power-Lab (ADInstruments, Oxford, UK).
6. Acetylcholinchlorid (ACh) 99% (Sigma-Aldrich, St. Louis, MO).
7. Indomethacin (Sigma-Aldrich, St. Louis, MO).
8. Glycerol trinitrate (GTN) (Nitrolingual) (Pohl-Boskamp Hohenlockstedt, Germany).
9. Prostaglandin $F_2\alpha$ (Ann Arbor, Michigan, USA).

2.5 Flow Cytometric Analysis of Aortic Lysates

1. MSZ5000-T-IL-TL stereo microscope (A.KRÜSS Optronic, Hamburg, Germany).
2. PBS Gibco with 2% FCS Gold.
3. HBSS +/+ or PBS +/+.
4. Liberase (1 mg·ml^{-1}) (Roche, Mannheim, Germany) or collagenase II (1 mg·ml^{-1}) (Gibco, Thermo Fisher scientific, Dreieich, Germany) and DNase I (50 μg·ml^{-1}) (Roche, Mannheim, Germany).
5. Razor: double edge blade, 1 mm thick.
6. Monoclonal antibodies (eBioscience, if not stated otherwise): example of staining.

   CD45-APC-eFluor® 780 (clone 30-F11), CD11b-PE (clone M1/70, BD), Ly6G-FITC (BD), Ly6C-PerCP-Cy5.5 (clone 1A8), F4/80-APC (clone BM8), TCR beta-PE-Cyanine5 (clone H57-597), Fixable Viability Dye eFluor® 506.
7. BD FACS CANTO II flow cytometer (Becton Dickinson, Franklin Lakes, NJ) and FACSDiva software (Becton Dickinson, Franklin Lakes, NJ).

3 Methods

3.1 Mouse Anesthesia and Surgery

1. All surgical procedures are performed under anesthesia. Anesthesia master mix (200 μl/30 g mouse; i.p. injection) contains following substances: midazolam (5 mg·kg^{-1}), medetomidine (0.5 mg·kg^{-1} body weight), and fentanyl (0.05 mg·kg^{-1} body weight). The mix to antagonize anesthesia ("antisedan mix", 200 μl/mouse in 1 ml syringe with 26 G needle) is s.c. injected and consists of Alzane (0.05 mg·kg^{-1}) and Flumazenil (0.01 mg·kg^{-1}). An opioid (buprenorphine, 100 μl/mouse, 0.075 mg·kg^{-1}) is injected subcutaneously after telemetry catheter surgery for analgesia, one injection before awakening and 2 other injections later (6 h after and 24 h after surgery).
2. All surgery procedures are performed on an operation field with a 39 °C warming platform using disinfectant: Braunol and octeniderm. Fur is removed with razors or hair removal cream and cotton swabs. Animal eyes are protected with eye ointment. All tools used are sterilized in a disinfection bath. Tools used are: standard straight scissors, thin spring scissors, straight and curved hemostat, straight and curved 0.3 × 0.25 mm forceps, shaving razor, 7-0 prolene suture.

3.2 Angiotensin II Pump Preparation and Implantation

1. Osmotic mini-pump needs to be filled up with ATII to deliver 1 mg·kg^{-1}·d^{-1} for 7 days. Amount of ATIIi is adjusted to the weight of each mouse and to the pump rate (see lot specific value in pump package). Needed amount of ATII is weighed

and diluted in sterile saline (*see* **Note 1**). Pumps of the control animals are filled only with sterile saline. Pumps are filled using a needle supplied by the manufacturer, once the pump is full of liquid the flow moderator is plugged to the top. Then the prepared pumps are kept in sterile saline at 37 °C for at least 4–6 h.

2. Once the animal is under complete anesthesia, which can be tested by the rear foot reflexes, the lower back is shaved and the skin is disinfected with octeniderm. A 1 cm incision is made perpendicularly to the spine. The pocket for the pump is created by inserting a strait hemostat into the incision and slowly opening and closing it. The pocket must be 1 cm longer than the pump and a little bit bigger to allow free movements (but not too big to avoid complete turnaround of the pump). Insert the pump into the pocket (side with the flow moderator first) and push it 1 cm deeper than the incision (it is possible to do this using the fingers over the skin). Then the wound is closed using sutures or clips (three should be enough) and the lesion disinfected with Braunol. Anesthesia is antagonized by s.c. injection of 200 μl antisedan mix to awake the mouse.

3.3 Blood Pressure Recording

1. Prior to surgery, the good health and condition of the animals is verified using the official stress score sheet (Table 1). Therefore, before surgery, animals should be monitored once per day for 2–3 days concerning general condition (appearance, posture, spontaneous behavior) as well as for body weight, food and water consumption (*see* **Note 2**).

Prior to implantation, the telemetric transmitters are first put in sterile saline. The transmitter serial number must be noted and associated with the respective mouse (this is crucial for the measurement).

Once the mouse is under complete anesthesia, the animal is placed in dorsal recumbence on a warmed (39 °C) surgical plate and the neck hairs are removed using the hair removal cream. Use the cotton swab to spread the cream and rub it 2 min until hairs start to fall. Then, wait for two more minutes and remove the cream and hairs with the spatula and disinfect with octeniderm. The eyes are protected with ointment during the entire procedure. Make sure working space and instruments are disinfected before use. Surgery is performed under a stereomicroscope with a complete disinfected bench (surgery can also be performed under laminar flow hood for even better aseptic conditions).

2. A 1–1.5 cm long incision in the skin is made longitudinally in the neck, next to the trachea. First the pocket for the telemetric transmitter is made by inserting a hemostat into the incision and slowly opening and closing it. The pocket must be placed next to the heart and not too deep to avoid movements that would stretch the catheter and impair the measurement. When

Table 1
Stress score sheet for animal health

Observation	Parameters	Score
Behavior	Attentive, active, social contacts, normal moves, curious	0
	Decreased reaction and moves, limited or excessive activity	1
	Crouch and partially segregated from the group, reduced moves and visible pain when walking	2
	Apathetic, no reaction or aggressiveness in handling, strong restricted movement, isolated	3
Appearance	Smooth and glossy fur, grooming, eyes shining	0
	Dull fur, grooming (limited or absent), eyes cloudy	1
	Partly shaggy, slightly ruffled fur, nasal discharge, eyes sunken, bonded body orifices	2
	Fully shaggy, dull coat, abnormal posture, curved back, eyes closed, cyanosis	3
Weight	In adult: constant. In growing animals: equal growing compared to the same genotype control group	0
	<10 % weight loss since the beginning of the experiment or compared with the growth curve	1
	>10 < 20 % weight loss since the beginning of the experiment or compared with the growth curve	2
	<20 % weight loss since the beginning of the experiment or compared with the growth curve	3
Breathing	Normal, uniform and regular	0
	Slightly more visible breathing	1
	Significantly enhanced breathing	2
	Cyanotic mucous membrane, gasping for air	3
Other criteria for immediate termination	Rectal prolapse	3
	Automutilation	3
Tumor	No tumor visible or palpable	0
	<1 cm diameter	1
	>1 cm < 1.5 cm diameter	2
	<1.5 cm diameter or ulcerating	3

Rating (additive)

0–1 = normal. 2–3 = low stress. 4–7 = medium stress, veterinarian or palliative measures should be taken (e.g., analgesics, glucose in drinking water, frequent inspection 4–7 $\geq$ 24 h). If these measures are ineffective, the animal is euthanized. 8 = immediately euthanize. If one of the parameters alone reaches the score of 3, the animal is immediately euthanized opening and closing, the hemostat must be kept close to the skin and not too deep into the tissues to not break brachial artery or other vessels. Once the pocket is made, 37 °C sterile saline is injected into it.

Then the left carotid artery is isolated and prepared. The area covering the left trachea is dissected using cotton swabs and 0.7–0.9 mm of the carotid artery is uncovered with thin curved forceps. It is important for the healing to avoid tissue damage. Once the carotid is free from surrounding tissues, the vagus nerve (a thin white line adjacent to the carotid) must also be removed from the vessel. The thin forceps can be closed and slowly opened to gently mobilize the nerve. Once the artery is completely clean, one forceps is positioned under the vessel and three 7-0 sutures of 10 cm each are placed under the vessel. The suture close to the head is closed with two knots, the two other knots are prepared but not closed. The suture proximal to the aortic arch is clamped and pulled to interrupt the blood flow. The catheter of the telemetric transmitter is held with a forceps with one hand while with the other hand a small incision is made into the vessel (*see* **Note 3**), then the catheter is inserted into the vessel and the middle suture knot is closed but not too strongly. The clamp suture is then released and the catheter is inserted deeper into the artery (the catheter can be pulled until a mark present on it). Once the catheter is in good position the three sutures (even the one closer to the head) are closed three times over the catheter to ensure complete immobilization (Fig. 1). The transmitter is then inserted into the pocket, the glands are put back over the trachea and the wound is closed with separate sutures.

One week after the telemetric transmitter implantation, once the mouse has recovered well (mouse health and wound healing must be checked every day), measurement of blood pressure can

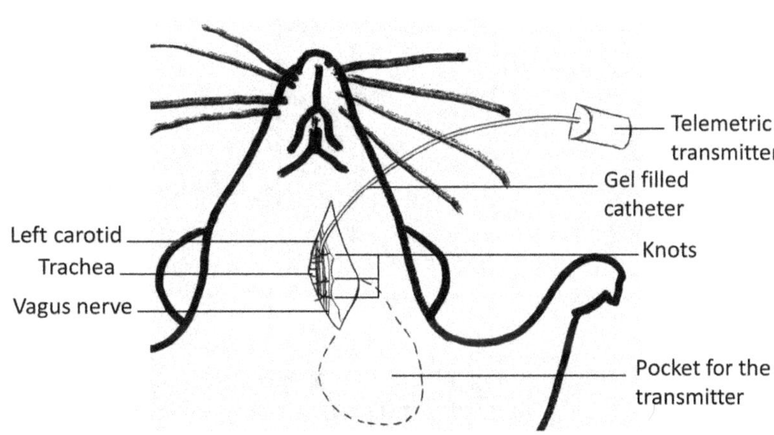

Fig 1 Implantation of a telemetric transmitter for blood pressure monitoring

be started. The mouse is placed over a receiver platform and the telemetric transmitter is enabled with a magnet (it is possible to check whether the transmitter is on or off with a small radio) (*see* **Note 4**). Then, preparation of the software is made by associating the transmitter with the receiver. If the DQ ART software is used the serial number of the transmitter that was noted during the surgery must be entered. If the newest Ponemah 6.00 software is used this association should be automatically done. The calibration parameters must be added into the software as well; they can be found on the front of the transmitter box. Calibration parameters are also automatically integrated into the software with Ponemah 6.00. Concerning the measurement parameters we recommend to set the system to a 10 s measurement every 15 min (depending on the purpose of the study it is possible to make continuous measurements). The control measurement is enabled for 1 week and then the ATII osmotic mini-pump is implanted for 1 week (*see* **Note 5**). Concerning the data analysis, the mean of each daily measurement is made in order to avoid daily variations (Fig. 2).

3.4 Organ Bath

1. Thoracic Aortas are explanted from mice sacrificed by isoflurane or CO_2 inhalation. Under a stereo microscope in a petri dish filled with KH buffer and on ice, fatty tissue surrounding the vessel is removed as well as blood inside the vessel. Fatty tissue removal is possible with small straight scissors and a thin straight forceps. It is very important to avoid stretching of the vessel during the cleaning process. Clean thoracic aortas are cut into ring segments of approximately 3-mm length and kept in KH buffer on ice.

In our studies we use the complete Radnoti Organ bath system combining the ADInstruments data acquisition system, Bridge

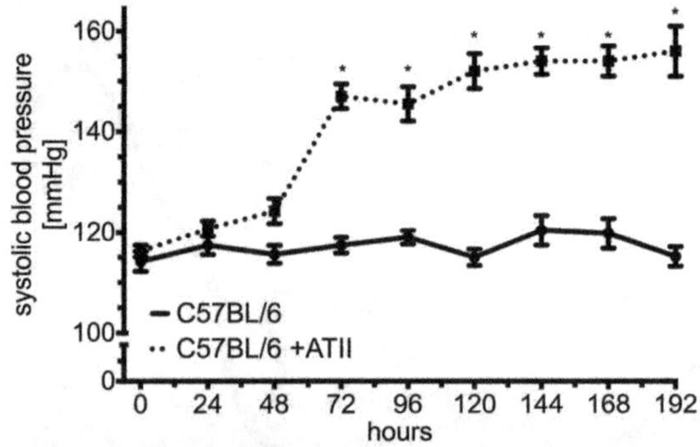

Fig 2 Summary of 384 h of telemetrically recorded systolic blood pressure (mmHg, millimeter mercury) in C57BL/6 mice measured at baseline for 192 h and then infused with ATII. $n = 4–5$ animals/group and results are expressed as mean ± SEM, $p < 0.05$ *, vs. C57BL/6 with 2-way ANOVA

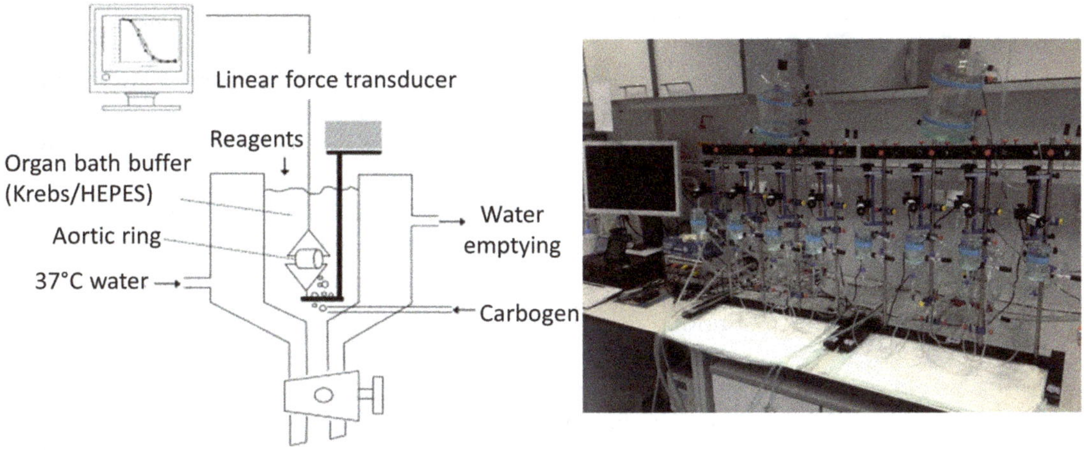

Fig 3 Organ bath setup for aortic ring reactivity measurement

Amplifier, Isometric Transducers and LabChart software with a Radnoti Tissue-Organ Bath Apparatus.

Once the organ bath chambers are completely filled (25 ml) with temperature-controlled (37 °C) buffer and the transducers are calibrated, the aortic rings are carefully mounted on triangle adapters (avoid stretching of the rings) and put in the organ chamber for isometric tension recording (Fig. 3). The solution is continuously gassed with 5% CO_2 in O_2 resulting in a physiological pH at 7.4.

2. The optimum resting tension for tone development in response to 80 mM KCl is 1.00 g, which is achieved by gradual stretching over 1 h (starting at 0.1 g, increase 0.2 g every 5–7 min). It is important for the analysis to precisely enter what you do into the LabChart software before every chemical addition or wash step (for example KCl 1, wash 1, ACh 10^{-9} M, GTN 10^{-4} M).
3. To test the contractile capacity of each vessel segment a constriction with KCl is performed by adding KCl at 80 mM final concentration (1 ml of 2 M KCl into 25 ml OB buffer). Then wait for 10 min, wash and wait again for 10 min. Washing steps are performed by emptying the chamber by opening the buffer outlet valve and adding new OB buffer from the reservoir. Repeat the KCl step a second time for 15 min and wash two times with 7 min intervals.
4. The next step is to start recording of dose response curves to different vasodilators. First, the vessels need to be preconstricted with prostaglandin $F_{2\alpha}$. Add 6 μl of prostaglandin $F_{2\alpha}$ (5 mg·ml^{-1} in methanol) into the 25 ml chamber (final concentration 3.4 μM), wait for 2 min and if nothing happens add another 3 μl and wait for 15 min for reaching the plateau. After preconstriction a concentration-response curve cumulative

increasing concentrations of the endothelium-dependent vasodilator ACh (1 nM to 3 μM) is recorded (2 min between every concentration). First prepare a serial dilution of ACh from a 2 mM ACh stock solution (stored at −20 °C). *See* Table 2 for instructions for the serial dilution preparation. Cumulatively add the ACh dilutions to the organ chamber following the instructions in Table 3. Always wait for 2 min in between steps until the plateau is reached. After adding the last concentration the chamber is washed two times with 7 min intervals.

5. Endothelium independent vasodilator GTN (1 nM to 30 μM) is used in the same way as ACh. After a preconstriction with prostaglandin $F_{2\alpha}$ the different concentrations of GTN are pipetted into the chamber every 2 min. *See* Table 4 for preparing GTN dilutions and Table 5 for instructions for addition of the dilutions to the organ bath chambers. After measuring the final concentration the organ bath chamber is emptied and washed.
6. Data are analyzed by LabChart software (ADinstruments). The maximal relaxations (Emax) to ACh or GTN are expressed as the percentage of the maximal concentration previously obtained by prostaglandin $F_{2\alpha}$-induced contraction (Fig. 4).

3.5 Flow Cytometric Analysis of Aortic Lysates

1. Freshly harvested aortas are cleaned from surrounding tissue like described in subheading 3.3, **step 1**. Length of clean aortas is measured and the aortas are kept in KH buffer on ice. Before enzymatic digestion aortas are scrambled thoroughly with a razor blade until very small pieces remain (*see* **Note 7**).
   - If the focus of the aortic FACS analysis lies on differentiation of different T-cell subpopulations, enzymatic digestion is performed with 1 mg·ml^{-1} collagenase II in HBSS +/+ (or PBS +/+) and 50 μg·ml^{-1} DNase.
   - If myeloid cells are in the focus of interest, enzymatic digestion is made with liberase (1 mg·ml^{-1}) in HBSS +/+.

Table 2
Serial dilution of acetylcholine (ACh)

Final concentration ACh dilution 10^{-x} [M]	Volume double distillated water [μl]	Volume ACh
−3	900	100 μl of −2 stock
−4	900	100 μl of −3 dilution
−5	900	100 μl of −4 dilution
−6	900	100 μl of −5 dilution

Table 3
Pipetting scheme for recording an acetylcholine (ACh) dose–response curve

	ACh dilution 10^{-x} [M] added in each step	Volume of ACh dilution added to chamber [μl]	Final concentration in 25 ml chamber 10^{-x} [M]
1	−6	25	−9
2	−6	50	−8.5
3	−5	17.5	−8
4	−5	50	−7.5
5	−4	17.5	−7
6	−4	50	−6.5
7	−3	17.5	−6
8	−3	50	−5.5

Table 4
Serial dilution of glycerol trinitrate (GTN)

Final concentration GTN dilution 10^{-x} [M]	Volume double distillated water [μl]	Volume GTN
−3	4632	1368 μl of nitrolingual solution (1 mg·ml)
−4	900	100 μl of −3 dilution
−5	900	100 μl of −4 dilution
−6	900	100 μl of −5 dilution

Table 5
Pipetting scheme of glycerol trinitrate (GTN) dose–response curve

	GTN dilution 10^{-x} [M] added in each step	Volume of GTN dilution added to chamber [μl]	Final concentration in 25 ml chamber 10^{-x} [M]
1	−6	25	−9
2	−6	50	−8.5
3	−5	17.5	−8
4	−5	50	−7.5
5	−4	17.5	−7
6	−4	50	−6.5
7	−3	17.5	−6
8	−3	50	−5.5
9	−3	175	−5
10	−3	500	−4.5

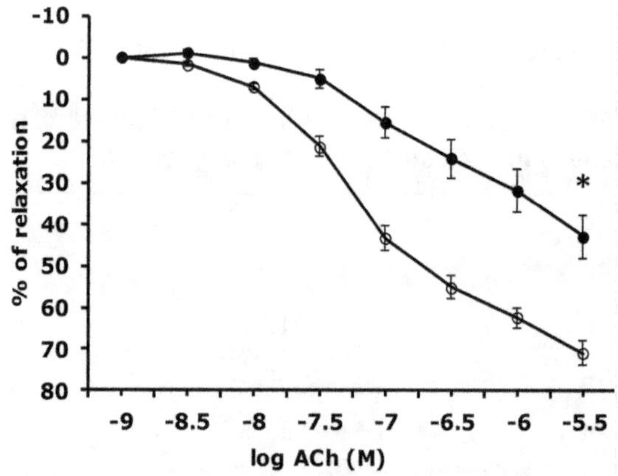

Fig 4 Concentration–relaxation curve in response to acetylcholine (ACh, endothelium dependent) of isolated aortic segments of C57BL/6 mice with (*full circles*) or without (empty circles) ATII for 7 days $n=4$ mice per group and results are expressed as mean ± SEM, $p<0.05$ *, vs. C57BL/6 with 1-way ANOVA of maximal relaxation

The pieces of the aortas are incubated together with the enzymatic mix (1 ml per aorta, 2 ml reaction tubes) at 37 °C, 500 rpm for 20–30 min. When aortic pieces are dissolved, digestion is stopped with ice cold PBS/2 % FCS (*see* **Note 6**) and stored on ice. Cell suspension is then pressed through a 70 μm strainer (Greiner) in a 50 ml Falcon tube. Cell mixture is divided in 15 ml Falcon tubes, cells are pelleted by centrifugation (300 × *g*, 6 min, 4 °C) and resuspended in 0.1 ml PBS/2% FCS. Cells are counted with trypan blue to estimate living cells. The cells are now ready for staining (Fig. 5).

2. Unspecific binding is blocked by adding 30 μl/aorta Fc block (anti-mouse CD16/32 eBioscience (5 $ng \cdot \mu l^{-1}$ in PBS/2% FCS). After 10 min wash once with PBS/2% FCS (300 × *g*, 6 min, 4 °C). Then the master mix is added (30 μl per aorta in PBS/2% FCS) and the cells are kept in the dark at 4 °C. Reaction is stopped with 100 μl PBS/2% FCS and cells are washed again with PBS/2% FCS. Cells are resuspended in 200 μl PBS + FCS before acquisition.
3. In our studies we use based on the aim of our study several different staining protocols (master mixes). In the material part we give an example of one of our standard protocols in which we focus on myelomonocyte cell infiltration into the aorta. For this staining we use a liberase digestion. First of all we always gate on single cells based on FSC-H/FSC-A and SSC-H/SSC-H scatter plots. Next we gate on living cell based on the staining with a Viability dye. In the next step we gate on $CD45^+$ overall leukocytes, then gate out T cells based on TCR beta

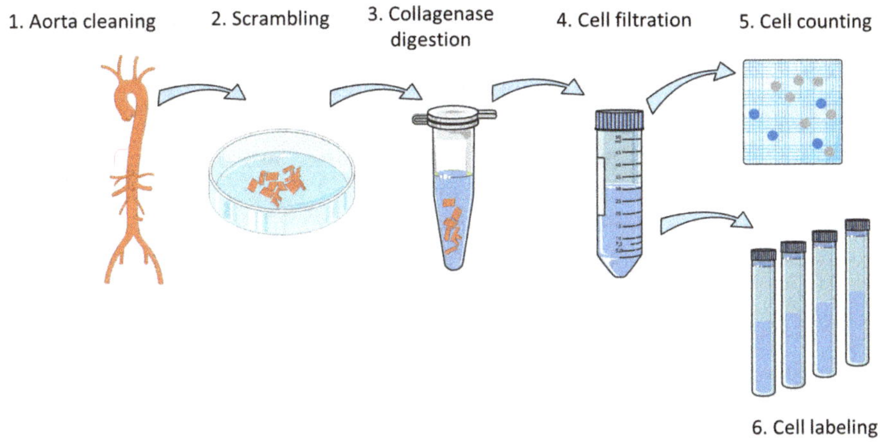

Fig 5 Aortic cell isolation steps

staining. To differentiate between neutrophils and different monocyte and macrophage population is gated first on CD11b$^+$ cells (all myeloid cells), followed by CD11b$^+$F4/80$^+$ (macrophages), Ly6G$^+$Ly6C$^+$CD11b$^+$ (neutrophils), Ly6C^{high}CD11b$^+$Ly6G$^-$ classical proinflammatory monocytes and Ly6C^{low}CD11b$^+$ Ly6G$^-$ nonclassical monocytes.

4. Data are analyzed by BDFACSDiva or FlowJo software (TreeStar). Number of each cell subpopulation is calculated based on viability staining and live cell counts and normalized to aortic length.

4 Notes

1. Repeated cycles of freezing and thawing of prepared stock aliquots of ATII diluted in sterile saline can lead to altered ATII responses. These problems can be avoided by preparing a fresh ATII solution for every new osmotic mini-pump that needs to be filled.
2. Implantation of a telemetric transmitter can be performed on small mice but, to have a good rate of success we recommend using mice that weigh at least 22 g.
3. Making an incision in a very small vessel to insert a catheter can be difficult. One easy way to insert a catheter is to use a 26 G needle with a 90° bend point. Once the point is inserted into the carotid artery the needle can be used to hold the vessel while introducing the telemetric transmitter catheter into the vessel.

4. Since the telemetric transmitter can be activated by magnets the storage must be done far from magnetic devices. Moreover it is important to check when unpacking the devices that none of them is activated.
5. The battery of the transmitter lasts for 2 months while the mice are already measured after 2 weeks; the transmitter can be carefully extracted (without stretching the catheter) and, given an undamaged state of the catheter, disinfected and reimplanted (sometimes the tip of the catheter must be refilled with gel).
6. The cell yield mainly depends on digestion efficacy. If the pieces of aorta are too big, digestion will be ineffective and therefore last longer, which will destroy a large number of cells.
7. Depending on the kind of analysis the number of aortas necessary can vary. One single aorta is enough to perform extracellular stainings, while a pool of 2–3 aortas might be necessary for intracellular stainings.

References

1. De Ciuceis C, Amiri F, Brassard P, Endemann DH, Touyz RM, Schiffrin EL (2005) Reduced vascular remodeling, endothelial dysfunction, and oxidative stress in resistance arteries of angiotensin II-infused macrophage colony-stimulating factor-deficient mice: evidence for a role in inflammation in angiotensin-induced vascular injury. Arterioscler Thromb Vasc Biol 25(10):2106–2113
2. Guzik TJ, Hoch NE, Brown KA, McCann LA, Rahman A, Dikalov S et al (2007) Role of the T cell in the genesis of angiotensin II induced hypertension and vascular dysfunction. J Exp Med 204(10):2449–2460
3. Harrison DG, Marvar PJ, Titze JM (2012) Vascular inflammatory cells in hypertension. Front Physiol 3:128
4. Weiss D, Kools JJ, Taylor WR (2001) Angiotensin II-induced hypertension accelerates the development of atherosclerosis in apoE-deficient mice. Circulation 103(3):448–454
5. Kossmann S, Schwenk M, Hausding M, Karbach SH, Schmidgen MI, Brandt M et al (2013) Angiotensin II-induced vascular dysfunction depends on interferon-γ-driven immune cell recruitment and mutual activation of monocytes and NK-cells. Arterioscler Thromb Vasc Biol 33(6):1313–1319
6. Cross M, Renkawitz R (1990) Repetitive sequence involvement in the duplication and divergence of mouse lysozyme genes. EMBO J 9(4):1283–1288
7. Drechsler M, Megens RTA, van Zandvoort M, Weber C, Soehnlein O (2010) Hyperlipidemia-triggered neutrophilia promotes early atherosclerosis. Circulation 122(18):1837–1845
8. Rotzius P, Soehnlein O, Kenne E, Lindbom L, Nystrom K, Thams S et al (2009) ApoE(−/−)/lysozyme M(EGFP/EGFP) mice as a versatile model to study monocyte and neutrophil trafficking in atherosclerosis. Atherosclerosis 202(1):111–118
9. Rotzius P, Thams S, Soehnlein O, Kenne E, Tseng C-N, Björkström NK et al (2010) Distinct infiltration of neutrophils in lesion shoulders in ApoE−/− mice. Am J Pathol 177(1):493–500
10. Wenzel P, Knorr M, Kossmann S, Stratmann J, Hausding M, Schuhmacher S et al (2011) Lysozyme M-positive monocytes mediate angiotensin II-induced arterial hypertension and vascular dysfunction. Circulation 124(12):1370–1381
11. Kossmann S, Hu H, Steven S, Schönfelder T, Fraccarollo D, Mikhed Y et al (2014) Inflammatory monocytes determine endothelial nitric-oxide synthase uncoupling and nitro-oxidative stress induced by angiotensin II. J Biol Chem 289(40):27540–27550
12. Wenzel P, Rossmann H, Müller C, Kossmann S, Oelze M, Schulz A et al (2015) Heme oxygenase-1 suppresses a pro-inflammatory phenotype in monocytes and determines endothelial function and arterial hypertension in mice and humans. Eur Heart J 36(48):3437–3446

13. Cave AC, Brewer AC, Narayanapanicker A, Ray R, Grieve DJ, Walker S et al (2006) NADPH oxidases in cardiovascular health and disease. Antioxid Redox Signal 8(5-6): 691–728

14. Swirski FK, Nahrendorf M, Etzrodt M, Wildgruber M, Cortez-Retamozo V, Panizzi P et al (2009) Identification of splenic reservoir monocytes and their deployment to inflammatory sites. Science 325(5940):612–616

Erratum to: Isolation and Characterization of Aortic Dendritic Cells and Lymphocytes in Atherosclerosis

Tae Jin Yun, Jun Seong Lee, Dahee Shim, Jae-Hoon Choi, and Cheolho Cheong

Erratum to:
Chapter 29 in: Björn E. Clausen and Jon D. Laman (eds.), *Inflammation: Methods and Protocols*, Methods in Molecular Biology, vol. 1559, DOI 10.1007/978-1-4939-6786-5_29

In the original version of this chapter, in page 421, the sentence "1 ml collagenase cocktail: 880 μl 1× HBSS, 100 μl collagenase type I (Sigma-Aldrich, C0130, 10× stock: 675 U/ml), 10 μl collagenase type XI (Sigma-Aldrich, C7657, 10× stock: 187.5 U/ml), 10 μl hyaluronidase type I-s (Sigma-Aldrich, H1115000, 10× stock: 9 U/ml) (*see* **Note 2**)" was published with inaccurate value of the components.

It has now been changed to "1 ml Collagenase cocktail: 600 μl 1X HBSS, 100 μl Collagenase type I (Sigma-Aldrich, C0130, 10X stock: 6750 U/ml), 100 μl Collagenase type XI (Sigma-Aldrich, C7657, 10X stock: 187.5 U/ml), 100 μl Hyaluronidase type I-s (Sigma-Aldrich, H1115000, 10X stock: 900 U/ml), 100 μl DNase I (Sigma-Aldrich, 11284932001, 10X stock: 900 U/ml) (*see* **Note 2**)" to reflect the accurate value of the components.

The updated online version of this chapter can be found at
https://doi.org/10.1007/978-1-4939-6786-5_29

Björn E. Clausen and Jon D. Laman (eds.), *Inflammation: Methods and Protocols*, Methods in Molecular Biology, vol. 1559,
DOI 10.1007/978-1-4939-6786-5_31,

Index

Björn E. Clausen and Jon D. Laman (eds.), *Inflammation: Methods and Protocols*, Methods in Molecular Biology, vol. 1559, DOI 10.1007/978-1-4939-6786-5, © Springer Science+Business Media LLC 2017

N

O

U

V

GPSR Compliance
The European Union's (EU) General Product Safety Regulation (GPSR) is a set of rules that requires consumer products to be safe and our obligations to ensure this.

If you have any concerns about our products, you can contact us on

ProductSafety@springernature.com

In case Publisher is established outside the EU, the EU authorized representative is:

Springer Nature Customer Service Center GmbH
Europaplatz 3
69115 Heidelberg, Germany

www.ingramcontent.com/pod-product-compliance
Lightning Source LLC
LaVergne TN
LVHW082027200926
848481LV00010B/2938
* 9 7 8 1 4 9 3 9 8 3 0 0 1 *